...th

through

discovery

GEORGE B. DINTIMAN • JERROLD S. GREENBERG

Virginia Commonwealth University   *University of Maryland*

 ADDISON-WESLEY PUBLISHING COMPANY

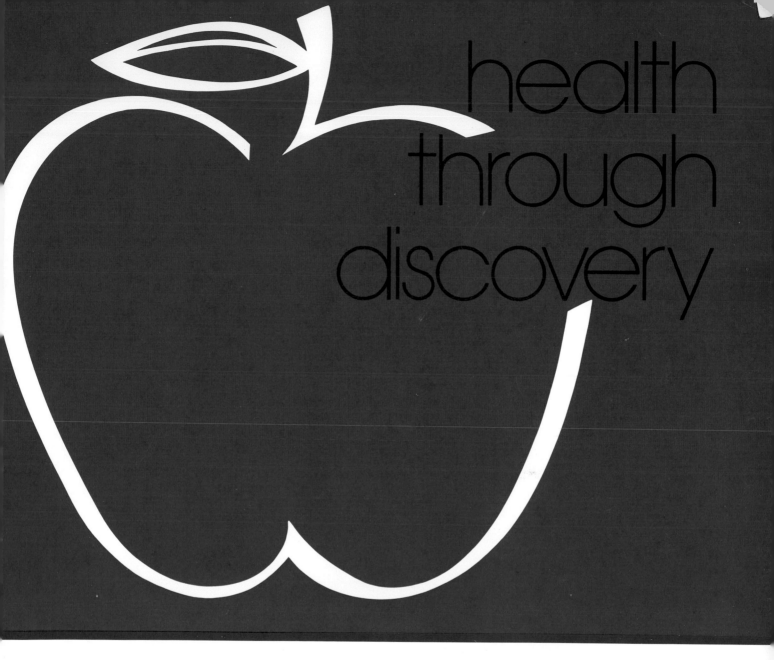

health through discovery

Second Edition

Reading, Massachusetts ● Menlo Park, California ● London ● Amsterdam ● Don Mills, Ontario ● Sydney

Sponsoring Editor: Ronald R. Hill
Developmental Editor: Kathe G. Rhoades
Production Editors: Mary W. Crittendon and Stephanie Argeros-Magean

Text and Cover Designer: Margaret Ong Tsao
Illustrators: Kristin Belanger and Oxford Illustrators
Cover Photographer: Marshall Henrichs
Art Coordinator: Kristin Belanger

Production Manager: Sherry Berg

The text of this book was composed in Optima by General Graphic Services.

Library of Congress Cataloging in Publication Data

Dintiman, George B.
  Health through discovery.

  1. Health.   2. Health attitudes.   I. Greenberg,
Jerrold S.   II. Title.
RA776.D57   1983   613   82-11421
ISBN 0-201-10370-2

Reprinted with corrections, June 1983

BCDEFGHIJ-HA-89876543
ISBN 0-201-10370-2

to our parents
George Byers and Gladys Blough Dintiman
and
David and Bess Greenberg

preface

During the twentieth century great advances have been made in the prevention and cure of disease. Infectious diseases that were of serious concern to earlier generations, such as polio, tuberculosis, smallpox, diphtheria, and measles, have either been virtually eliminated or are treated successfully with medicines. The health problems that concern us now are much more likely to be self-inflicted than to be ills over which we have no control. Heart disease, cancer, and stroke—the three leading killers of American adults—have been shown to be closely related to lifestyle factors, among them nutritional patterns, smoking, exercise or the lack of it, and stress, as well as to personality factors. These are all areas over which we as individuals have a great deal of control. Clearly, disease prevention, longevity, and wellness during the next decades will result not from medical discoveries but from adopting more healthy lifestyles. The potential for good health rests in large measure with each of us and the health-related decisions we make every day of our lives.

We believe that the responsibility for each person's health rests primarily with that individual. To become healthy, a person must be informed about health-related issues; equally important, that person needs to make conscious decisions about a variety of behaviors that can make a difference in his or her health status.

Our book is intended both to increase students' knowledge about health and to enable them to analyze their own attitudes and behaviors and, if necessary, alter them. The title we have chosen, *Health Through Discovery*, is intended to focus attention on the need for individuals to arrive at their own informed conclusions about how to take responsibility for their health. We feel this is the best way to involve them in the material. To make the task easier, we have strengthened this edition in several ways.

Each chapter has been thoroughly revised to assure that the content is in line with the latest research in the health field. For example, we discuss new advances in cancer treatment, new findings about high blood pressure, and toxic shock syndrome. We give more emphasis in this edition to aspects of mental health, including stress, marital and family relationships, mental problems, and aging. Topics of particular public concern in recent years have been added or strengthened: rape and incest, the male climacteric, child abuse, sexually transmitted diseases, parental bonding with infants, singlehood, and communication in relationships, to name some of the most pertinent. In response to users of the text, we have made some broad organizational changes and added more headings to improve the clarity of organization within chapters.

Features of This Edition

To enhance our "learning by doing" approach, we have strengthened several of the features of the first edition.

Each chapter contains from three to five *Discovery Activities* on topics ranging from *What do you know about suicide?* to *Contraceptive decision making* to *Do you want to change your smoking habits?* These activities are presented in a variety of formats, from simple questions to multiple choice quizzes to charts for students to fill in. The activities are carefully integrated with the text and are intended to help students analyze their own attitudes and behaviors in relation to the topic under discussion. Each acitivity has been given a title and a number for convenient reference.

Each chapter contains two *Issues in Health* which examine briefly the opposing arguments on controversial health-related topics. Students are asked to consider where they stand on the issues. New topics include *Should laetrile be legal?*; *Should minors who have a sexually transmitted disease be treated without parental consent?*; and *Children's health: who decides?*, which explores whether parents should always have the ultimate decision-making authority when their child's life may be at stake.

At the end of each chapter there are two Laboratory activities related to the chapter content. Some are to be completed individually; others are completed in small groups, which then report their findings to the rest of the class.

To help students focus on the pertinent points in each chapter, we include one-sentence *Concepts* set off from the text.

A new feature of this edition is the numbered chapter summary at the end of each chapter, which is intended to help students recall the basic points.

Important new terms are printed in boldface in the text and defined or explained in the glossary at the back of the book.

Finally, particular attention has been given to ensuring that the book's design and art program will help stimulate student interest in the text, as well as enhance the material visually. In addition to numerous charts and tables, many new photographs have been added and some pertinent cartoons.

We hope that the approach we've taken in writing this book will make it enjoyable and engaging, and we're confident that our coverage of the facts and findings in the health field will help students make health-related decisions that will enhance the quality of their lives, promote health and wellness, and prevent disease and premature death.

ACKNOWLEDGMENTS

We are grateful for the thoughtful criticisms and helpful suggestions of the following reviewers:

Robert Russell, Southern Illinois University

Mark Kittleson, Youngstown State University

Valerie Pinhas, Nassau Community College

James McIntyre, Kutztown State College

Russell Whaley, Slippery Rock State College

Linda Brown, San Francisco City College

Herb Jones, Ball State University

We also wish to thank Albert Barnes, Fred Browning, and Lawrence Cappiello for writing chapters related to their areas of expertise. They approached that task diligently and with exceptional aptitude.

In addition, we owe a debt of gratitude to the people at Addison-Wesley who committed themselves to our project and whose efforts helped us communicate our message better than we might otherwise. In particular, Kathe Rhoades challenged us to improve upon our first edition by asking for clarification, suggesting additional topics, and offering better ways for our written words to take on life and meaning. We are proud of this book, and Kathe's contributions are a good part of it. Our editor, Ron Hill, deserves special recognition. His encouragement in this project was a major influence in its fruition. He served as reviewer, advocate, cajoler, sympathizer, and generally kept us on track throughout. His help was vital in the production of *Health Through Discovery*.

Richmond, Virginia   G.B.D.
College Park, Maryland   J.S.G.
November 1982

to the instructor

Supplements

A number of supplements have been prepared for this edition to help make your teaching job easier. The Instructor's Manual, prepared by Professor Mark Kittleson, Youngstown State University, contains learning objectives, detailed chapter outlines, additional activities and issues, and approximately ten essay-type questions per chapter. The Test Item File, prepared by Judy B. Baker of East Carolina University, contains over 2,000 test items. Multiple choice, matching, true–false, and fill-in questions are provided for each chapter of the text. The Test Item File is available both in paperback and on magnetic tape along with the instructions necessary for your computer department to implement your testing program.

Customized Testing Service

Adopters of *Health Through Discovery* can take advantage of Addison-Wesley's customized testing service. We will prepare your tests for you if time or departmental resources are limited. Here's how the service works: You select the questions and problems from the Test Item File, circle the test item numbers on one of the order forms, and mail it to us. (We can prepare separate tests for multiple exams, but each test must appear on a different order form.) For even faster service, you can phone us your order directly. Within 24 hours we will mail you your exam master, numbered sequentially, along with an answer key for easy grading.

Film Policy

Addison-Wesley will assist in your use of films in the classroom. For every 100 copies of the text ordered prior to the term in which the film(s) will be used, we offer you the one-time use of any film from a list compiled by the Indiana University Film Library. This offer is free of charge except for the cost of return postage to the rental source. You can also rent a film not on the Indiana University list. In that case, for every 100 copies of the text ordered prior to the term in which the film(s) will be used, Addison-Wesley will grant you an allowance of up to $25.00 for film rental.

contents

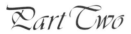

Part Two

HEALTH AND YOUR MIND

---

3 MENTAL HEALTH 43

---

4 STRESS 65

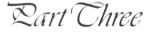

Part Three

HEALTH AND YOUR BODY

DRUGS AND YOUR HEALTH

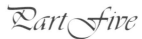

Part Five

SEX AND FAMILY LIFE

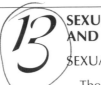

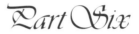

DISEASES

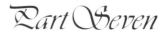

Part Seven

HEALTH AND SOCIETY

**19 HEALTH AND
THE CONSUMER** 453

20 CHOOSING MEDICAL SERVICES AND HEALTH INSURANCE   477

21 YOUR ENVIRONMENT   501

health behavior questionnaire

Throughout this book, we will ask you to make reference to your own health behavior. So before we begin, take a few moments to complete this questionnaire.*

BEFORE YOU TAKE THE TEST

This is not a pass-fail test. Its purpose is simply to tell you how well you are doing to stay healthy. The behaviors covered in the test are recommended for most Americans. Some of them may not apply to persons with certain chronic diseases or handicaps. Such persons may require special instructions from their physician or other health professional.

You will find that the test has six sections: smoking, alcohol and drugs, nutrition, exercise and fitness, control, and safety. Complete one section at a time by circling the number corresponding to the answer that best describes your behavior (2 for "Almost Always," 1 for "Sometimes," and 0 for "Almost Never"). Then add the numbers you have circled to determine your score for that section. Write the score on the line provided at the end of each section. The highest score you can get for each section is 10.

*SOURCE: U.S. Department of Health and Human Services, *Health Style: A Self Test* (Washington, D.C.: Public Health Service, 1981).

A TEST FOR BETTER HEALTH

 Cigarette Smoking

If you never smoke, enter a score of 10 for this section and go to the next section on *Alcohol and Drugs*.

	Almost Always	Sometimes	Almost Never
1. I avoid smoking cigarettes.	2	1	0
2. I smoke only low-tar and nicotine cigarettes *or* I smoke a pipe or cigars.	2	1	0

Smoking Score: _____

1

Alcohol and Drugs

Eating Habits

	Almost Always	Sometimes	Almost Never

1. I avoid drinking alcoholic beverages *or* I drink no more than 1 or 2 drinks a day.   (4)   1   0

2. I avoid using alcohol or other drugs (especially illegal drugs) as a way of handling stressful situations or the problems in my life.   (2)   1   0

3. I am careful not to drink alcohol when taking certain medicines (for example, medicine for sleeping, pain, colds, and allergies).   (2)   1   0

4. I read and follow the label directions when using prescribed and over-the-counter drugs.   (2)   1   0

Alcohol and Drugs Score: _____

1. I eat a variety of foods each day, such as fruits and vegetables, whole grain breads and cereals, lean meats, dairy products, dry peas and beans, and nuts and seeds.   (4)   1   0

2. I limit the amount of fat, saturated fat, and cholesterol I eat (including fat on meats, eggs, butter, cream, shortenings, and organ meats such as liver).   2   (1)   0

3. I limit the amount of salt I eat by cooking with only small amounts, not adding salt at the table, and avoiding salty snacks.   (2)   1   0

4. I avoid eating too much sugar (especially frequent snacks of sticky candy or soft drinks).   2   (1)   0

Eating Habits Score: _____

Exercise and Fitness

 Stress Control

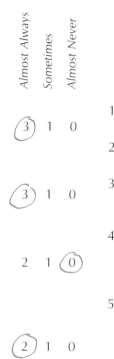

	Almost Always	Sometimes	Almost Never
1. I maintain a desired weight, avoiding overweight and underweight.	(3)	1	0
2. I do vigorous exercises for 15–30 minutes at least 3 times a week (examples include running, swimming, brisk walking).	(3)	1	0
3. I do exercises that enhance my muscle tone for 15–30 minutes at least 3 times a week (examples include yoga and calisthenics).	2	1	(0)
4. I use part of my leisure time participating in individual, family, or team activities that increase my level of fitness (such as gardening, bowling, golf, and baseball).	(2)	1	0

Exercise and Fitness Score: _____

	Almost Always	Sometimes	Almost Never
1. I have a job or do other work that I enjoy.	2	(1)	0
2. I find it easy to relax and express my feelings freely.	(2)	1	0
3. I recognize early, and prepare for, events or situations likely to be stressful for me.	2	(1)	0
4. I have close friends, relatives, or others whom I can talk to about personal matters and call on for help when needed.	(2)	1	0
5. I participate in group activities (such as church and community organizations) or hobbies that I enjoy.	2	(1)	0

Stress Control Score: _____

Safety

	Almost Always	Sometimes	Almost Never
1. I wear a seat belt while riding in a car.	2	(1)	0
2. I avoid driving while under the influence of alcohol and other drugs.	(2)	1	0
3. I obey traffic rules and the speed limit when driving.	(2)	1	0
4. I am careful when using potentially harmful products or substances (such as household cleaners, poisons, and electrical devices).	(2)	1	0
5. I avoid smoking in bed.	(2)	1	0

Safety Score: _____

YOUR HEALTH STYLE SCORES

After you have figured your score for each of the six sections, circle the number in each column that matches your score for that section of the test.

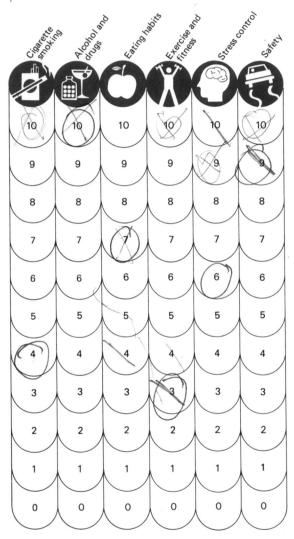

Remember, there is no total score for this test. Consider each section separately. You are trying to identify aspects of your lifestyle that you can improve in order to be healthier and to reduce the risk of illness. So let's see what your scores reveal.

WHAT YOUR SCORES MEAN TO YOU

Scores of 9 and 10

Excellent! Your answers show that you are aware of the importance of this area to your health. More important, you are putting your knowledge to work for you by practicing good health habits. As long as you continue to do so, this area should not pose a serious health risk. It's likely that you are setting an example for your family and friends to follow. Although you received a very high score on this part of the test, you may want to consider other areas where your scores could be improved.

Scores of 6 to 8

Your health practices in this area are good, but there is room for improvement. Look again at the items you answered with a "Sometimes" or "Almost Never." What changes can you make to improve your score? Even a small change can often help you achieve better health.

Scores of 3 to 5

Your health risks are showing! Would you like more information about the risks you are facing and about why it is important for you to change these behaviors? Perhaps you need help in deciding how to make the changes you desire. In either case, help is available.

Scores of 0 to 2

You may be taking serious and unnecessary risks with your health. Perhaps you are not aware of the risks and what to do about them. In this book you will find the information and help you need to improve your scores and, thereby, your health.

basic health concepts

concepts

Part one

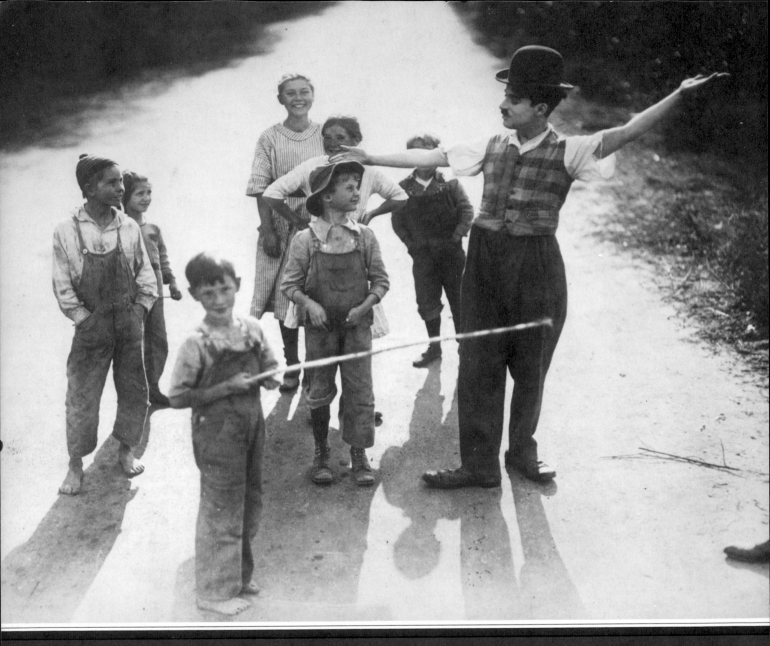

chapter **1**

the concept
of health

- *defining health*
- *theories of human behavior*
- *education about health*

Most of us assume we know what health is. Before proceeding with this chapter, write your definition of health:

_____

_____

_____

DEFINING HEALTH

Concept: How we define health affects how we conduct our lives.

How we define health determines, to a large extent, how we behave. This becomes clear when we realize that all of us want to be healthy. Whether we define health in terms of the quality of life or its quantity (length), all of our goals are related to health.

For example, if you define health as the absence of disease, illness, or injury, then you are probably a person who obtains regular medical examinations, drives an automobile with caution, and gets adequate sleep. If you define health as deriving satisfaction from life, then you may be a person who is willing to risk your physical health in order to achieve this satisfaction. You may, for instance, sky dive, drive fast, or ski for excitement, even though each of these activities poses some threat to your physical health. For most of us, both aspects of "health"—absence of disease *and* satisfaction from life—are important, and therefore in each situation we weigh the benefits of the risk involved against its dangers in deciding how to behave.

Concept: Health is multifaceted.

Look at the definition of health that you wrote. Does it pertain to physical well-being alone, or does it also include mental and emotional well-being? Most people consider only physical health in their definitions. Consider the case of an overweight man who enjoys his involvement in a gourmet club and decides to maintain that involvement even though he is doing

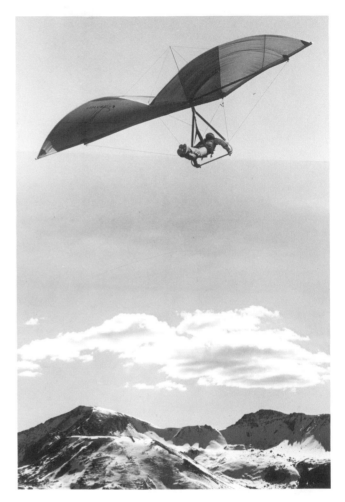

If the quality of life is important to one's definition of health, then the individual must always weigh the benefits of personal satisfaction against the risks involved in each situation.

apparent harm to his physical well-being by eating foods high in saturated fats. This man has chosen to enhance his social health at the expense of his physical health.

Obviously, it is hard to separate one aspect of health from another, and advocates of **holistic health** view the aspects of health as inseparable. Holistic health educators work with the total person on all of his or her health needs.

Wellness

Concept: Health and wellness may differ.

Depending on your definition, health may not be the same as wellness. For example, would you consider a diabetic healthy? Probably not. However, if that diabetic has adjusted his or her life so as to be happy and self-fulfilled, we'd probably say he or she has achieved a high level of wellness. Wellness concerns the quality of life; it means being in control of your life while at the same time recognizing that you can't control everything affecting you. It means living your life so that it is meaningful and satisfying. It is possible to be physically healthy but not have "wellness"; and it is possible to have wellness but not be physically healthy.

Health Is Dynamic

Health is a dynamic process. If we were to depict health on a continuum, it might appear this way:

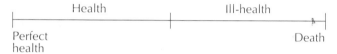

Health	Ill-health
Perfect health	Death

Before we could locate any individual on this continuum, we would have to assess each aspect of health— physical, mental, social, spiritual, and emotional—and then we would have to make some judgments regarding the relative importance of each. For example, in the case of the overweight gourmet, is the man healthier for having maintained his involvement in the club or is he less healthy? Your answer might depend on how important you consider social health in relation to physical health. If we were to complicate this example by including decisions regarding the man's spiritual and mental health, the point being made here would become more obvious; that is, it is impossible to classify anyone as healthy or unhealthy unless he or she is at an extreme end of the continuum. Different people would classify an individual in different ways depending on their values regarding health. And, of course, one's health status today can, and often does, differ from one's health status tomorrow. An accident, an

Issues in Health
SHOULD HEALTH CARE BE SPECIALIZED?

Few would suggest that physicians should not have specialized training. Cardiologists, neurosurgeons, endocrinologists, and the like are needed because our accumulated knowledge of the human body is too much for one person to know. However, in terms of health care, some argue that to treat a person's kidney while ignoring that person's psychological health is to work with blinders. Since the body is so affected by what goes on in the mind, and vice versa, both need care when a problem in either surfaces. We can't expect patients to take their medications in proper dosages at recommended intervals unless we consider the social implications of potential side effects (for example, some hypertensive drugs may cause impotency in male patients). To care for a person's heart after a heart attack without considering physical rehabilitation, exercise, and sexual activity is to treat the heart and not the person. There are those, then, who advocate a health care team approach. When a patient is treated, the physician, nurse, physical therapist, psychologist, patient educator, and others should all be involved. In this manner, the whole person will be treated.

Others argue that such health care is expensive and ineffective. To pay all these professionals for participation in treatment plans means the cost of health care will be beyond the reach of the masses. Either national health insurance will be required and taxes significantly increased or a caste system of the haves and have nots will develop. Further, when professionals collaborate in this manner, each tends to view his or her care as the most important. The result is bickering among the health care providers, which in turn means poorer health care for the patient.

What do you think? ●

argument with a friend, a success, or a failure could all affect health status in a short period of time.

The bottom line is: Are *you* happy with your health status? Discovery Activity 1.1 asks you to evaluate your satisfaction with your health status.

Health and Values

Concept: Health is a matter of values.

As we stressed above, health is perceived differently by different people, and these perceptions are a matter of **values**. Once again, consider the gourmet club member:

> A businessman might be 15 pounds overweight for no apparent reason other than careless eating habits, or an unawareness of the advantages of trim physique, and ignorance of the basic principles of weight control. This should be classed as a remedial health defect and one important indicator of reduced health status. However, let us compare this case with the case of another businessman, equally overweight, who happens to be a well-informed and enthusiastic amateur gourmet. His library of cookbooks includes directions for preparing many of the most popular dishes of other cultures. He spends many interesting hours in offbeat markets shopping for hard-to-get food items. The meals he prepares constitute focal points of an interesting and satisfying social life. This man realizes he is overweight; he knows how to reduce and control his weight; and he may even suspect that his coronary may arrive a year or two ahead of schedule, but he does not care. His overweight condition constitutes a health defect only in the absolute sense. When viewed in relation to his value system, it represents a logical concomitant to his particular pattern of good health.*

Clearly, our judgments of behavior as healthy or unhealthy depend on our values and the factors surrounding each situation. Our values contribute a great deal to our evaluation of situations.

*From Walter Greene, "The Search for a Meaningful Definition of Health," in *New Directions in Health Education: Some Contemporary Issues for the Emerging Age*, by Donald A. Read. Copyright © 1971, Donald A. Read. Used with permission.

Discovery Activity 1.1 ## *EVALUATING YOUR HEALTH STATUS*

In the space provided, evaluate your satisfaction with your health status. Include both strong points and weak points regarding your mental and physical health. After you have done this, choose one weak point of one component of health that you cited, and list three ways in which you could lessen the impact of or eliminate this weak point. Similarly, choose one strong point of one component of health that you cited, and list three ways in which you could make that strong point even stronger.

	Mental health	*Physical health*
Strong points:	1. 2. 3. 4.	
Weak points:	1. 2. 3. 4.	

Ways to eliminate weak point:

1. _____
2. _____
3. _____

Ways to strengthen strong point:

1. _____
2. _____
3. _____

THEORIES OF HUMAN BEHAVIOR

Concept: There are many different theories of behavior.

Why do people adopt certain health-related behaviors and not others? Although many theories have been proposed to explain why people behave as they do, no one knows for sure. The theories described below, however, are those often cited as most adequately explaining why some people smoke cigarettes and others do not, why some people abuse drugs and others do not, and generally why some people behave in a healthy way and others do not. This is no magic list, though. Your instructor or other sources can provide you with additional theories of human behavior.

Hierarchy of Needs

Abraham Maslow proposed that human beings behave in ways that seek to satisfy certain needs.[1] Further, there exist levels of needs, and the high-level needs do not emerge until the low-level needs are satisfied.

Figure 1.1
Maslow's hierarchy of needs.
From *Toward a Psychology of Being*, by Abraham Maslow. Copyright © 1962 by D. Van Nostrand. Reprinted by permission of Brooks/Cole Publishing Company, Monterey, California 93940.

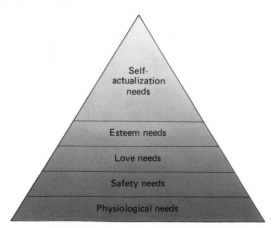

Self-actualization needs

Esteem needs

Love needs

Safety needs

Physiological needs

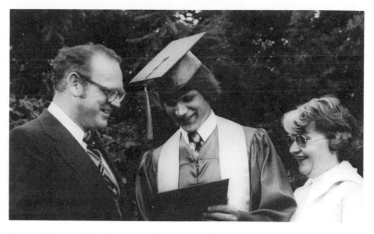

According to Abraham Maslow, complex psychological motives, such as the pursuit of intellectual achievement, become important only after more basic needs are satisfied.

Until your needs for hunger and thirst (physiological needs) are satisfied, you will not be concerned with safety. In fact, if you need food badly, you might even chase a lion away from a felled prey. Until you feel safe and secure (safety needs), you will not be concerned with others loving you. Until you are loved (love needs), you will not be concerned about whether others respect you (esteem needs). And until you are respected by others, you will not care whether you can achieve your potential (self-actualization needs).

In our society, most of these needs are met to some degree. However, the degree to which they are met varies and consequently our behavior varies. Some of us might behave in sexual ways contrary to our nature because of our need to have others love us. Others of us might conform to our friends' drug behavior because of our need for esteem.

Force Field Theory

According to Kurt Lewin,[2] human behavior is a constant tug and pull of driving and restraining forces. When one set of forces becomes stronger than another, you behave one way. When the other set of forces becomes stronger, you behave another way.

For example, you might want to lose weight but live with someone who nightly eats high-calorie foods. If the attraction of these foods is stronger than your desire to lose weight, your diet goes down the drain.

Issues in Health
SHOULD WE STOP TRYING TO FIND OUT WHY PEOPLE BEHAVE AS THEY DO?

There are those who believe it would be tragic if we were ever able to identify the reasons why people do the things they do. Theorists do not yet agree on one model of human behavior. If such a model were found, it would allow those most proficient with the model to influence other people's behaviors. Government leaders might use the model to manipulate us and gain more power than is healthy in a democratic society. Advertisers might use the model to influence us to buy their products. Military experts might use the model to convince us that war is necessary. Rather than wait for these abuses to occur and then respond, we should now stop funding research on theories of human behavior so that no such model is discovered.

Others believe this view is shortsighted. They separate the value of new knowledge from its use. Why is it not possible for a model of human behavior to be used to help people? If we knew with certainty how to influence people's behaviors, we could educate them to brush and floss their teeth, to exercise, to use drugs as prescribed, to manage stress, and to eat nutritionally balanced meals. What's wrong with that? Rather than less funding for the testing of theories of human behavior, we need more.

What do you think? ●

Adjustment Theory

Others believe that human beings are constantly striving to adjust to their environments. This adjustment is needed to maintain an equilibrium necessary for a healthy existence. When the environment places us in disequilibrium we behave in ways to right ourselves. Thus when a student enters college and leaves home for the first time, that student seeks to replace the family with close friends. To acquire these friends might mean joining college organizations, taking drugs, or other behaviors designed to reacquire equilibrium.

The Health Belief Model

One model of health behavior looks at what motivates people to behave as they do.[3] This theory states that people will adopt a health behavior if:

1. They consider it likely that they will contract a disease or illness if they don't (*susceptibility*).
2. The illness or disease they may contract is severe enough to be of serious concern (*severity*).
3. The health behavior, if adopted, can prevent the contraction of the severe illness or disease (*prevention*).
4. The barriers to performing the health behavior are not too difficult to overcome (*removal of barriers*).

Health educators have developed programs based upon this model. For example, consider an exercise program. One component of the program might be describing the likelihood (*susceptibility*) that those who don't exercise regularly will contract a serious illness such as coronary heart disease (*severity*). Exercise must then be demonstrated to be effective in *preventing* the development of coronary heart disease. Finally, any *barriers* to regular exercise must be removed or diminished. For example, exercise clothes (shorts, sneakers) should be placed on the dresser first thing in the morning to prepare for exercise after classes or work. Or arrangements can be made to exercise with a friend so that time is not taken from socializing.

Which health behaviors would you like to adopt? Why not use this health behavior model to adopt those behaviors successfully?

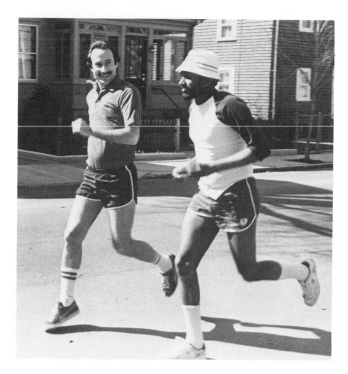

The health belief model is based on the premise that people will adopt health-related behaviors if they can be convinced the behavior will improve their health and prevent disease and if the barriers to starting the behavior are not too difficult to overcome.

EDUCATION ABOUT HEALTH

Concept: Health problems have changed.

The major causes of death in the United States have changed from what they were at the beginning of the century. What do you think the three major causes of death were in 1900? What are they today?

1900

1. _____
2. _____
3. _____

Today

1. _____
2. _____
3. _____

If you look at Table 1.1, you will see how greatly things have changed. In 1900 the three leading causes of death were communicable diseases. As a result of legislation pertaining to quarantine, inoculation, sewage disposal, and food and water sanitation, only one of these remains in the top ten today. Statistics prove that the government response was effective. But today the three leading causes of death are noncommunicable conditions that require responses of individuals rather than governments. Experts believe that if individuals have adequate exercise, proper nutrition, and periodic medical examinations, stop smoking, drive automobiles safely (and not while under the influence of alcohol), and keep medicines out of the reach of children, these precautions can have a dramatic effect upon the number of deaths from cardiovascular diseases (heart attacks and strokes), cancer, and accidents.

Table 1.1
LEADING CAUSES OF DEATH IN THE UNITED STATES: 1900 AND 1978

1900	1978
1. Tuberculosis	1. Heart disease
2. Pneumonia and influenza	2. Cancer
3. Enteritis, gastritis, colitis	3. Stroke
4. Diseases of the heart	4. Accidents
5. Stroke or apoplexy	5. Pneumonia and influenza
6. Kidney diseases	6. Diabetes Mellitus
7. Accidents	7. Cirrhosis of the liver
8. Cancer	8. Arteriosclerosis
9. Diseases of early infancy	9. Suicide
10. Diphtheria	10. Certain conditions of infants

SOURCE: U.S. Public Health Service.

The Objectives of Education about Health

Concept: Health education is defined as a "freeing process."

At this point, you might wonder why we even offer **health education**. If we cannot even define health, if it is really a matter of individual interpretation, if it is always changing, if people have different values that affect their health behaviors, and if we do not really know why people behave as they do, then it is reasonable to question the value of health education.

For purposes of this discussion, let us define health education as a process in which the goal is to free people so that they can make health-related decisions based upon *their* needs and interests, as long as these decisions do not adversely affect others.[4] The goal of this book, then, is to help you make informed health-related decisions. For the most part we are not attempting to get you to behave in certain ways that we declare are "healthy." Rather, we want to help you explore the consequences of your behavior and your needs and motivations as they relate to that behavior and to identify for you the various factors that might affect your decisions. In discussing most topics, we're going to encourage you to explore openly, make your own decisions, and exercise your freedom. Sometimes, however, there is compelling evidence that some choices are far more likely to enhance your health than others. When we discuss those topics we'll advocate our point of view openly, giving you "our side" as a balance to the "other side" which you get from friends, common sense knowledge, and similar sources.

Our definition of health education as a freeing process assumes that you are not now free. There is evidence, for instance, that feelings of inferiority,[5] hostility,[6] and alienation[7] are related to alcohol abuse; that socioeconomic status is associated with obesity;[8] and that emotional distress is related to cigarette smoking.[9] Evidently, people are not always as free to choose health-related behaviors as they might be. Health education aimed at diminishing these enslaving factors will make us freer to select health behaviors than we were before.

Other things that enslave us are ignorance (a lack of health knowledge and skills), poor self-esteem, poor problem-solving and communication skills, undue pressure from our peers, and lack of assertiveness. These issues will be discussed in more detail in Chapter 2. The purpose of mentioning them here is to explain how health education, and this book in particular, can help you become healthier as *you* define that term.

In summary, health education should provide:

1. knowledge about specific health behaviors and their physiological, sociological, psychological, and legal consequences and implications;

2. understanding of the motivations of yourself and others regarding health behavior;

3. help in acquiring health-related attitudes and behaviors that are consistent with your values;

4. learning experiences that will help you improve self-esteem, decrease alienation, develop a sense of personal control, and otherwise free you to make health-related decisions, thereby allowing you to achieve your full potential; and

5. assistance in developing decision-making, problem-solving, and communication skills.

Based on this model of health education as a freeing process, we will explore health behaviors that require a decision on your part. We want to help you to make decisions in such a way that you can realize your own potential. We will stress repeatedly that the decision is yours, but how you make it will be very important. Someone once said, "Give me a fish and I eat today, but teach me to fish and I eat forever." Throughout your reading of this book, focus on the *process* of decision making as well as the actual decision required.

Sources of Health Information

Concept: Health education takes various forms.

Health education occurs in so many subtle ways that we often don't recognize it for what it is. For instance, when an advertisement associates the ideal social life

Discovery Activity 1.2
HEALTH AND
THE MEDIA

Thumb through any popular magazine: *Redbook*, *Reader's Digest*, *People*, or the like. Briefly describe three advertisements related to health and the needs to which they appeal:

1. _____
   _____
   _____

2. _____
   _____
   _____

3. _____
   _____
   _____

with a bottle of beer, we are being taught to drink beer. The very purpose behind marketing research is to identify the consumer's personal needs and to develop advertising campaigns that represent a product as being able to satisfy those needs.[10] [11] Ads portray women in bikinis selling automobiles, "macho" men smoking cigarettes or using deodorants, and romantic evenings with handsome men and beautiful women sharing a bottle of liquor. Once you become attuned to these ploys, it is easier to identify the needs to which the advertisement is directed.

The point here is that we are encouraged by advertisers to satisfy our needs by purchasing a car, a cigarette, or a bottle of liquor—in other words, by consuming—by relying on external resources. We learn to rely on consumable products to solve our problems and satisfy our needs. This learning is, in a sense, health education.

Of course, education about health also takes place in more positive surroundings under more valid cir-

cumstances. Many newspapers and popular magazines publish articles related to health or even run a column in each issue that is concerned with the subject of health. Almost daily, television and radio programs consider health-related matters. However, all of these sources of health education must be carefully scrutinized before they can be regarded as authoritative.

Organized Health Education

More formal programs of health education, conducted by trained professional health educators, occur in school and community settings. Whether school teachers or

Many advertisements appeal to psychological needs such as the need to be loved and accepted. Thus their educational value must be judged cautiously.

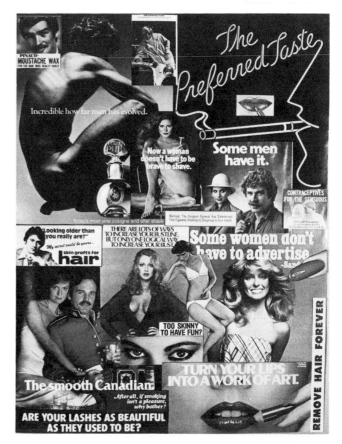

Discovery Activity 1.3
HEALTH-RELATED ARTICLES

Now return to the magazine in which you found the three advertisements you described earlier. List the titles of three articles in it that are in some way related to health:

1. _____
   _____

2. _____
   _____

3. _____
   _____

We also obtain health information by word of mouth. For instance, researchers have found that among college students the major source of information about sex is peers, rather than parents, books, films, or schools. Here, as well, information should be evaluated in terms of the expertise of the source. Too often, word-of-mouth is a case of the blind leading the blind. It is a good way to perpetuate misconceptions. ●

Discovery Activity 1.4
HEALTH PERCEPTIONS AND MISPERCEPTIONS

Try the following exercise. Read the list of health concepts presented below and decide which items are true.*

1. A person having a stomach ache should usually take a laxative.

*From Joseph G. Dzenowagis, P. V. McPherson, and Leslie W. Irwin, "Harmful Health and Safety Misconceptions of a Group of Tenth-Grade Girls," *Journal of School Health* 24 (1954): 240. Copyright, 1954, American School Health Association, Kent, Ohio 44240. Used with permission.

2. It is impossible to cure cancer.

3. There are certain remedies to cure the common cold.

4. A great deal of exercise can never hurt anyone.

5. Mental illness usually happens suddenly.

6. Most accidents cannot be prevented.

7. A good way to treat frostbite is to rub the frostbitten part in snow.

8. A daily bowel movement is necessary for a person to stay healthy.

9. Sugar diabetes is caused by eating too much sugar.

10. Most cases of baldness can be cured if treated early.

As it happens, all of the statements in Discovery Activity 1.4 are untrue. Nevertheless, such concepts are believed by many people. When one of the authors was teaching high school students, he administered a health misconceptions test like this one and found that of the 49 misconceptions he presented, over one-third of the students believed at least 10 of them to be true.[12] ●

public health educators, these professionals organize learning experiences for the dissemination of health information, the development of health-related attitudes, and the investigation of health-related behavior. Some of these health educators have as their focus **primary prevention**—the maintenance of good health and the prevention of disease. Others focus on **secondary prevention**—the early detection of illness and education regarding what the ill can do to return to optimal health. Health educators are trained in the educational process as well as in the subject of health.

CONCLUSION

Health relates to all aspects of our lives: from our physical well-being to our social interactions, our mental and emotional capacities, and even our spiritual lives. Defining how healthy we are at any one time involves assessing the very complex interaction of all of these facets of our health, as well as ordering them in terms of their value to us. It is meaningless, then, if not outright impossible, to assess someone else's health without involving that person in the assessment. The remainder of this book will help you to evaluate how healthy you are and provide you with guidance in improving those aspects of your health that *you* decide need improvement.

Good luck in this most important endeavor; your good health depends upon it.

SUMMARY

1. Our personal definitions of health largely determine how we behave. Those of us who define health as more than the absence of disease are concerned with the quality of our lives and not just with postponing death.

2. Advocates of holistic health view emotional, mental, social, spiritual, and physical health as intertwined and inseparable. To consider one component of a person's health without concurrently considering the other components is contrary to the practice of holistic health.

3. Wellness concerns the quality of life. Even if a person is not ill, he or she may not be happy or self-actualized and, therefore, may not have achieved a high level of wellness.

4. Health is a dynamic process. We move up and down the health continuum depending on the status of our emotional, mental, social, spiritual, and physical health at any particular time.

5. We view health through our value systems. If we value social health more than physical health we might smoke cigarettes because our friends do. If we value mental health more than social health we might not attend a concert with our friends because we have to study for an exam.

6. Many theories attempt to explain human behavior. When applied to health-related behavior, these theories elucidate the components of the decision-making process—for example, why some people take drugs and others do not.

7. The biggest health problems of the early 1900s were communicable diseases. Government legislation, such as quarantine and sanitation laws, was enacted to prevent the spread of these diseases. Today the major causes of death are noncommunicable and largely a function of our own health behavior.

8. Education about health should free people to make informed decisions and help them to evaluate sources of health information.

REFERENCES

1. Abraham Maslow, *Toward a Psychology of Being* (Princeton, N.J.: D. Van Nostrand, 1962).

2. Kurt Lewin, *Resolving Social Conflicts* (New York: Harper, 1948).

3. Marshall H. Becker, "The Health Belief Model and Personal Behavior," *Health Education Monographs* 2 (1974): 326–473.

4. Jerrold S. Greenberg, "Health Education as Freeing," *Health Education* 9 (1978):20–21.

5. James Calhoun and Stanley Zimmering, "Is There an Alcoholic Personality?" *Journal of Drug Education* 6 (1976):76.

6. Mary C. Jones, "Personality Correlates and Antecedents of Drinking Patterns in Adult Males," *Journal of Consulting and Clinical Psychology* 32 (1968):10.

7. Richard W. Warner, "Alienation and Drug Abuse: Synonymous?" *National Association of Secondary School Principals Bulletin* 59 (1971):55–62.

8. Werner J. Cahnman, "The Stigma of Obesity," *Sociological Quarterly* 9 (1968):283–299.

9. M.A. Jacobs et al., "Orality, Impulsivity, and Cigarette Smoking in Men: Further Findings in Support of a Theory," *Journal of Nervous and Mental Disease* 143 (1966):207–219.

10. Vance Packard, *The Hidden Persuaders* (New York: Simon & Schuster, 1957).

11. Wilson B. Key, *Subliminal Seduction* (Englewood Cliffs, N.J.: Prentice-Hall, 1973).

12. Jerrold S. Greenberg, "A Health Misconception Study," *High Points* 48 (1966):61–64.

Laboratory 1
HEALTH AND VALUES

Purpose To provide insight into the relationship between our values and our health.

Size of Group Small group of six students.

Equipment None.

Procedures

Each member of the group should individually rank order the facets of health listed below by placing a number 1 in the blank to the left of that facet of health believed to be most important, a number 2 to the left of that facet judged to be second most important, and so on.

_____ mental health _____

_____ social health _____

_____ physical health _____

_____ emotional health _____

_____ spiritual health _____

Next, add the rankings made by all of the members of the group for each of the facets of health and compute an average ranking. To do this, use the following formula:

$$\frac{\text{sum of rankings for mental health}}{\text{number of group members}} = \text{average ranking.}$$

By way of example, if the six rankings for mental health were 4, 2, 1, 4, 4, 3, the formula would be:

$$\frac{4 + 2 + 1 + 4 + 4 + 3}{6} = \text{average ranking for mental health,}$$

or

$$\frac{18}{6} = 3.$$

Write in the average rankings for all five facets of health in the space provided to the left in the Group Rankings column, in the Results section.

Next, each group member must describe the rationale behind his or her rank order of the facets of health. After each person in the group does this, the rank ordering is done once again. The rankings this time are placed in the blanks to the right of the facets of health. If any member's rationale is persuasive enough to have influenced the group, these second rankings will differ from the first.

Now compute the new group average rank orders, and write in the new rankings in the space provided to the right below.

Results

Group Rankings

Original   **Revised**

_____ mental health _____

_____ social health _____

_____ physical health _____

_____ emotional health _____

_____ spiritual health _____

Compute the change in group rankings for each aspect of health by subtracting the second ranking from the first and dropping the + or − sign. Write these in below.

Change in Group Rankings

_____ mental health

_____ social health

_____ physical health

_____ emotional health

_____ spiritual health

Discuss the following:

1. Did the group's ranking change? Why do you think it changed or didn't change?

2. If these rankings were made 20 years in the future, how do you think they would change?

3. If these rankings were made in 1900, how do you think they would differ from the rankings you came up with today?

Laboratory 2
HEALTH BELIEF MODELING

Purpose   To practice changing health behavior by using the health belief model.

Size of Group   Four students per group.

Equipment   None.

Procedure

1. Each student selects an unhealthy behavior he or she would like to give up.

2. Relative to the selected behavior, each student completes the following:

   a) The behavior is _____.

   b) The disease or illness this behavior makes me susceptible to or prevents is _____.

   c) This disease or illness is serious because ____
   _____.

   d) I can greatly diminish my chances of getting this serious illness or disease by _____.

   e) To change my behavior I would have to eliminate the following barriers:

      1. _____

      2. _____

   3. _____

   4. _____

3. Then the students form groups and share the results of the above. The group focuses on one student at a time, with other group members offering suggestions to help effect the behavioral change. For example, they may suggest ways to remove or diminish barriers to change.

Results

After all members of the group have been focused upon, they write contracts between themselves and the group. These contracts should include:

1. the behavior that will change,

2. how much of a change will occur in one week, and

3. how the change in behavior will be rewarded or how a lack of behavioral change will be punished.

One week later the group reconvenes and evaluates the members' attempts at behavioral change.

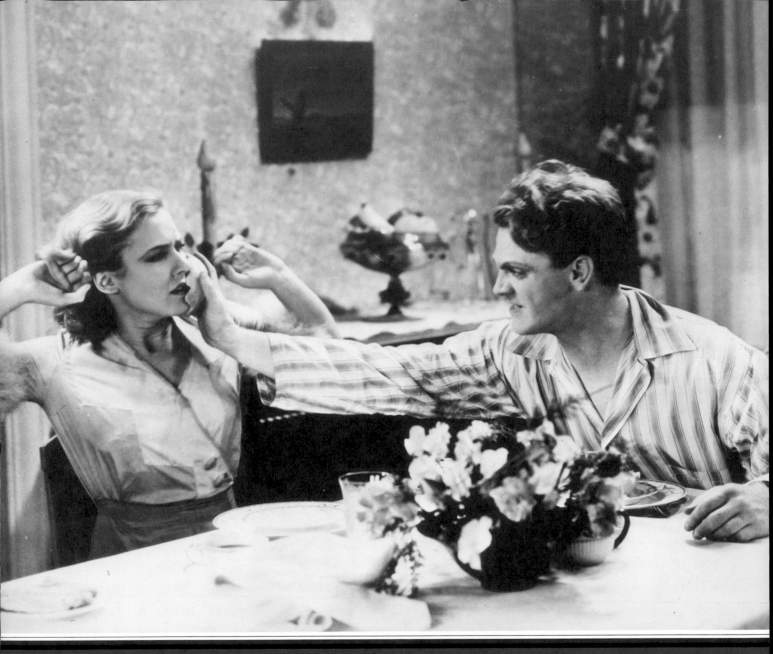

psychosocial
aspects of health

- *personal factors in health behavior*
- *social factors in health behavior*
- *other psychosocial influences*

The decisions we make about health are very complex. To illustrate, consider the apparently simple decision one might make to exercise. Exercise might be viewed as a simple solution to a concern about physical health. Most likely, however, there is more to it than this. The desire to present a pleasing physical appearance, to achieve athletic goals and thereby feel more competent, and to interact socially with others via sporting activities may also be involved in the decision to exercise. This chapter is concerned with our psychosocial reasons for behaving as we do. Throughout, you will have the opportunity to determine for yourself which psychosocial factors are influencing your own behavior.

PERSONAL FACTORS IN HEALTH BEHAVIOR

Self-Esteem

Discovery Activity 2.1
SELF-ESTEEM SCALE

For each of the statements in the Self-Esteem Scale,[1] check the letter that most accurately describes how you feel:

1. I feel that I'm a person of worth, at least on an equal plane with others.
   a) _____ Strongly agree
   b) _____ Agree
   c) _____ Disagree
   d) _____ Strongly disagree

2. I feel that I have a number of good qualities.
   a) _____ Strongly agree
   b) _____ Agree
   c) _____ Disagree
   d) _____ Strongly disagree

3. All in all, I am inclined to feel that I am a failure.
   a) _____ Strongly agree
   b) _____ Agree
   c) _____ Disagree
   d) _____ Strongly disagree

4. I am able to do things as well as most other people.
   a) _____ Strongly agree
   b) _____ Agree
   c) _____ Disagree
   d) _____ Strongly disagree

5. I feel I do not have much to be proud of.
   a) _____ Strongly agree
   b) _____ Agree
   c) _____ Disagree
   d) _____ Strongly disagree

6. I take a positive attitude toward myself.
   a) _____ Strongly agree
   b) _____ Agree
   c) _____ Disagree
   d) _____ Strongly disagree

7. On the whole, I am satisfied with myself.
   a) _____ Strongly agree
   b) _____ Agree
   c) _____ Disagree
   d) _____ Strongly disagree

8. I wish I could have more respect for myself.
   a) _____ Strongly agree
   b) _____ Agree
   c) _____ Disagree
   d) _____ Strongly disagree

9. I certainly feel useless at times.
   a) _____ Strongly agree
   b) _____ Agree
   c) _____ Disagree
   d) _____ Strongly disagree

10. At times I think I am no good at all.
    a) _____ Strongly agree
    b) _____ Agree
    c) _____ Disagree
    d) _____ Strongly disagree

You have just completed a **self-esteem** scale. To score the scale and thereby derive a measure of your self-esteem, follow these instructions:

1. The positive responses for questions 1–3 are:
   question 1: (a) or (b)
   question 2: (a) or (b)
   question 3: (c) or (d)

   If you answered two or three of these questions positively, give yourself one point.

2. The positive responses for questions 4 and 5 are:
   question 4: (a) or (b)
   question 5: (c) or (d)

   If you answered either one or both of these questions positively, give yourself one point.

3. If your answer to question 6 was (a) or (b), give yourself one point.

4. If your answer to question 7 was (a) or (b), give yourself one point.

5. If your answer to question 8 was (c) or (d), give yourself one point.

6. If your answer to question 9 or 10 or both was (c) or (d), give yourself one point.

   Add up all the points you gave yourself.

   The range of scores on this self-esteem scale is 0–6. The higher the score, the more positive your self-esteem. ●

The author of this scale defines self-esteem in the following way:

> . . . the individual respects himself, considers himself worthy, he does not necessarily consider himself better than others, but he definitely does not consider himself worse, he does not feel that he is the ultimate in perfection but, on the contrary, recognizes his limitations and expects to grow and improve.

People who do not feel good about themselves or respect themselves do not regard their own opinions and decisions as worthwhile. If we lack confidence in our own opinions and decisions, we are more apt to be influenced by others. Television advertisements, behaviors of respected peers, or adult models will unduly influence our health decisions. Thus self-esteem is a significant component of our health choices.

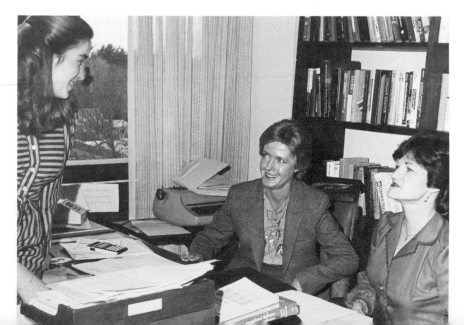

Self-esteem is an essential underpinning of healthy behavior.

To increase your self-esteem, focus on your good traits and your achievements, rather than on your poor traits and your failures. Too often we relive situations in which we "goofed" by playing them over and over again in our minds. We remember past embarrassments and actually feel them again by recalling what we did to make ourselves embarrassed. Those things are in the past. They've already happened. Learn from them, and then forget them.

On the other hand, we should make a conscious effort to pat ourselves on the back when we have succeeded at something or when one of our positive traits has been recognized. If you do well on an exam, tell others about it. You don't need to be boastful in a negative sense. You can say, "I'm proud about something, and I'd like to share it with you." When you have a spare moment, think about how well you did on that exam, rather than thinking about those on which you "bombed." Focus on the positive, on your good side. Build yourself up; don't rely on others to do it for you. You *can* be, your own best friend.

Alienation

Concept: How alienated you are affects your behavior.

Discovery Activity 2.2
ALIENATION SCALE

Below are some very general statements with which some people agree and others disagree. Indicate whether you agree or disagree with each item as it stands.[2] Check the appropriate blank, as follows:

_____ A (Strongly agree)

_____ a (Agree)

_____ U (Undecided)

_____ d (Disagree)

_____ D (Strongly disagree)

I   1. Sometimes I feel all alone in the world.

_____ A _____ a _____ U _____ d _____ D

P   2. I worry about the future facing today's children.

_____ A _____ a _____ U _____ d _____ D

I   3. I don't get invited out by friends as often as I'd really like.

_____ A _____ a _____ U _____ d _____ D

N   4. The end often justifies the means.

_____ A _____ a _____ U _____ d _____ D

I   5. Most people today seldom feel lonely.

_____ A _____ a _____ U _____ d _____ D

P   6. Sometimes I have the feeling that other people are using me.

_____ A _____ a _____ U _____ d _____ D

N   7. People's ideas change so much that I wonder if we'll ever have anything to depend on.

_____ A _____ a _____ U _____ d _____ D

I   8. Real friends are as easy as ever to find.

_____ A _____ a _____ U _____ d _____ D

P   9. It is frightening to be responsible for the development of a little child.

_____ A _____ a _____ U _____ d _____ D

N 10. Everything is relative, and there just aren't any definite rules to live by.

_____ A _____ a _____ U _____ d _____ D

I 11. One can always find friends if he or she acts friendly.

_____ A _____ a _____ U _____ d _____ D

N 12. I often wonder what the meaning of life really is.

_____ A _____ a _____ U _____ d _____ D

P 13. There is little or nothing I can do toward preventing a major "shooting" war.

_____ A _____ a _____ U _____ d _____ D

I 14. The world in which we live is basically a friendly place.

____ A ____ a ____ U ____ d ____ D

P 15. There are so many decisions that have to be made today that sometimes I could just "blow up."

____ A ____ a ____ U ____ d ____ D

N 16. The only thing one can be sure of today is that one can be sure of nothing.

____ A ____ a ____ U ____ d ____ D

I 17. There are few dependable ties between people any more.

____ A ____ a ____ U ____ d ____ D

P 18. There is little chance for promotion on the job unless a person gets a break.

____ A ____ a ____ U ____ d ____ D

N 19. With so many religions abroad, one doesn't really know which to believe.

____ A ____ a ____ U ____ d ____ D

P 20. We're so regimented today that there's not much room for choice even in personal matters.

____ A ____ a ____ U ____ d ____ D

P 21. We are just so many cogs in the machinery of life.

____ A ____ a ____ U ____ d ____ D

I 22. People are just naturally friendly and helpful.

____ A ____ a ____ U ____ d ____ D

P 23. The future looks very dismal.

____ A ____ a ____ U ____ d ____ D

I 24. I don't get to visit friends as often as I'd really like.

____ A ____ a ____ U ____ d ____ D

You have just completed an alienation scale. To score this scale, award yourself the number of points indicated for each response you made:

1.	4 A	3 a	2 U	1 d	0 D
2.	4 A	3 a	2 U	1 d	0 D
3.	4 A	3 a	2 U	1 d	0 D
4.	4 A	3 a	2 U	1 d	0 D
5.	0 A	1 a	2 U	3 d	4 D
6.	4 A	3 a	2 U	1 d	0 D
7.	4 A	3 a	2 U	1 d	0 D
8.	0 A	1 a	2 U	3 d	4 D
9.	4 A	3 a	2 U	1 d	0 D
10.	4 A	3 a	2 U	1 d	0 D
11.	0 A	1 a	2 U	3 d	4 D
12.	4 A	3 a	2 U	1 d	0 D
13.	4 A	3 a	2 U	1 d	0 D
14.	0 A	1 a	2 U	3 d	4 D
15.	4 A	3 a	2 U	1 d	0 D
16.	4 A	3 a	2 U	1 d	0 D
17.	4 A	3 a	2 U	1 d	0 D
18.	4 A	3 a	2 U	1 d	0 D
19.	4 A	3 a	2 U	1 d	0 D
20.	4 A	3 a	2 U	1 d	0 D
21.	4 A	3 a	2 U	1 d	0 D
22.	0 A	1 a	2 U	3 d	4 D
23.	4 A	3 a	2 U	1 d	0 D
24.	4 A	3 a	2 U	1 d	0 D

Alienation consists of three factors:

1. **Social isolation.** The lack of significant others (friends, relatives, etc.) in whom one can confide.
2. **Normlessness.** The lack of rules, regulations, and standards by which one chooses to live.
3. **Powerlessness.** The feeling of not being in control of one's own destiny.

To determine your scores on each of these three factors, add up separately the points for all the items preceded by an I (social isolation), an N (normlessness), and a P (powerlessness). The higher your score, the more you possess this factor.

When this scale was administered to male under-graduates, they averaged 36.64, with the following subscores:

social isolation—11.76,

normlessness—7.62,

powerlessness—13.65.

Undergraduate women averaged 36.25, with these subscores:

social isolation—14.85,

normlessness—7.63,

powerlessness—12.73.

If you scored higher than 37 you may be more alienated that the average college student. If that is the case, perhaps your health behavior is being influenced by your degree of alienation, and you might decide to do something about this. To begin, inspect your sub-scores. Is one subscore way out of line with the average scores reported above? If so, that is the component of alienation that needs attention. If it's social isolation, you may be conforming to other people's behaviors because you're lonely. To develop friendships, you might want to join a club on campus or get involved with the student newspaper, yearbook, or student government. If you scored high on normlessness or powerlessness, joining an organized group will also help. You will have a set of standards (the group's) to guide your be-havior and to which you can relate, and the sense of being unable to control your destiny can be diminished by working with others toward a common goal.

Researchers have found that alienation is related to health behavior. Harris, for instance, found that the use of marijuana was greater for college students who were highly alienated than for those less alienated.[3] Further, researchers have concluded that suicide, the second leading cause of death among college students, is di-rectly related to alienation. As one writer states:

> Of all the psychodynamic attributes associated with suicidal behavior, the factor of human isolation and withdrawal appears to be the single most effective distinction between those who kill themselves and those who do not. Numerous investigators have re-ported that youngsters who commit suicide invariably had no close friends with whom they could share confidences or receive psychological support.[4]

It seems evident, finally, that if you scored high in powerlessness, for instance, you might decide not to behave in a healthy manner since you would feel that you had little control over your health anyway.

Locus of Control

Concept: How much in control you think you are affects your behavior.

Discovery Activity 2.3
LOCUS OF CONTROL SCALE*

Read the statements below and circle the appropriate responses.[5]

1. Good health comes from being lucky.

   yes   no

2. There is nothing I can do to keep from getting sick.

   yes   no

3. Bad luck makes people get sick.

   yes   no

4. I can only do what the doctor tells me to do.

   yes   no

5. Getting sick just happens.

   yes   no

6. People who never get sick are just plain lucky.

   yes   no

7. It is my parents' job to keep me from getting sick.

   yes   no

*The Children's Health Locus of Control Scale is a copyrighted in-strument and permission must be obtained from Guy S. Parcel prior to using the scale for research or evaluation purposes.

8. Only a doctor or a nurse keeps people from getting sick.

   yes   no

9. I can make very few choices about my health.

   yes   no

10. Accidents just happen.

    yes   no

11. I can do many things to fight illness.

    yes   no

12. Only the dentist can take care of my teeth.

    yes   no

13. The only way I can stay healthy is to do what other people tell me to do.

    yes   no

14. I always go to the Student Health Service on campus if I get hurt at school.

    yes   no

15. It is the college's job to keep me from having accidents at school.

    yes   no

16. I can make many choices about my health.

    yes   no

17. If I feel sick, I have to wait for other people to tell me what to do.

    yes   no

18. Whenever I feel sick I go to the Student Health Service.

    yes   no

19. There is nothing I can do to have healthy teeth.

    yes   no

20. I can do many things to prevent accidents.

    yes   no

These items comprise a health **locus of control** scale. To score this scale, award one point for each "No" response *except* for items 11, 16, and 20. For those items, score one point for each "Yes" response. The range of scores is 0–20 with higher scores indicating internal health locus of control and lower scores indicating external health locus of control. ●

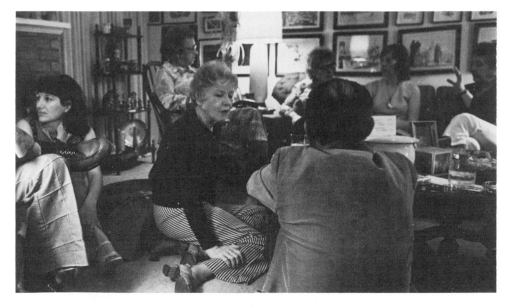

Participation in a self-help group such as Parents without Partners probably reflects an internal locus of control—the belief that you can influence the events in your life.

Internal locus of control refers to one's belief that he or she can influence events, whereas external locus of control refers to one's belief that he or she has very little influence over events. This scale relates locus of control to influences upon one's health. If you scored near 20, you feel that you can do things that can have an effect upon your health. If you scored near 0, you feel that your health is beyond your control. It stands to reason that those with an internal health locus of control would be more apt to adopt positive health behaviors than those with an external health locus of control.

Each of us is in control of much more of our lives than we may realize. Experiments with biofeedback equipment (discussed in Chapter 4) suggest that people can exert some control over their own blood pressure, brain waves, body temperature, secretions of acid in the stomach, and serum cholesterol level. We may not be able to control others or our environment, but we can control our reactions to these external stimuli. For example, consider people who say, "So-and-so got me angry." No one gets you angry. You *allow* yourself to be angered by so-and-so. The anger is your own doing. To prove this point, aren't there some days when you awake in a great frame of mind, the sun is shining, you anticipate an enjoyable day, and you tell yourself, "This day is so great, nothing can bother me today"? On those days, nothing will bother you even though things might happen that would drive you up a wall on any other day. You are in control on those days.

Of course, some things are beyond our control. We don't live on an island separated from the rest of the human race. Our environment places many demands upon us, as do other people about whom we care. In a very real sense we co-create our futures with external forces and events.

Unfortunately, many of us forget *our* impact on the future and on our health behavior. If we possess an external locus of control, we might decide not to work hard at giving up smoking. "After all, not everyone who smokes gets lung cancer. The air we breathe is so polluted it doesn't matter whether we smoke or not. It's a matter of luck or chance whether or not we get lung cancer." If we possess an internal locus of control, we might say: "Although I have no control over the air I breathe in, I don't have to contaminate that air further. I can give up cigarette smoking and decrease my chances of getting lung cancer. I can exercise some degree of control over my health."

Assertiveness

Concept: Assertiveness, or the lack of it, affects our health decision making.

Discovery Activity 2.4 ### *ASSERTIVENESS SCALE*

Using the code given below, indicate how characteristic or descriptive of you each of the following statements is.[6]

+3 Very characteristic of me, extremely descriptive

+2 Rather characteristic of me, quite descriptive

+1 Somewhat characteristic of me, slightly descriptive

−1 Somewhat uncharacteristic of me, slightly nondescriptive

−2 Rather uncharacteristic of me, quite nondescriptive

−3 Very uncharacteristic of me, extremely nondescriptive

_____ 1. Most people seem to be more aggressive and assertive than I am.

_____ 2. I have hesitated to make or accept dates because of "shyness."

_____ 3. When the food served at a restaurant is not done to my satisfaction, I complain about it to the waiter or waitress.

_____ 4. I am careful to avoid hurting other people's feelings, even when I feel I have been injured.

5. If a salesperson has gone to considerable trouble to show me merchandise that is not quite suitable, I have a difficult time in saying "No."

6. When I am asked to do something, I insist upon knowing why.

7. There are times when I look for a good, vigorous argument.

8. I strive to get ahead as well as most people in my position.

9. To be honest, people often take advantage of me.

10. I enjoy starting conversations with new acquaintances and strangers.

11. I often don't know what to say to attractive persons of the opposite sex.

12. I will hesitate to make phone calls to business establishments and institutions.

13. I would rather apply for a job or for admission to a college by writing letters than by going through with personal interviews.

14. I find it embarrassing to return merchandise.

15. If a close and respected relative were annoying me, I would smother my feelings rather than express my annoyance.

16. I have avoided asking questions for fear of sounding stupid.

17. During an argument I am sometimes afraid that I will get so upset that I will shake all over.

18. If a famed and respected lecturer makes a statement that I think is incorrect, I will have the audience hear my point of view as well.

19. I avoid arguing over prices with clerks and salespeople.

Issues in Health
HOW MUCH SHOULD PEOPLE BE "SOCIALIZED" TO FIT INTO OUR SOCIETY?

A high school student, so the story goes, wrote the following poem and left it on his desk at school just prior to taking his own life:*

*He always wanted to say things. But no one understood.
He always wanted to explain things. But no one cared.
So he drew.*

*Sometimes he would just draw and it wasn't anything. He wanted to carve it in stone or write it in the sky.
He would lie out on the grass and look up in the sky, and it would be only him and the sky and the things inside him that needed saying.*

*And it was after that, that he drew the picture. It was a beautiful picture. He kept it under the pillow and would let no one see it.
And he would look at it every night and think about it. And when it was dark, and his eyes were closed, he could still see it.*

And it was all of him. And he loved it.

When he started school, he brought it with him. Not to show anyone, but just to have it with him like a friend.

*It was funny about school.
He sat in a square, brown desk like all the other square, brown desks and he thought it should be red.
And his room was a square, brown room. Like all the other rooms. And it was tight and close. And stiff.*

(continued)

*Source unknown.

Issues in Health (continued)

*He hated to hold the pencil and the chalk,
with his arm still and his feet flat on the floor,
stiff, with the teacher watching and watching.
And then he had to write numbers. And they
weren't anything. They were worse than the
letters that could be something if you put
them together.*
*And the numbers were tight and square, and
he hated the whole thing.*

*The teacher came and spoke to him. She told
him to wear a tie like all the other boys. He
said he didn't like them, and she said it didn't
matter.*
*After that they drew. And he drew all yellow
and it was the way he felt about morning.
And it was beautiful.*

*The teacher came and smiled at him. "What's
this?" she said. "Why don't you draw
something like Ken's drawing? Isn't that
beautiful?"*
It was all questions.

*After that his mother bought him a tie, and he
always drew airplanes and rocket ships like
everyone else. And he threw the old picture
away.*
*And when he lay out alone looking at the
sky, it was big and blue and all of everything,
but he wasn't anymore.*

*He was square inside and brown, and his
hands were stiff, and he was like anyone else.
And the thing inside him that needed saying
didn't need saying anymore.*

*It had stopped pushing. It was crushed. Stiff.
Like everything else.*

Some would say schools are supposed to prepare people to function in society and that requires
giving up some individuality. Others believe society
can only develop and improve if people's individ-
ualities are nurtured.

What do you think? ●

_____ 20. When I have done something important
or worthwhile, I manage to let others know
about it.

_____ 21. I am open and frank about my feelings.

_____ 22. If someone has been spreading false and
bad stories about me, I see him or her as
soon as possible to "have a talk" about
it.

_____ 23. I often have a hard time saying "No."

_____ 24. I tend to bottle up my emotions rather than
make a scene.

_____ 25. I complain about poor service in a restaurant and elsewhere.

_____ 26. When I am given a compliment, I sometimes just don't know what to say.

_____ 27. If a couple near me in a theater or at a
lecture were conversing rather loudly, I
would ask them to be quiet or take their
conversation elsewhere.

_____ 28. Anyone attempting to push ahead of me
in a line is in for a good battle.

_____ 29. I am quick to express an opinion.

_____ 30. There are times when I just can't say anything.

You have just completed a scale that assesses **assertiveness**. To score this scale, first change the signs
(+ or −) for items 1, 2, 4, 5, 9, 11, 12, 13, 14, 15,
16, 17, 19, 23, 24, 26, and 30. Next add up all the
(+) items and all the (−) items. Now subtract the minus
total from the plus total. The possible scores range from
−90 to +90; the midpoint is zero. The higher the
score, the more assertive your behavior. ●

When this scale was administered to college students, they averaged 0.30. However, more important
than someone else's average is your own score. How
assertive are you? It stands to reason that if you have
difficulty asserting your own needs and desires, you
will be more likely to do what others expect of you
than what you think is right. You will have difficulty

asserting yourself in a job situation or resisting the pressure to behave in certain ways—for example, sexually.

It should be noted that assertive behavior differs from aggressive behavior. You can assert yourself firmly but nicely, rather than by being argumentative or belligerent. In any case, being submissive is not conducive to making the health-related decision that is right for you.

Some definitions seem in order here:

1. *Assertive behavior*—Expressing yourself and satisfying your own needs. Feeling good about this and not hurting others in the process.
2. *Nonassertive behavior*—Denying your own wishes to satisfy someone else's.
3. *Aggressive behavior*—Seeking to dominate others or to get your own way at their expense.

Assertiveness is not only a matter of *what* you say but also a function of *how* you say it. Assertive body language consists of: straight, steady posture and eye contact; speaking in a clear, steady voice that is loud enough to be heard; and speaking fluently, confidently, and without hesitation. In contrast, nonassertive body language is marked by: lack of eye contact (looking down or away), swaying and shifting of weight from one foot to the other, and whining and hesitancy when speaking.

Aggressive behavior can also be recognized by body language as well as words. Aggressive behavior often includes: leaning forward with glaring eyes, pointing a finger at the person to whom one is speaking, shouting, clenched fists, and hands on hips. ●

If you want to act assertively, you must pay attention to your body language. Practice and adopt assertive nonverbal behavior, while concentrating on eliminating signs of nonassertive and aggressive behavior. Even if you make an assertive verbal response, you will not be believed if your body's response is nonassertive.

As to *what* you say, an effective formula in helping people express themselves assertively is the DESC Form.[7] The verbal response is divided into four components: Describe, Express, Specify, and Choose. Each of these is described below:

1. *Describe:* Paint a verbal picture of the other person's behavior or the situation to which you are reacting. "When you . . ."; "When . . ."
2. *Express:* Relating your feelings regarding the other person's behavior or the situation you have just described. Use "I" statements here: "I feel . . ."
3. *Specify:* Identify several changes you would like to see in the other person's behavior or in the situation. Rather than saying, "You should . . .," again use "I" statements: "I would prefer . . .," "I would like . . .," "I want . . ."
4. *Choose:* Select the consequences you have decided to apply to the behavior or situation. What will you do if the other person's behavior or the situation changes to your satisfaction? "If you do . . ., I will . . ." What will be the consequences if nothing changes, or if the changes do not meet your needs? "If you don't . . ., I will . . ."

To demonstrate the DESC form of organizing assertive responses, let's assume Jim and Kathy are dat-

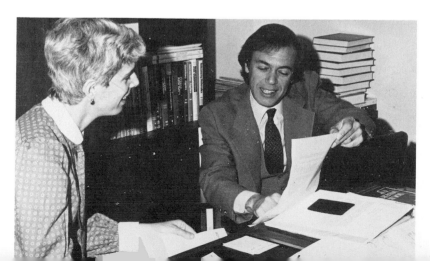

Being assertive without being aggressive can be crucial in many situations, such as a job interview.

ing. Jim wants Kathy to date him exclusively. Kathy believes she's too young to eliminate other men from her love life. Jim's assertive response to this situation might be:

"[Describe] When you go out with other men, [Express] I feel very jealous and have doubts about the extent of your love for me. [Specify] I would prefer that we only date each other. [Choose] If you only date me, I'll make a sincere effort to offer you a variety of experiences so that you do not feel you've missed anything. We'll go to nice restaurants, attend plays, go to concerts, and whatever else you'd like that we can afford and that is reasonable. If you do not agree to date me exclusively, I will not date you at all. The pain would be more than I'm willing to tolerate."

SOCIAL FACTORS IN HEALTH BEHAVIOR

Values

Concept: Your values affect your behavior.

In many situations people react quite differently from one another. One reason for this is that we all have different value systems. For instance, some people smoke cigarettes because they value the immediate pleasure it provides and are willing to risk the inherent long-term danger. Other people refrain from smoking cigarettes because they value physical fitness and abhor any insult to physical health. One student may seek sexual liaisons with as many partners as possible since he or she values pleasure; whereas another may limit sexual behavior to marriage since he or she has great respect for religious teachings. Of course, many factors lead to any one behavior, but values are important. The exercises below are designed to assist you in determining what your values are.

Peer Group Pressure

Concept: Friends have a profound influence on how we behave.

For most people, peer group pressure is a very powerful force. In particular, if you possess low self-esteem, an external locus of control, and little assertiveness, you are probably greatly influenced by your friends. The questions in the activity are designed to reveal for you just how important your friends' behaviors are in determining how you will behave.

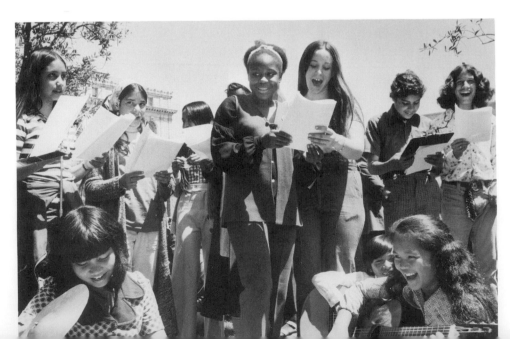

Peers have a strong influence on the kinds of behaviors and activities in which people engage.

Discovery Activity 2.5
VALUES

List ten of your material possessions:

1. _____
2. _____
3. _____
4. _____
5. _____
6. _____
7. _____
8. _____
9. _____
10. _____

Beside each possession listed, briefly write what you would like to have happen to it when you die.

- Why are these possessions valuable to you? What about your values is revealed by what you decided you'd like done with these possessions when you die?
- Would you rather be healthy, rich, or intelligent? Why?
- Would you rather smoke a pack of cigarettes each day, a joint of marijuana each day, or drink two bottles of beer each day? Why?
- Would you rather spend money on an annual medical examination, season tickets for a professional sports team, or membership in an athletic club? Why?
- Would you rather purchase medical insurance, dental insurance, or life insurance? Why?

What have your responses to these questions taught you about your values?

- Of all the people who ever lived, whom do you admire the most?

- Of all the parts of your body, which do you abuse the most? Which do you concentrate on developing the most? Do you value physical appearance more than physical health?
- What have you done for your mind lately? For your body? For your relations with others? For fun? For health?
- What could you do to live longer? Is it worth doing or does it take time away from something more important? Is quality of life more important to you than quantity or length of life? How do you know? What about your typical behavior leads you to answer this way?
- After you pay for the necessities (room and board and the minimum required clothing), how do you spend your money? What does this reveal about your values?

Write down what you have learned about your value system from these questions and exercises:

_____
_____
_____
_____

Discovery Activity 2.6
PEER INFLUENCE

Answer the following questions to determine to what degree you are influenced by peer pressure.

1. In what ways are you and your friends similar?
2. What qualities in your friends do you like best? Do you find yourself trying to emulate these qualities?
3. What qualities in your friends do you like least? Do you try to avoid assuming these qualities yourself?

Issues in Health
HOW INDEPENDENT SHOULD PEOPLE BE?

Some people believe that the focus of the 1970s upon the individual has been harmful. The emphasis on assertiveness, positive self-esteem, and being in control of one's destiny has led to more societal disharmony than necessary. The rate of divorce is increasing because people are focusing on their own needs and personal development rather than on the marital union. Out-of-wedlock pregnancies and sexually irresponsible behavior are prevalent because people are being taught that they have a right to have their needs met. More and more frustration is evident in people who, believing they can control their destinies, attempt to lose weight only to find that this behavior is beyond their control. Drug dependence, cigarette smoking, and sedentary lifestyles are other behaviors that people have difficulty controlling. We should teach people how to relate to and depend upon other people rather than to function independently, these observers of the 1970s would say. What's wrong with a little peer pressure to influence people to behave in a healthy manner?

Others believe independence is positive. People who have confidence in themselves, who can assert their needs, and who believe they have some measure of control over events that affect their lives are happier and healthier. Only when people feel good about themselves can they relate well with others. That people are helped to become more independent in their decision making does not mean they do not consider the opinions, feelings, and needs of others. Rather, independence allows for more objectivity in decision making, resulting in a better decision. As a consequence, marriages are improved, health behaviors are adopted that satisfy needs, and everyone is better in the long run. What do you think? ●

4. What kinds of health habits do your friends have? Do they smoke, drink, eat healthy food, exercise? Do their health patterns influence your own?

5. Do you stick to your guns when your opinions differ from those of your friends, or are you more likely to bow to the majority opinion?

6. Do you share the same interests as your friends? Are they interests you developed on your own, or did you develop them as a result of your friendships? ●

OTHER PSYCHOSOCIAL INFLUENCES

Concept: Many psychosocial factors influence health decisions.

Many psychosocial variables besides self-esteem, alienation, locus of control, assertiveness, Type A behavior pattern, values, and peer pressure influence health behavior. Fear of medical procedures or of becoming ill, anxiety, stress, and shyness may all be related to a person's health decisions. Certain sociological factors, such as education, age, religion, and race, have also been found to be related to health behavior and to health status. Access to health care and to health messages disseminated through various media also affect health behavior.

The list goes on and on. The point is that health status and health behavior are complex variables comprised of physiological components but greatly influenced by psychosocial factors. This point will become even clearer in Chapter 4 when we discuss stress.

CONCLUSION

In this chapter we have presented some of the myriad of psychosocial influences upon health decisions. More important, you have had the opportunity to determine how you might be influenced by these factors. The important question now is, how will you use this new awareness to become healthier?

Will you enroll in an assertiveness training course if you scored low on assertiveness?

Will you consciously seek ways to improve your self-esteem, for instance, by spending considerable time on those activities in which you have a reasonable chance of success?

Will you decrease your alienation by seeking out more friends and social contacts?

Will you use knowledge of your values to increase the satisfaction you derive from life?

Only you can answer these questions, for you have the most to gain by incorporating this new awareness into a pattern of living that will result in a healthier life.

SUMMARY

1. Our health behavior is influenced by our level of self-esteem. If we don't think well enough of ourselves, we might not have confidence in our own health decisions, and consequently we might be inordinately influenced by other people.

2. Alienation consists of three factors: social isolation, normlessness, and powerlessness. High levels of alienation are related to such behaviors as drug abuse and suicide.

3. Our perception of the degree of control we have over our own destiny has a significant impact on our health behavior. If we view the locus of control as external, we will not expect to have much influence over our health. If we consider the locus of control to be internal, we will tend to pay attention to our health behavior in the belief that we can influence our health status.

4. If we don't know how to state our needs and rights verbally, we are liable to behave in ways inconsistent with our real nature. Assertiveness helps us to be able to say yes and no as we desire. In this way our health behavior will be a result of our decisions.

5. Our health behavior is influenced by our values. When we choose to behave in certain ways, we are often deciding between two or more alternatives. The choice we make reflects our values.

6. Most of us are influenced by, and exert influence upon, our friends. We hold similar values, adopt similar behaviors, and even speak and dress similarly. It is not surprising that people are more likely to smoke cigarettes, for instance, if their best friends smoke.

7. Many other psychological factors are related to our health status and behavior. Some of these are sex, education, socioeconomic status, age, fear, anxiety, and stress.

REFERENCES

1. Morris Rosenberg, *Society and the Adolescent Self-Image* (Princeton, N.J.: Princeton University Press, 1965), p. 305. Copyright ©1965 by Princeton University Press; Princeton Paperback 1968. Reprinted by permission of Princeton University Press.

2. Dwight G. Dean, "Alienation: Its Meaning and Measurement," *American Sociological Review* 26 (1961):753–758. Reprinted by permission of the author.

3. Eileen Harris, "A Measurement of Alienation in College Student Marijuana Users and Non-users," *The Journal of School Health* 41 (1971):133.

4. Richard H. Seiden, "The Problems of Suicide on College Campuses," *The Journal of School Health* 41 (1971):244. Copyright ©1971, American School Health Association, Kent, Ohio 44240.

5. Adapted from Guy S. Parcel and Michael P. Meyer, "My Views About Health and Illness," personal communication, 1977.

6. Spencer A. Rathus, "A 30-Item Schedule for Assessing Assertive Behavior," *Behavior Therapy* 4 (1973):398–406. Reprinted by permission.

7. Sharon Bower and Gordon Bower, *Asserting Yourself* (Reading, Mass.: Addison-Wesley, 1976).

Laboratory 1
IMPROVING SELF-ESTEEM

Purpose   To provide ways in which each member in the class can improve his or her self-esteem.

Size of Group   Small group of four students.

Equipment   None.

Procedure

Recognizing that you can feel good about your physical self but feel badly about other aspects of yourself, rank order the list below by placing a number 1 next to that part of you that you feel best about, a number 2 next to that part you feel next best about, and so on until you reach that part of yourself that you feel least good about.

Your physical self   _____

Your intellectual self   _____

Your spiritual self   _____

Your social self   _____

Your family self   _____

Your emotional self   _____

Focusing upon one group member at a time, follow the procedure outlined below:

1. The group member explains his or her rationale for the number 6 ranking (that aspect that he or she believes is most in need of improvement).

2. The other group members ask questions directed toward clarifying the ranking rather than toward changing the individual's mind or making the individual feel better.

3. After ten minutes of discussion, the individual's chair is turned so that he or she is sitting facing away from the group. The individual is not allowed to talk at this time. The group discusses possible behaviors that he or she could adopt to improve that aspect of the self judged to be most in need of development. This discussion is limited to three minutes.

4. The individual then sits facing the group and in one minute reacts to the suggestions offered. The other group members must remain silent while the individual makes a commitment to trying one of the suggested behaviors.

5. The cycle is repeated until each group member has been the focus.

Results

After each group member has had ample time to try a suggested behavior (perhaps one or two weeks), the groups should be reconvened to discuss the results of attempts to improve aspects of self-esteem. Those feeling successful should be encouraged. Those not feeling successful should have other behaviors suggested to them by the group.

Laboratory 2
ASSERTIVENESS TRAINING

Purpose   To observe, analyze, and practice assertive behavior.

Size of Group   Total class.

Equipment   One table.
One tablecloth.

Procedure

Choose volunteers to act out the following parts:

1. A *waiter* in a restaurant. This waiter is rude, slow, and a male chauvinist with filthy hands.

2. A *female patron* seated with her boyfriend at a table that the waiter is serving.

3. The *boyfriend*. This man is shy and fearful. He has been stepped on all of his life and never reacts.

4. The *manager* of the restaurant. He wants the patrons of the restaurant to be satisfied so that they will return in the future. However, the waiter is his best friend.

The scene is set by the manager seating the patrons. The rest of the class observes the behavior of the female patron, who is charged with being assertive. Remember the differences between being assertive, submissive, and aggressive:

1. *Assertive behavior.* Expressing yourself and satisfying your own needs. Feeling good about this and not hurting others in the process.

2. *Submissive behavior.* Denying your own wishes to satisfy someone else's. Sacrificing your own needs to meet theirs.

3. *Aggressive behavior.* Seeking to dominate others or to get your own way at their expense. Not desirable behavior.

Results

After 20 minutes of role playing, a class discussion should revolve about these questions:

1. When was the female patron acting assertively? Submissively? Aggressively?

2. When should the male patron have been assertive?

3. How frequently is assertive behavior needed and how many of you are usually assertive?

4. Describe a situation in which you should have been assertive but were not.

5. Do either males or females need assertiveness training more than the other sex?

health and your mind

Part two

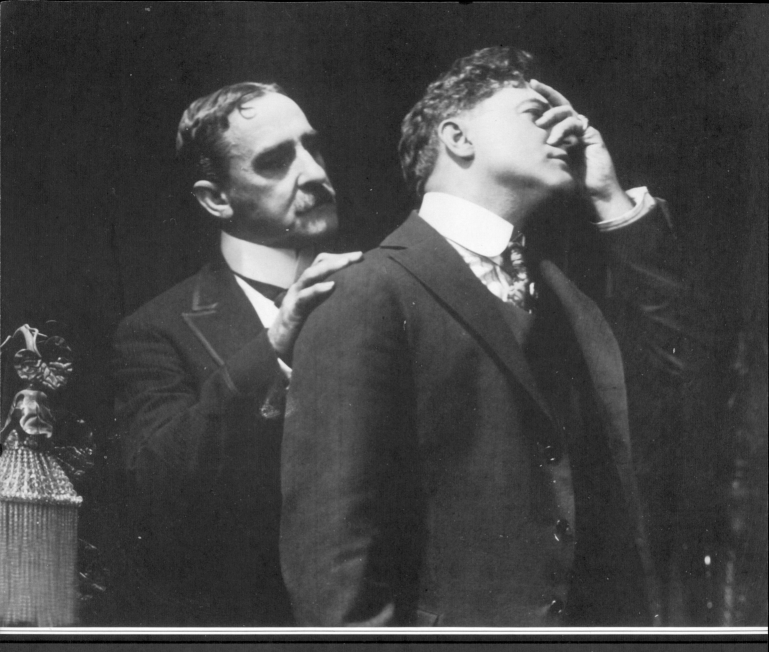

chapter 3

mental health

- *characteristics of emotional health*
- *personality development*
- *modes of coping*
- *coping with common problems*
- *mental disorders*
- *seeking help*

Mental health is a significant part of your well-being. You may not have a noticeable physical illness, but your ability to interact with other people may be limited. You may not have contracted a communicable disease, but your anger may be uncontrollable. You may not have any physical pain, but your inability to manage anxiety may be causing a great deal of hurt. Because our minds and bodies are inseparable—what happens to one invariably affects the other—the consideration of our mental health is of equal importance to the study of our physical health.

This chapter discusses such mental health topics as the characteristics of emotional health, personality development, modes of coping, common coping problems, mental disorders, and the types of help available for mental health problems.

CHARACTERISTICS OF EMOTIONAL HEALTH

Think of someone you know whom you would describe as emotionally healthy. This may seem premature when emotional health hasn't even been defined yet, but having someone in mind when the characteristics of emotional health are discussed will provide you with a model of these characteristics. Having this model in mind, it will be easier for you to emulate the emotionally health characteristics of this person so that you too can be emotionally healthy.

Emotional health includes the ability to deal constructively with reality. If things aren't going your way and you are emotionally healthy, you are probably making the best out of a bad situation. For example, suppose you meet a person with whom you would like to be friendly but who has another person as a best friend. You could mope around or act angrily toward the person with whom you would like to be friends. This behavior certainly wouldn't win the friendship, but it is how many people would act when not getting what they want. An emotionally healthy person would savor the time spent with the other person, however limited, and develop other friendships.

An emotionally healthy person also adapts to change and realizes that life would be dull without it. Rather than viewing changes as threatening and always attempting to maintain the status quo, an emotionally health person considers change an opportunity for new experiences and new challenges. Although change is not always for the better, an emotionally healthy person will recognize when change is inevitable and adjust to it as well as possible.

An emotionally healthy person exercises a reasonable degree of independence (not overly conforming but also not overly individualistic), has the ability to make long-range choices, and can work productively. In addition, the emotionally healthy individual can establish satisfactory relationships by showing concern and love for other people. These relationships provide companionship, love, someone with whom to share joys and sorrows, and a focus outside of the self. Developing such relationships requires the ability to live with emotions. The emotionally healthy can accept their own emotions as well as those of others. Fear, anger, insecurity, and love are accepted as part of living and do not incapacitate the emotionally healthy.

Now to return to that emotionally healthy person we asked you to think about: Does the description

An important criterion of emotional health is the ability to show love and concern for others.

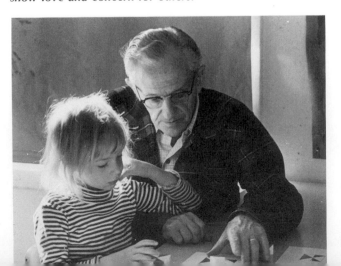

above characterize that person? No one has *perfect* emotional health, so no one will demonstrate all of these characteristics all the time. Generally, however, emotionally healthy people function as we have described. Which behaviors of your emotionally healthy model would you benefit from emulating? Would someone use you as a model of an emotionally healthy person? If so, what are you doing right? If not, what can you change to become more emotionally healthy?

PERSONALITY DEVELOPMENT

Our emotional health depends in large part on our socialization, which makes us the persons we are. To change our behaviors, we first need to understand these socializing influences on them. The theories of personality development discussed in this section offer various perspectives on socialization as it influences your emotional health and style of coping.

Concept: People's behaviors can be understood in the context of their personality development.

Freud's Theory

One well-known theory of human behavior is Sigmund Freud's analysis of psychosexual development. Freud proposed that the personality is composed of three basic elements: the id, the ego, and the superego. The **id** is the part of us that is always seeking pleasure. The **ego** is the part that is in touch with reality—the intellectual part. The **superego** represents our conscience—our sense of right and wrong. The ego uses defense mechanisms (discussed in the next section) to control the id. These three elements are constantly in conflict. We seek pleasure (id) but realize reality places limits on our pleasure seeking (ego). Our conscience (superego) then takes over and seeks the best course for that situation. The superego is like the rider pulling on the reins (ego) of the wild horse (id). For example, you might be tempted to get high on drugs (id) but realize that drug abuse is illegal and risky to your health (ego). Your conscience (superego) then decides to pull in the reins on your desire to get high, and you pass up the drugs.

Freud believed that we always seek pleasure but are controlled by our sense of reality and our conscience. Therefore, we are constantly trying to balance these forces and sometimes engage in unpleasurable activities that we believe are right or good for us.

Have you ever done this? When you find it difficult to cope, could you understand your behavior better by considering how the id, ego, and superego interact with one another?

Freud described five stages of psychosexual development. He believed that sexuality was the central motivator of human behavior and that personality was determined by whether or not the goals of each psychosexual stage of development were achieved. These stages are:

1. Oral stage. From birth to 18 months of age, sucking and other oral stimulation are extremely satisfying and important to the child. The conflict of this stage centers around receiving adequate oral gratification. Children who are weaned (taken off the breast or bottle) too early may experience frustration and become fixated (arrested) at this stage of development. Among the traits associated with an "oral" personality are dependency and excessive optimism or pessimism.

2. Anal stage. Beginning at approximately a year and a half and lasting until age three, control of anal functions develops, and satisfaction shifts from the mouth to the anus. According to Freud, those who do not achieve anal control or for whom this focus is prolonged or exaggerated may develop certain personality traits. For instance, children who are anal-retentive (who did not successfully give up their feces by achieving the goal at this stage) may become stingy, obstinate, or obsessively clean adults.

3. Phallic stage. Beginning at age three, the focus of attention is on the sexual organs. Pleasure is derived from handling and viewing these organs. In addition, Freud suggested, this stage is the one in which an unconscious sexual desire for the parent of the opposite sex and jealousy of the parent of the same sex develop. The goal of this stage is to resolve the **Oedipus** (boy-father) or **Electra** (girl-mother) **complex** and identify with the parent of the same sex. Those unsuccessful during this stage may be unable to establish close relationships with other people.

4. Latency stage. Appearing in schoolchildren, this stage is represented by social conformity and by repression of sexuality and sex. If personality development is successful at this stage, the individual will establish friendships with members of the same sex. The adult fixated at this stage may have difficulty developing close relationships with other people of the same sex.

5. Genital stage. This stage begins in puberty, when sexual maturity occurs, and is characterized by a renewed focus on the genitals as a source of pleasure. The genitals remain the focus of sexual satisfaction throughout life. However, fixation at this stage can lead to sexual permissiveness, adultery, excessive flirting, and a general overemphasis on sexual gratification compared to other kinds of satisfaction in adult life.

Before ending this discussion, it should be noted that Freud's theory is just that—a theory. Some people believe a major portion of it is valid, whereas others consider its emphasis on sexuality as the motivator of human behavior misplaced. The debate goes on.

Erikson's Theory

Psychoanalyst Erik Erikson, a student of Freud, proposed a theory of psycho-social stages of development. According to Erikson's theory of human behavior,[1] there are eight stages of life. In each of these stages we experience a crisis with which we must cope. Although Freud and Erikson differ on the particular tasks and crises at different stages, they agree that how the goals of each stage are handled determines a person's personality. Erikson's stages are:

1. Age 0–1. The crisis at this stage is *trust versus mistrust.* Trust is learned by interactions with parents and other primary caregivers. By being fed, comforted, and held, the infant learns that his or her needs will be met and that the world is a place that can be trusted. If the needs of the infant are not met consistently, that individual won't be able to trust others—an attitude that will affect relationships in later life.

2. Age 1–3. The crisis at this stage is *autonomy versus shame.* The child wants to be more independent (control of feces represents a major achievement of independence) but must also submit to control by parents. The individual who fails to achieve a balance between cooperation and autonomy will be either overly influenced by pressures to conform (cooperation) or insistent on getting his or her own way (autonomy).

3. Age 3–5. The crisis at this stage is *initiative versus guilt.* The child's interest in the parent of the opposite sex is channeled into acceptable behaviors, and the child begins to look outside the home and develop his or her own initiative. Through play, the child learns socially acceptable ways of relating with other people. Unless this crisis is satisfactorily resolved, the child's conscience may not develop fully, and as an adult, his or her behavior will be selfish or inhibited by feelings of guilt.

4. Age 5–12. The crisis at this stage is *industry versus inferiority.* The tasks of school are influential in the resolution of this crisis. Knowledge and skills develop rapidly, and the child craves recognition but is sensitive to criticism. Too much criticism or difficulty in acquiring knowledge and skills could result in feelings of inferiority.

5. Puberty and adolescence. From age 12 to 17 the crisis is *identity versus role confusion.* The task is to develop a sense of **identity.** Plans for the future are made and values identified at this stage. An inability to resolve this crisis could lead to **identity diffusion—** uncertainty about what one values, what one believes, how to spend one's time, etc.

6. Young adult years. From age 17 to 22 the crisis is *intimacy versus isolation*. Most people are forming sexual relationships during these years, but intimacy also refers to closeness with friends and relatives. If an ability to be intimate with others is not developed, you will not have others with whom to share your joys and sorrows. A lack of intimate relationships is related to the onset of physical and mental illness and certainly limits the quality of life.

7. Middle adult years. The crisis at this stage is *generativity versus stagnation*. This crisis involves focusing on a concern beyond oneself, such as devoting oneself to parenthood or a cause, versus satisfaction only of one's personal needs. An overemphasis on the self results in stagnation or lack of growth.

8. Older adult years. The crisis at this stage is *integrity versus despair*. The question here is whether one comes to accept the life one has lived or despairs about what might have been. One who successfully copes with this crisis develops a feeling of continuity with those who have come before and those who will come after. The individual develops an identification with all of humanity. Failure to resolve this conflict successfully may result in a sense of futility, that is, the feeling that life has been useless.

Do you recognize yourself as presently being in one of the last four stages? Do you recognize stages through which you've passed? Do you recognize others, such as parents or friends, in other stages? Can you identify the crises with which you and they are coping?

Behavioral Theory

Behaviorism is a psychological theory concerned with external dynamics rather than what goes on in the mind. Whereas Freud and Erikson focused upon personality development through stages of life and the consequences of success or failure with the tasks of each stage, behaviorists emphasize present behavior. Behaviorists believe people behave as they do because of conditioning. They believe that we grow up being rewarded for certain behaviors and ignored or punished for others. We repeat behaviors for which we are rewarded until they become part of our general behavior pattern. We do not adopt behaviors for which we are ignored or punished.

For example, if dieting to lose weight, the scale reinforces your behavior every time it records a lower weight. You therefore continue your diet. However, initial weight loss is mostly lost water, and the early stages of a diet often show a rapid loss of water. During the later stages of the diet, fat is lost, but more slowly. Consequently, the later stages of a diet are less rewarding and people often give up at that point.

Behavioral theory is more complex than it appears at first glance. For instance, you would think that a child who is repeatedly punished for interrupting conversations would stop this behavior. However, perhaps that child is really seeking attention. The attention the child gets from interrupting—punishment—is the reward the child sought. Therefore, the interruptions will continue.

If you want to change one of your behaviors, you can use behavioral theory and increase your chances

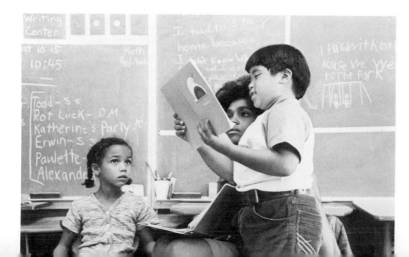

According to Erikson, the elementary school years are influential in resolving the crisis of industry versus inferiority.

of success. The first step is to identify a reward, which can be material, such as presents, or intangible, such as recognition or attention. Once you have chosen the reward, decide what frequency or degree of changed behavior will earn the reward. For example, if you're trying to give up cigarette smoking and now smoke 20 cigarettes a day, you could reward yourself when you smoke only 10. Reserve punishments for not reaching your target behavior. Ignoring undesirable behavior has been shown to be more effective than punishing it.[2]

MODES OF COPING

To survive anxiety-producing situations, we usually take one of two actions. We can defend ourselves against the threat by taking drugs, popping tranquilizers, or using some other external crutch in order to not deal directly with the anxiety-provoking stimulus. This solution is really not a solution at all, because the anxiety will return when the pills or drugs wear off. More subtle, but still a means of defending against rather than dealing with the anxiety producer, is the use of **defense mechanisms.** The second manner of coping with anxiety is to change the situation or avoid it in the first place. For example, if you have an important test next week, you can study for it and thereby decrease your anxiety by believing yourself to be more knowledgeable.

Concept: Coping can involve dealing directly with or defending against anxiety-provoking stimuli.

Defense Mechanisms

Sometimes people attempt to manage anxiety-provoking situations by unconsciously distorting reality. Freud described these defense mechanisms as affecting one's perceptions of reality rather than the actual situation. All of us could profit from perceiving some situations as less distressing. However, when this becomes a per-

Discovery Activity 3.1
DEFENSE
MECHANISMS

Can you recall using defense mechanisms? Briefly describe how you have used any of the following:

Compensation: _____

_____

Displacement: _____

_____

Intellectualization: _____

_____

Projection: _____

_____

Rationalization: _____

_____●

son's predominant coping strategy, anxiety is only temporarily relieved and returns when the defense mechanism is no longer used. In addition, defense mechanisms often involve other people in the self-deception and therefore tend to have a negative effect on interpersonal relationships.

Some common defense mechanisms include:[3]

1. *Compensation:* Covering up our weaknesses by emphasizing desirable traits or making up for frustration in one area by overgratification in another.

    Example: A man who feels inferior because he is short may strive to achieve a powerful position of leadership.

2. *Denial:* Protecting oneself from unpleasant reality by refusing to accept something that is obviously true.

    Example: A boy whose mother has died insists that she's going to be coming home soon.

3. *Displacement:* Shifting feelings, attitudes, and impulses from the original source to a different object or person.

   Example: I'm angry at my teacher, but I can't yell at her so I yell at my friend.

4. *Fantasy:* Gratifying desires that have been frustrated or cannot be achieved in reality by the use of imagination.

   Example: A little girl who has no friends pretends that her dolls are companions.

5. *Intellectualization:* Using logic, reason, and theory to detach oneself from an emotionally threatening situation.

   Example: A doctor treats the physical ills of his or her patients and avoids dealing with them on an emotional level.

6. *Isolation:* Detaching feelings from objects and people who produce anxiety.

   Example: A man who is going to have major surgery is unaware of any feelings of fear.

7. *Projection:* Attributing one's own unacceptable feelings and attitudes to others.

   Example: Sue is jealous of Joan but does not want to acknowledge this feeling in herself, so she insists that Joan is jealous of her.

8. *Rationalization:* Attempting to assign rational or desirable motives to our behavior so that we seem to have acted appropriately.

   Example: John fails a test he didn't prepare for and insists, "I failed the test because I went out last night."

9. *Reaction formation:* Preventing dangerous impulses from surfacing or being expressed by behaving in the opposite manner.

   Example: A man who is afraid of his sexual impulses becomes involved in a crusade against pornography.

10. *Regression:* Retreating to earlier developmental levels that involve less mature responses.

    Example: When a new baby is born in the family, the older child begins to wet his or her bed.

11. *Repression:* Preventing painful or undesirable feelings, memories, or impulses from entering consciousness.

    Example: A man whose wife was killed in a fire cannot remember the event.

Conscious Modes Of Coping

Some methods of dealing with anxiety are adopted consciously. The Discovery Activity entitled Coping With Difficult Situations will help you identify the conscious modes of coping that you use.

Generally speaking, there are three conscious modes of coping:

1. Submission: Avoiding the problem or situation. This mechanism may be appropriate when a problem is insurmountable. For example, consider the dilemma faced by a teacher employed in a school system that discourages teachers and their students from becoming too friendly with one another, yet the teacher believes that a good rapport between student and teacher is a necessary prerequisite to learning. The teacher might decide to leave the school system rather than attempt to change its philosophy of education. In other instances, submission may be inappropriate because it is based on a fear of facing a problem or situation. For instance, you may yearn to date a particular person but refrain from asking that person out because you fear rejection. In this case, you are withdrawing from a situation that it would have been better to face, despite the risk of rejection.

2. Aggression: Approaching the problem head on and working your hardest to resolve it in the way you think best. Like other coping behaviors, aggression can be adaptive (arguing or fighting for things that involve your values or ethical judgments) or maladaptive (always expecting to get your way). For instance, if you are waiting in line to enter a movie theater and someone slips into the line ahead of you and you punch that person in the nose, you have acted aggressively. Not only could this get you in trouble with the law, but it might also mean a fight and you might miss the movie.

Discovery Activity 3.2
COPING WITH DIFFICULT SITUATIONS

How do you cope with difficult situations? Choose one response to each of the situations described below and circle the letter of that response.[4]

1. If a salesgirl refuses to give me a refund on a purchase because I've lost the sales slip:

   a) I tell her, "I'm sorry—I should have been more careful," and leave without the refund.

   b) I tell her, "You're the only store in town that handles this brand of merchandise. I demand a refund, or I'll never shop here again."

   c) I say, "Look, if I can't have a refund, can I exchange it for something else?"

2. If I had irritated a teacher by questioning his theoretical position and he retaliated by giving me a D on an excellent paper:

   a) I wouldn't say anything; I would realize why it happened and be quieter in my next class.

   b) I would tell him he was dead wrong and that he couldn't get away with being so unfair.

   c) I would try to talk to him and see what can be done about it.

3. If I worked as a TV repairman and my boss ordered me to double-charge customers, I would:

   a) Go along with him; it's his business.

   b) Tell him he's a crook and that I won't go along with his dishonesty.

   c) Tell him he can overcharge on *his* calls, but I'm charging honestly on mine.

4. If I gave up my seat on the bus to an older woman with packages, but some teenager beat her to it:

   a) I would try to find the woman another seat.

   b) I would argue with the teenager until he moved.

   c) I would ignore it.

5. If I had been waiting in line at the supermarket for 20 minutes, then some woman rushed in front of me saying, "Thank you—I'm in such a hurry".

   a) I would smile and let her in.

   b) I would say, "Look—what do you think you're doing? Wait your turn!"

   c) I would let her in *if* she had a good reason for being in such a hurry.

6. If a friend was to meet me on a street corner at 7:00 one night and at 8:00 he still wasn't there, I would:

   a) Wait another 30 minutes.

   b) Be furious at his thoughtlessness and leave.

   c) Try to telephone him, thinking, "Boy, he'd better have a good excuse!"

7. If my wife (or husband) volunteered me for committee work with someone else she (or he) *knew* I disliked, I would:

   a) Work on the committee.

   b) Tell her she had no business volunteering my time . . . call the committee chairman and tell him the same.

   c) Tell her I want her to be more thoughtful in the future, and then make a plausible excuse she can give the committee chairman.

8. If my four-year-old-son "refused" to obey an order I gave him, I would:

   a) Let him do what he wanted.

   b) Say, "You do it—and you do it now!"

   c) Say, "Maybe you'll want to do it later on."

The responses provided above can be classified as either submissive, aggressive, or compromise. Using the key below, give yourself three points for each submissive response, two points for each compromise response, and one point for each aggressive response.

Question 1:	(a) submissive	(b) aggressive	(c) compromise
Question 2:	(a) submissive	(b) aggressive	(c) compromise
Question 3:	(a) submissive	(b) aggressive	(c) compromise
Question 4:	(a) submissive	(b) aggressive	(c) compromise
Question 5:	(a) submissive	(b) aggressive	(c) compromise
Question 6:	(a) submissive	(b) aggressive	(c) compromise
Question 7:	(a) submissive	(b) aggressive	(c) compromise

The range of possible scores is 8–24, with the higher scores respresenting a pattern of submission when conflict occurs, the lower scores representing a pattern of aggression, and scores near the middle of the range (14–18) representing a pattern of compromising. What you have learned about your style of coping? ●

3. Compromise: Fitting in; accepting things as they are. If you and a friend can't agree on which of two restaurants to eat at, you could be submissive and agree to your friend's choice, you could be aggressive and argue until you get your way, or you could compromise and go to a third restaurant that will please both of you.

The point worth reiterating in this section is that most coping behavior cannot be easily categorized as healthy or unhealthy. To evaluate a coping response, you need to know the specifics of the situation and the qualities of the person making the response. When you are faced with a problem or situation, stop to think of all possible actions and their consequences prior to deciding how to act. To practice this, choose a problem you anticipate having to cope with relatively soon. Then complete the questionnaire entitled Coping Analysis.

COPING WITH COMMON PROBLEMS

All of us face such problems as anxiety, shyness, jealousy, and frustration as well as many others. This section describes anxiety, shyness, and jealousy and discusses how to cope with them. Frustration is discussed

Discovery Activity 3.3
COPING ANALYSIS

The Problem
_____
_____

Possible Ways to Respond
A. _____
B. _____
C. _____
D. _____
E. _____

Things to Be Gained by Each Response Above
Response A: _____
Response B: _____
Response C: _____
Response D: _____
Response E: _____

Negative Aspects of Each Response
Response A: _____
Response B: _____
Response C: _____
Response D: _____
Response E: _____

Assume that you could subtract the weight of the negative aspects from the weight of the gains cited above. Which response (A, B, C, D, or E) would result in the greatest plus?_____ ●

in the first Laboratory Activity at the end of the chapter. These problems are common to people of all ages, and many people cope with them successfully.

Concept: There are effective means of coping with anxiety, shyness, jealousy, and frustration.

Anxiety

Anxiety refers to feelings of apprehension that may stem from either real or imagined concerns. We all know the symptoms of anxiety. We feel edgy and uncomfortable (afraid), our heart races, we perspire, and our muscles feel tense. Most of us learn to deal with anxiety by trying to discover what is causing it. When the cause is obvious, for example, in the case of anxiety over an upcoming test, it may be relatively easy to cope with anxious feelings. However, when the cause is more complex, we may need help in understanding it. Nevertheless, there are things you can do for yourself to cope with the anxiety you experience. These strategies include environmental planning, self-talk, relabeling, and systematic desensitization.

Environmental planning.   Sometimes it is appropriate to avoid the anxiety stimulus. Suppose you are afraid to fly in an airplane. If the quality of your life would not be diminished by never flying, it wouldn't be worth the effort to try to overcome this fear. However, if your fear of flying prevents you from visiting loved ones who live in different parts of the country, that anxiety is diminishing the quality of your life, and is therefore worth managing. Other adjustments in your environment may be appropriate. For instance, you might be able to move closer to loved ones so you don't have to fly at all or so often. How might you adjust your environment to manage your anxieties?

Self-talk.   That which we are most anxious about will probably never occur, or if it does occur, it won't be catastrophic. Have you experienced anxiety about taking tests? One way of overcoming it is by having a dialogue with yourself. The self-talk might go something like this:

I probably won't fail since I studied well and have been conscientious about my school work. But even if I do fail, that wouldn't be the end of the world. I can always repeat the course, or make up the grade on the next test. That won't be a good situation, but it's better than being so worried that I can't function.

Make up a self-talk to manage the anxious feelings you might have about interviewing for a job:

_____

_____

_____

Relabeling.   Everything has a positive and negative component to it. Even if things are terrible, you could tell yourself, "At least it can only get better from here." Relabeling uses this concept to manage anxiety. For example, rather than consider flying in an airplane as dangerous, closed in, and nerve-racking, you can label it as a chance to get away from a busy schedule where no one can bother you. Rather than label an examination a threat, you can consider it an opportunity to demonstrate how much you have learned. Which of your anxieties can be better managed by relabeling them?

Systematic desensitization.   Developed by psychiatrist Joseph Wolpe,[5] this technique assumes that

Which strategies might be most useful in coping with a frustration such as your car breaking down?

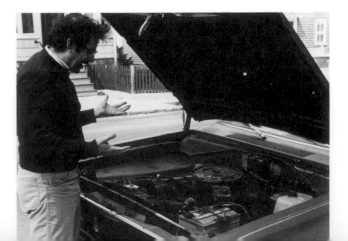

many forms of anxiety are learned and can therefore be unlearned. **Systematic desensitization** involves arranging anxiety-producing stimuli in a hierarchy or sequence according to the amount of fear they evoke. The anxious person proceeds very gradually through the hierarchy in an effort to face the anxiety-producing stimulus without fear. Suppose Jim is very fearful of receiving injections. His fear hierarchy might include such stimuli as a picture of a nurse holding a needle, a picture of the nurse aiming the needle toward someone's arm, and so on, with the final image being of the nurse giving the person an injection. Each time Jim looks at one of the pictures, he is encouraged to relax. When he is able to look at the picture without anxiety, the next picture is shown, until Jim is finally able to look at the slide that creates the most anxiety. Systematic desensitization has been used very successfully to help people overcome phobias—severe fears that include fear of enclosed spaces, fear of snakes, and the like. If you have a phobia, you might want to contact the school psychology department, where you can receive a referral to a behavior therapist who uses systematic desensitization.

Shyness

All of us feel shy at times. Shyness is fear of people, especially people who are emotionally threatening, strangers we want to impress, people who wield power and authority, and people in whom we are sexually interested. Shyness makes it hard to think clearly and communicate effectively, to meet new people, and to assert our opinions and needs. Because it is often accompanied by feelings of depression, anxiety, and loneliness, shyness prevents significant human interaction.

Although overcoming shyness requires a good deal of hard work, Philip Zimbardo, in *Shyness: What It Is and What To Do About It*, suggests taking the following steps:[6]

    1. Recognize your strengths and weaknesses and set your goals accordingly.

    2. Decide what you value, what you believe in, what you realistically would like your life to be like.

    3. Determine what your roots are. By examining your past, seek out the lines of continuity and the decisions that have brought you to your present place. Try to understand and forgive those who have hurt you and not helped when they could have. Forgive yourself for mistakes, sins, failures, and past embarrassments. Permanently bury all negative self-remembrances after you have sifted out any constructive value they may provide. . . .

    4. Guilt and shame have limited personal value in shaping your behavior toward positive goals. Don't allow yourself to indulge in them.

    5. Look for the causes of your behavior in physical, social, economic, and political aspects of your current situation and not in personality *defects* in you.

    6. Remind yourself that there are alternative views to every event. "Reality" is never more than shared agreements among people to call it the same way rather than as each one separately sees it. This enables you to be more tolerant in your interpretation of others' intentions and more generous in dismissing what might appear to be rejections or put-downs of you.

    7. Never say bad things about yourself; especially, never attribute to yourself irreversible negative traits, like "stupid," "ugly," "uncreative," "a failure," "incorrigible."

    8. Don't allow others to criticize *you* as a person; it is your *specific actions* that are open for evaluation and available for improvement—accept such constructive feedback graciously if it will help you.

    9. Remember that sometimes failure and disappointment are blessings in disguise, telling you the goals were not right for you, the effort was not worth it, and a bigger letdown later on may be avoided.

    10. Do not tolerate people, jobs, and situations that make you feel inadequate. If you can't change them or yourself enough to make you feel more worthwhile, walk on out, or pass them by. . . .

    11. Give yourself the time to relax, to meditate, to listen to yourself, to enjoy hobbies and activities you can do alone. In this way, you can get in touch with yourself.

    12. Practice being a social animal. Enjoy feeling the energy that other people transmit, the unique qualities and range of variability of our brothers and sisters. . . .

    13. Stop being so overprotective about your

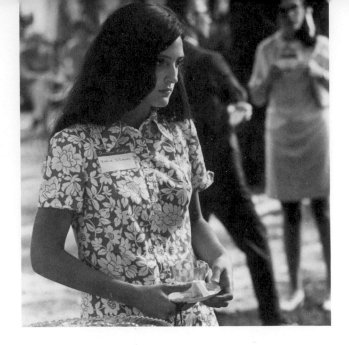

ego; it is tougher and more resilient than you imagine. . . .

14. Develop long-range goals in life, with highly specific short-range subgoals. Develop realistic means to achieve these subgoals. Evaluate your progress regularly and be the first to pat yourself on the back or whisper a word of praise in your ear.

Jealousy

Concept: Jealousy is a response to a threat to our pride or property.

Jealousy is a common emotion,[7] one that almost all of us experience at some point in our lives. Most theorists agree that jealousy has two basic components: (1) a feeling of battered pride, and (2) a feeling that one's property rights have been violated. Most of us respond to jealousy in one of two ways: We use either defense mechanisms or some conscious method of coping. For example, if you feel jealous because a coworker has been given a pay raise and you haven't, you might rationalize by saying, "Taxes would eat up most of any pay raise I received anyhow," or you might try harder to get a pay raise by taking work home with you.

How can you control jealous feelings? Just as in the case of anxiety, the first step is to find out exactly what is making you jealous. Usually something specific about a situation is bothering you. In the example above you may be jealous not because your coworker is getting extra money, but because your coworker is considered more valuable than you are. Key questions to ask are:

What was going on in the few moments before you started to feel this way?

What are you afraid of?

What rights of yours seem to have been violated?

Why is your pride hurt?

Next try to put your jealous feelings in perspective. Is it really so awful that your coworker received a raise and you didn't? Wouldn't you want that person to be pleased if you received a pay raise? Is it of any value to feel jealous and miserable? Questions like these will help you feel less jealous.

Jealousy in intimate relationships is quite common and can be very distressing. In addition to the suggestions above, jealousy in a love relationship can be managed by negotiating a contract—one that balances security and freedom for both partners. Counselors have also found that it is easier for couples to maintain a close but not excessively possessive love relationship if they maintain some separate friends and interests. Naturally, it's easier to have confidence in your desirability if you have an independent identity and if there are others who like and admire you. You are less likely to fear being abandoned by your partner, and it's much easier to cope if you are.

MENTAL DISORDERS

An individual who has severe problems and cannot cope effectively with them may develop a mental disorder. This section will discuss such disorders only briefly; to do so in detail would not be consistent with the theme of the chapter—mental health. However, a discussion of mental health is incomplete without a consideration of its counterpart—mental disorder.

Anxiety Disorders

Anxiety disorders are mental disturbances in which individuals experience high levels of anxiety. This category includes **phobic disorders** and **obsessive-compulsive disorders.** A phobic disorder is an abnormal fear of a particular situation or object; an obsessive-compulsive disorder is a disturbance involving constant repetition of particular acts in anxiety-producing situations.

Somatoform Disorders

Somatoform disorders are mental disturbances in which individuals experience physical symptoms that have no known organic cause. Included in this category are **conversion disorders,** which are disturbances involving one relatively severe symptom (e.g., blindness, paralysis, or deafness).

Schizophrenic Disorders

Individuals with **schizophrenic disorders** exhibit dramatic breaks with reality and severe distortion in thought and perception. Included in this category are **disorganized schizophrenia** and **paranoid schizophrenia.** Disorganized schizophrenia is characterized by hallucination, delusion, strange thought and behavior patterns, and occasional violent activity and gestures. Paranoid schizophrenia is characterized by general suspiciousness and mistrust of people, hallucinations, inappropriate emotional expressions, and occasional hostility and violence.

Personality Disorders

Personality disorders are mental disturbances in which individuals exhibit a set of inflexible behaviors or personality traits that impair their social functioning. This category includes **antisocial personality** and **paranoid personality.** Antisocial personality is a disturbance characterized by chronic antisocial behavior, a lack of long-range purpose and moral sense, and feelings of anxiety or guilt. The paranoid personality is characterized by a pervasive and unwarranted suspiciousness and mistrust of people.

Issues in Health
IS THERE ANY SUCH THING AS MENTAL ILLNESS?

The notion that abnormal or socially unacceptable behavior was a result of mental illness first became popular in the middle of the nineteenth century. People exhibiting deviant behavior were considered sick, and the mental health movement developed in response to such sickness. Further refining this approach, mental health professionals classified the different forms of mental illness (for example, psychoses and neuroses) and began talking about symptoms, diagnosis, and treatment.

Some experts have suggested that this medical model of mental illness is inappropriate when applied to abnormal behavior. Psychiatrist Thomas Szasz even suggests that there is no such thing as mental illness. Szasz believes abnormal behavior results from an inability to manage life's stresses. If abnormal behavior is viewed as symptomatic of an illness, people cannot be held responsible for their actions but rather can blame them on their sickness. Furthermore, a particular behavior may be abnormal and unacceptable in one society but common and accepted in others. Whereas cancer is cancer, regardless of the society in which it occurs, behavior must be viewed in its cultural context to be classified as appropriate or inappropriate. How then can behavior be illness?

Further complicating this issue is the legal definition of mental illness. For example, when is mental insanity a defense for criminal or otherwise illegal behavior and when isn't it? Is Russia's incarceration of dissenters in psychiatric hospitals because of socially unacceptable behavior a manifestation of the Russian definition of abnormal behavior (mental illness) or merely an excuse to eliminate dissent?

The debate, then, is whether there really is such a thing as mental illness. What do you think? ●

Affective Disorders

Individuals with **affective disorders** are inappropriately joyful, unrealistically sad, or both. This category includes **manic-depressive disorders,** which are characterized by sharp mood swings between severe depression or suicidal feelings and elation (often inappropriate).

Suicide

Approximately 200,000 suicides are attempted in the United States annually, and 25,000 of those attempts are successful. The actual number may be as high as 80,000, because of the many deaths that are suicides but cannot be established as such.[8]

Suicide is the second leading cause of death (after accidents and homicides) on college campuses. Approximately 1,000 college students take their own lives each year, and this figure is twice as high for college students as for people the same age but not in college.[9] The reason for these suicides is seldom difficulty with school work, although the pressure to perform well is often a contributing factor. Another factor in college suicide is the feeling of isolation that results from not being able to establish close personal relationships.

In addition to college students, the elderly have a high suicide rate, which is suspected to be a function of physical illness, death of loved ones, retirement, and having to be dependent on children and/or medical personnel. Women attempt suicide three times more often than men, but more men actually succeed in killing themselves, probably because men choose more lethal methods.

How much do you know about suicide? To find out, complete the Discovery Activity on suicide.

How can you tell if someone you know is contemplating suicide? Some of the more general signs include:

1. communication of feelings of hopelessness ("The world would be better off without me," "I can't see any reason to go on living");
2. actual threats to commit suicide;
3. a prior attempt to commit suicide;

4. making sudden gifts to others, especially of the person's most valued possessions;
5. exhibiting symptoms such as depression, withdrawal, weight loss, or apathy.

Discovery Activity 3.4
MYTHS ABOUT SUICIDE

There are many misconceptions about suicide.* To determine what you know about it, mark "True" or "False" in the space provided next to each of the items below:

_____ 1. People who commit suicide clearly want to die.

_____ 2. People who commit suicide are insane.

_____ 3. People who talk about committing suicide are unlikely to do it.

_____ 4. There is a higher incidence of suicide at certain seasons, under certain weather conditions, or at certain phases of the sun or moon.

_____ 5. People inherit suicidal tendencies.

_____ 6. Suicide is often committed without warning.

_____ 7. Suicide occurs more frequently in lower socioeconomic classes.

_____ 8. The motives for suicide are well known.

_____ 9. A person who improves after a depressive episode probably won't try to commit suicide.

_____ 10. Anyone who commits suicide is depressed.

*Adapted from E. S. Shneidman, "Suicide," in A. M. Freeman, H. I. Kaplan, and B. J. Sadock, eds., *Comprehensive Textbook of Psychiatry,* 2nd ed. (Baltimore: Williams & Wilkins, 1975).

You may be surprised to learn that all of these statements are false. Here are the facts:

1. Most people who commit suicide are ambivalent about their death.
2. Most people who commit suicide are rational and in touch with reality.
3. The great majority of people who kill themselves have communicated their intent beforehand.
4. There is no evidence to confirm a connection.
5. Although suicide does often run in families, there's no evidence of a genetic link.
6. Suicidal persons usually give many warnings, such as giving away valued possessions.
7. Suicide occurs across all socioeconomic classes in equal distribution.
8. We have a very poor understanding of the motives for suicide.
9. People often commit suicide after their spirits rise following a depression.
10. Some experts believe this is not so, and it is known that some people seem at peace after deciding to kill themselves. ●

Suppose you think your friend Mary may be suicidal. What can you do for her? First, try to talk to her. Suggest that she seek help from professionals, such as mental health counselors, and if possible, enroll in therapy with these resource personnel. You might also consider the crisis intervention technique, which can be outlined as follows:

1. Make contact at a feeling rather than a factual level; that is, show you care what happens to Mary.
2. Explore the problem as it presently exists.
3. Summarize the problem to Mary's satisfaction.
4. Focus on one aspect of the problem that can be improved.
5. Explore resources available in responding to this one aspect of the problem.
6. Make a contract with Mary regarding what she will do and what you will do.

Issues in Health
SHOULD PEOPLE HAVE THE RIGHT TO TAKE THEIR OWN LIVES?

Some say yes. They believe that some people exist under such adverse conditions or have such unsolvable problems that it is unrealistic to expect them to "muddle through." They suggest that it might be cruel to require them to live under such circumstances. Other people might be too sick or in too much pain to appreciate life and should be allowed the relief that death would provide.

Others would deny anyone the right to take his or her own life. Both religious teachings and our society's laws prohibit suicide or aiding someone in killing himself or herself. Opponents of the right to suicide contend that since it is a decision from which there is no retreat, it is unacceptable. They also cite the anguish suicide causes family and friends, and maintain that if conditions are so horrendous, help is available through social services and counseling to aid suicidal people. They believe that life is valuable and that no one should devalue it by contemplating suicide. There is always hope for improvement.

What do you think? ●

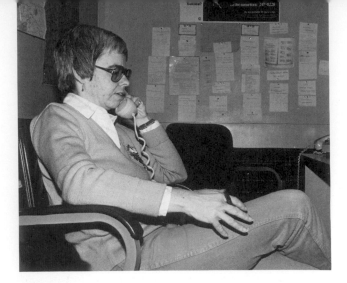

At suicide prevention centers trained volunteers encourage callers to talk out their problems. Would-be suicides are often referred for professional help.

The first step in crisis intervention is to accept the feelings of the suicidal person instead of evaluating or denying them. Rather than saying, "Things aren't that bad," you should say, "It must be terrible to feel so alone that you would contemplate killing yourself." This is the step most people have difficulty with, so you might want to practice giving feeling responses prior to actually talking with the suicidal person.

Once you have made contact at a feeling level, help the person to look at the problem in the here and now rather than talking about what might have been or might be. Then summarize the problem so the suicidal person appreciates that you really have been listening and that you understand. Now choose one part of the problem that you think the person can improve and explore resources that might help respond to this part of the problem. Obtain the suicidal person's agreement to work on that part of the problem, to meet again, and to contact you if he or she begins feeling worse. Remember, professional help is needed for a person who is suicidal, but you too can do much to help.

One last point regarding suicide: During times of social protest, such as occurred on campuses during the war in Vietnam and during the free speech movement at Berkeley in 1964, statistics indicate that suicides decrease in number.[10] A similar condition existed during both world wars. The point is that when people

develop a sense of community, regardless of the cause, they feel less alone and are less apt to take their own lives. As Seiden stated:

> Of all the psychodynamic attributes associated with suicidal behavior, the factor of human isolation and withdrawal appears to be the single most effective distinction between those who kill themselves and those who do not. Numerous investigators have reported that youngsters who commit suicide invariably had no close friends with whom they could share confidences or receive psychological support.[11]

SEEKING HELP

Concept: Help in coping is available.

An ancient Chinese proverb states:

> *That the birds of*
> *worry and care*
> *fly above your*
> *head, this you*
> *cannot change,*
> *But that they*
> *   build*
> *nests in your*
> *   hair,*
> *This you can*
> *   prevent.*[12]

If you recognize the signs and symptoms of mental illness in yourself or someone else, be comforted by knowing there are resources for coping with such disorders.

Where to Get Help

A good place to start is your college campus. The psychology department probably has a counseling clinic or can refer you to one. Your local or state health department probably also offers counseling services.

Of course, there are many private psychiatrists, psychologists, and mental health counselors. Many clinics and some private sources of counseling offer a sliding scale of fees so that those with little money pay low fees and those who are more affluent pay higher fees.

Types of Therapy

Many different types of therapy are available according to the nature and severity of the problem and the philosophy of the patient and clinician. Psychoanalysis, for example, would not be appropriate for specific behavior disorders that could be corrected relatively quickly, and transactional analysis would not be appropriate treatment for a schizophrenic patient. The major forms of therapy are:

Psychotherapy. Originally termed psychoanalysis and developed by Freud, **psychotherapy** is a long-term treatment (many years) requiring several visits a week with the therapist. The goal is to make the client aware of repressed material that unconsciously affects the client's behavior. Once this material is brought to consciousness, the client can better understand the problem and adjust his or her behavior.

Client-centered therapy. Sometimes termed Rogerian therapy after its founder Carl Rogers, **client-centered therapy** promotes the growth of the client by reducing destructive forces, such as anxiety. The therapist creates an atmosphere of "unconditional positive regard," empathy, and genuineness. This atmosphere

of total acceptance of the patient is designed to aid patients in accepting themselves as they are. The result will then be personal growth.

Behavior therapy. Whereas psychotherapists predominantly employ interpretation and client-centered therapists use acceptance and empathy, **behavior therapists** do not rely on one particular mode of treatment. They tailor a treatment program to the individual's needs in an effort to change behavior rather than feelings. Imagine a client afraid to speak before groups of people. The psychotherapist might view this fear as a function of poor self-esteem and try to find its roots in the client's childhood. A behavior therapist, however, might have the client speak before one other person, then two, and eventually before a group, rewarding the client at each step. The behaviorist would not work on the self-esteem of that client.

The behaviorist establishes specific behavioral goals for the client and uses techniques such as systematic desensitization (presented earlier in this chapter) to aid the client in achieving these goals. It is expected that once the behavior is changed, the feeling will change. The client who gradually learns to speak before groups of people will probably improve his or her self-esteem as a result of overcoming that fear.

Group therapy. The forms of therapy we have discussed so far have involved one therapist working with one client. **Group therapy** involves a therapist working with several clients at the same time. It was developed during World War II, when there was a

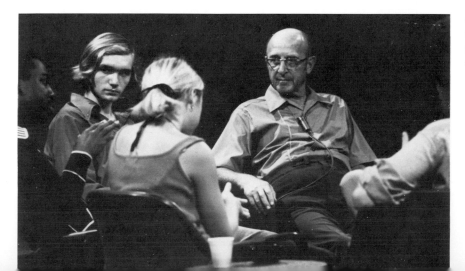

Client-centered therapy, developed by Carl Rogers, is based on the premise that individuals can learn to recognize and work out their own problems.

shortage of therapists. Although group therapy can take many different forms, usually one therapist meets with six to ten clients, and the cost to the client is less than in individual therapy. One advantage of group therapy is that clients can learn social skills, which are often retarded in people with mental disorders. In addition, knowing that others need help too, and seeing people at various stages of mental illness (some at the latter stages of therapy), provides comfort to those greatly concerned with their own disorders. The group therapist's task is to get the members of the group to help one another by establishing an atmosphere of acceptance and support. In addition, the therapist tries to draw comparisons between situations and interpretations that arise in group meetings and those that the members encounter in their lives outside the group.

Family therapy. One criticism of many forms of therapy is that the therapist works with the client for a relatively short period of time, and then the client returns to a dysfunctional family unit, which counteracts the benefits of therapy. **Family therapy** is based on the premise that unless the key people in a client's life also change, the client will not improve. A family therapist usually works with individual family members at some times and with the whole family unit at other times. The goal is to help each member of the family understand his or her effect upon the other members and upon the unit as a whole. An important ingredient of successful family functioning is effective communication, and improving communication skills in families is a major goal of family therapy.

Chemotherapy. Some clients are treated with medication: tranquilizers, lithium, antidepressants, and antianxiety drugs. These drugs are usually used to prepare the client for entering therapy, but they are also often used for extended periods of time. Tranquilizing drugs were developed in the 1950s to reduce "excitement, agitation, aggressive behavior, delusions, and hallucinations."[13] Before the development of tranquilizers, seriously disturbed patients were not as able to focus upon and profit from therapy. Lithium carbonate is used to treat manic-depressive disorders. It levels a person's moods and allows for more effective therapy. Antidepressant drugs are used for patients suffering from depression and are taken regularly rather than only when depression occurs, because these drugs work on a long-term, as opposed to an immediate, basis. Some therapists argue that antianxiety drugs, such as Valium, treat the symptom (anxiety) rather than the problem. Others believe anxiety must be reduced before the client can deal with its causes.

Alternative therapies. Many other therapies are available, most of them adaptations of the ones described above. **Hypnotherapy** involves hypnotizing patients and suggesting new forms of behavior. In **Psychodrama** the patient acts out events that cause problems, and then the actions and feelings experienced by the patient are analyzed. In **transactional analysis** interactions between people are analyzed in terms of ego—parent, child, and adult. **Rational emotive therapy** counsels the patient to adopt behaviors that will disprove his or her self-defeating thoughts. In **existential therapy** the therapist helps the patient choose behaviors consistent with the patient's values.

CONCLUSION

Throughout this chapter we have emphasized that although learning to cope with one's environment is a difficult task, there are ways to meet this challenge. However, should problems become so overwhelming that the usual coping techniques are not enough, help is available. It is unrealistic to choose to maintain a "stiff upper lip" rather than ask for help. Perhaps that sort of behavior actually increases the likelihood of problems becoming so severe that they cause illness, either mental or physical. The instructor in the course for which you are reading this book might be a good first contact. He or she may be able to refer you to someone who can help you cope. Ask for help if you need it.

SUMMARY

1. Emotional health includes the abilities to deal constructively with reality and to adapt to change, exercising a reasonable degree of independence, establishing positive relationships with other people, and being able to live with emotions.

2. Several different theories explain personality development, including Freud's stages of psychosexual development; Erikson's stages of crises; and behavioral theory, which is more concerned with external dynamics than with what goes on in the mind.

3. Defense mechanisms are unconscious attempts at coping with anxiety. They include compensation, denial, displacement, fantasy, intellectualization, isolation, projection, rationalization, reaction formation, regression, and repression.

4. The conscious means of coping with anxiety-provoking stimuli can be divided into three categories: submission (giving in or withdrawing from the stimulus), aggression (fighting to overcome the situation), and compromise (fitting in as a means of coping).

5. Some of the problems that we all must cope with are anxiety, shyness, jealousy, and frustration.

6. Anxiety can be managed by environmental planning, self-talk, relabeling, and systematic desensitization.

7. Shyness is fear of people, especially those we want to impress, those who wield power and authority, and those in whom we are sexually interested.

8. Jealousy has two basic components: a feeling of battered pride, and a feeling that one's property rights have been violated.

9. Mental disorders include anxiety disorders, somatoform disorders, schizophrenic disorders, personality disorders, and affective disorders.

10. Therapy takes various forms depending on the nature of the mental disorder and the philosophy of the therapist. Forms of therapy include psychotherapy, client-centered therapy, behavior therapy, group therapy, family therapy, chemotherapy, and such alternative therapies as hypnotherapy, psychodrama, transactional analysis, rational-emotive therapy, and existential therapy.

REFERENCES

1. Erik Erikson, *Childhood and Society* (New York: Norton, 1963).

2. Portia E. Perry, "Behavior Modification and Social Learning Theory: Application in the School," *Journal of Education* 53 (1971):20.

3. Adapted from Lila Swell, *Educating for Success: Theory Manual* (New York: Queens College, 1972), pp. 69–70. Reprinted by permission of the author.

4. Lila Swell, *Educating for Success: Workbook* (New York: Queens College, 1972). pp. 46–47. Reprinted by permission of the author.

5. Joseph Wolpe, *Psychotherapy by Reciprocal Inhibition* (Stanford, Calif.: Stanford University Press, 1958).

6. Philip G. Zimbardo, *Shyness: What It Is and What To Do About It* (Reading, Mass.: Addison-Wesley, 1977), pp. 158–160.

7. Adapted from Elaine Walster and G. William Walster, *A New Look at Love* (Reading, Mass.: Addison-Wesley, 1978), pp. 89–94.

8. Ralph Grawunder and Marion Steinmann, *Life and Health*, 3rd ed. (New York: Random House, 1980), p. 42.

9. Paul M. Insel and Walton T. Roth, *Health in a Changing Society* (Palo Alto, Calif.: Mayfield, 1976), p. 77.

10. Richard H. Seiden, "The Problem of Suicide on College Campuses," *The Journal of School Health* 41 (1971): 243–248.

11. Ibid., p. 244.

12. Stephen Maltz, *Workbook for College Health: Critical Issues* (Dubuque, Iowa: William C. Brown, 1970), p. 1. Reprinted by permission.

13. Valerian J. Derlega and Louis H. Janda, *Personal Adjustment: The Psychology of Everyday Life* (Morristown, N.J.: General Learning Press, 1978), p. 519.

Laboratory 1
COPING WITH FRUSTRATION

Purpose To experience and discuss how people cope with frustration.

Size of Group Five students seated around a table participating, while the rest of the class surrounds and observes them.

Equipment

1. Five envelopes.
2. An oak tag (manila) sheet of paper cut into pieces of various shapes as shown in Fig. 3.1.

Procedure

Five students volunteer to bring one friend each to class (five friends in total), all of whom are to be kept unaware of the purposes of this activity. The five guests sit around a table and each is handed one envelope containing parts of a puzzle. The envelopes should contain the following parts of the diagram:

Envelope 1: a, a, c

Envelope 2: a, j, d

Envelope 3: g, i, f

Envelope 4: b, e, f

Envelope 5: c, h, a

The instructor reads the following instructions:

As of this moment, you are not allowed to talk with one another nor communicate in any nonverbal fashion (no gesturing, making facial expressions, etc.). Take the pieces out of the envelope in front of you and place the envelopes to one side. Your group's task is to form five squares of equal size, one in front of each person. This is not a race, but the task is not completed until each person has before him or her a square equal in size to that of every other person.

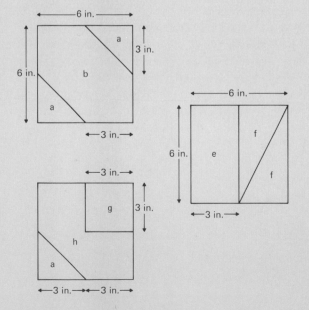

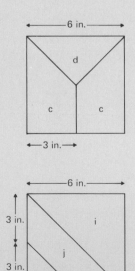

Figure 3.1

You are not allowed to take or ask for a piece of the puzzle that is in front of someone else. You *are* allowed to give someone else a piece of the puzzle in front of you.

The rest of the class stands around the participants and looks for signs of frustration, such as body posture or facial expressions.

Results

When the five squares are properly designed, discuss the following:

1. To the observers: What signs of frustration did you notice?

2. To the participants:
   a) Were you frustrated? When?
   b) What did it feel like to be frustrated?
   c) What did it feel like to be causing the others to be frustrated?
   d) How did you manifest your frustrations non-verbally?

3. To the total class:
   a) How do people generally cope with frustration?
   b) How do you personally cope with frustration?

Laboratory 2
SHOUTING FEELINGS

Purpose To experience and discuss feelings and the differences between feelings and thoughts.

Size of Group Total class.

Equipment None.

Procedure

1. Choose two student volunteers.

2. One volunteer stands in the front of the room and the other is in the rear. The volunteers should be facing each other, with the remainder of the students seated between them.

3. The volunteers then stand on a chair and tell the class their names.

4. On command from the instructor, one of the volunteers is asked to shout, as loud as he or she can, the name of the other volunteer. Then the second volunteer shouts the name of the first.

5. Last, the class shouts out the name of the first volunteer and, one minute later, the name of the second volunteer.

Results

1. At the conclusion of the activity the volunteers are asked to describe their feelings preceding, during, and after the shouting. Were they nervous prior to volunteering? Anxious? Curious? During the shouting were they surprised? Self-conscious? Afterward, did they feel relieved? Let down?

2. The other students are then asked to relate their feelings preceding, during, and after the activity.

3. The distinction between feelings and thoughts should be emphasized during this discussion whenever a student attempts to describe his or her feelings by discussing thoughts. For example, "I thought it was silly" is not the same as "I felt silly."

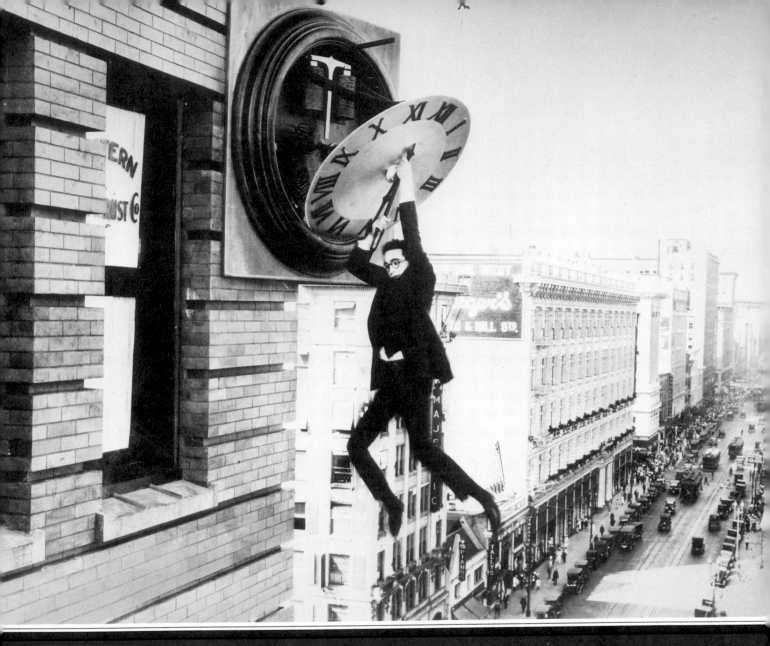

chapter 4

stress

There is an old saying: "a sound mind in a sound body." It is becoming increasingly evident, however, that this dichotomy between mind and body is more arbitrary than real. As both the functioning of the mind and the workings of the body are better understood, their effects upon one another become more evident. Nowhere has this mind-body relationship been better demonstrated than in the area of stress. Psychological stress can have a serious impact on the body, and bodily disease can affect the health of the mind. In this chapter we shall discuss stress, its effect on the body, stress-related diseases, and methods of stress management.

WHAT IS STRESS?

Bodily Expressions of Emotion

Concept: Emotions are evidenced by the body.

Stand before a mirror. Act out the following feelings with your face only: anger, joy, confusion. Now act out those feelings with the rest of your body as well. If you found this easy to do, it is because we do it all the time, though not always consciously. When unhappy we tend to slump our shoulders, frown, move our heads back and forth as if to say, "No, not me," and stare forlornly. When confused we squint our eyes, tilt one ear in the direction of the confusion (as if to comprehend better), and scratch the top of the head. The next time a class of yours meets, notice that if it's an interesting class the students will be leaning bodily toward the instructor or the center of the group. If it's dull, the students will be leaning against the backs of their chairs or away from the instructor or group. In addition, look at the faces of the students in this class. Pick out three classmates and guess whether they're interested or bored, then ask them after class.

There are other ways in which the body can be seen to demonstrate emotions. Individuals with low self-esteem tend to slump, don't smile much, and aren't very expressive with their arms when they talk. In contrast, individuals with high self-esteem "walk tall," talk animatedly, and smile a good deal. People exhibit hostility by a certain look, tense muscles, or an aggressive forward angle of the head, as if ready to charge.

You can probably think of other ways in which we express our emotions bodily. In fact, there are so many ways that many verbal expressions use body words to describe feelings. Examples are the term "no guts" and the phrase "stand on your own two feet." Try listing ten more such expressions in the spaces provided before looking below:

1. _____
2. _____
3. _____
4. _____
5. _____
6. _____
7. _____
8. _____
9. _____
10. _____

The Stress Response Pattern

Concept: Emotions result in stress.

Emotions, then, are manifested by the body. We shall soon see that emotions are a component of the stress response and as such have implications for our health.

One of the leading researchers in the area of stress is Hans Selye. Selye defines **stress** as "the nonspecific

Body expressions: stiff upper lip; can't stomach it; hair-raising; no backbone; yellow stripe down your back; tongue-tied; welcome with open arms; catch your eye; two left feet; spine-tingling.

66

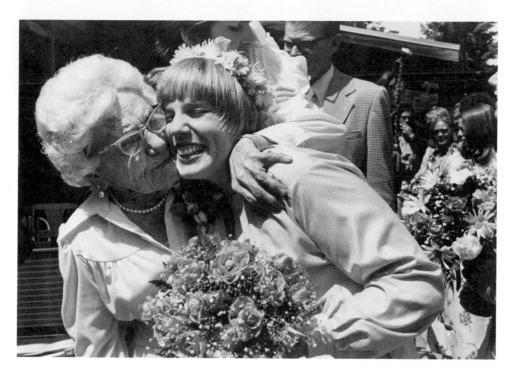

Happy events as well as negative ones produce the physiological response known as stress.

response of the body to any demand made upon it."[1] What this means, in effect, is that any change we encounter to which we must adapt results in stress. That change can be internal, such as the degeneration of a body organ, or external, such as having to speak in front of a large group of people. Selye found that although the stressful stimulus, or stressor, varies, the body's physiological response is generally the same. Thus an experience might result in feelings of joy or sorrow, but in either case the person would experience the same physiological response, or stress.

Selye termed the body's response to stress the **general adaptation syndrome** (GAS). The GAS occurs in three stages, as outlined below.

1. Alarm. The body exhibits physiological signs when it is first exposed to a stressor, such as rapid pulse, a tightening of muscles, sweaty palms, a knot in the stomach. At the same time, body resistance to the stressor is diminished, and if the stressor is sufficiently strong (severe burns or extreme temperature, for example), death may result.

2. Resistance. The bodily signs characteristic of the alarm reaction disappear. Now the task is to adapt to the stress and retain the normal internal state, which requires considerable energy.

3. Exhaustion. Following a long-continued exposure to the same stressor, to which the body has become adjusted, eventually the energy required to adapt to the stress may be exhausted. If this happens, the signs of alarm reappear. At this stage, however, they are irreversible, and the individual dies.[2]

Of course, we usually don't get to the exhaustion stage. We learn to adapt to change after a while, and in fact are even unaware that we are adapting. For example, a family moving into a new house near an airport might at first be bothered by the sound of planes overhead, but after several weeks they are unaware of the airplanes. They have become used to the sound of the airplanes, a process called **habituation,** and the noise no longer consciously bothers them. It should be noted here that even if habituated, you can still become ill from the stressor. However, in many cases, becoming used to a stressor is an effective means of coping with it. If you give many speeches, for example, you'll experience less stress than you did the first time you spoke to a large group.

Distress and Eustress

Concept: Stress can be either positive or negative.

If you accept an invitation to give a speech before a large number of people, you might expect to feel stress. If that stress manifests itself in such anxiety that a panic reaction results and you cannot get the words out during the speech, the stress is obviously dysfunctional. However, if the stress leads you to spend a great deal of time developing the speech, making it interesting and informative, then you are using the stress productively. Thus stress can be a helper or an inhibitor. The stress associated with physical danger, for instance, can be used to place reasonable limits upon the daredevil activities of a person who would otherwise get hurt. Conversely, stress could be used negatively by another person who withdraws from risk-taking activities that are stressful but that promote goal achievement and personal development.

Selye terms the negative use of stress **distress** and the positive use **eustress.** Some have described the use of stress as positive or negative by noting that the Chinese word for crisis is a combination of the symbols for the words danger and opportunity. Certainly a stressor can cause harm to one person but offer a tremendous opportunity to another. Further, within the same person one stressor will become distress whereas another stressor will result in self-fulfillment. We all experience stress often. Discovery Activity 4.1, Identifying Stressors in Your Life, is intended to help you recognize what has been stressful to you in the past month.

Stress and Life Changes

Many things, events, or people can be stressors. Bacteria can cause stress. So can noise. So can a person

Discovery Activity 4.1
IDENTIFYING STRESSORS IN YOUR LIFE

List ten events or stressors that you can recall having occurred in the past month.

1. _____
2. _____
3. _____
4. _____
5. _____
6. _____
7. _____
8. _____
9. _____
10. _____

Describe on a separate sheet of paper how you responded to five of the stressors you listed. Include both *positive* and *negative* responses.

Next, choose one response with which you are not completely satisfied and list other ways in which you could have responded. Do you think you'll respond differently next time? Why or why not?

Do you notice any consistencies in your reactions to stress? If yes, what are they? Why not ask a friend how he or she perceives your behavior when under stress? ●

whom you dislike. The realization that there are a vast number of stressors can be disheartening when it is further recognized that these stressors combine in their effects upon us. For instance, during an influenza epidemic the people who die are usually those with chronic illnesses. People who are highly stressed are more susceptible to a number of conditions, both physical and psychological. Can you recall a time when you were

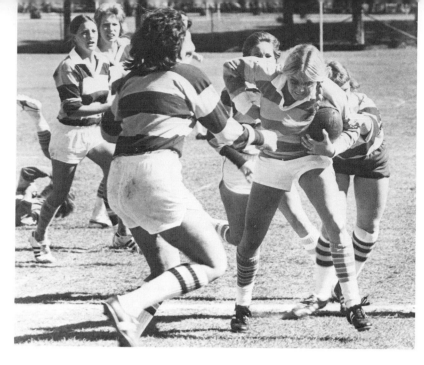

Stress that produces a positive outcome—such as motivating athletes to improve their performance—is known as eustress.

stressed (for example, during final exams) and then succumbed to another stressor (maybe you caught a bad cold)?

Two researchers have determined that certain life changes, when accumulated, can become significant stressors in people's lives. Thomas Holmes and Richard Rahe, specialists in the area of stress, compiled a list of typical events that occur in people's lives. They asked people of varying ages and occupations to rate these events on a scale of 1 to 100 according to how much adjustment they felt each event required. From the responses they determined that some events were considerably more stressful than others, and they weighted them accordingly. The resulting scale, called the Social Readjustment Rating Scale,[3] appears in modified form in Table 4.1. Check those events that you have experienced in the past year.

Completing this scale should underline for you the cumulative nature of stress—the more stressors, the higher you score. The significance of the scores has been determined through research studies conducted by the scale's developers. They found that a low score (below 150) indicated only a 37 percent chance of illness during the next two years, an average score (150–300) indicated a 50 percent chance of illness during the next two years, and a high score (over 300)

indicated a 90 percent chance of serious illness sometime during the next two years. On the modified version of the scale, which you just completed, a score below 128 is probably low, a score between 128 and 255 is probably average, and a score above 255 is probably high. A person scoring high on this scale should make a conscious effort to avoid, whenever possible, any further life changes for the rest of the year.

What was your score? Will you make any adjustments in your lifestyle as a result of this experience?

Stress and Personality

Some researchers believe that personality is an important indicator of whether or not a person will experience a greater or lesser amount of stress and of the effects stress will have on the person. Drs. Meyer Friedman and R. Ray Rosenman described two personality types, Type A and Type B. The **Type A** pattern is described by a complex of personality traits that includes "excessive competitive drive, aggressiveness, impatience, and a harrying sense of time urgency." Type A is a stressful pattern that has been found to be related to greater susceptibility to heart disease. Type B personality, by contrast, is characterized by patience, a relaxed attitude, and noncompetitiveness.

Table 4.1
MODIFIED SOCIAL READJUSTMENT RATING SCALE

Rank	Life event	Value	Your checks	Rank	Life event	Value	Your checks
1	Death of steady boy/girl friend	100	_____	19	Outstanding personal achievement	28	_____
2	Break up with boy/girl friend or divorce	73	_____	20	Boy/girl friend begins or stops school	26	_____
3	Separation with boy/girl friend (to see if you really love one another)	65	_____	21	Starting or finishing school	26	_____
				22	Change in living conditions	25	_____
4	Jail term	63	_____	23	Revision of personal habits	24	_____
5	Death of close family member	63	_____	24	Trouble with a faculty member	23	_____
6	Personal injury or illness	53	_____	25	Change in school hours, conditions	20	_____
7	Going steady, engagement, or marriage	50		26	Change in residence	20	_____
				27	Change in schools	20	_____
8	Flunk out of school or fired from work	47	_____	28	Change in recreational habits	19	_____
9	Reconciliation with boy/girl friend	45	_____	29	Change in church activities	19	_____
10	Change in family member's health	44	_____	30	Change in social activities	18	_____
11	Pregnancy	40	_____	31	Loan less than $10,000	17	_____
12	Sex difficulties	39	_____	32	Change in sleeping habits	16	_____
13	Change in financial status	38	_____	33	Change in number of family get-togethers	15	_____
14	Death of a close friend	37	_____	34	Change in eating habits	15	_____
15	Change in number of boy/girl friend arguments	35	_____	35	Vacation	13	_____
16	Loan over $10,000	31	_____	36	Christmas	12	_____
17	Change in school responsibilities	29	_____	37	Minor violation of law	11	_____
18	Trouble with boy/girl friend's parents	29	_____				

SOURCE: Based on Thomes H. Holmes and Richard H. Rahe, ''The Social Readjustment Scale''
Journal of Psychosomatic Research. Copyright © 1967, Pergamon Press, Ltd. Reprinted by permission.

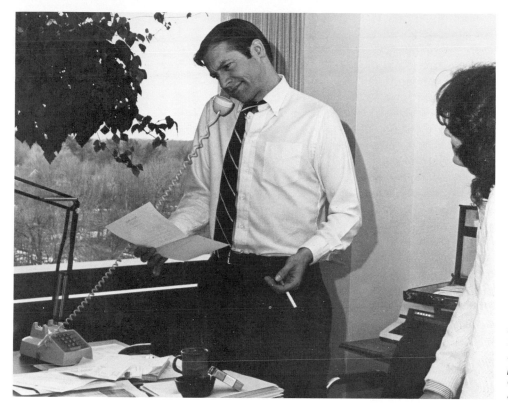

Personality type has been found to have a significant impact on health. The Type A personality is competitive, easily irritated, impatient, and always rushed.

If you find yourself answering yes to many of the following questions, you may possess the Type A behavior pattern:

1. Do you often do two things at the same time (for example, eat and read the newspaper)?
2. Do you speak rapidly?
3. Do you walk quickly?
4. Do you interrupt others?
5. Do you find it difficult to wait in line?
6. Do you feel guilty when you relax?
7. Are you overscheduled?
8. Are you overly worried about being late?
9. Do you drive your car too fast?
10. Is it difficult for you to watch people doing things more slowly than you know you can do them?

Intervening Variables

Although life changes and personality are important indicators of a person's chances of becoming ill from stress, a number of factors can help to reduce the chances of stress-related illness.

It has been found that social support, for instance, can act as a buffer between life change and illness.[4] That is, people who have "significant others" with whom to discuss their joys, concerns, and problems (such as close friends and parents) are less likely to become ill when experiencing stressful life changes than are individuals without social support. Some of the variables discussed previously also affect the degree to which stress will be harmful. These include self-esteem, alienation, assertiveness, and locus of control.

Thus, stress does not *necessarily* lead directly to illness and disease. It has the potential to do so, but many factors influence this relationship. If you lack assertiveness, for example, you will not have your needs met and you will experience more stress than an assertive person. To intervene between stress and disease, you should take an assertiveness training course. If you don't feel good about yourself—you have low esteem—you will find that state stressful. To intervene between stress and disease, you must work on improving the part of yourself that you hold in low esteem. Perhaps a diet will improve your physical self-esteem, maybe more reading will help you to feel better about your intellectual self, or a workshop on communication skills may improve your low opinion of your social self.

Stressors Related to College Life

Concept: College life can be stressful.

For most people, college life is an experience that is both enjoyable and fondly remembered, but it can also be very stressful. Many of the stressors affecting college students are health-related. The close living quarters shared by students residing in dormitories or apartments foster the rapid spread of communicable diseases. Influenza epidemics and bouts of mononucleosis are frequent visitors to college campuses. Other stressors, such as lack of sleep, examinations, and inadequate nutrition, also contribute to the spread of such diseases.

The psychological stressors associated with college life have to do with changes and decisions, which are normal and part of the maturing process. Students living away from home for the first time may find it difficult to make their own decisions, independent of the family. Who will do the laundry? Who will make the bed? Who will shop for food and cook? And will there be enough time left over for studying? Separation from people whom one has seen every day of one's life can be a strain as well, and for some students, homesickness is an intense stressor.

Of course, there are substitutes for the people one misses. Friends of the same and the opposite sex often

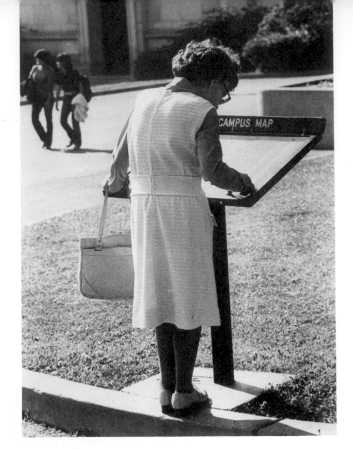

College life can be a stressor regardless of one's age.

replace the absent family members. The process of making friends in itself can be stressful, however, especially for people who fear they will fail at this task.

Of course, not all college students are young people. The older college student, who may be working while going to school, or returning to school after the children have left the home or after retirement, encounters stressors as well. One of the major stressors of adults returning to school is the fear of failure. However, older students do have more experience to draw upon than younger students do, and this can help them understand and apply the information learned in school. College campuses are changing today, and the older student population is increasing. In an effort to help older students manage the stressors they will encounter, many colleges offer counseling for career changes, methods of study, fear of failure, and test taking. In effect, these are stress education activities.

Discovery Activity 4.2
STRESSORS OF COLLEGE LIFE

List five things about college life that *you* find stressful.

1. _____
2. _____
3. _____
4. _____
5. _____

For each of the five stressors you listed, write how you have tried to deal with it.

1. _____
2. _____
3. _____
4. _____
5. _____

For each of the five stressors you listed, list another way in which you might have responded.

1. _____
2. _____
3. _____
4. _____
5. _____●

You have probably noticed that some responses to stress are healthier than others. For example, if you were lonely and were befriended by someone who spent a great deal of time at bars drinking alcohol, you might be tempted to drink alcohol to excess as well. The loneliness might be so unbearable that alcohol abuse would seem a small price to pay to alleviate it. A healthier response would be to join a club at which you could make friends, or a social service organization where you could make friends while doing something of value for others.

The decisions college students are required to make often have long-range significance. Your decision regarding what to do for the rest of your life may be especially stressful because it involves making a major, long-term commitment. There are other decisions you must also make, which may not seem significant in themselves, but when totaled they add to the stress you must manage. These decisions might include:

1. Do I join a group? Which one? Fraternity? Sorority? Athletic team? Campus newspaper? Student government?
2. Should I repair this old car or get a new one?
3. What should I study for this test?
4. Should I go on a vacation during spring recess or go home?
5. Should I go to summer school or take some time off?
6. Should I get engaged?
7. Should I join the demonstration?

Whereas all of life involves decision making, college life is somewhat different. It may be the first time that some people are required to make decisions relatively independently—decisions of real importance, that is. The fact that suicide is the second leading cause of death among college students can be better understood when the stresses of college life are considered. Some college students experience alienation and have a low sense of self-worth resulting from the pressure to make new friends and the fear of failing at this task, as well as confusion regarding important decisions that must be made. Add to this the need to succeed and the effect that failure can have upon self-esteem, and the stresses of college life become clear.

Life's Other Stressors

Other aspects of life in the twentieth century create stress with which we must deal. One of these stressors is stress on the job. Occupational stress usually occurs as the result of role overload, role ambiguity, role insufficiency, or role conflict. **Role overload** occurs when too much work is required in too little time, **role am-**

Discovery Activity 4.3
MAKING DECISIONS

You might be asking yourself, "How do I go about making major decisions?" To gain practice, think of an important decision you are facing now or expect to face in the future. Now write out responses to the following points.

1. Specify the reason a decision is needed.

2. Brainstorm a list of as many possible decisions as imaginable.

3. List the pros and cons of each decision you might choose.

4. Choose one decision and try it.

5. Evaluate how well that decision has worked.

6. If satisfied, fine. If not, try a different decision and evaluate that one. Repeat this process until you have made a decision with which you are satisfied.

If you're trying to resolve a problem, try the form below:[5]

1. A problem I have that needs a solution is _____
   _____

2. More specifically, this problem entails _____
   _____

3. Possible solutions are
   a. _____
   b. _____
   c. _____
   d. _____
   e. _____

4. The best possible solution is _____
   _____

5. I will try this solution (when?) _____

6. After trying the solution, I found that _____it worked _____it didn't work.

7. If the solution didn't work, I will next try to _____
   ●

biguity occurs when aspects of the job are unclear, **role insufficiency** is a situation in which a worker's background (education and training) is not adequate to accomplish the job, and **role conflict** entails two supervisors having different and conflicting expectations of a worker. If severe enough, job-related stress can result in illness or disease.

Another stressor, which is increasingly common in our society today, is the dual-career family, in which both husband and wife work. Whether the reasons are financial or related to career satisfaction the dual-career family can create problems: how best to care for the children, how to make sure time is provided for one's spouse, and the like. Family responsibilities often conflict with job demands—for example, when a child is sick and must be cared for at home.

Urban life has its own complement of stressors. Those of you who have been stuck in rush hour traffic, couldn't get a reservation at a restaurant, have been bothered by city noises, or feel crowded by too many people and buildings have firsthand experience with these stressors. If you're afraid for your safety or if you can't stand the smell of automobile exhaust whenever you're in the city, you are experiencing an urban stressor.

The physiological and psychological consequences of ignoring stress or responding to it inappropriately can be severe. However, there are ways to handle such stresses and to prepare for others that will inevitably occur. We will discuss some of these methods later in the chapter. First, let's consider what is known about how stress affects us both physically and psychologically.

THE PHYSIOLOGY OF STRESS

Concept: The body responds to stress in a specific manner.

When your brain perceives something as stressful, the hypothalamus of the brain responds by releasing corticotropin-releasing factor (CRF), which in turn acti-

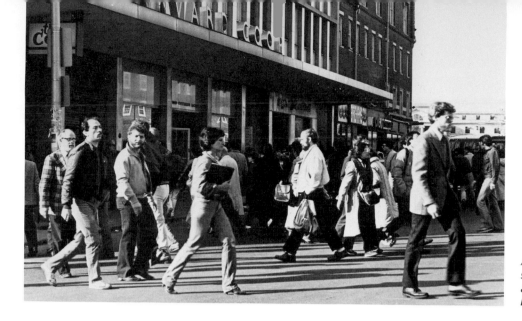

Among the more prominent stressors related to urban life are noise, crowding, and a hurried pace.

vates the pituitary gland to secrete adrenocorticotropic hormone (ACTH) into the circulatory system. ACTH signals the adrenal glands to secrete the hormone cortisol from their cortex (outer section), while a direct nervous pathway from the brain to the adrenal medulla (inner section) stimulates secretion of epinephrine (adrenalin) and norepinephrine (noradrenalin). Table 4.2 lists the effects of these adrenal secretions.

The endocrine system is not the only system activated by stress. Secretions occur in the digestive system, the autonomic nervous system (sympathetic and parasympathetic) changes body processes, the circu-

latory system and heart speed up, the brain emits certain brain waves, and the skin releases perspiration. Figure 4.1 depicts the physiological stress reaction.

Figure 4.1
Stress reaction.

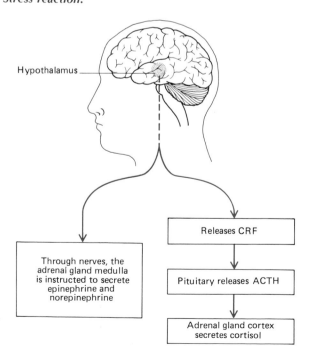

Table 4.2
EFFECTS OF ADRENAL HORMONES

Cortisol	Epinephrine and Norepinephrine
1. Increases glucose	1. Increase heart rate
2. Increases blood fats	2. Increase blood pressure
3. Reduces protein stores	3. Increase contractility of heart
4. Reduces white blood cell count	4. Increase cardiac output
5. Increases body-core temperature.	5. Cause copious sweating

SOURCE: Adapted from a handout entitled "Stress," given in a course conducted by Dr. Richard Yarian at the State University of New York at Buffalo, Summer 1976.

To test your understanding of these physiological changes, take the test in Discovery Activity 4.4, Self-test of Your Understanding of the Physiology of Stress. Understanding the physiology of stress is important to the success of the stress-reducing techniques that we will discuss later in this chapter.

Discovery Activity 4.4
SELF-TEST OF YOUR UNDERSTANDING OF THE PHYSIOLOGY OF STRESS

Directions: Match each of the following *numbered* items with the *lettered* item that most pertains to it:

Correct Letter	Numbered Item	Lettered Item
_____	1. Adrenal cortex	a) A hormone that increases glucose
_____	2. Pituitary gland	b) Activates the adrenal gland
_____	3. Cortisol	c) Secretes epinephrine
_____	4. Hypothalamus	d) Secretes ACTH
_____	5. Adrenal medulla	e) Stimulates the pituitary gland
_____	6. ACTH	f) Secretes cortisol
_____	7. Epinephrine	g) Releases CRF
_____	8. CRF	h) Adrenalin

STRESS AND DISEASE

Concept: Stress has been associated with several diseases and illnesses.

Most researchers agree that stress is associated with the psychosomatic diseases. A **psychosomatic disease** is a physical disorder that has its origin in or is worsened by psychological or emotional processes. In other words, in a psychosomatic disease, the mind affects the condition of the body to cause or to worsen an illness.

Psychosomatic Conditions

The following psychosomatic conditions have been related to stress:

1. Ulcers. A fissure or open sore on the stomach lining is called a peptic ulcer. It is thought that the condition is associated with increased secretion of the acid juices that aid in digestion. An ulcer can result in severe stomach pain, heartburn, nausea, and a bloated-stomach sensation. Approximately 5 percent of Americans develop a peptic ulcer and each year about 10,000 die of it.[6] Ulcers have been produced in mice by subjecting them to psychological stress.

2. Ulcerative colitis. This condition is characterized by a deterioration of the membrane of the colon so that it bleeds a great deal and may eventually perforate. Studies have found that people who suffer from this condition have a deep feeling of helplessness. Many believe that this feeling creates stress and contributes to the development of ulcerative colitis.

3. Diarrhea and constipation. "Both are centered in the colon, which, like the stomach, is designed to work intermittently, not continuously. When it overworks, the result is diarrhea; when it underworks, constipation; and stress is often the culprit in both."[7]

4. Allergies. Since stress affects the immunological response of the body, it has been cited as a cause of allergies. An asthmatic child, or the parent of one, does not need scientific data, however, to be convinced that emotional situations can precipitate an asthmatic reaction. Similarly, hay fever attacks often follow or immediately precede emotional excitation.

5. Migraine headaches. Headaches are the cause of more than half the visits to physicians' offices in the United States. One type of severe headache is the migraine, in which the blood vessels in the scalp are dilated. The victim feels a painful pounding in the head and experiences nausea. The patient with a migraine is usually an individual who feels a great deal of pressure to succeed and works very hard. A migraine attack generally occurs when the stress is relieved rather than during moments of stress.

6. Tension headache. Another type of headache resulting from stress is termed a tension headache. This occurs as a result of chronic muscle tension, most often a result of stress, in the neck and scalp. Did you ever wonder where the expression "pain in the neck" came from? Have you ever had one?

7. Mental illness. Many researchers believe that stress can cause various forms of mental illness. One can escape a stressful existence by escaping from reality. We all know the recuperative value of vacation periods in which we "get away from it all." The mentally ill person may be unable to rejoin a world that he or she finds too stressful.

Psychosomatic Conditions over Which There Is Debate

The conditions cited above are but a few of those associated with stress, and ones about which there is little disagreement. The conditions listed below are controversial in that some experts believe stress is an important factor in their etiology, whereas others discount its significance.

1. Hypertension. Perhaps as many as 33 percent of adults in the United States are hypertensive, meaning that their blood pressure is abnormally high. **Hypertension** is accepted as a factor in both coronary heart disease and stroke and has been associated with stress. Some physicians are working with stress-reducing techniques as an aid to control this condition.[8] Hypertension is discussed in more detail in Chapter 16.

2. Coronary Heart Disease. Some researchers believe that stress is a significant factor in heart attacks and in the blockage of the arteries supplying the heart.

While acknowledging the importance of physical activity, levels of serum cholesterol, cigarette smoking, sex, and family history as factors in heart disease, Friedman and Rosenman, who advanced the theory of Type A Behavior Pattern, regard stress as the pervasive underlying cause.

3. Stroke. **Stroke** is a rupture of a blood vessel in the brain and can result in paralysis, loss of speech, or death (see Chapter 16). Stroke is related to hypertension, and hypertension is related to stress. Thus it is logical that stroke is also related to stress.

4. Cancer. Though such factors as viruses, chemicals, and radiation are suspected of causing **cancer,** there is a growing belief that stress also may play a role. It is believed that cancerous mutations occur in us all, but since our immunological system destroys the mutant cells before they can multiply, most of us do not develop cancer. Likewise, it is suspected that a lowering of one's immune defenses will allow such cancerous cells to multiply. According to one theory, "Stress helps to cause cancer because it depresses the immune response, the body's only real means of defending itself against malignant cells. It does this through the action of the adrenal cortex hormones, which particularly affect the T-lymphocytes. Searching out foreign antigens in the body is one of the tasks of these T-lymphocytes, and significantly they measure at low levels in the tissues of most cancer patients."[9] Further, some have theorized that the blood's increased coagulability, a result of stress, "causes deposits of fibrin to form on the walls of blood vessels which may snag passing cancer cells. The cells then take up residence and begin growing in surrounding tissues."[10]

5. Diabetes mellitus. Stress has the effect of increasing sugar in the blood. Because the body is preparing for "fight-or-flight" when stressed, the sugar is designed to provide energy for either of these two reactions. Some researchers believe that chronically high levels of blood sugar, brought about by chronic stress, will diminish the ability of the pancreas to develop the insulin needed to metabolize the sugar (glucose) resulting in a permanent insulin deficiency.

Other conditions in which stress is suspected of being a factor include obesity, rheumatoid arthritis, and accidents. Have you developed one of the conditions related to stress? How might you change your lifestyle to prevent these conditions from developing or from getting worse?

COPING WITH STRESS

Before we begin looking at ways of managing stress, let's first consider a model of the manner in which stress results in illness or disease.

How Stress Can Lead to Illness

Figure 4.2 describes a road down which a stressed individual may travel to illness or disease. The journey begins with a *situation* to which one has to adjust. As an example, let's assume that several of the major life changes discussed earlier have occurred. A couple has

Figure 4.2
A stress consequence model.

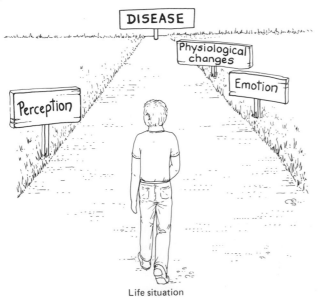

Life situation

just moved to a new town where they both are starting new jobs. These stressors alone will not result in disease. They must first be *perceived* as distressing.

Suppose the husband is extremely concerned about how he will do in his new job. Instead of perceiving it as a challenge, he worries that he will make many mistakes, that he's not up to the demands he's going to face. He's concerned that if he loses the job, his wife's salary won't cover the mortgage payments on the new house.

If he perceives his new job as a threat, the husband has certain *emotional* reactions. He's tense, feels anxious, and is extremely insecure. These emotional reactions lead to *physiological* changes—increased heart, respiratory, and perspiration rates; increased muscle tension and beta brain waves; increased blood pressure and serum cholesterol; a knot in the stomach; and the other fight-or-flight responses. If these physiological changes occur often, are prolonged, or go unabated, he may experience an *illness or disease.*

Stress Management: Setting Up Roadblocks

The management of stress is based upon this model. Stress management entails setting up roadblocks so that the progression we have described does not reach the illness or disease level. If we could eliminate or block all potentially distressing life situations, the journey down the road would never begin. Of course, this is not only impossible, it is undesirable, because life would be extremely dull if we did not have to adapt to change.

On the other hand, there are numerous adjustments that we all could make in our lives to eliminate *unnecessary* stressors. Can you think of some stressors you could eliminate from your life?

Some stressors will sift through to the next level, which is perception, so the stress management techniques we employ will have to relate to our perceptions of these stressors. One way to perceive a stressor as less distressing is to find and focus upon the positive component of the situation. Rather than focusing on the possibility of failure, the husband in our example could concentrate his attention on the positive opportunities his new job provides. This is an important approach to take toward minor stressors as well. For example, if you usually get irritated by having to wait in line, say to yourself, "Seldom in my busy day do I get a chance to do nothing. I'm going to take this opportunity to slow down. The telephone can't ring here and no one can barge in." In this manner, by not perceiving the situation as stressful, you may be able to prevent it from becoming so. You cannot control everything that happens to you, but you can certainly be in control of how you perceive those things, what you think about them, and how you behave in response to them.

Relaxation Techniques

Recognizing that some stressors will still be perceived as distressing, you can use various techniques to control your responses at the emotional level. One set of techniques results in a relaxation response, as opposed to a fight-or-flight response. Relaxation techniques, as these are known, include meditation, autogenic training, progressive relaxation, and the use of biofeedback equipment.

Meditation. **Meditation** has been popularized in the Western world by Maharishi Mahesh Yogi's teaching of transcendental meditation (TM). This form of meditation requires 40 minutes a day (20 minutes in the morning and 20 minutes in the late afternoon). The meditator, who is seated in a quiet location, repeats a Sanskrit word (mantra) and when other thoughts come to mind gently returns to the repetition of the mantra. Researchers have found that during meditation people experience a lowering of metabolic rate, respiratory rate, pulse rates, oxygen consumption, and blood pressure. This state is the opposite of the physiological condition that occurs in reaction to stress.

Dr. Herbert Benson, a heart specialist, suggests that a similar technique is just as effective in eliciting the physiological reaction to meditation. That physiological reaction is termed the relaxation response, and involves the following steps:

1. Sit quietly in a comfortable position.
2. Close your eyes.
3. Deeply relax all your muscles.
4. Breathe through your nose and say the word "one" each time you breathe out.
5. Do this for 20 minutes maintaining a passive attitude; that is, don't try to bring about the desired physiological reaction.[11]

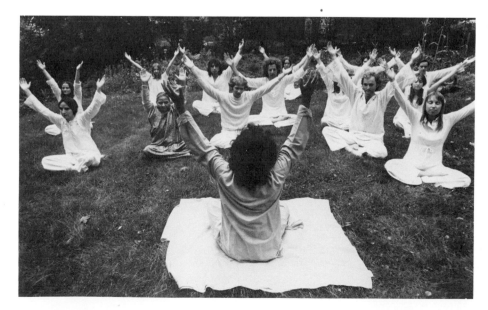

A stress-reduction technique that has helped many people is meditation.

Issues in Health
WILL PEOPLE WHO ENGAGE IN RELAXATION TECHNIQUES BE LESS PRODUCTIVE?

Some researchers believe that stress spurs people on to do their best. They argue that in response to stress the body prepares for action and has greater energy than it does when at rest. This extra energy can be used to do a better job than would otherwise be possible. Advocates of the usefulness of the stress response believe that the fight-or-flight response is necessary in order to prepare people *both* physiologically and psychologically to perform their best. They believe that hormonal secretions, increased muscular tension, increased respiratory rate, increased cardiac output, and higher serum sugar levels are positive reactions to a situation requiring an effective response. To engage in relaxation exercises would negate the body's natural reaction—a reaction developed through evolution over hundreds of thousands of years.

Others believe that physiological and psychological reactions to stress are dysfunctional, that the fight-or-flight response has served us well to a point, but is now harmful. They advocate the regular practice of relaxation techniques, arguing that the reactions of both the body and the mind to stress get in the way of effective action. How can one pay attention to a task and do one's best at it if the muscles are too tense, the hands are slippery from perspiration, and the mind can't focus upon the task? Those who favor relaxation techniques argue that people who use them regularly do not become hermits, are not amotivational or apathetic, but will be better able to think rationally and arrive at the most appropriate behavior under stressful circumstances. What do you think? ●

Autogenic Training. Developed by Dr. H. H. Shultz,[12] a German psychiatrist, the **autogenic training** method of relaxation involves self-hypnosis. Using imagery and suggested feelings of heaviness and warmth in the limbs, the subject learns to recognize a relaxed state and call upon it when needed. Autogenic training has been found to result in decreased respiratory and heart rates, decreased muscle tension, and an increase in alpha brain waves.

The following are typical instructions for autogenic training:

> Sitting with your hands rested on your thighs (not touching each other), back straight against the chair, head hanging loosely forward, and both feet flat on the floor, close your eyes.
>
> Imagine you've just come from a long walk and you're very tired. Your legs are most tired.
>
> Feel the heaviness in your legs. They are very heavy. Just let your legs weigh themselves down.
>
> Now they are feeling very warm. Just relax them, but feel how heavy and warm they are.
>
> Enjoy this feeling. Retain it.[13]

The idea of autogenic training is similar to many of the stress-reducing (relaxation) exercises; it is to provide the individual with the feeling of relaxation so that it can be called upon during times of stress.

Use a tape recorder now to record the instructions for autogenic training or make up your own. Or just sit back and think of a pleasant scene. Once relaxed, try to notice the heaviness and warmth you are feeling.

Progressive relaxation. Developed by Dr. Edmund Jacobson,[14] a physician, the **progressive relaxation** method requires the participant first to tense and then to relax muscles in the body in order to learn to recognize tenseness and to learn to relax during periods of stress. It is termed progressive because it starts with muscles in one part of the body and progresses to all the other parts. Here is an example of instructions for progressive relaxation:

> Sitting in your seat with your eyes closed, extend your right arm, with the palm upward, to the right. Now make a fist and bend your arm at the elbow and contract your biceps. After ten seconds just stop contract-

ing all at once and the whole arm should fall to your side. Experience the muscle tension when the muscle is contracted, and the relief when it is relaxed. Learn to recognize both feelings and to be able to call upon either when desirable.[15]

Try progressive relaxation yourself. Start with your feet and move from one muscle group to another until you relax your frontalis muscle (in your forehead). Don't rush it. Don't miss any parts of your body.

Biofeedback. Some people do not trust subjective measures of relaxation and need objective measures to verify their relaxed state. **Biofeedback** is used to control functions of the body usually considered involuntary—such as brain waves, muscle tension, and skin temperature—by measuring physiological events and instantaneously reporting them back to the person. For example, electromyographic (EMG) feedback instrumentation records the amount of contraction of a particular muscle. Electrodes connected to the EMG machine are attached to the skin covering the muscle whose tension is being measured. The woman hooked up to an EMG machine in the picture on this page is having the tension of her frontalis (forehead) muscle measured, because this muscle gives the best indication of general body relaxation. The machine itself does not produce the relaxed state; its function is to enable the subject to recognize and control her own responses.

One of the advantages of biofeedback training over some of the other relaxation techniques is the speed with which the participant learns the relaxation response. The disadvantage is that it involves the use, and sometimes purchase, of sophisticated equipment that is usually only available on college campuses or in clinical settings. You might be able to locate biofeedback equipment on your campus (in the psychology, physiology, or health education department) and make arrangements for biofeedback training.

Physical Activity

Another means of diminishing stress is to engage in vigorous physical activity and use the built-up stress products, such as muscle tension and increased heart

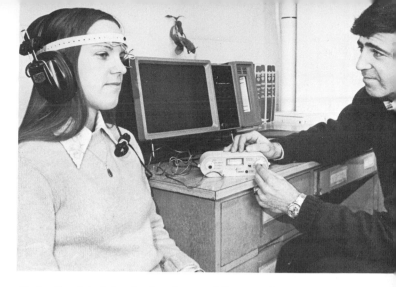

Biofeedback training is aimed at enabling people to control functions of the body that are usually considered involuntary, such as brain wave pattern and muscle tension.

rate. Joggers and long-distance runners have reported experiencing a meditativelike state, and it is suspected that the repetition of the sound of the foot on the ground serves as a mantra. Many kinds of exercise and sport serve this purpose, but a caution is advised. If you are so competitive that you must win, these activities may produce stress rather than reduce it. Get into the activity itself—not the end result of the activity. Enjoy doing it—not having won it. If you are highly competitive and winning is important, try such physical activities as backpacking, hiking, cross-country skiing, or canoeing. Activities other than sports can also reduce stress. Working on a car or in a garden can serve the same purpose.

Which type of physical activity is best suited to your purposes? Will you do it regularly? Don't wait. Set up a schedule to begin it now.

Other Techniques

There are many other ways to relieve stress. Religion is a source of strength for some to overcome stressful events. Philosophies and practices such as yoga, Sufism, and Zen can also serve the same purpose. You probably already employ some ways to relieve stress that are unique to you. What are they? Do they work? When did you last use one?

Issues in Health
SHOULD STRESS MANAGEMENT PROGRAMS BE ELIGIBLE FOR THIRD-PARTY REIMBURSEMENT?

Stress management programs can be costly, and some people argue that those enrolling in them represent the socioeconomic elite of society. Some programs cost hundreds of dollars, and others require membership in organizations, which can also be expensive. If stress management programs are effective in preventing illness and disease, is it ethical for a society to allow only the socioeconomically advantaged to benefit from them? Shouldn't the government offer such programs free of charge to those who can't afford them? Further, if these programs are effective in preventing illness and disease, shouldn't health insurance carriers, such as Blue Cross/Blue Shield or health maintenance organizations, reimburse those whom they insure for enrollment in such programs? Insurance companies lower insurance premiums for people who have enrolled in driver education courses because they believe education can prevent automobile accidents and thereby decrease the amount of claims they have to pay. Wouldn't stress management programs decrease the amount of payments insurance carriers have to pay by teaching people how to stay healthy?

Others argue that the cost for reimbursing people for enrollment in stress management programs would be excessive. Further, education itself won't reduce the incidence of illness and disease. People must change their behavior to do that. How can health insurance carriers be sure people are eliminating stressors in their lives, are meditating, or are exercising? Even if stress management does lower the incidence of illness, should the rest of the taxpayers or the other enrollees in the health insurance plan have to pay for that? The benefit is to the individual, therefore the individual should pay it.

What do you think? ●

CONCLUSION

We have seen how our bodies manifest our emotions, how our emotions result in stress, and how stress can build up within us. Further, we have noted how stress operates physiologically and how it causes disease states. Last, and most important, we described some ways to reduce the negative effects of stress. The bottom line, however, is whether you decide to use this knowledge about stress to improve your health. You *can* eliminate some stressors in your life. You *can* perceive some stressors differently so as to make them less distressing. You *can* regularly practice a relaxation technique: meditation, autogenic training, or progressive relaxation. You *can* exercise at least every other day in order to use the built-up stress in your life. You *can* prevent illness and disease and, what's more, feel better about each day.

SUMMARY

1. Emotions are expressed by the body. For example, individuals with low self-esteem slump and are not very expressive; individuals with high self-esteem walk tall and talk animatedly.

2. The stress response pattern has three stages: alarm, resistance, and exhaustion. This response was first identified by Hans Selye, one of the leading researchers in the area of stress.

3. Stress can be positive or negative. Positive stress is called eustress. Negative stress is called distress. The stress response is the same, regardless of the type of stress experienced.

4. Stress results from changes in life—the more changes one experiences, the more susceptible one is to illness or disease. However, certain intervening variables, such as social support, can serve as a buffer between stress and illness or disease.

5. Stress is associated with college life and situations outside the school setting. College stressors include disease-causing bacteria and viruses that are spread by close contact among individuals, the pressure to get good grades, being independent, and making a new set of friends. Other stressors are urbanization, the dual-career family, and job stress.

6. Stress physiology begins with the hypothalamus, which perceives a stressor and releases CRF, which in turn signals the pituitary gland to release ACTH. The ACTH activates the adrenal gland cortex to secrete cortisol. At the same time, the hypothalamus, through nerve pathways, directly activates the adrenal gland medulla to secrete epinephrine and norepinephrine. The result of these hormonal secretions is an increase in the heart beat, respiratory rate, muscle tension, serum cholesterol, and perspiration, and a decrease in white blood cells, surface body temperature, and digestive processes.

7. Stress has been associated with such conditions as ulcers, ulcerative colitis, diarrhea and constipation, allergies, migraine and tension headaches, mental illness, hypertension, heart disease, stroke, cancer, and diabetes mellitus.

8. Stress can be depicted as beginning with a change in a life situation that is perceived as distressing. Emotional reactions to this change lead to the physiological stress response. If this physiological response is chronic, prolonged, or goes unabated, illness or disease may result.

9. Stress can be managed by eliminating the stressors one encounters, perceiving stressors as less distressing, exercising to use up stress products, and regularly practicing a relaxation technique. Relaxation techniques include meditation, autogenic training, progressive relaxation, and biofeedback training.

REFERENCES

1. Hans Selye, *Stress without Distress* (New York: J. B. Lippincott Company, 1974), p. 14. Copyright © 1974 by Hans Selye, M.D.

2. Ibid. p. 27.

3. Thomas H. Holmes and Richard H. Rahe, "The Social Readjustment Scale," *Journal of Psychosomatic Research* 11 (1967):213–218.

4. Stanley Cobb, "Social Support as a Moderator of Life Stress," *Psychosomatic Medicine* 38 (1976):300–314.

5. Clint E. Bruess and Jerrold S. Greenberg, *Sex Education: Theory and Practice* (Belmont, Calif.: Wadsworth, 1981), p. 162.

6. Kenneth Lamott, *Escape from Stress: How to Stop Killing Yourself* (New York: Putnam, 1974), p. 61.

7. Walter McQuade and Ann Aikman, *Stress* (New York: Bantam, 1975), p. 42.

8. Excerpt "hypertension . . . United States" and abridgment and adaptation of the relaxation response in *The Relaxation Response* by Herbert Benson, M. D., p. 19. Copyright © 1975 by William Morrow and Company, Inc. By permission of the publishers.

9. McQuade and Aikman, *Stress*, p. 76.

10. Ibid., p. 77.

11. Excerpt "hypertension . . . United States" and abridgment and adaptation of the relaxation response in *The Relaxation Response* by Herbert Benson, M. D., pp. 162–163. Copyright © 1975 by William Morrow and Company, Inc. By permission of the publishers.

12. W. Luthe, "Autogenic Training: Method, Research, and Application in Medicine," *American Journal of Psychotherapy* 17 (1963):174–195.

13. Jerrold S. Greenberg, *Student-Centered Health Instruction* (Reading, Mass.: Addison-Wesley, 1978), p. 202.

14. Edmund Jacobson, *Progressive Relaxation* (Chicago: University of Chicago Press, 1938).

15. Greenberg, *Student-Centered Health Instruction*, p. 202.

Laboratory 1
THE EFFECTS OF STRESS

Purpose   To observe the effects of stress.

Size of Group   Class is divided in half.

Equipment   Record player.
Record—rock music with lyrics.

Procedure

1. Determine your pulse rate. Do this with your first two fingers (not the thumb) and find the pulse either on your wrist (palm up, side away from body) or in the carotid artery (in the neck just above the collar bone). Pulse should be taken for 30 seconds while seated and then doubled to arrive at a rate per minute. This is the resting heart rate.

2. Write your pulse rate per minute in large numbers on a sheet of paper. Hold the paper at chest level so everyone can see everyone else's. Wander about the room and pair up with someone whose pulse rate is within four numbers of yours.

3. Next, divide your class into two groups, you joining one group and your partner joining another. One group goes to another room while the other stays in the classroom. This procedure will assure that the two groups have approximately the same average pulse rates.

4. Groups A and B, as they will be called, should each be divided into thirds: one third will solve the mathematical task described below, another third will take the pulse of the problem solvers, and the last third will observe.

Group A

1. Problem solvers
This subgroup should be seated and asked to do the following *as fast as possible:*

   a) Add 57329, 4351, 76740, 86152, 7212, 5472, 12471, 99865, 9876, 457320, 87310, 76547, 55698, 22439, 7549, 67923.

   b) Divide that sum by 2398.

   c) Then multiply by 789.

2. Pulsetakers

   a) Pair up with one problem solver and record that person's resting pulse rate for 15 seconds prior to the mathematical computation.

   b) Keep monitoring the pulse rate by holding the wrist of the hand not needed by your partner (e.g., left wrist for right-handed person).

   c) Record the pulse rate of your partner as specified below. *Pulse should be taken for 15 seconds each time.*

   1. Resting pulse rate   _____
   2. 30 seconds into task   _____
   3. $1\frac{1}{2}$ minutes into task   _____
   4. 2 minutes into each task   _____
   5. 3 minutes into task   _____
   6. At conclusion of task   _____

3. Observers
Choose a student doing the computational task, observe him or her, and look for signs of stress, such as perspiration, moving around in the seat, angry or frustrated facial features. Observable signs of stress should be written on a sheet of paper.

Group B

The same procedure should be followed as for Group A except that the record should be played very loudly in this room and the observers should try to distract the problem solvers by talking to them, calling out numbers, dancing, turning on and off the lights, and other such activities. However, be sure not to touch the students doing the computation.

Results

1. Compare the pulse rates for each group. Did the students in the stressed group (B) have higher pulse rates during the activity? Discuss.

2. Compare the observations of stress recorded for each group. Discuss.

3. Ask the students who did the mathematical computing to relate how they felt during the activity. Compare these feelings for each group. Discuss.

Laboratory 2
RELAXATION

Purpose   To note the physiological reactions to relaxation.

Size of Group   Small group of four students.

Equipment   Each group will need a stethoscope and a sphygmomanometer.

Procedure

1. Choose one student to meditate for 20 minutes.

2. Choose another student to take the pulse of the mediator. Take the pulse at the wrist of the left arm (the one not being monitored for blood pressure).

3. Choose another student to note respiratory rate by placing hand on the chest of the meditator and noting the number of times the chest moves up (expands) per minute.

4. Choose another student to monitor the blood pressure of the meditator. Place the cuff just above the right elbow with the stethoscope just over the brachial artery (feel for pulse in the inside of the el-

bow). Pump up cuff after turning knob to prevent air from escaping. Stop pumping when pulse is not heard through the stethoscope. Then turn knob and release air *slowly* recording the reading (on the column of mercury) when the pulse first returns and then when it can't be heard any longer. An average reading is 120/80.

5. Pulse, respiration, and blood pressure should be taken just prior to, and then 15 minutes into, meditating.

Results

	Prior to Mediating	15 Minutes into Meditating
1. Pulse	_____	_____
2. Respiration	_____	_____
3. Blood Pressure	___/___	___/___

Discuss each group's results with the total class.

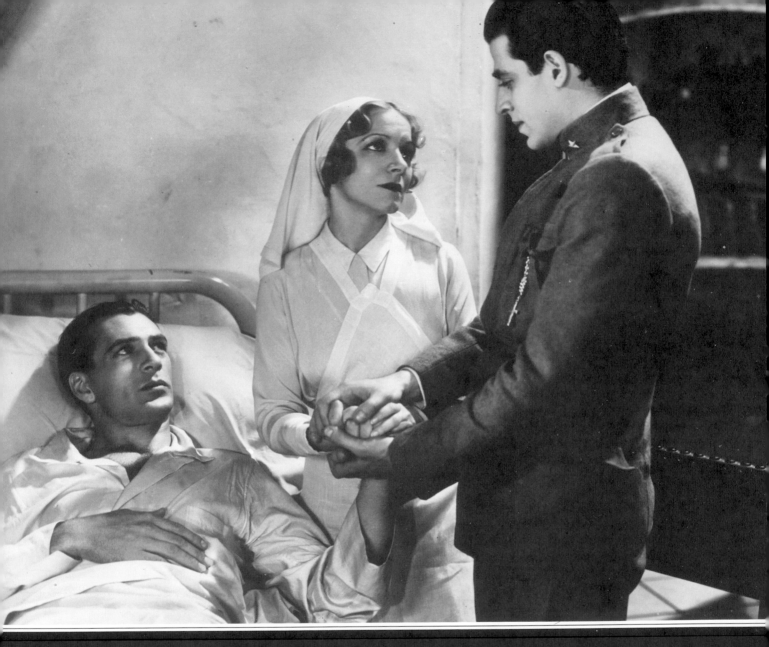

chapter 5

aging, dying, and death

For most people in the United States, aging, dying, and death are difficult topics. Understanding and accepting old age and death are not easy for the average American, who minds losing what our culture associates with youth: health, beauty, sexual attractiveness, strength and vitality, employment, long-range goals, hopes, and dreams.

The emphasis placed on youth in the United States is clearly excessive and emotionally unhealthy. Aging is a natural process. In many cultures older individuals are respected for their experience, intelligence, and advice. In the United States, however, older people often reduce their social interaction in spite of their need and desire for it; they gradually withdraw as they lose their influence in society. Fortunately, with the steadily increasing number of individuals over age 65, groups of elder activists, such as the Gray Panthers and the American Association of Retired People, have emerged to work toward raising the status of the elderly. As people are better informed about aging and death,

perhaps our society's view of these life passages will become more healthy. In this chapter we present some of the health issues—both physiological and psychological—related to aging, and we consider some of the ways in which people can cope with death and dying.

Discovery Activity 5.1
HOW DO YOU VIEW THE ELDERLY?

Take a few minutes to think about the elderly people with whom you are associated: relatives, friends, or old people in the park or walking on the streets. For each set of descriptions, mark a number from 1 to 5, with 1 indicating that you think the description in the left-hand column is most accurate and 5 indicating that the description in the right-hand column is most accurate.

Personal Qualities of the Elderly 1 2 3 4 5	
Friendly and warm	Unfriendly and cold
Happy	Unhappy
Very capable intellectually	Less capable intellectually
Openminded and adaptable	Oldfashioned and inflexible
Physically active	Physically inactive
Sexually active	Sexually inactive
Healthy	Sick or incapacitated

If you selected mostly numbers 4 and 5 for each set of characteristics, your view fits the popular stereotype of old people: white-haired, inactive people who are losing their intellectual abilities, are inflexible in their thinking, and are unhappy. This description of the elderly has been found to be inaccurate in most cases. Why do you think it is so persistent? ●

Activist Maggie Kuhn of the Grey Panthers has helped focus attention on the particular concerns of aging Americans.

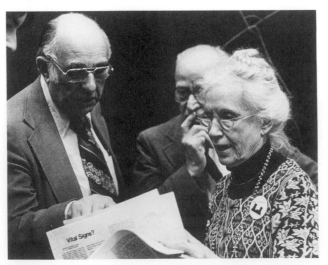

AGING

Theories of Aging

Concept: Although numerous biological theories of aging exist, there still is no "fountain-of-youth" formula.

"Primary" aging is biological, rooted in genetics and inevitable, regardless of health and daily routine. This biological process occurs at different rates for different people and may be modified or delayed through exercise, drugs, and changes in lifestyle. But the end result remains the same in time—aging and death. "Secondary" aging refers to disabilities resulting from degenerative diseases, such as arthritis, atherosclerosis, diabetes, and heart disease.

Several theories have been proposed to explain the reasons for the aging process.

1. *The genetic theory* suggests that we inherit cell make-up, which in turn controls aging. Some experts even hypothesize that organisms possess aging genes which control the rate of tissue degeneration throughout the body.

2. *The defective DNA or genetic material theory* proposes that somehow the DNA becomes defective, thereby causing the synthesis of defective protein, until the organism is unable to function properly and deteriorates.

3. *The errors theory* implies that the body, at some point, begins to make errors in protein synthesis and produces changed proteins. As the body's immune system reacts against these changed proteins, cells are destroyed and body functions impaired, resulting in aging.

4. *The theory of aging hits* views aging as a result of random events, accumulating errors that affect the body several times each year throughout life, which in turn affect cell life.

5. *The theory of accumulation of deleterious material* suggests that the body builds up unstable and harmful material that produces various detrimental biological changes, such as alterations in chro-mosomes, build-up in pigment, and alterations in macromolecules.

6. *The theory of a stress-stimulated response of the adrenal glands* proposes a relationship between aging and exercise. It is known that exercise stimulates both the adrenal cortex and the medulla, and this theory suggests that a cellular mechanism is responsible for increased life span through exercise.

7. *The theory of loss of nerve cells in the brain* suggests that aging is directly related to the nerve cells in the brain responsible for keeping body tissues finely tuned. Since nerve tissue neither divides nor is replaced, it is believed to be more prone to aging.

8. *The hormone imbalance theory* suggests that aging is strongly linked to the hormones.

9. *The cross-linking of molecules theory* suggests that aging occurs when giant molecules in cells, such as DNA, link together with other molecules, which then become unable to function properly. Exactly what causes this phenomenon is unknown.

Physiological Changes: You Do Have Some Control

Concept: The rates at which we age vary and are affected by a number of controllable factors.

The theories of aging concern bodily processes that we as individuals can't control. However, several bodily changes that occur with aging can be altered by exercise and diet.

1. Excess body weight often accumulates with age; excess weight contributes to cardiovascular disease and early death. Proper diet and exercise can help regulate body weight.

2. The percentage of body fat (ratio of body fat to muscle mass) increases with age. The average percentage of body fat has been estimated at about 10.3 percent at age 20, 20.0 percent at age 40,

and 25.0 percent at age 55. Proper diet and exercise can help control this rise.

3. The walls of the coronary arteries thicken with age, increasing the risk of high blood pressure and heart disease. There is about a 25 to 35 percent reduction in the area open to blood flow in the 40 to 50 age group, compared to the 20 to 29 age group. Increasing evidence demonstrates that people who have engaged in aerobic exercise for several years have a larger area open to blood flow than those who have been inactive.

4. Maximum oxygen uptake (the ability to take in atmospheric oxygen, diffuse it into the blood, and utilize it at the tissue level) decreases with age (see Chapter 6). However, the rate of decline has been shown to be much less rapid in individuals who are engaged in aerobic exercise.

Although continuous aerobic exercise throughout life delays the decline of bodily functions, there is as yet no concrete evidence linking exercise to increased longevity. Several studies have demonstrated that programs of lifelong physical activity improve the life expectancy of laboratory animals, but this link has not been verified for humans. However, it is anticipated that similar evidence for humans will be forthcoming, particularly in view of recent research indicating that aerobic exercise protects against early heart disease.

Improving Longevity

Life expectancy in the United States has risen from about 54.1 years in 1920 to 73.3 years in 1979. Much of the increase can be attributed to reduced infant mortality rates and control of childhood diseases. The majority of deaths in the age range of 10 to 70 years are accidental or due to degenerative diseases. Because degenerative diseases are related to lifestyle, many believe that changes in lifestyle can lead to a significant increase in longevity.

What are the lifestyle contributors to early death? Among the most important are overweight and obesity, smoking, poor nutritional habits, excessive stress, and inactivity. Overweight is a particularly important con-

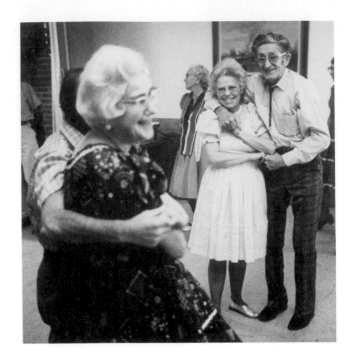

Physical activity throughout life can be an important factor in improving longevity.

tributor to artery damage, and the process of clogging of the arteries can start very early in life. Fat deposits that lead to hardening of the arteries and related age-associated diseases, such as stroke, senility, and coronary heart disease have been identified in children as young as 10 years of age.

Inactivity as a lifestyle factor in early death is especially prevalent among Americans. The average American leads a sedentary life throughout adulthood. Although aerobic exercise such as tennis and racquetball, and other healthy activities are becoming increasingly popular, it is still true that fewer than 50 percent of the American people exercise at least twice per week.

Heredity is another significant factor in longevity. A reporter once asked a 103-year-old man the question, "If you had your life to live over again, would you do anything differently?" "Well," pondered the old man, "if I'd known I was going to live to be 103, I sure would have taken better care of myself." By "choosing the right parents," many people live long lives regardless of their lifestyle. But for most of us there are other, more practical ways of improving our chances of living a long life.

Concept: Although there are no guarantees of longer life, you can improve your chances by making certain lifestyle changes.

The following suggestions, if followed, should increase the likelihood that the individual will be free from certain types of diseases and able to live a healthier, perhaps longer life.

1. Engage in an aerobic exercise program (see Chapter 6) at least three times weekly throughout life.

2. Avoid smoking cigarettes or using tobacco in any form (see Chapter 11).

3. Eat a balanced diet and drink alcohol only in moderation (see Chapters 7 and 10).

4. Control body weight and maintain minimal body fat (see Chapter 8).

5. Control high blood pressure and diabetes (see Chapters 10 and 17).

6. Reduce excessive emotional stress (see Chapter 4).

7. Remain socially active throughout life, keeping mentally alert and involved as much as possible.

8. Use all body systems; the cliché "use it or lose it" has implications for all systems, including sexual activity and mental functions.

9. Adopt a lifestyle conducive to the prevention of chronic and degenerative diseases (see Chapter 17).

10. Learn to live with yourself and accept your limitations (mental, physical and economic).

THE CHALLENGES OF AGING

Sexuality

One of the most notable signs of aging for women is the cessation of menstruation and ovulation. These events, referred to as menopause or "change of life," may cause emotional and physical problems in some women. Skin may become dry and less elastic. Lubrication secretions in the vagina may be reduced. Some women experience sudden sensations of heat (hot flashes). But only about 25 percent of women experience disturbing symptoms that require a physician's care. The loss of fertility may place considerable stress on some women. However, research suggests that for most, middle age may bring a sense of freedom from worry about pregnancy and a heightened interest in sexual activity.

While some men experience reduced sexual drive during middle age, similar reproductive changes do not occur. The average man remains fertile and capable of sexual relations throughout life. However, men do require longer to achieve erections as they grow older, and they ejaculate with less force.

Sexuality in old age is more problematic. While some older individuals continue to be sexually active during their later years, others who are still healthy and have a healthy partner fail to do so because of societal attitudes. The myth is still prevalent that old people are not supposed to have sexual feelings and that to continue sexual activity in old age is shameful. These attitudes arise long before people reach old age. Your present attitude and your own sexual adjustment are probably the best indicators of whether or not you'll continue to be sexually active in your later years. It is a choice you can make.

Retirement

Retirement means different things to different people. In our youth-oriented society, many people look upon retirement as a signpost of old age. It is often assumed that retired people have difficulty adjusting to the loss of their primary role in life—that of productive worker. How true this is depends on several factors. People who have been forced to retire before they want to may indeed feel a sense of rejection and loss. However, there are many others who look forward to retirement at 65 or even earlier as a chance to experience new challenges or simply to enjoy a more relaxing lifestyle.

One important factor in how people feel about retirement is income. Studies suggest that many people retire voluntarily before the age of 65 if they are financially solvent. It is often concern about their financial future that keeps people on the job until the age of 65. Another factor in how people view retirement is whether or not they have planned for it. The adjustment is much easier for individuals who have planned for their retirement in terms of finances, activities, and the like.

We noted in Chapter 4 that various life changes contribute to stress. One of these is a change in financial status. Recently retired individuals tend to have significantly lower scores on measures of life satisfaction. Part of the reason for this is that the newly retired often experience a sudden drop in income. Fortunately, within a year or so after retirement, many find a way to supplement their income. Not surprisingly, then, people with low life satisfaction scores just after retirement score as well as nonretired people when tested a year or so after retirement.

What can be done to help people prepare for retirement? One important need is for a change in attitude on the part of our society as a whole. We believe that people should not be forced to retire before they are ready. It is time for Americans to begin to value older individuals, utilize their talents, and treat them with respect and dignity. Similarly, older persons should stop viewing themselves as useless and should perform useful activities throughout life. This means developing a healthy involvement and positive attitudes from childhood on. What does retirement mean to you? What can you do to prepare yourself for this life passage? Do you want to retire early or work as long as you can? Why? How will you handle it if you are forced to retire before you want to?

Remarriage

In general, older widows tend not to remarry and seek other widows as friends, whereas older widowers remarry within one year of the death of their spouses. Widows who remarry do so an average of seven years after the death of their husbands. Widowers have many more women to choose from in their age group but are more apt to marry younger women. The widow is less likely to marry a younger man because this is not as accepted in our society.

Most widows and widowers marry old friends, childhood lovers, or former neighbors. The majority of marriages that occur late in life are successful; few end in divorce.

It is becoming more common for older couples to seek alternatives to marriage. Living together provides love, security, comfort, and companionship; it also prevents a reduction in Social Security benefits or in a widow's pension.

Widowhood

Of the 12 million widowed men and women in the United States in 1975, 11 million were widows. Women outlive men by 10 or more years. Assuming that the 10-year difference in lifespan between men and women will continue, approximately 75 percent of wives will be widowed at some time in their lives. The average age of widows is 56 and the probability of remarriage is quite low. The first year after the death of a mate is the most difficult; there is a high death rate for the surviving spouse and an increased susceptibility to suicide. Both widows and widowers find adjustment difficult. Widows are more likely to suffer from chronic disabling physical ailments and face financial difficulties due to reduced income. In addition, widows find that they are often excluded from gatherings, have no one to escort them to social functions, are viewed with suspicion by some married women, and often can find friends only among other widows. Widowers are particularly susceptible to coronary heart disease, and they suffer a number of simultaneous role changes, such as loss of job, reduced income, loss of spouse, loss of health, and inability to assume the domestic responsibilities shouldered by the wife during the marriage. Widows, on the other hand, generally established more independent midlife roles when children left home.

Adjustment requires replacement of lost roles, such as sexual companion and friend. Those who have fewer roles to replace or who quickly reestablish former roles are less apt to experience difficulty adjusting. Elderly couples may also benefit from planning for death and widowhood by reviewing financial affairs, discussing funeral arrangements, purchasing a burial plot, and planning other such critical decisions in advance.

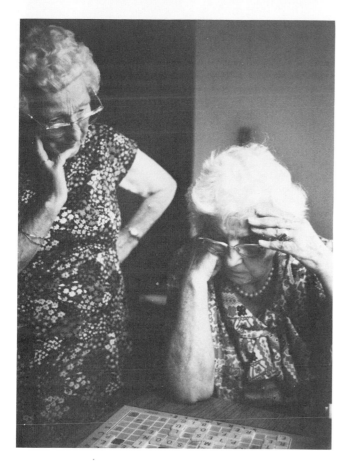

Women may have an easier time adjusting to widowhood than men because they are more likely to have established roles independent of the wife role when their children left home and because they generally have a network of friendships.

DYING

Concept: More attention is being paid to the needs of the dying.

Most people do not fear death as much as the process of dying—particularly if dying is accompanied by pain. "Sixty-seven percent of the people who die in the United States have chronic degenerative diseases which usually include a prolonged period of dying."[1] Consequently, more and more attention is being directed at ways to ease the fear and pain of dying people. Drugs such as LSD and marijuana have been used in research

This new environment can be traumatic as one leaves many years of friendship behind. Retirement communities also separate the elderly from the rest of society and perpetuate the myth that the old are misfits and have no significant contribution to make. Suddenly, retired individuals are faced with a totally new environment, new friends, and new roles, and are completely isolated from the society in which they worked and played for 60 years or more. So many drastic changes, it is argued, may be too much for some individuals to handle. In addition, many of these communities are too expensive for individuals who rely on Social Security benefits for their financial support.

What do you think? ●

1. Provide medical care for the continuing control of symptoms, such as pain and nausea;

2. Concentrate on bedside nursing to provide comfort, close attention to easing physical distress, interpersonal interactions, attention to feeding, emotional support, etc.;

3. Focus on the family unit and allow the patient and family to use the assets of their lifestyle to cope with the situation;

4. Include both the patient and the family by developing open communications;

5. Involve community volunteers, many of whom are widows or widowers, in such varied activities as assisting with patient care, gardening, working in the day-care center, and helping in the business office;

6. Provide spiritual care through ecumenical services, discussion groups, and an atmosphere of love and concern;

7. Provide a comprehensive program of outpatient and inpatient care to meet a variety of patient/family needs;

8. Foster a spirit of friendliness and encourage individuals to participate in life in a facility that is more homelike than a hospital; and

9. Establish built-in supports for staff and volunteers so that they can carry on their demanding work.[3]

settings to control the pain (both physical and psychological) experienced by dying patients. Many hospitals now offer counseling services for dying patients and their families.

In addition to these and other practices, a whole new environment in which to die is becoming established. Over 70 percent of all people die in institutions, where care is often expensive and dehumanizing. A study that attempted to determine where people would want to die found that 75 percent of the respondents did not want to die in a hospital and 82 percent did not want to die in a nursing home; 63 percent preferred to die at home.[2] A new system of care for terminally ill patients of all ages is attempting to meet the needs people have expressed to be able to die in a loving environment, close to their family.

The Hospice System

The **hospice**, meaning care to travelers (in this case, on the way to death), is a special facility that cares for dying patients. Hospices are intended to perform the following functions:

Understanding the Stages of Dying

Another means of meeting the needs of dying people is to recognize and respond to the stages of the dying process. The work of psychiatrist Elisabeth Kübler-Ross is often used as a guide in recognizing the stages of dying. Dr. Kübler-Ross identified five phases that dying people usually experience: *denial* of impending death; *anger* at having to die; *bargaining* (for example, "If I could have one more month I'd spend it doing only good"); *depression*; and, finally, *acceptance* of death.[4]

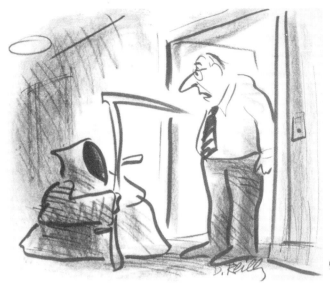

"Somehow I always expected someone tall and thin."

Reproduced by special permission of *Playboy Magazine;* copyright © 1979 by Playboy.

At the denial stage, the family can help the patient by discussing the medical evidence at hand. Perhaps a second opinion will verify the patient's condition. Family members can acknowledge the value of denial as a protective device: "It must be difficult to accept that you're going to die."

At the anger stage, families can let patients know that they have a right to be angry and that their anger will have an outlet—it will not be suppressed but rather encouraged. After all, wouldn't you be angry if you learned you would soon die?

Bargaining is a way of not accepting the inevitable. Death is imminent, regardless of the deals one makes, and the family needs to help the patient realize that: "I too, wish I could give one month of my life so you could live that much longer, but unfortunately neither of us can make such a deal." Such statements will help the patient recognize the futility of bargaining.

Depression, too, is understandable. As with anger, the patient should be encouraged to discuss feelings of depression with family members, and the family should accept these emotions. Too often, the family attempts to make the patient feel better by denying expressions of depression: "Come on, you don't really feel like that." It would be more valuable to acknowledge these feelings: "What a heavy burden you must bear. I can understand you're feeling depressed. I'm sure I would too. Do you want to talk about it?"

Acceptance of death is the goal of the terminally ill; not all such patients reach this stage. For those who

Discovery Activity 5.2
IDENTIFYING YOUR FEELINGS ABOUT DEATH[6]

To identify some of your thoughts and feelings about death and dying, complete the following sentences:

1. Death is _____

2. I would like to die at _____

3. I don't want to live past _____

4. I would like to have at my bedside when I die

   _____

5. When I die, I will be proud that when I was living I _____

6. My greatest fear about death is _____

7. When I die, I'll be glad that when I was living I didn't

   _____

8. If I were to die today, my biggest regret would be

   _____

9. When I die, I will be glad to get away from ____

   _____

10. When I die, I want people to say _____

What can you learn about your life from the sentences you have just completed? ●

do, the family should be ready to help them organize their affairs so that they feel everything is in order. The will should be updated if necessary, a list of bank accounts drawn up, health and life insurance policies at hand, and funeral and burial arrangements made.

People move through these stages at different rates and may move back and forth between stages or not go through all of them, but they do describe a process that the terminally ill commonly experience. The obvious implication is that dying people need different types of communications and relationships at different stages. In any case, not to discuss the condition of the dying person may do him or her a disservice. Family, friends, and caregivers should help the dying person through these stages by listening to and encouraging the individual and by respecting his or her special needs. The dying person has several basic needs:

1. The need to participate in one's own death—to know one is dying. Even though terminally ill patients may act as though they do not know or do not want to know that they are dying, the tone of conversation with loved ones and the medical staff all but shouts, "You are dying!" Denial is generally unhealthy and interferes with meaningful communication with loved ones—the best medicine available at this point.

2. The need to live to the end with dignity.

3. The need for hope (not necessarily hope for the preservation of life, but the hope that accompanies faith and meaningful living).

4. The need to work through and ventilate feelings of guilt, denial, jealousy, anguish, and other coping emotions.

5. The need to be listened to without censure or anger and to be accepted, regardless of the defense mechanisms used.

6. The need to feel valued as a person.

7. The need to give and be given to long after he or she is able to give.

8. The need not to be forgotten.

9. The need to function at some level, even if it's only deciding what to have for dinner.

10. The need for meaningful communication (not necessarily verbal).

11. The need for family and friends to resolve their own defense mechanisms and not to inflict unrealistic expectations on the dying person. Those who cannot face their own death can hardly help a dying person accept it calmly.

12. The need to maintain self-confidence, security, and self-esteem.

13. The need of some terminally ill people to receive permission from their loved ones to die.[5]

DEATH

American Attitudes Toward Death

Concept: The denial of death is unhealthy.

Only a few decades ago, sex was a taboo topic not discussed in mixed company. Today, in much the same way, death is not considered appropriate for conversation. The denial of death is implicit in the way we treat people dying. Since few people die at home, we seldom come in contact with the dead. We idolize youth and vilify old age. Face lifts are in, wrinkles out. Many adults dress in as youthful a style as possible. Children are seldom taken to funerals and seldom visit a graveyard. Dumont describes this attitude of denial when he writes, "When I am, Death is not. . . . When death is, I am not. Therefore we can never have anything to do with death."[7]

Even our terminology for death is indicative of this attitude. We refer to the dead as "passed away," "departed," "gone to heaven," and "laid to rest." In the end, they all mean the same. We will all be confronted by death at some time in our lives, therefore to deny it, or never to consider its significance in a rational manner, seems unhealthy. An educational council known as Concern for Dying has developed the Living Will (see Figure 5.1). This document is designed to protect the terminally ill from having their lives extended by the use of medical technology when they are no longer able to participate in the decision making.

Concept: The way you live your life may be a result of your attitude toward death.

Our attitudes toward our individual deaths . . . affect not only the way we view death, but also the way in which we live our lives. If one views his death with horror, he may have considerable difficulty in mustering the courage necessary to cross a street in heavy traffic. If, on the other hand, death is conceived as a pleasurable and exciting experience, one may not hesitate to walk a tightrope or go over Niagara Falls in a barrel. Furthermore, as at least one writer in the area of death research has suggested, the type of immortality we seek affects our behavior. If we seek biological immortality (through our children) or social immortality (through works or deeds that testify to our existence and live on in the minds of others), our philosophy toward life may be *carpe diem* . . . seize the day (live it up). On the other hand, if we seek a transcendental immortality (life hereafter), we may try to live a life of good deeds, so that we will be judged favorably after death by the supernatural forces.[9]

Death educators believe that the study of death and dying may provide clues to our behavior. The amount of risk we are willing to take may be a function of our conception of death. And, as we noted previously, during the latter years of our lives we strive for a feeling of continuity; that is, we try to achieve a sense of identification with all of humanity.

How do you conceptualize death? How does this conceptualization affect your behavior?

A Definition of Death

Concept: Death is not easily defined.

Thus far our discussion of death has assumed that we share a general understanding of what the term means. But how do we decide that someone is dead? The definition of death has been greatly complicated by the technological sophistication we have developed: we can keep people "alive" (that is, breathing, with a detectable heartbeat) for long periods of time. The use of this equipment, however, is controversial. Not only is

Discovery Activity 5.3 ## *ATTITUDES TOWARD DEATH*

What are your attitudes regarding death? Circle the number to the left of each item below with which you agree:[8]

249 The thought of death is a glorious thought.

247 When I think of death I am most satisfied.

245 Thoughts of death are wonderful thoughts.

243 The thought of death is very pleasant.

241 The thought of death is comforting.

239 I find it fairly easy to think of death.

237 The thought of death isn't so bad.

235 I do not mind thinking of death.

233 I can accept the thought of death.

231 To think of death is common.

229 I don't fear thoughts of death, but I don't like them either.

227 Thinking about death is overvalued by many.

(continued)

To My Family, My Physician, My Lawyer and All Others Whom It May Concern

Death is as much a reality as birth, growth, maturity and old age—it is the one certainty of life. If the time comes when I can no longer take part in decisions for my own future, let this statement stand as an expression of my wishes and directions, while I am still of sound mind.

If at such a time the situation should arise in which there is no reasonable expectation of my recovery from extreme physical or mental disability, I direct that I be allowed to die and not be kept alive by medications, artificial means or "heroic measures". I do, however, ask that medication be mercifully administered to me to alleviate suffering even though this may shorten my remaining life.

This statement is made after careful consideration and is in accordance with my strong convictions and beliefs. I want the wishes and directions here expressed carried out to the extent permitted by law. Insofar as they are not legally enforceable, I hope that those to whom this Will is addressed will regard themselves as morally bound by these provisions.

Signed_____

Date _____

Witness_____

Witness_____

Copies of this request have been given to _____

_____

_____

_____

---

225 Thinking of death is not fundamental to me.

223 I find it difficult to think of death.

221 I regret the thought of death.

219 The thought of death is an awful thought.

217 The thought of death is dreadful.

215 The thought of death is traumatic.

213 I hate the sound of the word death.

211 The thought of death is outrageous.

To determine your attitude toward death, disregard the first digit of the numbers (2), place a decimal point between the remaining two digits, and average all the circled responses. The average will correspond to an attitude statement or will fall between two attitude statements. This represents your attitude toward death. For example, if you circled numbers 241, 235, and 215, the computation would look like this:

4.1 + 3.5 + 1.5 = 9.1

9.1 ÷ 3 = 3.0 (to the nearest tenth)

Your attitude would fall between the attitude statements 231 and 229 on the above scale, because there is no item numbered 230.

If you discuss the results of this exercise with your classmates, you will find that attitudes toward death vary greatly. ●

To make best use of your LIVING WILL

1. Sign and date before two witnesses. (This is to insure that you signed of your own free will and not under any pressure.)

2. If you have a doctor, give him a copy for your medical file and discuss it with him to make sure he is in agreement.

   Give copies to those most likely to be concerned "if the time comes when you can no longer take part in decisions for your own

future". Enter their names on bottom line of the Living Will. Keep the original nearby, easily and readily available.

3. Above all discuss your intentions with those closest to you, NOW.

4. It is a good idea to look over your Living Will once a year and redate it and initial the new date to make it clear that your wishes are unchanged.

IMPORTANT

Declarants may wish to add specific statements to the Living Will to be inserted in the space provided for that purpose above the signature. Possible additional provisions are suggested below:

1. a) I appoint _____
      to make binding decisions concerning my medical treatment.
      OR
   b) I have discussed my views as to life sustaining measures with the following who understand my wishes

      _____,
      _____,
      _____,

2. Measures of artificial life support in the face of impending death that are especially abhorrent

to me are:
   a) Electrical or mechanical resuscitation of my heart when it has stopped beating.
   b) Nasogastric tube feedings when I am paralyzed and no longer able to swallow.
   c) Mechanical respiration by machine when my brain can no longer sustain my own breathing.
   d) _____

3. If it does not jeopardize the chance of my recovery to a meaningful and sentient life or impose an undue burden on my family, I would like to live out my last days at home rather than in a hospital.

4. If any of my tissues are sound and would be of value as transplants to help other people, I freely give my permission for such donation.

Figure 5.1
The Living Will.
Reprinted with permission from Concern for Dying, 250 West 57th Street, New York, N.Y. 10107.

---

it extremely expensive, but many believe that there is no real value in prolonging the "life" of an individual who is unaware of anything happening outside the self or even within his or her own body or mind.

The need for a reliable definition becomes even more urgent when we recognize that someone might be waiting for a donor's organ—the heart, for instance. Do we let the donor in this deathlike state die so that the waiting patient can receive the donor's heart, or do we use modern technology to keep the donor breathing and the heart beating? Clearly, a definition of death that goes beyond maintaining people in a vegetablelike state is needed. A Harvard Medical School committee developed a definition that is referred to as "brain death." The four criteria of brain death are:

1. *Unreceptiveness and unresponsiveness*—A total unawareness of externally applied stimuli and inner need accompanied by complete unresponsiveness. Even the most intensely painful stimuli evoke no vocal or other response, not even a groan, withdrawal of a limb, or quickening of respiration.

2. *No movements or breathing*—Observation covering a period of at least one hour by physicians is adequate to satisfy the criteria of no spontaneous muscular movements or spontaneous respiration.

3. *No reflexes*—Swallowing, yawning, etc. Pupils are fixed and dilated and do not respond to a direct source of bright light.

4. *Flat electroencephalogram*—No brain waves for at least 10 to 20 full minutes.[10]

Signed by the donor and the following two
witnesses in the presence of each other:

_____
DATE SIGNED   DATE OF BIRTH
                     OF DONOR
_____
STREET

_____
CITY   STATE

_____
SIGNATURE OF DONOR

_____
WITNESS

_____
WITNESS

This is a legal document under the Uniform Anatomical Gift Act or similar laws.

UNIFORM DONOR CARD

OF _____
        Print or type name of donor

In the hope that I may help others, I
hereby make this anatomical gift, if medically acceptable to take effect upon my
death. The words and marks below indicate my desires.
   For the purpose of transplantation,
therapy, medical research or education, I
give:

(U)_____Any needed organs or parts
(KE) _____Kidneys and Eyes Only
(K)_____Kidneys Only
(E) _____Eyes Only

Limitations or
special wishes,
if any: _____

_____

Figure 5.2
Sample donor card.

The committee recommends that all of the above tests be repeated at least 24 hours later. If no change has occurred, the physician may pronounce the patient dead.

Organ Donor Cards

One way people can feel better about dying is by contributing to life. More and more people are donating their organs at death. These organs (for example, eyes, heart, kidneys) can give life to someone else. An example of a donor card, which is carried by one wishing to donate his or her organs, appears in Fig. 5.2.

Grief and Mourning

Concept: Grief runs a predictable course.

The death of a loved one causes profound grief. In Chapter 4 we saw that this is one of the most stressful of life's events. The grieving process runs a predictable course, as described in Table 5.1. Each of the stages of ordinary grief is necessary, and together they serve to return the bereaved person to a normal life. The first stage is shock and disbelief. The grieving person may feel numb and weep for several days after the death. The second stage is a sense of profound sadness and longing for the deceased. The grieving person may be preoccupied with thoughts of the deceased and may even sense the presence of the dead person. Sadness, crying, loss of appetite, an apathetic attitude, and difficulty in sleeping all characterize the second stage of grief. In the third stage the grieving person becomes more accustomed to the reality of the death and fewer episodes of sadness occur. This stage marks a return to normal activities, and the bereaved person learns to live with the fact of the death.

Psychologists recommend three steps for working out one's grief:

1. facing up to the death and not denying it,
2. breaking bonds with the deceased (for example, disposing of his or her clothes), and
3. finding new interests in activities and relationships.

Table 5.1
STAGES OF ORDINARY GRIEF

Timetable	Manifestations
Stage 1	
Begins immediately after death; lasts one to three days	Shock Disbelief, denial Numbness Weeping Wailing Agitation
Stage 2	
Peaks between two to four weeks after death; begins to subside after three months; lasts up to one year	Painful longing Preoccupation Memories Mental images of the deceased Sense of the deceased being present Sadness Tearfulness Insomnia Anorexia Loss of interest Irritability Restlessness
Stage 3	
Should occur within a year after death	Resolution Decreasing episodes of sadness Ability to recall the past with pleasure Resumption of ordinary activities

SOURCE: Robert B. White and Leroy T. Gathman, ''The Syndrome of Ordinary Grief,'' *American Family Physician* 8 (1973):98. Reprinted with permission.

It is not easy to follow these steps, and grief needs to run its course before the bereaved can resume a normal life.

Sometimes the grieving person needs professional assistance in getting through the stages of grief, in which case a psychologist or psychiatrist, clergyman, or close relative may be able to help. Psychiatrists may prescribe sleeping pills for the bereaved, but they caution that daytime sedatives or tranquilizers may ''interfere with the natural course that grief must run.''[11] Extended psychotherapy may be required for the bereaved person who remains fixated at the first or second stage of grief. Since grief can result in physical illness as well, care should be taken to prevent or respond quickly to such conditions. The bereaved should be encouraged to maintain a nutritionally balanced diet, get enough sleep, etc.—in other words, to take care of their own health in spite of how depressed they feel.

Death is loss of life, loss of existence. However, we also grieve for other types of losses. One can lose a friend and grieve for that loss, even though it is caused by moving away rather than death. Graduation from high school, and everything associated with it, was probably a significant loss for you. What other losses have you had to grieve for?

1. _____

2. _____

3. _____

4. _____

5. _____

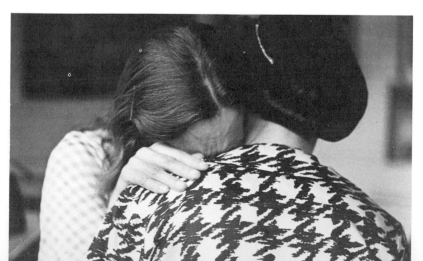

Studies of grieving persons indicate that people who have experienced the loss of a loved one go through a series of predictable stages in their feelings of grief. Most people need about a year's time to fully readjust.

As you grow older and more independent, your parents lose you; that is, they lose your dependence upon them, your actual presence in the home, or part of your time and love when you meet someone with whom you fall in love. Though it is perhaps not readily obvious, they mourn this loss; and if they don't have something in which they can take an active interest (work, a hobby, etc.) they may dwell on this loss so that it affects their health.

How can you help your parents, or the parents of someone close to you, deal with this loss?

1. _____

2. _____

3. _____

Discovery Activity 5.4
DEATH QUESTIONS AND DECISIONS

If you were to die today, what would you want people to say about you? Imagine you are a reporter for your local newspaper and write your obituary:

_____

_____

_____

_____

_____

Who would you want to read this obituary?

_____

List below your most valued material possessions:

1. _____

2. _____

3. _____

4. _____

5. _____

Beside each possession listed, write the name of the person you would like to see receive this possession upon your death. Who will miss you most when you die? Why?

_____

_____

_____

What do you want done with your body when you die? Why?

_____

_____

_____

Would you like to donate your organs for research? Why or why not?

_____

_____

Do you want your life sustained regardless of your condition? Why or why not?

_____

_____

_____

Funerals

Concept: Funerals seem to serve a deep-seated human need.

Every society memorializes the death of a person with some sort of ceremony. The ritual seems to satisfy deeply felt human needs. The family closeness and the support of friends and clergy aid the living in dealing with their grief. This group support is very important to the bereaved.[12]

In the United States most people choose burial as the means of disposing of the body. Although a growing number of people are selecting cremation, for most there is a desire to preserve the remains and mark the spot of burial for surviving family members.

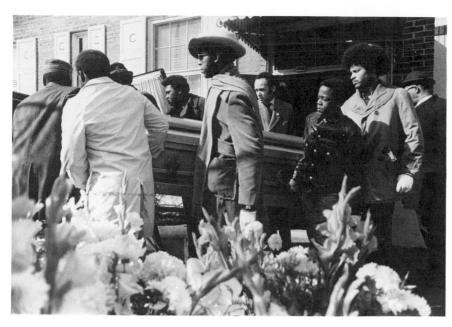

Funeral rites help to memorialize the dead person as well as provide comfort and support for the living.

The typical funeral in our society costs over $2,000. It isn't surprising, then, that there is now a trend toward more simple funerals. Regardless of the type of funeral chosen, certain services are provided. The funeral home will transport the body, provide facilities for the eulogy and/or viewing of the body, use their equipment to embalm it, acquire the death certificate, place the body in a casket for burial, and assist the family in filing the necessary papers to receive whatever death benefits they are entitled to (for example, Social Security or Veterans Administration benefits).

Several decisions are required when arranging for a funeral. For example, caskets vary greatly in price and, if the body is to be cremated, may not even be required. If cremation occurs, the same consideration applies to urns, which also vary greatly in price.

With the casket, cemeteries require a grave liner—a concrete container that lines the grave to prevent the earth from caving in when the casket deteriorates. An option to the grave liner is the vault. However, vaults have no advantage other than appearance—the body and casket still deteriorate—and they are very expensive. Some cemeteries require the grave marker to be purchased from them, others do not. However, the cemetery's charge to install a grave marker purchased elsewhere may be excessive.

Often a decision has to be made about embalming, that is, treating the body with various chemicals in an embalming fluid, which replaces the blood to make the body appear more presentable. If there will be no viewing of the body, embalming may be unnecessary; it will only postpone deterioration of the body for several days, not prevent it. Certain states require embalming under particular circumstances: if the body is to be transported over state lines, if the person died of a communicable disease, or if the body is to be held for over 24 hours before burial or cremation and adequate refrigeration facilities are not available.

Other costs associated with funerals are the cost of clergy, the cost of the cemetery plot, and the cost of opening and closing the grave.

Because several decisions need to be made—embalm or not, type of casket or urn to purchase, where to bury, where to get the grave marker, burial or cremation, which funeral home to use—it is wise to make funeral arrangements before the death, if possible. These decisions can then be given careful consideration rather than being made hastily and at a time of great emotion.

Issues in Health
LIFE CELEBRATIONS OR FUNERALS?

Some people believe funeral costs are excessive and funeral ceremonies useless. They argue that it is senseless to spend $2,000 to say good-bye to someone who won't even know about it. Rather than spend the money, make elaborate funeral arrangements, and present touching eulogies after someone has died, they believe life should be celebrated. A life celebration honors the person while still alive, allowing friends and family to express their gratitude to the person being honored. Life celebrations replace funerals and can be much less costly.

Others believe that funerals serve a useful purpose. While not so much an honor to the dead person, the funeral helps family and friends say good-bye to a deceased loved one. It provides a vehicle for those close to the dead person to gather together and support one another. Without funerals, they argue, the living will feel the death to be incomplete. Further, the benefit of seeing the casket lowered into the grave helps the living to accept that the death has occurred and the dead person will never be seen again.

Life celebrations or funerals? Which do you prefer? Why? ●

CONCLUSION

Aging, dying, and death are topics that need to be discussed and studied. We need to improve both the way people die and the way they live their lives. A study of aging, dying, and death can help to serve both these needs. Your conception of death influences your decisions and behavior in life. To come to grips with your death, your mortality, is to make better sense of your life and make you better able to help those who are dying. To appreciate the role of grief is to be better able to help the bereaved. And through an understanding of the aging process, you can improve the quality of your later years in life.

SUMMARY

1. Aging is a natural process, and many cultures respect the aged for their experience, wisdom, and advice. Elder activists—for example, the Gray Panthers—are working toward increasing the status of the elderly in the United States.

2. Several theories attempt to explain the aging process: the genetic theory, the defective DNA theory, the errors theory, the theory of aging hits, the theory of accumulation of deleterious material, the stress-stimulated response theory, the theory of loss of brain nerve cells, the hormone imbalance theory, and the cross-linking of molecules theory.

3. Exercise and diet can influence the aging process by controlling weight, body fat, the thickening of arterial walls, and maximum oxygen uptake.

4. Some of the lifestyle contributors to early death are overweight and obesity, smoking, poor nutrition, excessive stress, and inactivity.

5. Retirement is viewed differently by different people. Some consider it the end of their productivity,

whereas others look forward to retirement as an opportunity for new experiences.

6. Older widows tend not to remarry, whereas older widowers tend to remarry within one year of the death of their spouses.

7. Approximately 75 percent of wives will be widowed at some time in their lives. The average age of widows is 56.

8. Most people know they are dying, and most wish to die at home, yet over 70 percent of Americans die in institutions, and 67 percent die of degenerative diseases.

9. The hospice—meaning care to travelers—is a special facility that cares for dying persons.

10. The five stages of the dying process described by Elisabeth Kübler-Ross are denial, anger, bargaining, depression, and acceptance.

11. Our view of death affects how we live our lives. If we think death is the end of everything, we might live to experience as much of life as possible; if we think there is an afterlife whose quality depends on how we live this life, we might be especially kind and charitable.

12. Grief has been described as occurring in three stages. The first stage is one of shock and disbelief, the second stage consists of painful longing for the deceased, and the third stage is marked by a return to normal activities and acceptance of the loss.

13. Funerals can take many different forms and vary greatly in cost, depending on which services are included.

REFERENCES

1. J. Reed Nelson, "Hospice: An Alternative Solution to the Problem of Caring for the Dying Patient," *Colloquy* 7 (1974): 22–23. Copyright 1974 by United Church Press.

2. Ibid.

3. Ibid.

4. Elisabeth Kübler-Ross, *On Death and Dying* (New York: Macmillan, 1969).

5. Adapted from Brent Q. Hafen, "Death and Dying," *Health Education* 8 (1977):7.

6. Jerrold S. Greenberg, *Student-Centered Health Instruction: A Humanistic Approach* (Reading, Mass.: Addison-Wesley, 1978), p. 236.

7. Richard Dumont and Dennis Foss, *The American View of Death: Acceptance or Denial?* (Cambridge, Mass.: Schenkman Publishing Co., 1972), p. 104.

8. Dale V. Hardt, "Development of an Investigatory Instrument to Measure Attitudes Toward Death," *The Journal of School Health* 45 (February 1976):96–99. Copyright, 1976, American School Health Association, Kent, Ohio 44240. Reprinted by permission.

9. Edgar N. Jackson, "Grief," in Earl A. Grollman, ed., *Concerning Death: A Practical Guide for the Living* (Boston: Beacon Press, 1974), p. 9.

10. Report of the Ad Hoc Committee of the Harvard Medical School to Examine the Definition of Brain Death. "A Definition of Irreversible Coma," *Journal of the American Medical Association* 205 (1968):337–340. Copyright 1968, American Medical Association.

11. Robert B. White and Leroy T. Gathman, "The Syndrome of Ordinary Grief," *American Family Physician* 8 (1973): 97–98. Reprinted with permission.

12. Paul E. Irion, *The Funeral: Vestige or Value?* (New York: Abingdon Press, 1966), p. 99.

Laboratory 1
LIFE GOALS*

Purpose   To rank order one's goals so that a sense of death leads to sense in life.

Size of Group   Small groups of four students.

Equipment   None.

Procedure

1. Each group member should identify at least one goal for each decade of his or her life. Use the form below:

Decade	Goal
0–10	
11–20	
21–30	
31–40	
41–50	
51–60	
61–70	
71 +	

*Jerrold S. Greenberg, *Student-Centered Health Instruction: A Humanistic Approach* (Reading, Mass.: Addison-Wesley, 1978), pp. 237–238.

2. Next, rank these goals in order of importance by placing a number 1 to the left of the most important goal, a number 2 next to the goal that is second in importance, and so on.

3. Cross out the goals already achieved.

4. Place an X next to those goals that would *not* be accomplished if you were to die 10 years from now.

5. How many of the goals that would not be accomplished 10 years from now are ranked in the top four in importance? _____

6. Can the goals be reorganized so that those more important to you can be achieved earlier in your life? Place the letter E next to any such goals.

7. Are there goals you would like to add? If so, where would you place them in terms of decades of your life? Write these goals next to the appropriate decade in the space provided above.

Results

After each group member has gone through all the procedures, the group should discuss how people could accomplish more with their lives if they were to contemplate their deaths.

Laboratory 2
DEATH AND LIFE'S HUMAN RELATIONSHIPS*

Purpose   To make better use of human relationships by considering them finite.

Size of Group   Total class.

Equipment   None.

Procedure

1. List 15 people with whom you like to spend time.

2. Place an O next to anyone older than 50.

3. Place a Y next to anyone younger than 10.

4. Place a D next to the 5 people most likely to die first.

5. Place a T next to the 5 people you would most trust in a life-and-death situation.

6. Think of your three most valuable possessions. Place a G next to the 3 people to whom you would give one of these possessions if you were to die today.

7. If you were told you were dying and could only say goodbye to 5 of the people on your list, who would they be? Place an M next to these people.

Results

Silently contemplate your responses to each of the questions below:

1. Can you think of other people you would like to add to your list? Who are they? Why did you not include them originally?

2. Do you enjoy spending time with younger people, people your own age, or older people? Why?

3. Relative to the 5 people you identified as most likely to die first:

   a) Are they the oldest on your list?

   b) Do you now want to spend more time with them?

   c) What do you want to do with them before they die?

   d) Do you think they would guess that you would include them on such a list? Should you tell them you did?

4. If you were dying in a hospital would you want any of the 5 people you designated as the ones you most trust to decide when to "pull the plug?" Or is there someone else to whom you would rather assign that responsibility?

5. How would you feel giving one of your most valued possessions to the people you designated with a G now rather than when you are dying? Would the meaning behind the gift be more valuable to you than the possession itself?

The class should then discuss what they have learned from this activity and how their behavior will be changed (if at all).

*Jerrold S. Greenberg, *Student-Centered Health Instruction: A Humanistic Approach* (Reading, Mass.: Addison-Wesley, 1978), pp. 246–247.

health
and
your body

Part three

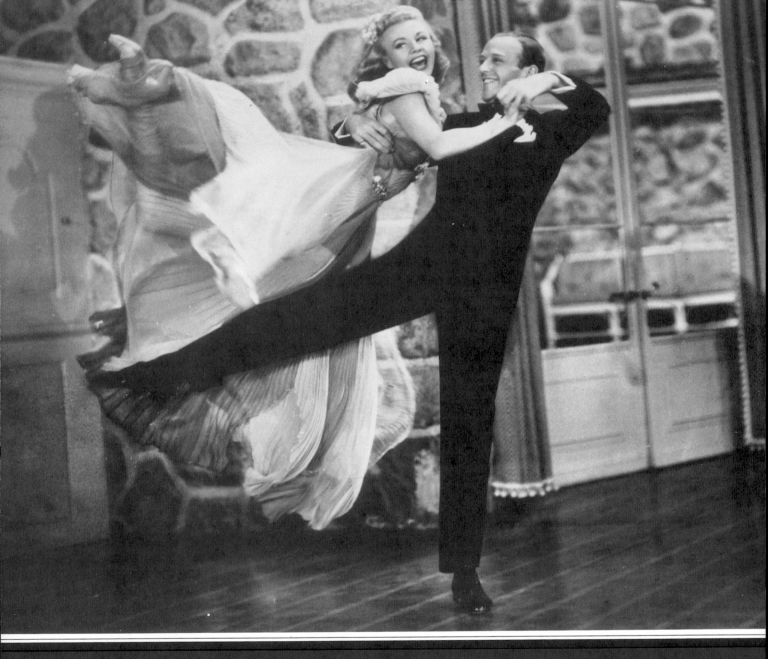

chapter

6

fitness

- *benefits of exercise*
- *principles of conditioning*
- *selecting an exercise program*
- *sleep*

Each year more and more Americans engage in regular exercise. According to a 1973 survey conducted by the President's Council on Physical Fitness and Sports, 55 percent of American adults were engaged in some type of physical activity. A 1979 national survey revealed that 35 percent of the age group 18–35 exercised regularly, and a 1980 study identified nearly 70 million people, or over one-half the adult population, who were practicing self-improvement through exercise.

Racquetball, cycling, jogging and running, aerobic dance, and swimming continue to attract people each year. More women are engaging in road racing and marathon running; health clubs are flourishing;

and Americans crave knowledge on exercise, nutrition, and healthy lifestyles. The exercise boom is apparently here to stay. Millions of Americans have discovered what it can do for their energy level, appearance, and health.

Unfortunately, the majority of the American people are still not very fit. Many people engage in the wrong kinds of activity and are irregular and unstematic in their approach. This chapter presents an overview of exercise and health so that you can evaluate your current fitness and make wise exercise choices that will meet your interests and health needs. Regular exercise is the best and least expensive approach to health insurance.

Discovery Activity 6.1
HOW FIT ARE YOU?

You can roughly evaluate your fitness level in just a few minutes. Test yourself in each of the areas described below to estimate your body fat, aerobic fitness, flexibility, muscular strength, and muscular endurance.

What did you discover? How fit are you? Regular exercise can bring about tremendous improvement in each of the test areas and in your health. ●

Test	Purpose	Procedure	Scoring
Pinch test	Measure body fat	Using the thumb and index finger, take a deep pinch of skin and fat on the back of the upper arm, thigh, back of upper leg, and the abdomen (to the right of the umbilicus).	A pinch of more than an inch at any site indicates excess fat.
60-second sit-up	Determine abdominal strength and endurance	Lie on your back with the knees bent and feet drawn up to the buttocks. On the signal, "go," raise your upper body until your chest touches both knees; return to the starting position. Continue as rapidly as possible for 60 seconds.	Adequate (men) 17–29—42 or more 30–39—33–41 40–49—28–32 Adequate (women) 17–29—33 or more 30–39—29–32 40–49—24–28
Toe touch	Determine lower body flexibility	With the feet together and knees straight, bend forward at the hips and touch the thumbs to the floor. Bend slowly without bouncing.	Adequate—floor contact with any part of the hand

BENEFITS OF EXERCISE

Concept: Regular exercise improves both physical and mental health.

With the exception of nutrition, more fallacies exist in the area of exercise than in any other area of health. Some of the common misperceptions are that exercise makes no difference, is dangerous (see Issues In Health), will enlarge your heart, or make a woman less feminine. As we will see, exercise does make a difference in body weight and fat, personal appearance, and health. It is the lack of exercise that is dangerous, not exercise itself. Although the heart will increase in size following an aerobic exercise program, this is a healthy condition because it increases the efficiency of the heart. There is absolutely no reason for a healthy individual to avoid regular exercise.

The idea that exercise has significant health benefits is supported by research. Research findings show that exercise:

1. Is related to life expectancy, along with other health habits;
2. Produces organic changes in the lungs and circulatory system that improve normal functioning and protect against stress and strain;
3. Maintains normal blood pressure;
4. Results in a more rapid return to normal heart rate and blood pressure, as well as other body functions, following exercise;
5. Strengthens the heart muscle;
6. Helps maintain a healthy heart and prevent cardiovascular disease, and lessens the severity of a heart attack, as well as speeding recovery;
7. Increases the **stroke volume** of the heart (amount of blood ejected per contraction);
8. Produces a lower resting pulse;
9. Decreases blood fat levels (triglycerides and cholesterol);
10. Improves respiratory efficiency and brings about a slower, deeper respiration than that of the sedentary individual;

Issues in Health
IS EXERCISE DANGEROUS?

Orthopedic surgeons and physicians have expressed concern about the hazards of jogging (back injuries, knee deterioration, feet and ankle problems) and the potential dangers to females who exercise. Many opponents of exercise argue that it is potentially dangerous to everyone in the early stages of a program and almost always results in injuries in the later stages from too much exercise and overtraining. It is true that the potential for injury or serious illness does exist for individuals who exercise haphazardly. Overtraining, exercising without preconditioning, neglecting a physical examination if you are over 35 or a high-risk individual—all these factors increase the danger.

Exercise proponents argue that the dangers of injury are exaggerated and that those who believe exercise is dangerous tend to cite isolated, well-publicized cases of celebrities who died while exercising. Such accounts often fail to reveal significant facts, such as previous heart or other health conditions, drugs found in the body, or congenital disorders. Exercise gets the blame, reinforcing the sedentary living habits of millions of Americans.

What do you think? ●

11. Improves the efficiency of the digestive system by accelerating the peristaltic action, increasing the efficiency of food absorption;
12. Is a significant factor in delaying the aging process;
13. Increases muscle strength and endurance, and improves muscle tone and posture;
14. Aids in weight reduction;
15. Improves appearance and imparts a feeling of vitality;
16. Increases body weight and vitality in children;

17. Assists in reducing mental tension, anxiety, and depression through release of emotions in a socially accepted manner;

18. Assists in reducing, withstanding, and adapting to psychological stress;

19. Improves sleeping habits.

PRINCIPLES OF CONDITIONING

Concept: To improve fitness you must apply certain principles of conditioning to your exercise program.

Mere participation in an exercise program or sport is no guarantee that you will become more physically fit. By keeping some simple records and applying a few basic conditioning principles, however, you can make tremendous gains in fitness with little risk of injury or illness. Fitness involves five basic elements: heart-lung endurance (cardiovascular and cardiorespiratory efficiency), muscular endurance, muscular strength, body fat (see Chapter 8), and flexibility. You can show improvement in each of these components of fitness by following the conditioning principles discussed in this section.

Work Hypertrophy

Concept: Improvement in the capacity of the human body to perform work is based on the concept of work hypertrophy.

Any improvement in the capacity of the human body to perform work is based on the concept of **work hypertrophy.** Let's examine what happens to your body when you first begin an exercise program. You start that program with a certain functioning or conditioning level (level A in Fig. 6.1). During and immediately after your first workout, this conditioning level temporarily declines (to point B). You are now actually in worse shape (physically) than you were before you exercised.

During the recovery phase, however, tissue will rebuild beyond the original level of conditioning (D) to point C. You are now able to perform more work than before with no more strain or effort. You are now (24 hours later) in better condition than before you completed your first workout.

Repetition of this simple process will lead to continued improvement of conditioning levels, as indicated by A–2, A–3, and A–4, providing certain basic principles are followed: (1) exercise must be sufficiently strenuous to cause an initial decrease in the conditioning level—the depth of the valley is in proportion to the intensity and duration or difficulty of the workout; (2) sufficient time must be allowed for the recovery; improvement will not occur and conditioning will suffer if your second workout is performed before the recovery phase is complete (48 hours for weight training and 18 to 24 hours for other workouts); (3) the next workout must occur within 36 to 48 hours—a greater time lapse will cause you to return to your original level or lower; and (4) each workout must be progressively more strenuous than the previous one to ensure a deep valley, continued progression, and increased capacity to perform exercise. If you apply these four principles to any training program, improved conditioning is guaranteed.

Law of Overcompensation

Vigorous exercise results in destruction of muscle constituents. As the lost materials are replaced, nature

Figure 6.1
Concept of work hypertrophy: (A) preexercise functioning level; (B) functioning level following exercise; (C) elevated functioning level following recovery; (A-2) elevated functioning level at the proper point to reconvene exercise.

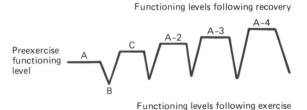

overcompensates in order to prepare the body for still more strenuous efforts. The degree of overcompensation is in direct proportion to the severity of the exercise.

Intensity, Duration, and Frequency

Although results can be attained without lengthy training periods, there are no short cuts to improving conditioning levels. Ten-second contractions, massage, mechanical devices, steam baths, three-minute slimnastic programs, and other such approaches vary from slightly effective to worthless.

Exercise intensity (work per unit of time) should be such that sweating is evident in the early stages of the workout. More important, exercise must be intense enough to cause you to reach your critical threshhold or target heart rate (see Discovery Activity 6.2, p. 118).

Exercise duration is affected by intensity. Obviously, you cannot sprint at near maximum effort for 15 minutes. If aerobic conditioning is your goal, the exercise session should maintain your target heart rate for 15 to 30 minutes. If the purpose of your program is cosmetic—to lose body weight and fat and to trim up—duration is the key. Long, slow runs are preferable to short, fast runs. A five-mile slow jog at a pace of 10 to 12 minutes per mile, for example, will burn about the same number of calories as a five-mile run at 6 minutes per mile.

Exercise frequency or regularity is the key to the success of your program. Exercising three to five days a week rather than doing one hard workout per week will greatly increase your chances of meeting your training objectives. It is important to start slowly (low intensity) and gradually work up to your target heart rate and 15 to 30 minutes of continuous exercise.

Alternate Light and Heavy Days

The body responds best to a conditioning program that alternates light and heavy workouts. This approach reduces the risk of injury, provides several emotionally relaxing exercise sessions each week, and allows the body to repair fully between workouts. Consider the following suggestions:

1. Do stretching exercises at the beginning of every workout.
2. Alternate hard and easy days; never train very hard on consecutive days.
3. Exercise hard no more than three times weekly.
4. Schedule one extra hard workout each week.
5. Know your body and allow it to direct you; if pain continues or worsens or your legs feel heavy, stop, regardless of whether it is a light or heavy day.

Warming Up

The purpose of warming up is to improve performance and prevent muscle injury. The theory behind warm-up is that muscle contractions depend upon temperature, and increased muscle temperature improves work capacity. Warm-up increases muscle temperature and the amount of fluid in the knee. It also improves oxygen intake, so that the amount of oxygen needed for exercise is reduced.

Research findings suggest the following facts about warm-up:

Stretching exercises are a good way to warm up for activities such as running; they are also a good way to cool down after strenuous activity.

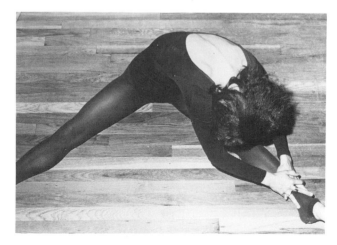

1. Warm-up of a vigorous nature should be used for 10 to 15 minutes prior to strenuous activity.
2. Only a few minutes should elapse from completion of the warm-up until the start of the activity.
3. A longer warm-up period is required in a cold environment to allow the body to reach the desired temperature.
4. Warm-up will not cause early fatigue or hinder performance.

Cooling Down

Blood returns to the heart through the veins, and is pushed along by the contraction of the heart and the "milking" action of the muscles. The veins are contracted or squeezed through muscular action, which moves the blood forward against the force of gravity while valves prevent the blood from backing up. If you stop exercising suddenly, the milking action of the muscles, which occurs only through muscle contraction, will stop; the blood return will drop quickly and may cause blood pooling in the extremities (blood remains in the same area) leading to deep breathing. The deep breathing in turn lowers the level of carbon dioxide, and muscle cramps can develop.

You should cool down (also called warm-down) following strenuous activity. Stretching exercises, walking, or swimming at an easy pace are good ways to cool down.

Training for Strength

Strength is defined as the amount of force you can apply with a particular muscle group at one time, such as the amount of weight you can lift over your head once. Among Americans of all ages, upper body strength (arms and shoulders) is generally poor.

To gain strength, muscles must be exercised against gradually increasing resistance. Loads that are increased beyond the demands regularly made on the organism determine the ultimate effectiveness of a strength training program, such as weight training. The overload principle is applied in exercise programs by increasing the resistance (amount of weight to be lifted or moved), increasing the number of repetitions (num-

ber of times you lift the weight), increasing the speed of contraction (speed at which you perform one repetition), and/or decreasing the rest interval (amount of rest between exercises). The closer a muscle is worked to maximum capacity, the greater the increase in strength.

Training for Heart-Lung Endurance

Respiration (oxygen absorption and elimination of carbon dioxide) and heart efficiency (ability to deliver oxygenated blood to tissues) form the foundation of any sound exercise program. Programs that improve efficiency of the heart and lungs also bring about improvements in general health. If heart-lung endurance is your training objective, your exercise program must result in your reaching a **target heart rate** (target HR), in terms of heart beats per minute, during exercise and maintaining this rate for 15 to 30 minutes. Only sustained, nonstop programs are strenuous enough to do this, such as vigorous walking (4 miles per hour or faster); jogging and running; lap swimming; bicycling; rope jumping; aerobic dance; and such sports as soccer, cross-country skiing, field hockey, lacrosse, and rugby. Immediately after your workout, before cooling down, take your heart rate. If your heart rate has not reached the target rate, you need to increase the intensity of the workout. Remember, this target heart rate is the minimum level at which cardiovascular improvement begins to occur. Your task is to work up slowly to continuous exercise for 15 minutes or more that elevates your heart rate to this minimum level.

Training for Flexibility

The range of motion that is possible at any joint is determined by bone structure, the state of the connective tissue maintaining a particular joint, the soft tissues, and the state of the muscle itself. The last two qualities can be altered significantly by stretching procedures that increase the total range of movement in a specific joint. Flexibility in the major joints can be improved in a relatively short period of time (2 to 3 weeks) through *static* (steady pressure applied at the extreme range of motion in a particular joint) exercises. Static procedures have been found to relax the muscles being stretched, reduce the probability of injury, and reduce the like-lihood of soreness. Increased flexibility will be maintained following periods of inactivity for a period of 8 to 16 weeks and indefinitely when exercise is continuous. Flexibility is extremely high in the early years of life and tends to diminish with age and lack of exercise. This quality can be retained in later years through stretching exercises.

Training for Weight and Loss of Body Fat

To lose weight and body fat, you must burn more calories than you consume. The key to successful weight and fat loss through exercise is *volume*, not intensity. It is much more beneficial, in terms of caloric expenditure, to engage in long workouts at a slow pace than to engage in short workouts at a fast pace. A five-mile walk burns almost as many calories as a five-mile run and many more calories than a fast one- or two-mile run. Few individuals with weight problems can run five miles, so it makes more sense to walk that distance than to concentrate on shorter runs that burn fewer calories. Likewise, five quick laps in the pool, sprint cycling, or short bouts of aerobic dance will burn fewer calories than long, slow workouts in these activities. A

Sustained, nonstop activities such as rowing can help to build heart-lung endurance.

more detailed discussion of weight and fat loss through exercise is provided in Chapter 8.

Training for Maintenance

It is possible to alter your training program to maintain the level of conditioning you have acquired. Strength, for example, can be maintained by doing one hard weight training workout weekly. Maintaining heart-lung endurance requires three to four workouts weekly.

SELECTING AN EXERCISE PROGRAM

Concept: The one best method for improving physical fitness has not been developed.

Any basic exercise program for people of all ages should emphasize development of the heart and lungs through aerobic training. The primary objective of an aerobic exercise program is to increase the amount of oxygen that can be processed by the body within a given period of time. An exercise program is judged according to the demand it places upon the heart and lungs and its

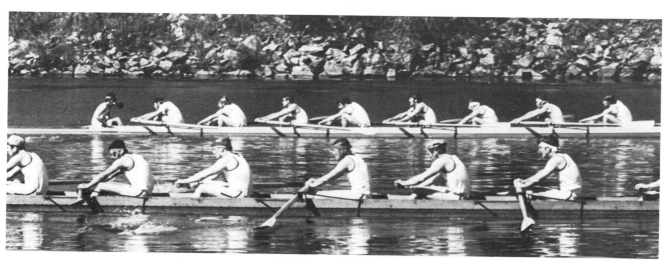

Discovery Activity 6.2
DETERMINING YOUR TARGET HEART RATE

Your target heart rate is equal to 60 percent of the distance between your resting heart rate (HR) and your maximum heart rate (maximum rate your heart can beat if you exercise to exhaustion).

Steps:

1. Find your resting HR. Use the radial pulse by locating the beat at the wrist, just below the base of the thumb. Record the beats per minute.

2. Find your maximum heart rate. This is an estimate of the highest possible number of beats per minute possible for your age during severe exercise. Subtract your age from 220.

3. Locate your target heart rate. Subtract your resting HR from your maximum HR. Multiply this figure by 60 percent. Add that figure to your resting HR.

   EXAMPLE: Brenda Jean, age 25
   Resting HR = 60
   Maximum HR = 220 − 25, or 195
   Target HR:
       195 − 60 = 135
       135 × 60% = 81
       60 + 81 = 141 (target HR). ●

caloric expenditure. You should select an exercise program according to your physical objectives, the amount of time you can devote to exercising, and your particular interests. Table 6.1 compares characteristics of various exercise programs.

Aerobic Programs

The term **aerobic** means "with oxygen" and describes extended vigorous exercise that stimulates heart and lung activity enough to produce a training effect. The primary objective of such a program is to increase the amount of oxygen processed by the body within a given time period (maximum oxygen uptake). Workouts and activities are classified according to the demands they place upon the heart and lungs and their caloric expenditure; an aerobic point value is assigned to each workout.

Any of the following types of sustained, vigorous exercises can be selected for achieving aerobic fitness: running, cycling, aerobic dance, rope jumping, walking, swimming, tennis (singles), handball, raquetball, basketball, and the like.

Discovery Activity 6.3
DETERMINING YOUR AEROBIC CONDITIONING LEVEL

If you are at home, measure off approximately 1.5 miles with your automobile. If you are near a one-quarter-mile track, use that facility. Your first task is to self-administer the 1.5-mile run/walk test and determine your fitness category from Table 6.2. If you have been inactive or are over 30 years of age, don't take the 1.5-mile test for six or seven weeks; instead begin a walking program at Level I (see Table 6.3). The run/walk test can be dangerous for older individuals and those who have been inactive, are overweight or obese, or have high blood pressure. If in doubt, don't take the test and begin at Level I.

If you score in the "Poor" or "Very poor" category, begin the walking program described at Level I in Table 6.3. If you score in the "Fair," "Good," or "Excellent" category, continue with your current exercise program. It would also be helpful to secure a good book on aerobics, such as *The New Aerobics* by Dr. Kenneth Cooper, and follow the progression for your fitness category. ●

Table 6.1
EVALUATION OF EXERCISE PROGRAMS

Characteristics of the Ideal Program	Aerobic Dance	Anae-robics	Calis-thenics	Cycling	Rope Jumping	Running Programs	Sports[b]	Walk-ing	Swimming (lap)
Easily adaptable to individual's exercise tolerance	P	Y	Y	Y	Y	Y	P	Y	Y
Applies the progressive resistance principle	Y	Y	Y	Y	Y	Y	P	Y	Y
Provides for self-evaluation	Y	Y	P	Y	Y	Y	P	Y	Y
Practical for use throughout life	Y	N	N	N	Y	Y	P	Y	Y
Scientifically developed	Y	Y	P	Y	Y	Y		Y	Y
Involves minimum time	Y	P	N	Y	Y	Y	N	Y	Y
Involves little or no equipment	P	Y	Y	N	Y	Y	N	Y	Y
Performed easily at home	N	N	Y	Y	Y	Y	N	Y	Y
Widely publicized	Y	N	N	Y	Y	Y	Y	Y	Y
Accepted and valued	Y	P	N	Y	Y	Y	P	Y	Y
Challenging	Y	Y	N	Y	Y	Y	Y	Y	Y
Firms body	Y	Y	Y	Y	Y	P	P	Y	Y
Develops flexibility[a]	Y	N	Y	N	Y	Y	Y	N	P
Develops muscular endurance	Y	Y	Y	Y		Y	Y	Y	Y
Develops cardiovascu-endurance: prevents heart disease	Y	N	Y	Y	Y	Y	Y	P	Y
Develops strength	P	P	Y	P	P	Y	Y	P	P
High caloric expenditure: weight loss	Y	P	P	Y	Y	P	Y	Y	Y

Note: Y = yes, P = partially, N = no provision, U = unknown. (Referring to meeting ideal characteristics)

[a]Flexibility can be improved only if the complete range of movement is performed in each exercise, applying static pressure at the extreme range of motion before returning to starting position.

[b]The value of the sports approach depends upon the activity and the level of competition.

Adapted from John Unitas and George B. Dintiman, *Improving Health and Fitness in the Athlete* (New York: Prentice-Hall, Inc., 1979).

Table 6.2
1.5-MILE TEST FOR MEN AND WOMEN

Fitness Category	Under 30	30–39	40–49	50+
Men				
I Very poor	16:30+	17:30+	18:30+	19:00+
II Poor	16:30–14:31	17:30–15:31	18:30–16:31	19:00–17:01
III Fair	14:30–12:01	15:30–13:01	16:30–14:01	17:00–14:31
IV Good	12:00–10:16	13:00–11:01	14:00–11:31	14:30–12:01
V Excellent	10:15	11:00	11:30	12:00
Fitness Category	**Under 30**	**30–39**	**40–49**	**50+**
Women				
I Very poor	17:30+	18:30+	19:30+	20:30+
II Poor	17:30–15:30	18:30–16:31	19:30–17:31	20:30–18:31
III Fair	15:30–13:01	16:30–14:01	17:30–15:01	18:30–16:31
IV Good	13:00–11:16	14:00–12:01	15:00–12:31	16:30–13:31
V Excellent	11:15	12:00	12:30	13:30

SOURCE: From *The Aerobics Way* by Kenneth H. Cooper, M.D., M.P.H. Copyright © 1977 by Kenneth H. Cooper. Reprinted by permission of the publishers, M. Evans and Company, Inc., New York, N.Y. 10017.

Table 6.3
AEROBIC TRAINING BY FITNESS CATEGORIES ON THE 1.5-MILE TEST

Rating	Week	Program	Comment
I Very poor II Poor III Fair	Initial workout	On a track, begin running at a comfortable pace until you sense the onset of fatigue (mild). STOP IMMEDIATELY and note distance covered. Walk at an average pace until fatigue symptoms subside. Note the distance walked. Return to running until fatigue symptoms reappear. STOP. Record the total distance covered during the two running phases and one walking phase. This is your first "target." Until you can run this entire distance nonstop, do not add any mileage to your workout.	This is a run/walk workout. Do not overdo it on the first day. After several weeks you should be able to run the target distance nonstop.
	Third week	Begin LSD (long-slow-distance) training—Use a pace that permits a pleasant conversation and causes only mild distress. Continue running nonstop for as long as possible. Rather than walk, slow the pace and attempt to finish the workout pleasantly tired but not exhausted. Do not be concerned about time.	Continue LSD training, add 30 seconds to one minute to each workout until you can run nonstop for at least 20 minutes.

Rating	Week	Program	Comment
	Sixth week	Test yourself in the 1.5-mile run again. If your category has changed, move on to the program for Rating II. If there was no change, continue LSD training until you can run 30 minutes nonstop.	
II Poor	First week	Use LSD training described above, covering a minimum of one mile each workout (nonstop) for several weeks before walk/running one to two additional miles at the end of each workout.	Increase the number of weekly workouts to four.
	Third week	Begin to time each mile, running at a pace of 8 minutes per mile for as long a distance as possible. Attempt to achieve two miles in 16 minutes or less.	Run a minimum of 6 miles weekly.
	Sixth week	Test yourself in the 1.5-mile run, moving to Rating III if you qualify. If there was no change, continue LSD training until you can run one mile in 7 minutes, 45 seconds and two miles in 15 minutes, 30 seconds.	
III Fair	First week	Continue LSD training at 8:00 pace.	Increase weekly mileage volume to 10–12 miles.
	Third week	Increase nonstop run to 3 miles.	
	Sixth week	Retake the 1.5-mile test, moving to Rating IV if you qualify. If you do not qualify, continue to increase weekly mileage volume by 2–3 miles.	
IV Good	First week	Continue LSD training at 8:00 pace, increasing nonstop run to 3.5 miles.	Increase weekly mileage to 16–28 by adding 2 to 2.5 miles per week. Continue running a minimum of 4 times weekly. Substitute sport workout for one run if desired.
	Third week	Increase nonstop run to 4–5 miles.	
	Sixth week	Retake the 1.5-mile test, moving to Rating V if you qualify. If you do not, continue LSD training for two additional weeks.	
V Excellent		Continue with whatever program you have been using if this was your original test category. If it was not, increase your nonstop run to 5–10 miles, depending upon your training objectives (shorter 5-mile runs for health-related objective and longer runs for competitive road racing). Take the 1.5-mile test once a month to judge the success of your maintenance program.	Continue training a minimum of 4–5 times weekly; alternate light and heavy days (short and long distances).

Note: At all levels, each workout begins with a slow one-mile run/walk and ends with a three-quarter to one-mile slow warm-down.

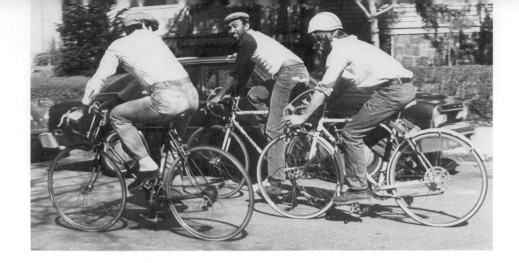

Cycling. Cycling has several advantages over jogging and running as an aerobic exercise: joint trauma (ankles, knees, and hips) is only mild and rarely results in injury; associated back problems are uncommon; and mild cycling can be used while recovering from certain types of injuries to the back, feet, or arms. A road bike is expensive and requires special protective head gear. Target heart rates can be reached and held for 15 to 30 minutes with either a road or stationary bike. Your task is to locate the speed that elevates your heart rate to the target level; in most cases, this requires rather vigorous pedaling as opposed to slow, recreational cycling. When performed correctly, cycling can be one of the best aerobic fitness choices for all age groups.

Aerobic dance. Aerobic dance (movement to music aimed at increasing aerobic fitness) can be an excellent form of aerobic exercise for attaining your target heart rate. Formal classes by certified instructors provide continuous activity and careful monitoring of the exercise heart rate. However, many classes that are called aerobic dance do not monitor heart rate carefully or record progress. You need to be certain your instructor is well qualified before signing up for classes in aerobic dance.

Calisthenics. Calisthenic exercises are designed to develop and maintain muscular strength, muscular endurance, and flexibility. A specific movement that utilizes the body as resistance is one of the oldest forms of conditioning in existence. Exercises such as situps, toe touching, trunk rotation, jumping jacks, and push-ups must be performed with many repetitions, because the resistance (body weight) is relatively low. Moreover, resistance remains constant, so the number of repetitions must be gradually increased, the rest interval between exercises decreased, the speed or rate

Calisthenic exercises are particularly useful in developing and maintaining flexibility.

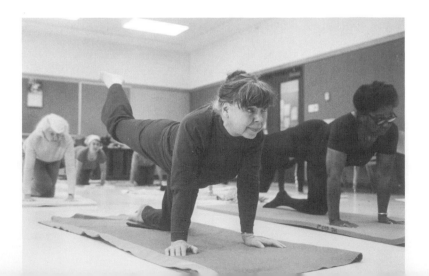

122

of execution increased, and the duration of the workout increased. In other words, you must perform more work each day through a longer, faster workout with less rest between each exercise. A sound practice is to add two to four repetitions every workout to each calisthenic exercise. With little or no rest between exercises, aerobic conditioning will also improve.

Rope jumping. Jumping rope is an inexpensive, effective way to develop aerobic fitness by elevating and maintaining the heart rate at the target level. You can easily stop jumping during your workout, take a radial pulse, compare this exercise pulse rate to your target rate, and adjust the intensity of the rope jumping accordingly. For variety, the type of jump and rope manipulation can be altered. By counting the number of jumps per minute, regulating the rest period between different jumps, and using some difficult high-energy jumps, a program can be designed that will improve both agility and aerobic endurance. During the first week or two it may be helpful to warm up by jogging in place 50 to 100 easy steps. The program below includes three warm-up jumps (to be completed slowly) and five basic jumps (to be completed at the rate of 70–75 jumps per minute). Locate your level on the sample ten-week program shown in Table 6.4 and begin at that point, progressing each week as indicated. The boxer's shuffle and single-foot jumps are performed at a rate of 70–75 per minute; the double jump is restarted when missed and continued for the specified number of repetitions.

Warm-up jumps:

- Two-foot jump with an intermediate jump (double beat)—After the rope passes under the feet, a small hop is taken before jumping again to clear the rope.
- Two-foot jump (single beat)—No intermediate jump is taken.
- Single-foot hop (single beat)—The left foot is used for a specified number of jumps, followed by the right foot.

Issues in Health
DMSO: QUICK CURE OR QUACK TREATMENT OF EXERCISE INJURIES?

As more and more individuals engage in regular aerobic exercise, the number of muscle and joint injuries they sustain increases. Sprained ankles, shin splints, knee pain, tennis elbow, shoulder pain, lower back pain, and other similar injuries are increasingly common. Many people are turning to a treatment promising quick recovery and return to regular exercise in the form of DMSO (dimethyl sulfoxide), a drug that has stirred considerable controversy. To date the Federal Drug Administration (FDA) has not approved DMSO for general use on humans.

Dimethyl sulfoxide surfaced publically on CBS-TV's "60 Minutes" in late 1979. Users of the drug claimed that it cured or relieved sprains, joint inflammation, arthritis, black eyes, muscle bruises, burns, athelete's foot, gum conditions, infections, painful breast conditions, and muscle pulls. Numerous athletes said they had used DMSO for more than 10 years and testified to its "miracle" effect in relieving joint pain and speeding recovery.

DMSO, in liquid or gel, is produced in strengths of 50 to 100 percent. It is actually a derivative of lignin, a by-product of wood pulp, and has been around for a long time. Paper manufacturing companies use it full strength as an industrial solvent. Veterinarians apply it topically at 90 percent strength to affected areas of horses and dogs to reduce swelling. In two states DMSO at 50 percent strength is used legally to treat a type of human bladder condition. However, in most states it is illegal to use DMSO for human conditions at concentrations as high as 70 percent.

DMSO is applied topically to the skin and rapidly absorbed. Within 15 to 20 minutes it can be found in practically any organ in the human body. It produces a garlic-like taste in the mouth and gives off a similar odor from the skin.

(continued)

Issues in Health (continued)

Proponents of DMSO argue that it is safer than aspirin and produces no serious side effects other than the garlic taste and skin redness in some users. They cite testimony from thousands of users over more than 10 years as proof of its effectiveness on traumatized joints and muscles. Some physicians who favor DMSO state that they have used it safely and effectively on their patients. It has so many uses, the argument goes, that opponents of the drug don't understand it. In addition, it is so inexpensive to produce that approval of the drug would result in little profit for drug companies. This fact, proponents believe, accounts for the lack of interest on the part of the FDA and pharmaceutical companies in having the drug approved. Some physicians charge that the FDA has scientific evidence of its safety and effectiveness but has not made that evidence known.

Opponents of DMSO point out that the rapid absorption of anything through the skin is dangerous because any impurities in the drug or on the skin are carried into the blood stream. Industrial DMSO is not purified and may contain pesticides and other impurities. They also point to side effects, such as nausea, headaches, skin rash, and possible eye damage. Opponents cite evidence from tests performed on rabbits, dogs, and pigs that DMSO made the lenses of their eyes dense and left them nearsighted. Opponents also express concern for hypersensitive people who could suffer serious consequences. Finally, opponents stress that the enthusiasm for DMSO use in humans comes largely from testimonials. Before the drug is approved, there should be adequate, controlled testing on human subjects to establish its safety and effectiveness.

What do you think? ●

Basic program:
- Boxer's shuffle (single beat)—Use alternate right and left foot jumping as the rope passes under.
- Running forward (single beat)—Jump while running forward; repeat running backward to starting position.
- Cross-overs (double beat)—Jump with the rope turning forward, cross the rope by fully crossing the arms as the rope clears your head, repeat with rope turning backwards.
- Single-foot hops (single beat)—Same as warm-up jump; progress from slow to fast or pepper jumping.
- Double jumps (double beat)—The rope must pass under the feet twice while in the air. Perform one double jump, one single jump, one double jump, alternating until completing the specified number.

On the first workout day, locate your level on the sample ten-week program and begin at that point, progressing each week as indicated. The boxer's shuffle and single-foot jumps are performed as rapidly as possible; the double jump is restarted when missed and continued for the specified number of repetitions.

Swimming. Swimming is one of the best overall aerobic exercise programs. The combination of cardiovascular development, muscular strength and endurance, and freedom from injury makes it superior in many ways to other forms of exercise. Initially you may find any stroke difficult to sustain for 15 to 30 minutes. The side, breast, and elementary back strokes can be used as resting strokes so movement can be continuous as you swim laps using either the front or back crawl stroke. Again, your task is to swim for 15 to 30 minutes at a pace that maintains your target heart rate. Slowly add one to two laps each workout over a period of several months, depending upon your conditioning level, until you are capable of 30 minutes of continuous swimming.

Walking. Walking can be an excellent form of aerobic exercise for people of all ages. To elicit your target heart rate, you will have to walk at a pace of 3.5 to 4 miles per hour (15-minute mile). Slowly, over a

Table 6.4
SAMPLE TEN-WEEK ROPE-JUMPING PROGRAM

Week	Exercises	Sets[a]	Number of Jumps	Rest between Jumps
First week	Warm-up jumps	1	15	Continuous
	Basic five jumps	1	15	2 minutes
	Practice session	1		15 minutes to learn jumps
Second week	Warm-up jumps	1	20	Continuous
	Basic five jumps	1	20	2 minutes
	Practice session	1		15 minutes to learn jumps
Third week	Warm-up jumps	1	25	Continuous
	Basic five jumps	1	25	90 seconds
Fourth week	Warm-up jumps	1	25	Continuous
	Basic five jumps	2	15	90 seconds
Fifth week	Warm-up jumps	1	25	Continuous
	Basic five jumps	2	20	90 seconds
Sixth week	Warm-up jumps	1	25	Continuous
	Basic five jumps	2	25	60 seconds
Seventh week	Warm-up jumps	1	25	Continuous
	Basic five jumps	2	35	60 seconds
Eighth week	Warm-up jumps	1	25	Continuous
	Basic five jumps	3	40	60 seconds
Ninth week	Warm-up jumps	1	25	Continuous
	Basic five jumps	3	45	30 seconds
Tenth week	Warm-up jumps	1	25	Continuous
	Basic five jumps	3	50	15 seconds

[a]Number of times the specified jumps are completed. A one-minute rest period is permitted between sets when multiple sets begin in the fifth week.

period of several months, add one-fourth to one-half mile to each workout until you are capable of walking for 3 to 5 miles at this brisk pace. With this approach you will expend a high number of calories and improve heart-lung endurance.

Anaerobics

Concept: A high level of anaerobic fitness is important to participants in sports that require repeated, short, all-out sprints.

The term **anaerobic** means "without oxygen" and describes short, all-out exercise efforts, such as a 100-meter dash, 200-meter dash, or 400-meter dash. An-aerobic metabolism comes into action at the beginning of any type of exercise as the immediate energy source for all muscle work. The energy source, called ATP (adenosine triphospate) is formed in the muscles through the metabolism of carbohydrates and fats. Every muscle needs ATP to perform its work. The process is termed anaerobic because ATP is metabolized without the need for oxygen. For short sprints, the heart and lungs cannot deliver oxygen to the muscles fast enough; anaerobic energy sources therefore must provide the fuel. The very second that the amount of oxygen breathed in is not enough to supply active muscles, oxygen debt occurs. In the absence of oxygen to fire working muscles, anaerobic metabolism comes into play. After exercise stops, this oxygen debt is repaid.

Table 6.5
Rating of Sports

Sport	Endurance	Agility	Leg	Abdomen	Arm and Shoulder	Age Range Recommended
Archery	L	L	L	M	H	All ages
Badminton singles or doubles	H–M	H	H	M	M	Singles under 50
Baseball (hard)	M	H	H	M	M	Under 45
Basketball	H	H	H	L	L	Under 30
Bicycling	M	L	H	L	L	All ages
Bowling	L	L	M	L	M	All ages
Boxing	H	H	H	H	H	Not recommended
Canoeing and rowing recreational	M	L	M	M	H	All ages
competitive	H	L	H	M	H	Under 30
Field hockey	H	H	H	M	M	Under 30
Football	H	H	H	H	H	Under 30
Golf	L	L	M	L	L	All ages
Handball singles or doubles	H–M	H	H	M	H	Singles under 45
Heavy apparatus tumbling	L	H	H–M	H	H	Under 45
Hiking	M	L	H	L	L	All ages
Horseshoes	L	L	L	L	M	All ages
Judo	H	H	H	H	H	Under 30
Lifesaving	H	M	H	H	H	Under 45
Skating speed	H	M	H	M	L	Under 45
figure	M	H	H	L	L	All ages
Skiing	H	H	H	M	M	Under 45
Soccer	H	H	H	M	L	Under 45
Softball	L	H	M	M	M	Under 50
Swimming recreational	M	L	M	L	M	All ages
competitive	H	M	H	M	H	Under 30
Table tennis	L	M	M	L	L	All ages
Tennis singles or doubles	H–M	H	H	M	M	Singles under 45
Touch football	H	H	H	M	M	Under 30
Track distance	H	L	H	M	M	Under 45
jumps	L	H	H	H	M	Under 45
sprints	M	M	H	M	M	Under 45
weights	L	M	H	M	H	Under 45
Volleyball	L	M	M	L	M	All ages
Wrestling	H	H	H	H	H	Under 30

Note: H = high; M = medium; L = low.

SOURCE: Arthur H. Steinhaus, *How to Keep Fit and Like It* (Chicago: George Williams College, 1963).

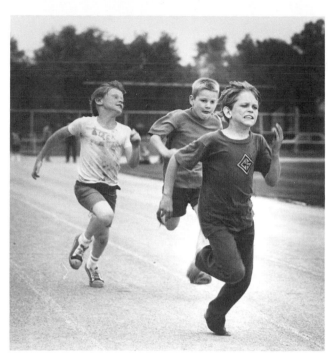

Anaerobic exercise refers to short, all-out efforts such as are required in sprints. Studies have shown that sustained aerobic exercise is less dangerous and produces better fitness than anaerobic exercise.

Skill Learning and Fitness

Concept: Sports can be an effective fitness choice.

Learning or improving an athletic skill is an excellent method of attaining and maintaining fitness, provided you select an appropriate sport. People who are skilled in a particular sport tend to participate in it throughout life, because they feel an inner motivation once they have attained a certain level of skill. Surprising as it may seem, however, mere participation in a sport often contributes little to fitness, weight loss, improved appearance, or general health. Sports such as golf, archery, bowling, croquet, horseshoes, and shuffleboard do not require sustained and vigorous effort, and therefore do little to improve conditioning. Select activities from Table 6.5 to meet your conditioning objectives.

SLEEP

Concept: The basic sleep cycle recurs many times nightly and moves through distinct stages.

Adequate sleep has been identified as one of several factors associated with longevity and good health. Although not much is known about the purpose of sleep, it does seem to have a restorative function. Thus, sleep is the counterpart of activity and exercise.

Sleep occurs in stages (see Figure 6.2). Stage 1 involves a transition from wakefulness to sleep and lasts about five minutes. In stage 2 breathing rate, heart rate, body temperature, and metabolism decrease significantly. Several minutes later, stage 3 begins. Sleep becomes deeper until, finally, the deep sleep of stage 4 arrives. The sleeper now returns to stages 3 and 2 before reaching REM (rapid eye movement) sleep.

Practically all dreams occur during the REM stage of sleep. Heart and breathing rates increase and be-

Figure 6.2
The stages of sleep, with brain wave patterns indicated for each stage. Dreams occur during REM sleep.

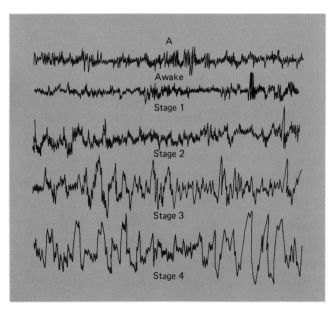

come irregular, and the eyes dart from side to side. The initial REM sleep lasts about 10 minutes, with later periods lasting for as long as an hour. The ratio of REM to other stages of sleep is approximately 20:80 in adults, whereas a 50:50 ratio is more common for babies. Most people dream every night, some in full color, with little recall unless awakened during the REM sleep. There is evidence to indicate that dreams that occur during REM sleep have some problem-solving value and help us adapt to stressful situations. Considerable research is now underway in the area of REM sleep.

From birth, the number of hours we sleep slowly decreases. Newborn babies average approximately 16 hours daily, decreasing to 12 hours by age 3, 11 by age 5, and 7.5 by age 19. The typical person over 50 years of age sleeps only 6.5 hours nightly, and in the elderly, stages 2 and 4 practically disappear from the sleep cycle.

Most adults need from 6 to 9 hours of sleep per 24-hour cycle. This period is critical to the organization of our lives, regeneration of body cells, and restoration of energy. Deviations from one's regular sleep pattern (too little or too much sleep) generally decrease performance and produce mood changes.

The cycle of sleep and wakefulness revolves around a period of 24 to 25 hours and is known as the **circadian rhythm**. Some people are more efficient early in the morning, others in the afternoon or evening.

Sleep Difficulties

Concept: Approximately 60 to 80 percent of all sleeping problems have psychological roots.

Chronic sleep difficulties fall into four main categories:

1. *Disorders of initiating and maintaining sleep (DIMS).* **Insomnia** (inability to sleep) is the term for this type of disorder, which may involve being unable to sleep, having difficulty remaining asleep throughout the night, or waking prematurely.

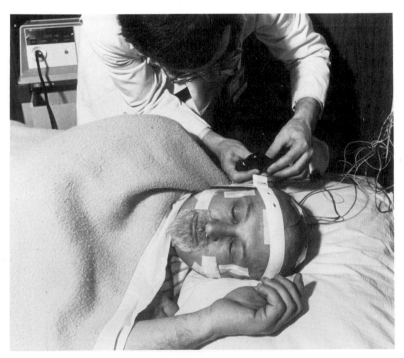

Sleep disorder centers assist in diagnosing and treating individuals who have sleep-related problems such as severe difficulties falling asleep or staying asleep at night, or staying awake during the day. The technician in this photo is preparing a subject for an all-night polysomnographic evaluation, which monitors the organization of sleep by recording patterns of brain waves, eye movements, and muscle activity, as well as breathing, heart activity, and body movements.

2. *Disorders of excessive somnolence (DOES).* **Hypersomnia** (sleeping too much) is the main manifestation of this disorder.

3. *Disorders of the sleep-wake schedule.* Problems of jet lag and work shift changes fall into this category.

4. *Dysfunctions associated with sleep, sleep stages, or partial arousals.* This category includes nightmares, sleepwalking, and sleep-related bed wetting.

The most widespread symptom of sleep problems is insomnia. Up to 90 percent of insomnia patients suffer from depression and anxiety. More than half of the sleep irregularities diagnosed at sleep centers, however, involve hypersomnia. Many such sufferers are afflicted with **narcolepsy**, which often starts toward the end of puberty. Narcolepsy victims may fall asleep many times daily with no apparent warning. The condition is incurable; however, the number and severity of attacks can be reduced.

Over the past 15 years, clinical scientists have been studying sleep disorders. Seventeen accredited, highly specialized facilities have been established for the treatment of severe sleep disorders at major hospitals and medical centers. In 1975 the Association of Sleep Disorder Centers was organized to begin training "somnologists" and "polysomnographers." Sleep disorder centers do not use pills as a part of their treatment approach. Practically all sleep medications lose their effectiveness quickly, and some are dangerous or addictive. Instead, treatment evolves from a complicated diagnostic procedure that measures and records physiological changes during sleep.

Almost everyone experiences some degree of insomnia on occasion. Worry, alcohol, depression, or several other factors may be responsible. However, this is not chronic insomnia requiring treatment. To improve your sleeping habits, try the following:

1. Avoid sleeping pills.
2. Avoid drinking too much alcohol.
3. Exercise on a regular basis in the morning or afternoon (moderate to heavy).
4. Avoid late, heavy meals.
5. Eliminate bothersome sounds and lights.
6. Avoid drinks containing caffeine (cola, tea, coffee, chocolate).
7. Relax your muscles by taking a 5- to 10-minute hot bath prior to bedtime, and
8. Keep regular sleeping hours.

CONCLUSION

It is evident that the choice of an exercise program depends upon the outcomes desired, as well as on pressures of time, available equipment, and personal qualities. The degree to which a program contributes to the development of physical fitness depends upon both the activity selected and the extent to which the principles of conditioning are applied. In terms of overall fitness, aerobic programs are the most desirable choice for adult men and women. They offer the advantages of high caloric expenditures for weight control, heart-lung development, and possible protection from early heart disease. In addition, the time required to follow aerobic programs of exercise is relatively limited.

SUMMARY

1. The majority of Americans are still unfit, and fewer than 50 percent engage in regular aerobic exercise.

2. Overall fitness is associated with limited body fat, heart-lung endurance, muscular strength and endurance, and body flexibility. Each of these components can be improved with regular exercise.

3. Regular aerobic exercise has been shown to contribute to both physical and mental health.

4. To continue to improve your conditioning level, you must perform more work in each exercise session.

5. Aerobic fitness is attained by following an exercise program that maintains your target heart rate for 15 to 30 minutes, three to four times weekly.

6. The key to weight loss through exercise is volume (length of workout); long, easy workouts expend more calories than short, intense sessions.

7. Sufficient warm-up and cool-down periods are needed to prevent muscle injuries.

8. Once you have attained your desired fitness objective, three to four workouts weekly will maintain this level.

9. Aerobic dance, cycling, rope jumping, running and jogging, swimming, and fast walking are excellent forms of aerobic exercise.

10. Anaerobic training is important for individuals who participate in sports requiring repeated short sprints (tennis, racquetball, squash, handball, football, baseball, basketball).

11. Attaining a high level of aerobic fitness through participation in recreational sports is difficult but possible if you select the right activity.

12. Adequate sleep is essential to fitness and good health.

13. Sleep needs vary from individual to individual and change with age.

14. The most common sleep disorders are insomnia; hypersomnia; disorders of the sleep-wake schedule; and dysfunctions associated with sleep, sleep stages, or partial arousals. Sleep clinics are successfully treating patients with these disorders.

Laboratory 1
ABDOMINAL AND SHOULDER/ARM STRENGTH EVALUATION

Purpose   To determine the strength of the abdominal muscles. To determine the strength of the arm and shoulder muscles.

Size of Group   Unlimited.

Equipment   Watch with second hand, chinning bar.

Procedure

1. Administer the modified sit-up test, as described in Table 6.6 in the classroom. Pair each student with a partner, one performing the test while the other holds the subject's feet at the ankles and counts. With the instructor as the timer, the entire class can be tested in less than five minutes.

2. Administer the pull-up (men) and flexed-arm (women) tests as described in Table 6.7.

Results

1. Find your percentile score in Table 6.7 and indicate the percentile below:

   _____ Modified sit-up test

   _____ Pull-ups or flexed-arm hang

2. Is a training program indicated (less than 50th percentile) to strengthen one or both of these areas?

   _____ Yes   _____ No

3. Devise a six-week program of exercises to improve the muscle strength in both areas. Show day-to-day progression, including the number of repetitions and rest between each exercise.

Table 6.6
TEST OF ABDOMINAL STRENGTH FOR MEN AND WOMEN—MODIFIED SIT-UPS

Equipment:	None
Validity:	Not reported
Reliability:	0.91 and up
Procedure:	The number of sit-ups completed in 30 seconds is recommended in preference to counting the maximum number of repetitions with no time limit for several reasons: (1) the timed and untimed measures are highly correlated, (2) test administration time is saved, (3) the effects of motivation are minimized, and (4) extreme muscular soreness often accompanying maximum effort testing is avoided.
Test administration:	Subjects lie on their backs, hands clasped behind the neck and the knees bent enough to allow a partner to place one fist underneath. A helper holds the feet down as the subject curls up off the floor and touches the right elbow to the left knee, alternating each sit-up. One sit-up includes the cycle from the prone position with elbows behind the neck to the specified upright position.
	Avoid use of straight-leg sit-up or leg-lift test. The iliopsoas muscle is the primary mover in the initial lifting of the trunk in these exercises, particularly when the back is arched during execution. Subjects should curl upward in the initial movement.

Table 6.7
TESTS OF UPPER-BODY STRENGTH FOR MEN AND WOMEN—PULL-UPS (MEN), FLEXED-ARM HANG (WOMEN)

Equipment:	Horizontal metal or wooden bar approximately 1.5 inches in diameter placed high enough for a student to hang off the floor with both arms and legs fully extended. Rings attached to a bar can also be used and permit a natural twisting of the wrists to occur.
Procedure:	From a hanging position, subject raises the body until the chin clearly surpasses the bar before lowering and completely extending the arms. The maximum number of legal pull-ups in 30 seconds constitutes the official score.
Test administration:	Use near arm to prevent swinging action and encourage only vertical movement. Enforce exact form, eliminating all incorrect repetitions.
Special rules:	To initiate the pull-up test, a forward grip (pronated) and a hanging position in which both the arms and legs are fully extended must be used. Swinging, jerking, kicking, partial extension of the chin over the bar, and flexed elbows prior to starting to another repetition are violations that invalidate the attempt. Subjects should be encouraged to perform in continuous action and avoid attempted rest periods while hanging motionless because this tends to induce rapid fatigue. To initiate the *flexed-arm hang*, adjust the bar at the subject's height. The bar is grasped with palms facing away from the body. Subject is then lifted to a position with chin just above the bar (chin may not contact bar), where she hangs for as long as possible. The score is the elapsed time subject remains in the proper hanging position.
Scoring tables:	Used in the combined scores of Roger's Physical Fitness Index. See also AAHPER Physical Fitness Test for Men (Chapter 3, "The Developmental Program," of the *Activities Manual*), Edwin A. Fleishman, *Examiner's Manual for the Basic-Fitness Tests* (Englewood Cliffs, N.J.: Prentice-Hall, 1964), p. 45.
Modifications of the test:	If the subject fails to extend the arms fully or raise the chin completely above the bar, half credit is awarded for that attempt.

Standards for Pull-Ups (College Men)				Standards for Flexed-Arm Hang (College Women)			
Percentile	*Pull-ups*	*Percentile*	*Pull-ups*	*Percentile*	*Seconds*	*Percentile*	*Seconds*
100	20	45	5	100	75	45	7
95	12	40	5	95	40	40	6
90	10	35	4	90	30	35	5
85	10	30	4	85	21	30	5
80	9	25	3	80	18	25	4
75	8	20	3	75	16	20	4
70	8	15	2	70	14	15	3
65	7	10	1	65	10	10	2
60	7	5	0	60	9	5	0
55	6	0	0	55	9	0	0
50	6			50	8		0

Laboratory 2
EVALUATION OF CARDIORESPIRATORY FITNESS

Purpose To determine heart-lung efficiency (aerobic capacity).

Size of Group Groups of 10–15 each, or assign each student the task of self-testing during free time.

Equipment Watch with second hand, area marked off to 1.5 miles.

Procedure

1. Warm up properly (see warm-up section of this chapter) with light jogging.

2. Run/walk 1.5 miles (three laps around a 1.5-mile track) for time.

3. When groups of 10–15 run simultaneously, the timer calls out times to the nearest second as runners cross the finish line. Each runner is responsible for reporting back to the instructor with the correct time.

4. Unconditioned students who are not accustomed to regular aerobic exercise should take caution not to overextend and walk if extreme breathlessness, chest pain, or nausea occurs.

Results

1. Determine your aerobic capacity rating from Table 6.2.

   _____ Very poor _____ Poor _____ Fair

   _____ Good _____ Excellent

2. Is an aerobic training program indicated (Poor or Very poor rating)?

   _____ Yes _____ No

3. Devise a progressive program of aerobic training that begins at the rating level indicated for your 1.5-mile time.

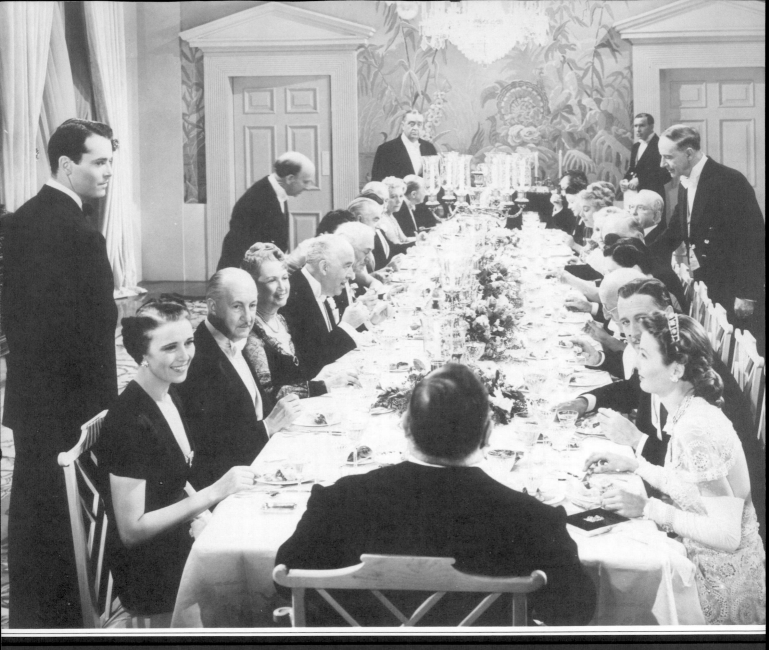

chapter 7

nutrition

- *basic food components*
- *regulating your diet for good health*
- *a look at selected foods*
- *nutrition and exercise*
- *nutrition myths*

What is the relationship between nutrition and health and nutrition and performance? The old cliche "you are what you eat" is taking on new meaning as evidence mounts associating dietary practices with health and longevity. The volume of information available on nutrition is almost over-whelming. As a result, it is often difficult for individuals to determine what constitutes a healthy diet for their particular needs. This chapter attempts to offer enough basic information so that you can make appropriate choices.

BASIC FOOD COMPONENTS

Concept: Six kinds of nutrients satisfy the body's basic needs.

Six categories of nutrients (water, minerals, vitamins, carbohydrates, fats, and proteins) satisfy the basic body needs: (1) energy for muscle contraction, (2) conduction of nerve impulses, (3) growth, (4) formation of new tissue and tissue repair, (5) chemical regulation of metabolic functions, and (6) reproduction. The body's use of these nutrients is called **metabolism.**

Water

The most critical nutrient is *water*. The body requires water for energy production, temperature control, and elimination. Inadequate water intake will decrease endurance, cause early fatigue, and restrict the function of all body systems.

Vitamins

Vitamins are essential in helping chemical reactions take place in the body. They are required in very small amounts. Vitamins are divided into two major categories. **Water-soluble vitamins** (vitamin C and the B complex vitamins) are those that are easily eliminated from the body if consumed in larger quantities than

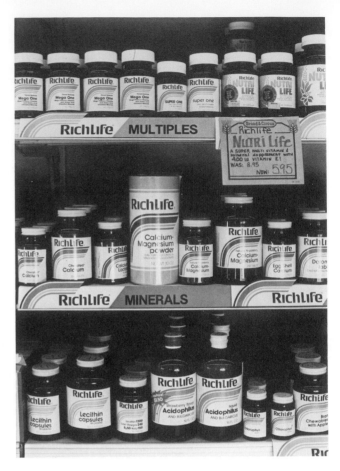

Although Americans spend millions of dollars annually on vitamin supplements, the evidence indicates that they would do better to eat a well-balanced diet instead.

necessary. **Fat-soluble vitamins** (vitamins A, D, E, and K) cannot be eliminated if consumed in excess; instead they are stored in the fatty tissues, where they may build up to produce a toxic reaction. Tables 7.1 and 7.2 list the functions of the 14 known vitamins and the diseases that may occur from a deficiency of water-soluble vitamins or an excess of fat-soluble vitamins.

Many people take large doses of vitamin supplements, believing that they cannot get enough vitamins from their diet or that vitamins will cure a variety of ills. The fact is that a well-balanced diet will provide most of the vitamins needed for good health.

Overconsumption of some vitamins has been shown to be dangerous. The Food and Drug Administration has restricted the quantity of Vitamin D that may be added to products, because it has been found that excessive amounts of this vitamin can produce toxic effects and tissue damage.

Vitamin C has been the focus of considerable controversy ever since Dr. Linus Pauling proposed that, taken in massive doses, it can prevent or cure the common cold. Many studies have tested this theory, but so far the results have been inconclusive. Vitamin E also generated considerable interest when it was claimed that it could improve sexual potency and alleviate several other problems. There is no evidence to support these claims.

Minerals

Minerals are present in all living cells. They serve as key components of various hormones, enzymes, and other substances that aid in regulating chemical reactions within cells. Mineral elements play a part in the body's metabolic processes, and deficiencies can result in serious disorders. There are two major categories of minerals. **Macrominerals** are those needed by the body in large amounts (such as sodium, potassium, calcium, phosphorus, magnesium, sulfur, and chlorides). **Trace minerals** are those needed by the body in small amounts. A minimum of 14 trace minerals must be ingested for optimum health; iron, iodine, copper, fluorine, and zinc appear to be the most important to proper body function. The body is composed of approximately 31 minerals, 24 of which are considered essential for sustaining life. A well-balanced diet will include the essential mineral elements.

Iron. **Iron** is one of the body's most essential minerals. Approximately 85 percent of our daily iron intake is used to produce new hemoglobin, with the remaining 15 percent used for the production of new tissue or held in storage. Iron deficiency results in loss of strength and endurance, rapid fatigue during exercise, shortening of attention span, loss of visual perception, impaired learning, and numerous physical disorders. Despite its importance, many people do not get enough

Issues in Health
ARE VITAMIN SUPPLEMENTS NECESSARY?

Proponents of vitamin supplements argue that because vitamin deficiencies decrease physical performance, and a little of something (in this case, vitamins) is good, it seems logical that a lot of the same (megavitamins) is better. Vitamins administered in excess may do nothing to improve physical performance or aid in the prevention of disease, but the removal of vitamin *deficiencies* in some areas does just that. Some vitamin deficiencies, such as thiamine, are common because our diet contains so many highly processed foods. A vitamin supplement can repair a deficiency of this sort. In any event, some feel that a balanced diet is more difficult to achieve in our world of fast-food chains. A vitamin supplement guarantees the daily intake of needed vitamins.

Opponents argue that a balanced diet solves the problem and is the only safe approach, because some vitamins are toxic and can produce nasty side effects when taken in excess. An excess of vitamin A, for instance, can lead to feet and ankle swelling, eye hemorrhages, and weight loss. An excess of vitamin D can lead to weight loss, calcium deposits in the kidney or heart, and thirst and vomiting. And an excess of vitamin K can lead to jaundice in infants. The use of megavitamins can also result in the rapid depletion of financial stores. The multimillion-dollar vitamin industry, say the opponents, does not need your contribution.

What do you think? ●

Table 7.1
WATER-SOLUBLE VITAMINS

Vitamins	Deficiency Syndrome		Physiological Role	Food Source	Recommended Daily Allowance*	
	Disease	*Symptoms*				
C (Ascorbic acid)	Scurvy	Rough, scaly skin; anemia; gum eruptions; pain in extremities; retarded healing	Collagen formation and maintenance; protects against infection	Citrus fruits, tomatoes, cabbage, broccoli, potatoes, peppers	Men: Women:	60 55
B₁ (Thiamine)	Beriberi	Numbness in toes and feet, tingling of legs; muscular weakness; cardiac abnormalities	Changes glucose into energy or fat; helps prevent nervous irritability; necessary for good appetite	Whole-grain or enriched cereals, liver, yeast, nuts, legumes, wheat germ	Men: Women:	1.4 1.0
B₂ (Riboflavin)	Ariboflavinosis	Cracking of the mouth corners; sore skin; bloodshot eyes; sensitivity to light	Transports hydrogen; is essential in the metabolism of carbohydrates, fats, and proteins; helps keep skin in healthy condition	Liver, green leafy vegetables, milk, cheese, eggs, fish, whole-grain or enriched cereals	Men: Women:	1.6 1.5
Niacin	Pellagra	Diarrhea; skin rash; mental disorders	Hydrogen transport; important to maintenance of all body tissues; energy production	Yeast, liver, wheat germ, kidneys, eggs, fish; can be synthesized from the essential amino acid trypotophan	Men: Women:	18 13
B₆ (Pyridoxine)	—	Greasy scaliness around eyes, nose, and mouth; mental depression	Essential to amino-acid and carbohydrate metabolism	Yeast, wheat bran and germ, liver, kidneys, meat, whole grains, fish, vegetables	Men: Women:	2.0 2.0
Pantothenic acid	—	Enlargement of adrenal glands; personality changes; low blood sugar; nausea; headaches; muscle cramps	Functions in the breakdown and synthesis of carbohydrates, fats, and proteins; necessary for synthesis of some of the adrenal hormones	Liver, kidney, milk, yeast, wheat germ, whole grain cereals and breads, green vegetables	Not known	
Folacin (Folic acid)	—	Anemia yielding immature red blood cells; smooth, red tongue; diarrhea	Necessary for the production of RNA and DNA and normal red blood cells	Liver, nuts, green vegetables, orange juice	Men: Women:	0.04 0.04
B₁₂ (Cyanocobalamin)	Pernicious anemia	Drop in number of red blood cells; irritability; drowsiness and depression	Necessary for production of red blood cells and normal growth	Meat, liver, eggs, milk	Men: micrograms Women: micrograms	5.0 5.0
Biotin	—	Scaliness of skin; pain in muscles; sensitivity to light; can possibly lead to eczema	Important in carbohydrate metabolism and fatty-acid synthesis; probably essential for biosynthesis of folic acid	Same as other B vitamins	Not known	

Table 7.1 (continued)

| Vitamins | Deficiency Syndrome | | Physiological Role | Food Source | Recommended Daily Allowance* |
	Disease	Symptoms			
Choline	—	None observed and identified in man	Synthesis of protein and hormones of adrenal gland; important in maintenance of normal nerve-impulse transmission	Brains, liver, yeast, wheat germ, egg yolk	Not known

SOURCE: Values are taken from *Recommended Dietary Allowances,* 7th ed. (Washington, D.C.: National Academy of Sciences Publication 1964, 1968).

*Values are given for men and women ages 18 to 22 (in milligrams unless otherwise indicated).

Table 7.2
FAT-SOLUBLE VITAMINS

Vitamin	Deficiency	Excess	Physiological Role	Food Source	Recommended Daily Allowance (International Units)	
A	Night blindness; growth decrease; eye secretions cease	Swelling of feet and ankles; weight loss; lassitude; eye hemorrhages	Maintenance of epithelial tissue; strengthens tooth enamel and favors utilization of calcium and phosphorus in bone formation	Milk and other dairy products, green vegetables, carrots, animal liver; carotene in vegetables is converted to vitamin A in the body	Men: Women:	5,000 5,000
D	Rickets; a softening of the bones causing bow legs or other bone deformities	Thirst, nausea, vomiting; loss of weight; calcium deposits in kidney or heart	Promotes absorption and utilization of calcium and phosphorus; essential for normal bone and tooth development	Fish oils, beef, butter, eggs, milk; produced in the skin upon exposure to ultraviolet rays in sunlight	Men: Women:	400 400
E	Increased red cell destruction	—	May relate to oxidation and longevity, as well as a protection against red blood cell destruction	Widely distributed in foods: yellow vegetables, vegetable oils, and wheat germ	Men: Women:	30 25
K	Poor blood clotting (hemorrhage)	Jaundice in infants	Shortens blood-clotting time	Spinach, eggs, liver, cabbage, tomatoes; produced by intestinal bacteria	Not known	

SOURCE: Values are taken from *Recommended Dietary Allowances,* 7th ed. (Washington, D.C.: National Academy of Sciences Publication 1964, 1968).

Table 7.3
SUMMARY OF IRON NEEDS

Group	Daily Needs	Daily Loss	Comments
Nongrowing adult men	10 mg	1 mg	Little need for iron; body absorbs 10 percent of iron ingested.
Women during childbearing years	18 mg	5–45 mg*	Great need for iron; body absorbs 20 percent of iron ingested.
Adolescent boys and girls	18 mg		Slightly greater need than categories above.
Growing children	16–18 mg		Additional iron needed during periods of growth (infancy and childhood).

*Loss during menstrual period.

iron in their diet. Iron intake has been reduced due to the removal of iron-containing soils from the food supply and the diminished use of iron cooking utensils. Whereas animals can ingest iron from muddy water and soil, we humans are concerned with cleanliness, so our intake is restricted to selected foods.

Iron needs vary according to age and sex. Table 7.3 summarizes these variables. Many children do not get enough iron. As a result, doctors sometimes suggest that they be given iron-fortified cereals, such as oatmeal or farina. Women need almost twice as much iron as men throughout the childbearing years. When a woman is pregnant or lactating, she is usually advised to take an iron supplement to replace the iron her body is using up. Iron supplements should only be taken on the advice of a doctor.

Iron is absorbed from meat, fish, and poultry more easily than from vegetables. Twice the volume of vegetable iron is absorbed when vegetables and meats are consumed in the same meal. The best sources of iron are liver (pork, lamb, chicken, beef), oysters, dried apricots, roast turkey, prune juice, dried dates, pork chops, and beef. Iron is also present in most other meats and vegetables.

Women need almost twice as much iron as men throughout the childbearing years.

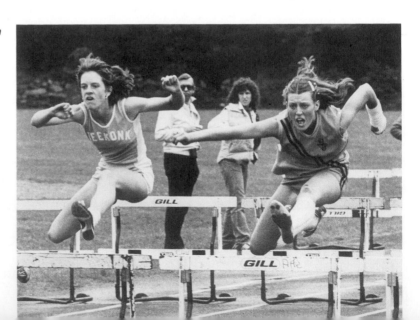

Carbohydrates

Carbohydrates provide a continuous supply of energy in the form of **glucose** to the trillions of body cells. There are three types of carbohydrates: sugars that occur naturally in such foods as vegetables and fruit, refined sugar made from cane or beet sugar, and naturally occurring complex carbohydrates. The complex carbohydrates are chains of sugar molecules that are linked together. The most important of these is **starch,** found in vegetables, fruits, and whole grains. About 50 percent of the American diet is composed of carbohydrates.

Carbohydrates are broken down into six simple carbon sugar molecules to permit absorption into the bloodstream. After food is eaten, the blood sugar level is elevated and there is an increase in glucose transported to the cells. Excess sugar is converted to **glycogen** and stored for future use. Once maximum storage capacity is reached, excess sugars are converted to fat and stored as adipose tissue under the skin.

In the past 75 years, the percentage of starch intake in the American diet has decreased by 30 percent and the percentage of sugar intake has risen by about the same amount. Unlike sugars, starches are the body's chief source of fuel. Their reputation as fattening comes from the fact that they are normally eaten with fat, such as butter on bread or potatoes. Sugar, on the other hand, provides empty calories and contributes to weight gain, tooth decay, and the development of some diseases. Complex carbohydrates should comprise approximately 50 percent of the American diet; sugar intake should be reduced by at least 50 percent.

Fats

Fats store energy for the body and store and transport vitamins A, D, E, and K. Fats are present in body tissues, with bone marrow containing 96 percent, adipose tissue 83 percent, nerve tissue 2 percent, liver 2.5 percent, and blood 0.5 percent. In the human body fatty deposits can be both helpful and harmful. Fatty tissue supports body organs, cushions organs from injury, and aids in the prevention of heat loss. However, too much fatty tissue and high blood lipid (fat) levels can shorten life and make the individual more vulnerable to various chronic and degenerative diseases, such as heart disease.

Dietary fats can be classified as **saturated** (fats derived from animal sources: meat, milk, butter), **polyunsaturated** (liquid vegetable oils, such as corn, soybean, and safflower oils), and **monounsaturated** (peanut and olive oils). Excessive consumption of saturated fats has been associated with high cholesterol levels and early heart disease (see Chapter 16). The amount of saturated fat in the American diet is increasing and now exceeds 40 percent of our food intake. For optimum health, saturated fat intake should be reduced to 15 to 20 percent.

Protein

Protein, from the Greek word *proteios,* or "primary," is critical to all living things. In the human body it is used to repair, rebuild, and replace cells. More specifically, protein aids in growth, fluid balance, salt balance, acid-base balance, and in providing needed energy when carbohydrates and fats are insufficient or unavailable. Protein is produced in the body through protein building blocks called **amino acids.** Some amino acids are produced in the body; others are derived from food sources. The body needs all amino acids, in the proper proportions, to function well. Animal protein (meats, eggs, poultry, fish, milk, and cheese) are complete sources of amino acids. Vegetable protein (beans, peas, nuts, and grains) are valuable sources but are incomplete. Approximately 54 grams of protein are recommended daily for males and 46 to 48 grams for females in the 15–65 age group. Excessive protein intake, common to the American diet, leads to consumption of excessive calories and cholesterol. Protein is not stored and the result is often the elimination of extra (and expensive) protein through urination. One way to regulate protein intake is to plan at least two meatless meals weekly, reduce egg consumption to two or three weekly, and cut down on the consumption of dairy products.

The principal sources and functions of the nutrients discussed in this section are summarized in Table 7.4.

Table 7.4
NUTRIENTS: THEIR SOURCES AND FUNCTIONS

Nutrient and Important Sources	Some Major Physiological Functions		
	Provide energy	*Build and maintain body cells*	*Regulate body processes*
Carbohydrate: Cereal, potatoes, dried beans, corn, bread, sugar	Supplies 4 calories per gram. Major source of energy for central nervous system.	Supplies energy so protein can be used for growth and maintenance of body cells.	Unrefined products supply fiber—complex carbohydrates in fruits, vegetables, and whole grains—for greater elimination. Assists in fat utilization.
Fat: Shortening, oil, butter, margarine, salad dressing, sausages	Supplies 9 calories per gram.	Constitutes part of the structure of every cell. Supplies essential fatty acids.	Provides and carries fat-soluble vitamins (A, D, E, and K).
Vitamin A: Liver, carrots, sweet potatoes, greens, butter, margarine		Assists formation and maintenance of skin and mucous membranes that line body cavities and tracts, such as nasal passages and intestinal tract, thus increasing resistance to infection.	Functions in visual processes and forms visual purple, thus promoting healthy eye tissues and eye adaptation in dim light.
Vitamin C: Broccoli, orange, grapefruit, papaya, mango, strawberries		Forms cementing substances, such as collagen, that hold cells together. Strengthens blood vessels, hastens healing of wounds and bones, and increases resistance to infection.	Aids utilization of iron.
Thiamine (B_1): Lean pork, nuts, fortified cereal products	Aids in utilization of energy.		Functions as part of a coenzyme to promote utilization of carbohydrate. Promotes normal appetite. Contributes to normal functioning of nervous system.
Ribflavin (B_2): Liver, milk, yogurt, cottage cheese	Aids in utilization of energy.		Functions as part of a coenzyme in the production of energy within cells. Promotes healthy skin, eyes, and clear vision.
Niacin: Liver, meat, poultry, fish, peanuts, fortified cereal products	Aids in utilization of energy.		Functions as part of a coenzyme in fat synthesis, tissue respiration, and utilization of carbohydrate. Promotes healthy skin, nerves, and digestive tract. Aids digestion and fosters normal appetite.
Calcium: Milk, yogurt, cheese, sardines and salmon with bones, collard, kale, mustard, and turnip greens		Combines with other minerals within a protein framework to give structure and strength to bones and teeth.	Assists in blood clotting. Functions in normal muscle contraction and relaxation, and normal nerve transmission.
Iron: Enriched farina, prune juice, liver, dried beans and peas, red meat	Aids in utilization of energy	Combines with protein to form hemoglobin, the red substance in blood that carries oxygen to and carbon dioxide from the cells. Prevents nutritional anemia and its accompanying fatigue. Increases resistance to infection.	Functions as part of enzymes involved in tissue respiration.

SOURCE: Adapted from National Live Stock and Meat Board data, 1964.

Fiber

Fiber is a nonnutritive substance that serves an important function in digestion. Chemically it is composed of cellulose and other compounds that are complex carbohydrates. Although the body cannot digest these substances, fiber binds other waste products with water to form stools that are easily passed from the body.

Food groups high in fiber include breads (whole wheat, whole grain, crackers), cereals (unprocessed bran, concentrated bran, 100 percent bran, shredded wheat, oatmeal), flours (wheat germ, wild rice, cornmeal, buckwheat, millet, rice bran), fruits (fresh with skin: apples, figs, apricots, peaches, pears, plums; bananas and berries; dried fruits), vegetables (raw: cauliflower, carrots, celery, lettuce, spinach, tomatoes, radishes, mushrooms, cabbage; and steamed in small quantities of water), nuts, and popcorn.

Recommended Daily Dietary Allowances

Every five years the Food and Nutritional Board of the National Academy of Sciences' National Research Council reviews for possible revision the recommended daily dietary allowances (RDAs) of certain essential nutrients. The RDAs are categorized separately for infants, children, males, and females. You can use Table 7.5 in conjunction with the tables in Appendix C to determine whether your basic nutritional needs are being met. Table 7.6 provides a recommended daily pattern of servings from the basic food groups for various categories of people. Consult this table to determine whether you are eating foods from each of the basic categories.

Calories

Food has energy potential, which is measured in **calories.** Since one calorie is too small a unit to be convenient, nutritionists use a large calorie, or "kilocalorie," as a measure. One kilocalorie is equal to 1000 small calories. In most of today's literature, the term calorie is used when reference is really being made to a large calorie, or kilocalorie. One calorie (kilocalorie)

Issues in Health
SHOULD THE AMERICAN DIET CONTAIN MORE FIBER?

The association between low fiber in Western diets and increases in colon cancer and diverticular and cardiovascular diseases has focused attention on our fiber intake. Research suggests that South Africans, who have a high-fiber diet, are relatively free of these diseases. While there is no clear-cut cause-and-effect relationship and no guarantee that high-fiber diets will eliminate these health problems, some experts believe that the argument for more fiber is valid. In Western cultures large numbers of the population are to some degree affected by diverticulosis, the ballooning of pockets in the digestive tract that may collect food particles. Proper fiber intake may offer some prevention and treatment of this condition. Proponents of the high-fiber diet also argue that fruits, vegetables, and whole grain cereals provide excellent sources of fiber and that some cereals that claim to have a high fiber content would be more appropriately labeled "softage," judging from their breakdown in contact with milk and digestive juices.

Opponents of high-fiber diets are concerned about an overreaction on the part of the general public. There is a danger in going overboard and adding large daily amounts of concentrated fiber, such as whole-wheat bran. Excessive fiber intake decreases the time it takes food to pass through the digestive tract, with some components of the fiber binding with trace minerals and rushing them through the system without a chance for absorption. Excessive fiber intake can lead to diminished absorption of needed calcium and zinc.

What do you think? ●

Table 7.5
RECOMMENDED DAILY DIETARY ALLOWANCES,[a] REVISED 1974

	Years from up to	Weight (kg)	Weight (lbs)	Height (cm)	Height (in)	Energy (kcal)[b]	Protein (g)	Fat-Soluble Vitamins: Vitamin A activity (RE)[c]	Vitamin A activity (IU)	Vitamin D (IU)	Vitamin E activity[d] (IU)
Infants	0.0–0.5	6	14	60	24	kg × 117	kg × 2.2	420[d]	1400	400	4
	0.5–1.0	9	20	71	28	kg × 108	kg × 2.0	400	2000	400	5
Children	1–3	13	28	86	34	1300	23	400	2000	400	7
	4–6	20	44	110	44	1800	30	500	2500	400	9
	7–10	30	66	135	54	2400	36	700	3300	400	10
Males	11–14	44	97	158	63	2800	44	1000	5000	400	12
	15–18	61	134	172	69	3000	54	1000	5000	400	15
	19–22	67	147	172	69	3000	54	1000	5000	400	15
	23–50	70	154	172	69	2700	56	1000	5000	—	15
	51+	70	154	172	69	2400	56	1000	5000	—	15
Females	11–14	44	97	155	62	2400	44	800	4000	400	10
	15–18	54	119	162	65	2100	48	800	4000	400	11
	19–22	58	128	162	65	2100	46	800	4000	400	12
	23–50	58	128	162	65	2000	46	800	4000	—	12
	51+	58	128	162	65	1800	46	800	4000	—	12
Pregnant						+300	+30	1000	5000	400	15
Lactating						+500	+20	1200	6000	400	15

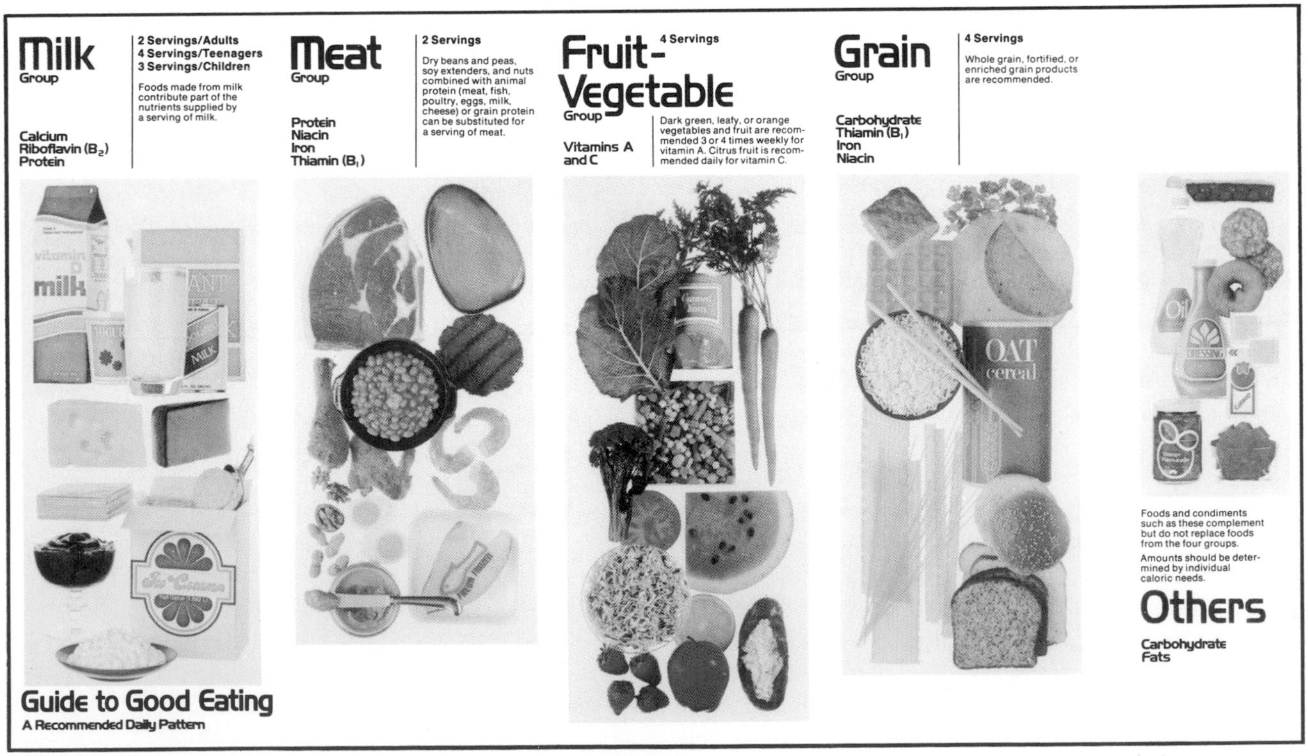
Milk
Group
2 Servings/Adults
4 Servings/Teenagers
3 Servings/Children
Foods made from milk contribute part of the nutrients supplied by a serving of milk.
Calcium
Riboflavin (B2)
Protein
Meat
Group
2 Servings
Dry beans and peas, soy extenders, and nuts combined with animal protein (meat, fish, poultry, eggs, milk, cheese) or grain protein can be substituted for a serving of meat.
Protein
Niacin
Iron
Thiamin (B1)
Fruit-Vegetable
Group
4 Servings
Dark green, leafy, or orange vegetables and fruit are recommended 3 or 4 times weekly for vitamin A. Citrus fruit is recommended daily for vitamin C.
Vitamins A and C
Grain
Group
4 Servings
Whole grain, fortified, or enriched grain products are recommended.
Carbohydrate
Thiamin (B1)
Iron
Niacin
OAT cereal
Foods and condiments such as these complement but do not replace foods from the four groups.
Amounts should be determined by individual caloric needs.
Others
Carbohydrate
Fats
Guide to Good Eating
A Recommended Daily Pattern

Table 7.5 (continued)

Water-Soluble Vitamins							Minerals						
Ascorbic acid (mg)	Folacin[e] (µg)	Niacin[f] (mg)	Riboflavin (mg)	Thiamine (mg)	Vitamin B_6 (mg)	Vitamin B_{12} (µg)	Calcium (mg)	Phosphorus (mg)	Iodine (µg)	Iron (mg)	Magnesium (mg)	Zinc (mg)
35	50	5	0.4	0.3	0.3	0.3	360	240	35	10	60	3
35	50	8	0.6	0.5	0.4	0.3	540	400	45	15	70	5
40	100	9	0.8	0.7	0.6	1.0	800	800	60	15	150	10
40	200	12	1.1	0.9	0.9	1.5	800	800	80	10	200	10
40	300	16	1.2	1.2	1.2	2.0	800	800	110	10	250	10
45	400	18	1.5	1.4	1.6	3.0	1200	1200	130	18	350	15
45	400	20	1.8	1.5	1.8	3.0	1200	1200	150	18	400	15
45	400	20	1.8	1.5	2.0	3.0	800	800	140	10	350	15
45	400	18	1.6	1.4	2.0	3.0	800	800	130	10	350	15
45	400	16	1.5	1.2	2.0	3.0	800	800	110	10	350	15
45	400	16	1.3	1.2	1.6	3.0	1200	1200	115	18	300	15
45	400	14	1.4	1.1	2.0	3.0	1200	1200	115	18	300	15
45	400	14	1.4	1.4	2.0	3.0	800	800	100	18	300	15
45	400	13	1.2	1.0	2.0	3.0	800	800	100	18	300	15
45	400	12	1.1	1.0	2.0	3.0	800	800	80	10	300	15
60	800	+2	+0.3	+0.3	2.5	4.0	1200	1200	125	18+[g]	450	20
60	600	+4	+0.5	+0.3	2.5	4.0	1200	1200	150	18	450	25

SOURCE: Food and Nutrition Board, National Academy of Sciences—National Research Council.

[a]The allowances are intended to provide for individual variations among most normal persons as they live in the United States under usual environmental stresses. Diets should be based on a variety of common foods in order to provide other nutrients for which human requirements have been less well defined. See text for more-detailed discussion of allowances and of nutrients not tabulated.

[b]Kilojoules (kJ) = 4.2 × kcal.

[c]Retinol equivalents.

[d]Assumed to be all as retinol in milk during the first six months of life. All subsequent intakes are assumed to be one-half as retinol and one-half as β-carotene when calculated from international units. As retinol equivalents, three-fourths are as retinol and one-fourth as β-carotene.

[e]The folacin allowances refer to dietary sources as determined by *Lactobacillus casei* assay. Pure forms of folacin may be effective in doses less than one-fourth of the RDA.

[f]Although allowances are expressed as niacin, it is recognized that on the average 1 mg of niacin is derived from each 60 mg of dietary tryptophan.

[g]This increased requirement cannot be met by ordinary diets; therefore, the use of supplemental iron is recommended.

is the amount of heat required to raise the temperature of one kilogram (approximately one quart) of water one degree Celsius. As an example, the energy in one peanut can add one degree of heat to two gallons of water.

Your **basal metabolism,** or **metabolic rate,** is the number of calories burned while at rest but not sleeping. Your body is in a state of caloric balance when food intake in calories is exactly equal to food expenditure and elimination through basal metabolism, activity, and calories lost in excreta. In this state no weight gain or loss will occur.

Caloric needs depend upon age, height and weight, metabolism, and activity patterns (work and play). We will discuss how to estimate your caloric needs and achieve caloric balance in Chapter 8.

Discovery Activity 7.1
HOW NUTRITIOUS IS YOUR DIET?

Record the foods you eat today (or on a typical day) from the time you awake until you go to bed. Use the chart below and the Guide to Nutritive Value in Appendix C to determine the nutritional value of your diet. Be certain to estimate proportions accurately and to record everything you eat.

Evaluate your eating habits for the day. Did you consume food from each of the basic food groups? Did you get the percentage of U.S. RDA you need for each food group? In what areas was your intake of nutrients insufficient? ●

Food	Amount	Percentage U.S. RDA You Consumed — Protein, Vitamin A, Vitamin C, Thiamine, Riboflavin, Calcium, Iron	Percentage U.S. RDA You Need
Milk and milk products			
Vegetables			
Fruits			
Meat, fish, poultry, eggs, legumes			

Cereal products

Other

Table 7.6
A RECOMMENDED DAILY PATTERN

| Food Group | Recommended Number of Servings | | | | |
	Child	Teen-ager	Adult	Pregnant woman	Lactating woman
Milk 1 cup milk, yogurt, or calcium equivalent: $1\frac{1}{2}$ slices ($1\frac{1}{2}$ oz) cheddar cheese* 1 cup pudding $1\frac{3}{4}$ cups ice cream 2 cups cottage cheese*	3	4	2	4	4
Meat 2 ounces cooked, lean meat, fish poultry, or protein equivalent: 2 eggs 2 slices (2 oz) cheddar cheese* $\frac{1}{2}$ cup cottage cheese* 1 cup dried beans, peas 4 tbsp peanut butter	2	2	2	3	2
Fruit-Vegetable $\frac{1}{2}$ cup cooked or juice 1 cup raw portion commonly served such as a medium-size apple or banana	4	4	4	4	4
Grain, whole grain, fortified, enriched 1 slice bread cup ready-to-eat cereal $\frac{1}{2}$ cup cooked cereal, pasta, grits	4	4	4	4	4

*Count cheese as serving of milk or meat, but not simultaneously.

''Others' complement but do not replace foods from the four food groups. Amounts should be determined by individual caloric needs.

The recommended daily pattern provides the foundation for a nutritious, healthful diet. The recommended servings from the four food groups for adults supply about 1200 calories. The chart gives recommendations for the number and size of servings for several categories of people.

Table 7.7

COMPARISON OF THE CHARACTERISTICS OF GOOD NUTRITION AND MALNUTRITION

Item	Good Nutrition	Malnutrition
Body	Well developed	Undersized, poorly developed; presence of physical defects
Weight	About average for height	Usually thin, but may be normal or overweight
Muscles	Well developed and firm	Small and flabby
Skin	Healthy color	Loose, pale, waxy, or sallow
Subcutaneous fat	Good layer	Usually lacking
Mucous membrane (eyelids and mouth)	Reddish pink	Pale
Hair	Smooth and glossy	Often rough and without luster
Eyes	Clear and without dark circles underneath	Dark hollows or blue circles under eyes
Facial expression	Alert, but without strain	Drawn, worried, old—or animated but strained
Posture	Good, head erect, chest up, shoulders flat, abdomen in	Fatigue posture: head thrust forward, chest flat and narrow, shoulders rounded, abdomen protruding
Disposition	Good natured and full of life	Irritable, overactive—or phlegmatic, listless
Sleep	Sound and restful	Difficult to get to sleep; sleep restless
Digestion and elimination	Good	Subject to nervous indigestion and constipation
Appetite	Good	Finicky about food, lacks appetite
General health	Excellent	Lacks endurance and vigor

SOURCE: Jean Bogert, *Nutrition and Physical Fitness*, 7th ed. (Philadelphia: Saunders, 1960), p. 593. Used by permission.

Evaluating Your Nutrition

Concept: You can be malnourished whether you are of normal body weight, overweight, or obese.

Nutrition is best evaluated by careful analysis of one's weekly food intake. One can suffer from malnutrition without being thin; the physical signs of nutrition are somewhat more complicated than mere weight. The consequences of eating too many "empty" foods or not eating enough nutritious foods are not reflected by one physical body type. Table 7.7 provides some guidelines for determining whether you are well nourished or malnourished.

Discovery Activity 7.2 *ARE YOU WELL NOURISHED?*

Take a moment to analyze your nutritional status. Using Table 7.7 as a guide, evaluate your body for indications of good nutrition or malnutrition. What did you discover? Do signs of malnutrition exist? ●

REGULATING YOUR DIET FOR GOOD HEALTH

Managing Fat and Cholesterol Consumption

Concept: Total fat consumption can be managed to help reduce blood serum cholesterol levels.

Blood cholesterol levels have been strongly linked to early heart disease; therefore it is important to regulate your dietary intake of cholesterol in the form of animal fats (saturated fats). To reduce cholesterol intake significantly and manage fat consumption, three measures are recommended: (1) cut total fat consumption, (2) reduce saturated fat intake, and (3) increase the ratio of polyunsaturated to saturated fat.

Some examples of high-fat foods that you should consume only in limited quantities are whole milk; butter; and meats such as bacon, ham, beef, hot dogs, pork, lamb, and lunch meat. In place of these meats, use more fish and poultry.

Although milk is a vital source of calcium and an excellent source of potassium, whole milk is a high-fat food. Each quart of whole milk contains approximately 34.14 grams of fat, or 47 percent of the total calories. More than half of whole milk is saturated fat. The Commission for Heart Disease Resources recommends that we consume no more than 10 percent of our total calories in the form of saturated fat and no more than 300 mg of cholesterol. One quart of whole milk contains 110 mg.

One solution is to switch to fortified skim (nonfat) milk, which provides the following benefits: (1) 25 percent fewer calories; (2) additional calcium, protein, and vitamins (with the exception of vitamin A); and (3) less saturated fat (30 percent of total calories rather than 47 percent). Skim milk is also slightly less expensive than whole milk. Another solution is to eat uncreamed cottage cheese. It contains little fat (3 percent of calories) and cholesterol (15 mg in 3.5 ounces). All other cheeses are high in cholesterol and fat content. Butter is all fat, with over half the contents saturated fat. Margarine has a similar number of calories but contains no cholesterol, and some brands contain limited saturated fat. Thus, using margarine in eating and cooking is preferable to using butter, if you are concerned with reducing your fat intake.

Some other foods that are particularly high in cholesterol are eggs, organ meats, and shellfish. To manage your cholesterol intake, eat them in moderate amounts. For example, eat only three eggs per week, and eat shellfish and organ meats such as liver only occasionally.

Many cooking oils are high in saturated fats. Avoid those that are labeled hydrogenated or partially hydrogenated, and substitute polyunsaturated oils, such as sunflower or sesame oil.

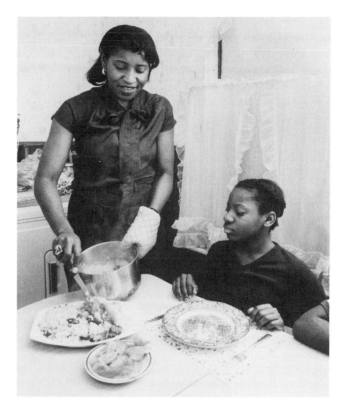

A nutritious diet is one that is moderate in calories, high in protein from lean meat and fish, and low in saturated fats, cholesterol, and foods with high sugar or salt content.

The Prudent Diet

Concept: The Prudent Diet is a wise choice for proper nutrition, reduced fat intake, preventing heart disease and weight maintenance.

The Prudent Diet is endorsed by the American Heart Association. It is a balanced diet that is low in saturated fats and cholesterol, low in calories (2400 per day compared to the American average of 3200), and low in fats (35 percent compared to the national average of 40 to 50 percent). It contains an increased portion of protein and reduced amounts of carbohydrates and salt. The Prudent Diet has the following special features:

1. Neither excessive consumption nor complete omission of any food is advocated. Individuals may treat themselves occasionally to any type of food. However, foods high in calories, sugar, fat, or salt should not be a regular part of the daily menu.

2. Excessive intake of fat meats, high-fat dairy products, eggs, hydrogenated shortenings, and foods with these ingredients is discouraged.

3. Consumption of more fish and of lean meats and poultry is recommended.

4. Polyunsaturated vegetable oils and margarines are substituted for butter, lard, hydrogenated shortenings, and other saturated fats.

5. Meat, poultry, and fish should be prepared by boiling, broiling, and baking rather than deep frying. Vegetables should be flavored with herbs, lemon, or beef bouillon cubes rather than butter. Consumption of fatty desserts and snacks (ice cream, cake, pie, potato chips) should be curtailed, as should red meats, organ meats, and fatty luncheon and variety meats (sausages, salami, and the like).

The Prudent Diet is not difficult to follow; however, it requires a change in purchasing habits, some meatless dinners, more fish, and consumption of dessert and fattening foods as an occasional treat rather than a daily ritual.

Regulating Sugar Intake

Sugar is consumed in four forms: sucrose, glucose, fructose, and lactose. Annual cane and beet sugar (sucrose) intake in the United States exceeds 100 pounds per person; 20 to 25 pounds of sugar syrups (glucose and fructose) are also consumed, bringing the total to 120 to 125 pounds of yearly sugar intake per person. Consumed in these large quantities, sugar contributes to dental cavities, excessive weight, and indirectly to such degenerative diseases as heart disease and diabetes.[1]

As you can see from Table 7.8, it is not unusual for a person to consume the equivalent of 50 teaspoons of sugar per day. Sugar intake should be managed beginning in infancy. Infants begin to show a preference

Table 7.8
SUGAR CONTENT OF COMMON FOODS AND DRINKS

Food	Size	Approx. Content in Teaspoons
Beverages	12 oz	
Sodas		5–9
Sweet cider		$4\frac{1}{4}$
Jams and Jellies	1 tbsp	4–6
Candies		
Milk choclate	$1\frac{1}{2}$ oz	$2\frac{1}{2}$
Fudge	1 oz	$4\frac{1}{2}$
Hard candy	4 oz	20
Marshmallow	1	$1\frac{1}{2}$
Fruits and canned juices		
Dried raisins, prunes apricots, dates	3–5	4
Fruit juice	8 oz	$2\frac{1}{2}$–$3\frac{1}{2}$
Breads		
White	1 slice	$\frac{1}{4}$
Hamburger/hotdog bun	1	3
Dairy Products		
Ice cream cone	single dip	3
Sherbet	one scoop	9
Desserts		
Pie (fruit, custard, cream)	1 slice	4–13
Pudding	$\frac{1}{2}$ cup	3–5

for sweet foods by 12 to 18 months of age, and it is not until early adulthood (around age 19 or 20) that the desire for sugar slowly decreases. To control a child's sugar intake so that the desire for sugar does not become a problem, parents can serve desserts high in sugar as an occasional treat rather than as part of every meal. It is not necessary to eliminate all foods high in sugar from the diet, only to limit their use. You can reduce your own daily sugar intake by reading the labels for sweeteners and sugars in products you are considering buying (the terms sucrose, glucose, dextrose, fructose, corn syrups, corn sweeteners, natural sweeteners, and invert sugar all mean that the product contains sugar), substituting water and fruit juices for sodas and punches, buying fruit canned in its own juice, cutting back on desserts, purchasing cereals low in sugar, reducing the amount of sugar called for in recipes, and avoiding sweet snacks.

Regulating Salt Intake

Concept: Daily salt intake should be regulated.

The U.S. dietary goals recommend restricting salt (sodium chloride) intake to 5000 mg (2000 mg of sodium) daily. The American diet typically contains between four and five times this amount. Some experts associate high salt intake with high blood pressure and increased risk of coronary heart disease. In addition, salt intake must be reduced for those who already suffer from heart, liver, or kidney disease.[2] To reduce salt intake, you should reduce consumption of cured meats (bacon, ham), luncheon meats, sausages, canned fish (crab, salmon, tuna), American cheese, instant potatoes, and table salt. Salt may be mildly habit-forming, and some people develop a craving for it. Because eating habits established in the early years tend to carry over into adult life, extra salt in the diet of children may become a difficult habit to shed later in life. "Lite" or diabetic salt may be indicated for some individuals. To discourage the salt habit, parents can serve their children unsalted foods beginning in infancy. The only time salt may be needed is when a child's salt and other mineral loss (potassium, chloride) is high due to heavy work or athletics.

A LOOK AT SELECTED FOODS

Dry Cereals

Concept: Breakfast cereals should be chosen that are low in sugar and high in fiber and vitamins.

Many dry cereals have been found to be nutritionally worthless. Findings of one study indicated that the consumer should "throw away the cereal and eat the boxes." Until recently, this would have been good advice. Cereal manufacturers have counted on the fact that children, not parents, choose the brand. Therefore, sales often are more dependent upon catch names, items to be purchased with box tops, and sweet taste—everything but nutrition.

A careful study of the contents listed on cereal boxes can help you identify good-tasting, nutritious cereals. Some provide nearly 100 percent of daily vitamin and mineral needs with one serving. Look for the presence of vitamin B (thiamine), because a deficiency of this vitamin is common in highly processed foods. Presweetened cereals with sugar as the leading ingredient are not a good source of nutrition. (Unfortunately, low-calorie cereal is also nutritionally unsound.) Cereal manufacturers defend their practice of presweetening by claiming to be controlling the amount of sugar, because cereal eaters use sugar anyway. The popular and expensive granolas also have no special nutritional value, are high in sugar, and contain 75 to 90 percent fewer key vitamins and minerals than some other cereals.

Vitamin C

Concept: The intake of large quantities of vitamin C (ascorbic acid) as protection against or cure for disease needs additional study and research.

Numerous claims appear in the research literature suggesting that vitamin C is a miracle vitamin for the prevention or cure of practially any disease, ranging from high blood pressure, heart disease, tumors, hepatitis, and varicose veins to the common cold. While most of this research is conducted by reputable scientists, there still does not exist any concrete evidence to support the value of taking high dosages of vitamin C, nor does it take any special effort to prevent vitamin C deficiency. A balanced diet containing fruits and vegetables is sufficient. Vegetables should not be overcooked, fruits should not be chopped into tiny pieces, and juices should not be left uncovered. Because vitamin C is susceptible to heat and air, and it dissolves in cooking water, each of these practices results in considerable loss of vitamin C content.[3]

Caffeine

Concept: Coffee, tea, cola, and cocoa are potentially dangerous when used in excess.

Coffee, tea, cola, and cocoa drinks have one common ingredient: caffeine. Tea contains theophylline and cocoa contains theobromine, both drugs related to caffeine. All three drugs have a similar effect: They stimulate the nervous system, particularly the brain. They also affect the kidneys, heart, blood pressure, digestion, and metabolism. Their use is accompanied by the following physiological changes:

1. Increase in resting heart rate.
2. Increase in metabolism of body cells by 10 to 25 percent, accelerating the burning of food for energy and requiring more oxygen. The heart is also required to work harder.
3. Decreased appetite.
4. Rise in blood pressure in sensitive people.
5. Stimulation of the formation of acid-pepsin digestive juice. Excessive amounts of acid digestive juice lead to peptic ulcers. The flavor oils in coffee also irritate the digestive track and may cause diarrhea. Tannin in tea has the opposite effect and may cause constipation.
6. Constriction of arteries to the brain and head region, which aids in relieving headaches, which in many cases are caused by overdilated arteries that stretch the small nerve fibers to the artery walls.

A recent study established a relationship between pancreatic cancer and coffee. The incidence of this disease has doubled in the last 20 years and now kills 20,000 Americans annually. British researchers have also noted that pancreatic cancer is more common in countries where coffee consumption is high. In contrast, low rates of pancreatic cancer have been found among Mormons and Seventh-Day Adventists, who abstain from coffee. It is estimated that drinking two cups of coffee daily increases the risk 1.8 times, and drinking three cups daily triples the risk in comparison with the

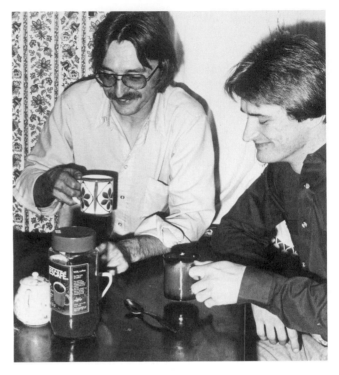

Caffeine, the stimulant present in coffee, tea, and many soft drinks, affects not only the brain but other organs and bodily processes as well.

noncoffee-drinking population. Some researchers suggest that coffee drinking could account for as much as one-half of all cases of pancreatic cancer. Although the evidence on coffee drinking and pancreatic cancer is incomplete, the studies that have been done suggest that coffee drinking may pose a substantial health risk.

Natural Foods

Concept: Organic foods do not guarantee improved nutrition.

Organic, or so-called "natural," foods are those that are grown in soil enriched with natural rather than chemical fertilizers. These foods are never sprayed with pesticides, and no artificial substances are added to the soil in which the foods are grown. Nevertheless, even organically grown products have traces of artificial chemicals. Food plants break all fertilizers (chemical or natural) into the same organic components. Consequently, organic foods are no more nutritious than foods grown with chemical fertilizers; in fact, chemical fertilizers help produce more nutritious food by improving the nutrients in the soil. There is no evidence that taste or nutritional quality is affected by the nature of the fertilizer. In addition, locally grown and marketed organic foods are not subject to the safety regulations applied to commercially grown foods.

Food Additives

Concept: Food additives are closely regulated by law and appear at safe levels in most foods.

Two basic kinds of additives appear in foods: intentional (used to improve nutrient content, shelf life, or quality), and incidental (such as pollutants). Food additives are used to protect against the spread of infection and food poisoning, lengthen the storage time of food, change the taste of food to improve sales, change the color of food to make it more appealing, and change the texture of food. Hundreds of additives fall into such categories as multipurpose additives, anticaking agents, chemical preservatives, emulsifying agents, nutrients and dietary supplements, sequestrants, stabilizers, flavoring agents, coatings, and films.

Manufacturers may legally use any additive that has been approved by the FDA, including GRAS (Generally Recognized as Safe). In 1975 food additives were rated sixth and last among the main areas of hazards identified by the FDA, behind food-borne infection, malnutrition, environmental contaminants, naturally occurring toxicants in foods, and pesticide residues. The fear that additives are an increasing hazard may not be unwarranted. The FDA 1958 Food Additives Amendment to the Food, Drug, and Cosmetic Act requires extensive testing on the chemistry, use, function, and safety of an additive before it is approved for use

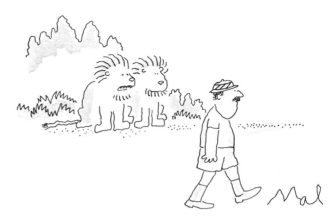

"Don't eat one of them—they're loaded with additives and preservatives!"

Reproduced by special permission of
Playboy Magazine; copyright © 1979 by Playboy.

in food. If an additive is found to be a carcinogen (cancer-causing agent) in any test on animals or humans, it is discarded (Delaney Clause). Additives that involve risk are permitted only at levels 100 times lower than those at which the risk may occur. This margin of safety of 1/100 appears quite adequate, because it is known that potentially harmful, naturally occurring substances appear at levels with a margin of safety of only 1/10. Moreover, toxicity has been found not to be additive; a 1/100 dose of 100 different compounds still results in a 1/100 toxic dose. The distinction between **toxicity** and **hazard** is very important. Toxicity refers to the potential capacity of a chemical to harm living organisms, and hazard is the potential of a chemical to produce injury under conditions of use. Most substances are potentially toxic but only hazardous if consumed in very large quantities. For an even greater margin of safety, individuals should avoid consumption of any one additive (such as drinking six to eight diet drinks with saccharin daily) by consuming a variety of foods and drinks from the basic four food groups. A quick look at the label will also reveal how much of the product is food and how much is artificial color, preservative, and other additives.

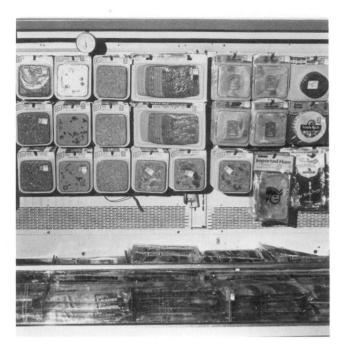

Some food additives have definitely been found to be dangerous. Nitrites, used to preserve processed meats, convert in the body to carcinogens known as nitrosamines.

Concept: Some additives used in food have been found to be potentially harmful to human health and life.

Several food additives remain controversial. Saccharin is one example. In 1977 the FDA proposed a ban on the use of saccharin as an artificial sweetener. Critics of this proposal argued that saccharin is a very weak cancer-producing agent and is useful to certain individuals, such as diabetics, who need to reduce their sugar and calorie intake. Consequently, saccharin is back on the market.

Nitrites and nitrates, used in bacon, sausages, and luncheon meats to prevent botulism and improve flavor, are potentially dangerous. Cooking at high heat and the digestive process convert nitrites to nitrosamines, a potential carcinogen. Nitrates and nitrites also occur naturally in vegetables in amounts higher than those added to bacon, sausages, and luncheon meats.

The controversy over saccharin, nitrites, and nitrates hinges on the issue of risk vs. benefit and whether the decision should be left up to the FDA or the individual. If a benefit of an additive is purely esthetic, the FDA imposes much more stringent restrictions. An example is FDA removal of all food color additives that are not thoroughly investigated. For additives serving valuable functions, however, the decision is not quite so clear, and some potentially hazardous additives remain on the market because of their benefit in preventing food poisoning and in helping certain individuals with specific medical problems.

NUTRITION AND EXERCISE

Need for Water During Exercise

The exact amount of water needed daily depends upon the individual and such factors as body weight, activity patterns, sweat loss, loss through expired air and urine, and the amount of liquid consumed through food and drink. Your body contains about 10 gallons of water. Loss of only 10 percent, or about one gallon, is disabling, and a 15 to 50 percent loss can cause death. A minimum of six to eight glasses (1.5 to 2 quarts) of water should be consumed daily. Water should also be consumed freely during exercise.

Regardless of the availability of water, most athletes do not consume enough to prevent a water deficit on hot, humid days. It has been shown that male athletes who are acclimated to the heat rarely drink more than two-thirds the fluid lost in sweat. It seems that fluid balance can only be maintained by taking frequent drinks, whether thirsty or not, prior to and during exercise, without reaching the point of discomfort. Forced drinking when no thirst sensation exists should mini-mize upset of body homeostasis during exercise, result in more efficient performance, and delay fatigue.[4]

Drinking too much water is not a problem; ob-viously water is not toxic, and the kidneys will excrete it efficiently. The kidneys are also capable of conserv-ing water when the body is deprived of it by excreting more highly concentrated urine.

Exercise After Eating

Concept: Exercise following a meal is not harmful.

Most of us were taught as children to avoid exercise after eating because it was supposed to hinder digestion and bring on stomach cramps. It is true that vigorous exercise slows acid secretion and peristaltic move-ments of the stomach during exericse and for a short time afterward (about one hour). Following this period, there is increased activity in these areas beyond the normal state. With mild exercise, however, gastric mo-tility and acid secretion actually increase. In the final analysis, exercise has little effect on the entire digestive process. Performance could be hindered, however, by discomfort due to overeating, a psychological feeling of lethargy or sickness, or a stomach fullness that does not allow the diaphragm to descend completely during inhalation.

Swimming After Eating

Concept: Swimming following a meal does not increase the possibility of drowning due to stomach cramps.

For over a hundred years, parents have warned against swimming immediately after eating. The fear of stom-ach cramps and drowning, supposedly caused by eat-ing, continues to keep many swimmers out of the water for one to two hours after eating. The truth is that stom-ach cramps are not common. One researcher who stud-ied 30,000 swimmers did not observe even one case of stomach cramps.

NUTRITION MYTHS

Concept: No special health food will prevent or cure any disease or affect one specific body part.

More than half a billion dollars are spent each year for the purchase of special health foods. Some people be-lieve that such foods will prevent and cure practically any illness. Some eat fish eggs, raw oysters, organic foods, or flavored insects as brain foods or foods that will nourish a specific body part. The truth is that eating a balanced diet of foods from the basic four food groups will supply you with the proper vitamins and minerals and make special foods unnecessary.

There are hundreds of food fallacies and miscon-ceptions that you may encounter. Here are some com-mon misbeliefs:

1. *The best food plan is a vegetarian diet.* It is difficult to get enough cell-building protein without eating some meat, fish, or poultry. For vegetarians who avoid dairy products and eggs, which are good protein sources, the difficulty is even greater. Cer-tainly too much meat, particularly beef, can in-crease the risk of heart disease. A good compromise is to eat fish, poultry, and cheese as sources of protein.

2. *Special "energy" foods, such as honey, improve your strength and vitality.* Honey, candy, and other highly sugared products are a form of quick en-ergy, but they will not improve your overall vital-ity. Only a balanced diet and exercise can do that. In fact, if an excess amount of sugar is ingested (an entire candy bar, for example), an insulin re-action occurs that removes sugar from the blood

and may leave you with less quick energy that you would have had without the sugar.

3. *Pasteurized milk is not very nourishing.* Pasteurization makes milk safe from harmful bacteria. In this process the only nutrient lost is vitamin C, and raw milk before pasteurization has very little vitamin C anyway.

4. *Yogurt is a health food providing special nutrition.* Yogurt is made from cultured whole milk evaporated to two-thirds its original volume, forming a solid that can be eaten with a spoon. It is neither more nor less nourishing than milk.

5. *White eggs are more nourishing than brown eggs.* Eggshell color depends on the breed of the hen and has nothing to do with nutritive value.

6. *The modern practice of food processing robs foods of their nutritional value.* Food is processed for our protection, and processed food is the most nutritious food possible.

7. *Steak is essential when performing hard physical labor.* Protein can be secured from a number of sources other than steak, and in any case, the source, whether steak, legumes, or eggs, is unimportant. In fact, Americans consume too much protein in their diet.

No Fountain of Youth

Concept: There is no "fountain of youth" diet that can prevent the aging process.

No one wants to grow old in our society. Americans spend large sums of money on special youth foods and treatments that claim to delay the aging process. There is no evidence that any of these products are the slightest bit effective. The best protection against premature aging is proper nutrition, adequate exercise and rest, wholesome and meaningful work, and good mental-emotional health.

CONCLUSION

Adequate nutrition is essential to proper body function and freedom from numerous diseases associated with excesses and deficiencies in vitamins, minerals, protein, carbohydrates, and fats. Nutritional needs vary for each individual, depending upon age, sex, weight, metabolism, and lifestyle. The typical American diet is currently too high in calories, too high in fats, too high in protein, too high in salts, too high in sugar, and too low in fruits and vegetables and water. The real secret to good nutrition is not multiple vitamins, organic foods, special diets, miracle foods; it is a balanced diet coupled with wise food purchasing and adequate rest, sleep, and exercise.

SUMMARY

1. Six nutrients are needed daily to satisfy the body's basic needs: water, minerals, vitamins, carbohydrates, fats, and proteins.

Discovery Activity 7.3
YOUR NUTRITION BIASES

Do you purchase any special foods with the hope of receiving particular health benefits from them? If so, list them here. Then ask your instructor to discuss whether these foods really do have special benefits.

Food or Drink   **Reason for Purchase**

1. _____

2. _____

3. _____

4. _____

5. _____ ●

2. For optimum health, the amount of carbohydrates, roughage, and water in the American diet should be increased and the amount of sugar, salt, and protein decreased.

3. Food energy is measured in units, called calories; one kilocalorie is equal to 1000 small calories and represents the amount of heat required to raise the temperature of one kilogram of water one degree Celsius.

4. Iron intake should be increased at certain times in our lives (adolescence, early childhood, and during pregnancy and while lactating).

5. Even the overweight and obese can be malnourished.

6. Total fat consumption should be carefully managed throughout life by reducing the intake of saturated fats and increasing the intake of polyunsaturated fats. Such an approach tends to lower blood cholesterol levels and the risk of early heart disease.

7. There is no evidence that the intake of large quantities of vitamin supplements improves health or prevents disease.

8. Water should be consumed freely before, during, and after exercise to delay fatigue and prevent dehydration.

9. No special foods prevent or cure disease, nor do any special diets improve health or cause rapid weight loss.

REFERENCES

1. Eva May Hamilton and Eleanor Whitney, *Nutrition Concepts and Controversies* (St. Paul, Minn.: West Publishing Co., 1979).

2. *Nutrition and Your Health: Dietary Guidelines for Americans*, Science and Education Administration/Human Nutrition, U.S. Department of Agriculture (Washington, D.C.: Government Printing Office, 1981).

3. Ronald M. Deutsch, *Realities in Nutrition* (Palo Alto, Calif.: Bull Publishing Company, 1976).

4. Ellington Darden, *Nutrition for Athletes* (Winter Park, Fla.: Anna Publishing Inc., 1978).

Laboratory 1
SOUND MEAL PLANNING

Purpose   To analyze personal eating habits.

Size of Group   Five to seven in each group

Procedure

1. Each group chooses one of the following meal or snack times:

   breakfast

   lunch

   dinner

   evening snacks

2. Each group compiles a list of the foods and portions they commonly eat for the meal or snack time selected.

3. Meals are analyzed for caloric content, saturated fat, polyunsaturated fat, sugar, ingredients from the basic four food groups, and water consumption.

4. Meals are then altered to accomplish the following nutritional objectives:

   Reduce saturated fat,

   Reduce sugar,

   Reduce caloric intake,

   Increase polyunsaturated fat intake,

   Consume a variety of foods from the basic four food groups each day,

   Consume a minimum of six glasses of water per day.

Results

1. Each group summarizes its findings and gives a brief presentation to the entire class.

2. Basic suggestions are given to change eating patterns at each meal time.

3. Students are asked to follow the altered meal for at least one week and report to the instructor, in writing, their findings: how they feel, difficulty in preparing, weight changes, etc.

Laboratory 2
A SURVEY OF NUTRITIONAL MYTHS

Purpose To uncover nutritional myths in your institution.

Size of Group Five in each group.

Equipment None.

Procedure

1. Each group chooses one of the following subject areas:
   a) Nutrition and sport,
   b) Nutrition and disease prevention and cure,
   c) So-called magic foods,
   d) Vitamin and mineral supplements,
   e) Food additives.

2. Each group develops a one-page questionnaire (open-ended) to guide interviews concerning nutritional beliefs and practices in its subject area.

3. Each group devises a plan for randomly selecting subjects on the college campus. The questionnaire and random selection procedure must be approved by the instructor before proceeding.

4. Each student in every group interviews 25–50 subjects. An interview should take less than five minutes.

Results

1. Summarize your data and give a brief presentation to the class.

2. Evaluate the soundness of the nutritional knowledge of those interviewed.

3. Identify the nutrition myths on your campus and their extensiveness.

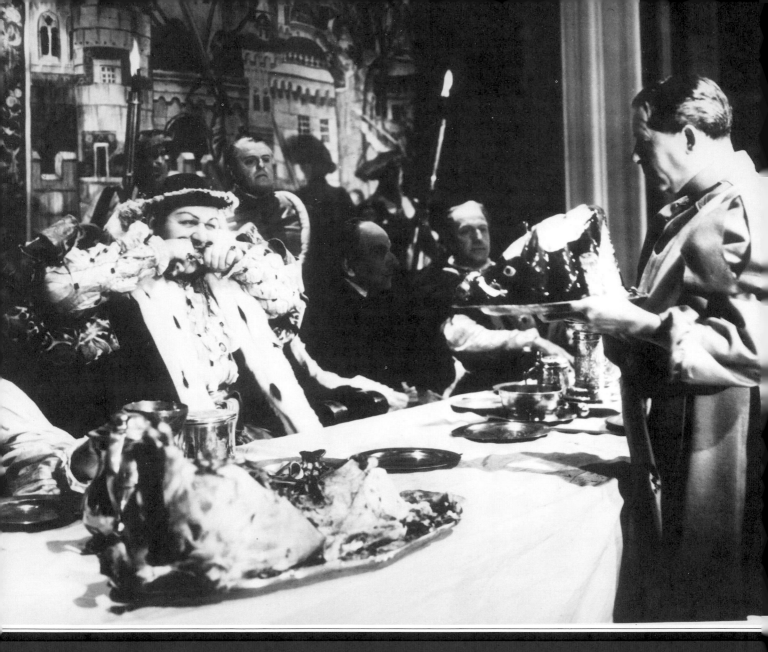

chapter 8

weight control

- *overweight and obesity*
- *weight control and nutrition*
- *weight control and exercise*
- *behavior modification and you*

Judging from television, magazines, and books, no topic is more important to Americans than weight control. Dieting has become a national obsession as people of all ages strive to be thinner and thus more "attractive." Many Americans are indeed overweight, but some of the techniques they use to reduce are unsound or potentially harmful to health. In this chapter we present the problems of being overweight, obese, and underweight and suggest how a healthy diet, combined with regular exercise, can set you on the right course.

OVERWEIGHT AND OBESITY

There are two basic methods of determining whether you are overweight, obese, underweight, or of normal weight. The most common procedure is to use a standard chart (see Table 8.1) to compare your body weight to the suggested ranges. You are considered overweight if you weigh 20 percent more than the suggested range for your height and frame, obese if you weigh 30 percent more, and underweight if you weigh 20 percent less. As we will discover later in this chapter, however, this method is crude and often inaccurate. A second method is to determine your percent of body fat (see Fig. 8.1). If you possess more than 15 percent (men) or 20 percent (women) body fat, you are considered to be overweight; more than 20 percent (men) or 25 percent (women) classifies you as obese, and less than 5 percent (men) or 10 percent (women) as underweight or thin.

Prevalence of Obesity in the United States

Overweight and **obesity** are serious problems in our society. Consider the following findings:

1. Fifty percent of males between 30 and 39 years of age are at least 10 percent overweight.

Table 8.1
DESIRABLE WEIGHTS FOR MEN AND WOMEN 25 YEARS AND OLDER

Height[a] (feet)	(inches)	Small Frame	Medium Frame	Large Frame
Men[b]				
5	2	112–120	118–129	126–141
5	3	115–123	121–133	129–144
5	4	118–126	124–136	132–148
5	5	121–129	127–139	135–152
5	6	124–133	130–143	138–156
5	7	128–137	134–147	142–161
5	8	132–141	138–152	147–166
5	9	136–145	142–156	151–170
5	10	140–150	146–160	155–174
5	11	144–154	150–165	159–179
6	0	148–158	154–170	164–184
6	1	152–162	158–175	168–189
6	2	156–167	162–180	173–194
6	3	160–171	167–185	178–199
6	4	164–175	172–190	182–204
Women[b,c]				
4	10	92– 98	96–107	104–119
4	11	94–101	98–110	106–122
5	0	96–104	101–113	109–125
5	1	99–107	104–116	112–128
5	2	102–110	107–119	115–131
5	3	105–113	110–122	118–134
5	4	108–116	113–126	121–138
5	5	111–119	116–130	125–142
5	6	114–123	120–135	129–146
5	7	118–127	124–139	133–150
5	8	122–131	128–143	137–154
5	9	126–135	132–147	141–158
5	10	130–140	136–151	145–163
5	11	134–144	140–155	149–168
6	0	138–148	144–159	153–173

SOURCE: Courtesy Metropolitan Life Insurance Company.
[a]Height is with shoes on: 1-in. heel for men; 2-in. heel for women.
[b]Weight is in pounds, according to frame, in indoor clothing.
[c]For women between 18 and 25, subtract 1 pound for each year under 25.

2. Sixty percent of males between 50 and 59 years of age are at least 10 percent overweight, and 33 percent are at least 20 percent overweight.

3. The percentage of overweight women under age 40 is lower than that of men; it is identical for ages 40–49; and more women are obese than men in the over-49 category.

4. Approximately 10 percent of the school population is obese (in some high schools, this figure reaches approximately 20 percent).

5. In the past ten years the average weight of men and women of various ages and heights has increased between seven and ten pounds.

Figure 8.1
Location of skinfold measures for men and women.

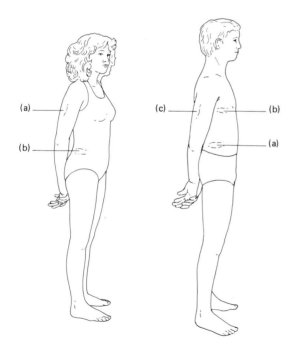

Women	Men	
(a) ((	(a) ≃	(c) ((
(b) ≃	(b) ≃	

This merely shows the direction of the skinfold after being grasped between the tester's thumb and index finger at the proper location.

Obesity is associated with a number of disorders, including atherosclerosis, high blood pressure, diabetes, heart/lung difficulties, early heart attacks, and other ailments. One long-term follow-up study of 5 million insured persons revealed that the death rate of obese men between the ages of 15 and 69 was 50 percent greater than that of normal-weight persons and 30 percent greater than that of persons classified as overweight. In addition, obese individuals are subjected to discrimination and prejudice and have fewer social interactions.

Causes of Obesity

Concept: The most common cause of obesity is inactivity combined with overeating.

Numerous studies reveal little difference in food intake between the obese and those of normal weight. The difference lies in degree of activity—obese people spend considerably less time in physical activity. Thus both overeating and lack of exercise contribute to obesity.

Social, genetic, and psychological factors are associated with obesity. Glandular and other physiological disorders are related to weight problems in only a small percentage of cases. Studies investigating the role of heredity and environment in obesity show that children of normal-weight parents are obese as youngsters in only about 7 to 8 percent of the cases studied; with one parent obese, this figure rises to 40 percent, and with both parents obese, it rises to over 80 percent. Studies of identical twins separated at birth and reared in different environments also indicate that heredity, more than environment, determines obesity.

Early eating patterns. Most experts agree that eating habits formed in infancy and childhood carry over to later life. An experiment with rats suggests the importance of early habits. In this experiment the milk of one mother was shared with four babies (plenty of milk for each), while the milk of other mothers was shared with as many as twenty-two babies (enough for only small quantities for each). Rats from the smaller litters were fatter and healthier in appearance at weaning. After weaning, all rats had unlimited food available. The rats who were accustomed to eating less continued to eat less, and the rats of small litters continued to eat more. After a short period of time, the thin rats overtook the fat rats in growth, showed much less heart and vessel disease, and outlived the fat rats.

Most experts agree that environmental forces influence eating patterns more than physiological forces, such as hunger. Negative eating behavior may begin in infancy. Some researchers feel that bottle feeding predisposes infants to obesity. Approximately three times more bottle-fed than breast-fed babies are overweight. The researchers suggest that bottle feeding fails to pro-

Heredity is a powerful factor in obesity. A study of obesity found that in 80 percent of cases in which both parents were obese, their children were also obese.

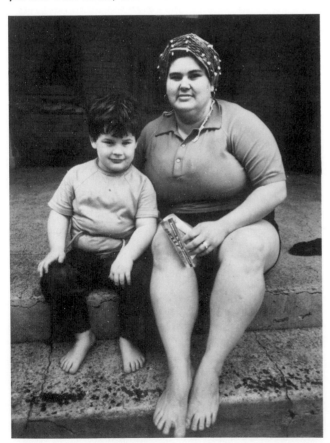

vide the solace of breast feeding, and an unsatisfying bottle produces anxiety, which provokes overeating. Breast-fed babies also learn to stop feeding after removing the richest portion of the milk (the highest fat content). The bottle does not provide such a natural mechanism, so that bottle-fed babies require more calories to satisfy hunger.

Perhaps a more important problem is feeding babies solid foods too early. Researchers believe that starting solid foods early in infancy contributes to the production of excess fat cells. They recommend that parents not start their infants on solid foods before the age of six months (a month or two earlier for very large or fast-developing babies). Another behavior that may continue long after infancy is the general parental tendency to foster overeating. Many children are forced to clean their plate after they are full.

Fat cells and overweight. Our **fat cells** are formed early in life and may increase in both size and number until puberty. Although research is inconclusive, it appears that diet decreases only the size of the fat cells, not the number. With a large number of fat cells formed, return to an overweight condition is much easier. This explains why adults who were heavy babies have difficulty keeping their weight down. These extra cells also may affect metabolism and result in the need for fewer calories to maintain normal weight than are needed by someone who has always maintained normal weight.

The number of fat cells in the human body grows rapidly during three stages of development: (1) the last trimester of pregnancy, (2) the first year of life, and (3) the adolescent growth spurt. Fat is acquired by storing larger quantities of fat in existing adipose cells (hypertrophy) and by new fat cell formation (hyperplasia). It is doubtful that new fat cells are formed after age 21 or so.

There is a large difference in the number of fat cells in different individuals. A nonobese person has approximately 25 to 30 million fat cells, and an extremely obese person has as many as 260 billion cells. A formerly obese person is never "cured," because weight loss does not change the number of fat cells. Research indicates that fat cell size (anytime in life) and number (before adulthood) can only be reduced by

THE WIZARD OF ID by Brant parker and Johnny hart

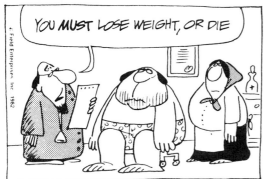
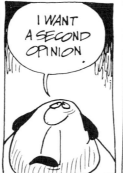
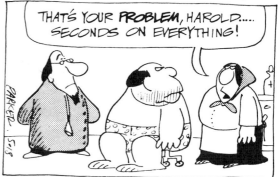

YOU MUST LOSE WEIGHT, OR DIE

I WANT A SECOND OPINION.

THAT'S YOUR **PROBLEM**, HAROLD..... SECONDS ON EVERYTHING!

By permission of Johnny Hart and Field Enterprises, Inc.

modifying nutrition and exercising regularly. Prevention of excessive fat cells centers around developing healthy eating and exercise habits early in life and during the growth spurt. Children who exercise have been found to develop fewer and smaller fat cells. In the adult the same approach will successfully reduce the size of existing fat cells and cause weight and fat loss.

Weight and Longevity

The Metropolitan Life Insurance Company developed charts of so-called ideal weight (later referred to as desirable weights) for men and women based upon data associating average weights by height and age with longevity. Early figures indicated that those who weighed up to 20 percent less than average lived longer. These charts, which became the national guide for determining overweight and obesity, were used to advocate the theory that "the greater the weight, the greater the risk of death." Recent research has cast doubt upon the validity of such data. Findings from one study suggest that individuals of less-than-average weight have health risks as great as those who are overweight and that the American preoccupation with being thin is not a health advantage. Even more dramatic results were found by a team of researchers from Northwestern University Medical School. Overweight (but not obesity) was found to be associated with longevity. In fact, subjects with the greatest longevity were as much as 20 to 25 percent above the Metropolitan chart's ideal weight. As Alfred

Harper, Chairman of the National Academy of Sciences Food and Nutrition Board, states, "The man in the street certainly deserves to know that desirable weights have been underestimated by 10 to 15 pounds." New charts are being developed that will add approximately 10 pounds to each weight category.

Estimating Body Fat

Concept: The most accurate indicator of obesity is body fat (adipose tissue), not body weight.

Weight charts, such as Table 8.1, provide only a rough guide to the determination of desirable weight and entail several pitfalls:

1. It is possible to be within the range of suggested weight and still possess excessive fat. The key to obesity is not total body weight but total fat. Weight charts fail to reveal the presence of fat.

2. It is possible to be classified as overweight or obese (10 or 20 percent above suggested ranges) when you are at a desirable weight and possess little fatty tissue. Among thick-muscled athletes with low body fat, this is common.

3. Some charts allow you to gain weight with age, suggesting that it is fine to be fat at age 30, 40, or 50, but not at age 20. Actually, weight should decrease slightly with age. If you weigh the same

now as you did 20 years ago, you may be over-weight. Loss of muscle mass from earlier active years is now made up by an increased proportion of fatty tissue. Ideally, you should be five to ten pounds lighter at age 50 than your ideal weight at age 25.

4. The three categories of small, medium, and large frame (on some charts) encourage cheating. Very few individuals take their recommended weight from the small- or medium-frame range; yet not everyone has a large frame.

Several methods of determining body fat are more accurate than weight charts. **Skinfold measures** are the most practical for home and school use. Since most body fat lies just under the skin, it is possible to pinch certain body parts, measure the thickness of two layers of skin and the connected fat, and refer to two charts to estimate the percent of body fat (see Laboratory 1 for cut-out fat calipers).

Discovery Activity 8.1
ESTIMATING BODY FAT

Administer the two tests described below to obtain a quick estimate of your body fat.

1. *The pinch test.* Using the thumb and forefinger, take a fold of skin and subcutaneous fat in these sites: back of arm, back below the shoulder blade, thigh, back of the calf, and abdomen. A fold greater than one inch indicates excessive body fatness.

2. *The ruler test.* For an individual who is not fat, the slope of the abdomen, when lying on the back, between the flare of the ribs and front of the pelvis is flat or slightly concave. A ruler placed on the abdomen along the midline should touch both ribs and the pelvic area.

What did you discover? Does there appear to be excess fat present? ●

All measurements are taken on the right side of the body. The skin is pinched firmly between the thumb and index finger and lifted upward. The calipers are then placed about $\frac{1}{16}$ of an inch under the pinch.

The proper location of each measure is shown in Fig. 8.1 (p. 163). For women and girls, only two locations are needed:

1. *Tricep measure.* The skin is pinched on the back of the arm exactly halfway between the tip of the shoulder and elbow. The pinched skin will run vertically toward the shoulder and elbow. Two separate measures are taken with the average score recorded in millimeters.

2. *Iliac crest.* Find the pelvic bone on the right side and take a deep pinch. Place the calipers $\frac{1}{16}$ of an inch behind the fingers toward the back. The pinched skin will run horizontally toward the stomach and back. Record the average of two measures.

For men and boys, three measures are used:

1. *Abdominal measure.* Take a deep pinch approximately one inch to the right of the navel; place the calipers $\frac{1}{16}$ of an inch behind the pinch and record the average of two measures. The pinched fat will run horizontally.

2. *Chest measure.* Pinch the skin approximately one inch to the right of the right nipple. Place the calipers $\frac{1}{16}$ of an inch behind the pinch and record the average of two measures. The pinched skin will run horizontally.

3. *Tricep measure.* Same as for women.

Estimating Your Caloric Needs

Concept: The exact number of calories needed daily depends upon the individual.

An individual's weight, age, sex, and activity patterns determine how many calories he or she needs daily. Certainly, if you experience no weight gain or loss, you are consuming an appropriate number of calories.

Table 8.2 shows the recommended daily dietary allowances of calories by age, weight, and height. Table 8.3 shows the recommended number of calories per pound per day for males and females of various age groups. To estimate your caloric needs, complete Discovery Activity 8.2.

Discovery Activity 8.2
ESTIMATING YOUR CALORIC NEEDS

Estimate your daily caloric needs by using the formula below:[1]

$$\overline{} \times \overline{}$$
Desirable Weight Calories per pound

$$= \overline{}$$
Calories per day

To find your desirable weight, refer to Tables 8.1 and 8.2. The recommended number of calories per pound is shown in Table 8.3. Use these tables as guides only. You may know from experience that you'll gain or lose weight by consuming a certain number of calories. What's right for you will also depend upon your metabolism and exercise habits. ●

Table 8.2
RECOMMENDED DAILY DIETARY ALLOWANCES BY AGE, WEIGHT, AND HEIGHT

Age (years)	Weight (pounds)	Height (inches)	Calories
Males			
10–12	77	55	2500
12–14	95	59	2700
14–18	130	67	3000
17–22	147	69	2800
25 and over	147	69	2500
Females			
10–12	77	56	2250
12–14	97	61	2300
14–16	114	62	2400
16–18	119	63	2300
18–22	128	64	2000
25 and over	128	64	1900

Table 8.3
RECOMMENDED CALORIES BY AGE

Age (years)	Calories per Pound per Day	
	Males	*Females*
10–24	32	29
12–14	24	23
14–18	23	21
18–22	19	19
25 and over	17	15

Caloric balance. You can determine whether you are in a state of caloric balance (food intake not excessive) by weighing yourself once a week. Weigh yourself at exactly the same time of day and under the same conditions (preferably in the morning upon rising). When the total daily caloric intake is equal to energy costs or expenditure and calories lost in excreta, a caloric balance has been attained and no weight loss or gain will occur. When you eat more calories than you use, these excess calories are stored as fat. With the accumulation of approximately 3500 excess calories, one pound of fat is stored. Remember, the body is extremely thrifty. Every unused calorie is stored as fat. Often, a change to an alternative food or drink will cause weight loss. An individual who drinks three glasses of whole milk daily (165 calories per 8-oz glass), for example, takes in nearly one pound of fat per week (3485 calories). A change to skim milk (85 calories per glass) results in a weight reduction of one-half pound weekly or two pounds monthly.

Once unused calories are placed in your fat bank, they cannot be withdrawn at a moment's notice. It takes weeks of deprivation and suffering to remove them. To top it off, you have to carry the bank around with you until a withdrawal is made.

Underweight: The Other Side of the Coin

Concept: Gaining weight requires very careful planning.

To gain weight, you must take in more calories each day than your body needs for energy. The body will store all calories that are not needed, but if food energy is not available, the body will turn to its fat supply for energy and you will lose weight.

A thin person expends fewer calories to exercise than a heavy person does, but the only real solution for the person who wants to gain weight is a large increase in daily food intake, with no increase in activity. If there is no existing medical condition affecting metabolism, the result will be a weight gain.

Our advice to the underweight is to have patience. Do not expect instant results. The following suggestions will assist in making your weight-gaining program a success:

1. Have a thorough physical examination to uncover any medical reasons for being underweight.

2. Maintain accurate records on the calories consumed over a period of six to ten days. Compare daily intake to needs for someone of your weight and activity patterns. You are probably not eating enough.

3. Increase your food consumption by eating more high-calorie foods, larger portions, seconds, and snacks. Become familiar with the high-calorie foods that you like and eat them daily.

4. Plan your diet around familiar foods and avoid foods (even high-calorie ones) that you don't like.

5. Avoid having too many between-meal snacks. Carbohydrates elevate the blood-sugar level and provide a sensation of "fullness." In this way, snacks can destroy your appetite for meals when consumption should be high.

6. Avoid drinking with meals. This will allow you to consume more food before feeling full.

7. Cut down on bulky foods, such as lettuce, carrots, apples, celery, and fresh fruits.

8. Always eat dessert, a second helping whenever possible.

9. Add a fourth meal just before bedtime; however, do not overeat, which might cause discomfort and difficulty in sleeping.

10. Get proper rest, increasing sleeping time to ten hours and using early afternoon naps to conserve energy.

11. Continue exercising to maintain proper muscle tone. Reduce your exercise volume.

WEIGHT CONTROL AND NUTRITION

A Sensible Approach to Dieting

Concept: Low-calorie diets offer a sensible way to lose weight.

Weight loss should occur gradually (no more than 2 to 4 pounds per week for a fairly heavy person) over a period of months and in combination with exercise. Such an approach is more likely to produce a permanent change in eating habits and result in a high proportion of fat loss and little loss of lean muscle tissue. A nutritious low-calorie diet is well rounded and consists of foods chosen from each of the basic four food groups. It is a diet scaled down in calories but not in nutrition. You can tailor your diet to your own needs. Healthy dieting involves learning how to gauge portion sizes, estimate calories closely, and create a daily calorie deficit. When a deficit of approximately 3500 calories exists, you will lose one pound. Most low-calorie

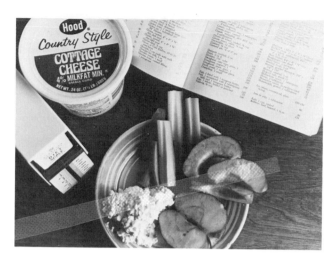

Using a diet scale to determine portion size and counting calories are helpful in creating the daily calorie deficit necessary to lose weight.

diets recommend approximately 1000 to 1200 calories per day for women and 1200 to 1500 for men. This represents a daily deficit of approximately 800 to 1700 calories, depending upon your weight, metabolism, and activity patterns. It also represents a potential weight loss of 2 to 4 pounds per week, as shown below:

Caloric Deficits Daily (minus calories from reduced food intakes and exercise expenditure − 3500 = 1 lb fat)	Approximate Weekly Weight Loss (in lbs)
250	$\frac{1}{2}$
500	1
750	$1\frac{1}{2}$
1000	2
1250	$2\frac{1}{2}$
1500	3

Follow the suggestions below for a healthy approach to a low-calorie diet:

1. Determine how much you should weigh for your height, frame, and age. If your desired weight loss exceeds 5 percent of your body weight or if you have any health problems, consult your physician before beginning a diet. Determine the number of calories you must cut out daily to reach this desired weight gradually. Count calories carefully and eat only this number daily. Weight loss will occur with reduced calories regardless of the diet's percentage of carbohydrates, fats, and proteins.

2. Eat three meals a day from the four basic food groups. Choose the foods from each group that you enjoy and can continue to eat over a period of several months.

3. Drink a minimum of six glasses of water daily.

4. If your doctor recommends it, take one multiple vitamin per day.

5. Combine dieting with exercise in an activity or aerobic program you enjoy. Exercise three times weekly, at least 30 minutes each time

6. Gear your program to a weight loss of between 2 and 4 pounds weekly, and stay with it until you reach your goal.

7. Make your evening meal your light meal, consuming less than 30 percent of your daily calories at this time. Research suggests that those who eat a big traditional evening meal gain more weight and do not lose as much weight as those who eat lightly. In fact, four or five light meals (total calories must conform to your desired weight) will produce the greatest weight loss.

8. Do not skip a meal.

9. Premeasure each portion.

10. If you snack, eat low-calorie snacks, such as carrots or celery.

Fats and Carbohydrates: Reduce, Don't Eliminate

Concept: Fats and carbohydrates should not be completely eliminated from the diet.

There is no doubt that too much fat in the diet contributes to obesity. However, people try so hard to minimize the amount of fat in their diets that it is easy to overlook the fact that fat does serve a valid function. Up to 65 percent of caloric intake should come from carbohydrates, 10 to 15 percent from protein, and the remainder from fats. Fat plays a vital part in digestion and the transportation of vitamins, and it is the main fuel for some muscle fibers in most muscle groups. Fat intake should therefore be reduced but not eliminated.

Similarly, starches and naturally occurring sugars have an important place in the diet. They should be restricted, not eliminated. Exercise, for example, draws from available carbohydrate supply for energy. If the supply is limited, the body must resort to fat for fuel, resulting in loss of fatty tissue. As a result, more fat will be present in the blood vessels, thereby increasing the risk of heart disease. In women, too little fat may lead to ammenorrhea. A constant supply of glucose is also needed by the brain. This need is so essential that the body has a built-in mechanism to convert protein to carbohydrates when the supply is absent.

Discovery Activity 8.3
FOODS AS REWARDS

All of us have been rewarded with food, and we often reward ourselves with food. Describe three occasions on which you rewarded yourself with food and try to explain why you did so.

1. _____
2. _____
3. _____

Now list three nonfood rewards you could substitute:

1. _____
2. _____
3. _____ ●

Snacking: It Can Have a Place

Concept: Snacking can be a very pleasant part of a nutritious diet and actually help you eat less.

Between-meal and late-evening snacking is a leading cause of obesity and overweight. Yet it is unrealistic to expect people to avoid snacking altogether. In fact, planned snacking on the right foods can help you control hunger and eat less.

Snacks likely to be low in calories are those that are:

Thin and watery, such as tomato juice;

Crisp but not greasy (celery, carrots, radishes, cucumbers, broccoli, cauliflower, apples, berries, and other fresh fruits and vegetables); and

Bulky, such as salad greens.

No Place for Sugar

Concept: Sugar that does not occur naturally in foods can be eliminated from the diet without any consequences.

As an important source of energy, as fuel for cell building, or as an aid to the functioning of body systems, sugar is nearly worthless. And as a by-product, it can lead to a pattern of eating that will encourage obesity in the future.

Most of the body's need for sugar can be supplied by eating foods that are naturally high in sugar, such as fruit. A common mistake people make is to reward children (or themselves!) with candy or other sweets. This establishes the fallacy that sweets are better than other foods. In addition, it associates warmth and love with food—a link that remains throughout life. Therefore it is wise to avoid establishing a pattern of using foods as rewards.

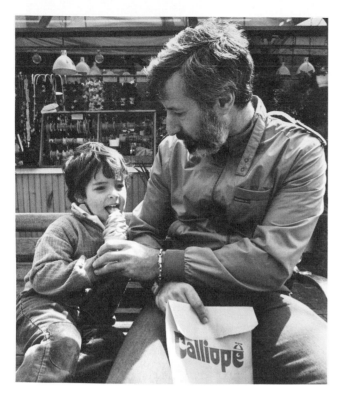

Parents can help their children limit their sugar intake by making sweets an occasional treat rather than an everyday occurrence.

The Need for Water

Concept: Six to eight glasses of water daily are critical to weight control and proper body functioning.

As we stated in Chapter 7, water is essential to the proper functioning of every body system. In addition, it is helpful to weight loss because it serves as a diuretic. About 80 percent of excessive weight is fat, not water. Thus, a person on a diet should not expect to lose weight by reducing water intake.

During the past ten years, we have moved toward a "waterless" society, drinking more sodas, beer, and other high-calorie drinks. Consuming four glasses of orange juice or beer daily provides 120 to 150 calories

IS IT DANGEROUS TO ENTER A STATE OF KETOSIS WHEN DIETING?

Most diets are high in protein and low in carbohydrates (if they do not forbid them altogether). A decrease in carbohydrate intake leads to an elevation of blood glucose. When the renal threshold of approximately 170 mg/100 ml of blood is attained, glycosiuria (a condition in which sugar or glucose is excreted in the urine) appears and polyuria (excessive urine secretion) and thirst develop. Stored fat is now made available for energy, causing a greatly increased production of ketone bodies by the liver. This process, called **ketosis,** is conducive to fat loss. A 24- to 48-hour fast will cause the urine to show ketones.

Proponents of this approach to weight loss maintain that short periods of ketosis are not harmful in any way. They claim that keeping an obese individual in a state of ketosis through a high-protein, low-carbohydrate diet expedites loss of body fat. Carbohydrates cause the obese individual to release excess amounts of insulin, which drive the carbohydrates into the fatty tissue cells and also inhibit the release of fat from the cells. While the individual is in a state of ketosis, insulin production is decreased and fat vacates the fat cells more freely.

Opponents maintain that a prolonged state of ketosis may damage the kidneys. In addition, low blood-sugar levels produce several additional undesirable symptoms, such as headache and low energy levels. According to the American Medical Association, this is a dangerous way to lose body weight and fat.

What do you think? ●

per 12-ounce glass. This can add approximately 8400 calories to the diet each week, or two pounds of fat. Water, on the other hand, can help to reduce hunger without adding a single calorie.

Fluid Retention

Concept: Dieting causes a temporary retention of fluids.

People in the early stages of dieting (first one-to-four weeks) frequently experience a temporary retention of water, which obscures their actual weight loss. This temporary water retention can be discouraging and cause the scales to record only moderate weight loss even when strict dieting has been observed. Nevertheless, actual weight loss has occurred and will be more apparent in terms of reduced pounds following this period. The problem is that vacated fat cells retain fluids. Many unhappy dieters discontinue the diet before this phase runs its course.

Some sound diets require the consumption of large quantities of water in order to prevent water retention; as we've already noted, increasing water consumption actually results in the elimination of water. A more accurate measure of weight loss during the initial stages of a diet is the reduction of adipose tissue in fatty body areas. Both observation and pinching fatty tissue or the skinfold measures described previously will reveal benefits even in the early stages.

Controlling Hunger

Concept: Hunger can be controlled by consuming noncaloric and low-calorie food and drink at the proper time.

There are two basic approaches to the control of hunger: (1) keeping the stomach relatively full, or (2) raising the body's blood-sugar level. Both are effective. Several of the following suggestions help most dieters:

1. Keep busy at work.
2. Increase fluid intake (particularly water) both between meals and at mealtime.
3. Eat small amounts of candy, such as one chocolate square, 20 to 30 minutes before meals (this raises the blood-sugar level and provides a sensation of "fullness").
4. Eat slowly to provide for the blood-sugar level to elevate before you complete the meal (20 to 30 minutes). This will reduce the temptation to overeat or have dessert.
5. Eat bulky foods between meals and at mealtime: lettuce, carrots, apples, celery, fresh fruits.
6. Take numerous breaks during the day. Drink water, diet soda, or other low-calorie beverages.
7. Space allotted calories over five small meals instead of three larger ones to prevent hunger.
8. Season food with lemon, lime, onion, garlic, celery, saccharin, and grapefruit.
9. Go to bed early to avoid the urge for a midnight snack brought on by lowered blood sugar as the evening meal is digested.

The Best Times to Diet

There are particular times when dieting is likely to be more successful. For example, controlled eating after splurges (such as eating out or parties) can prevent the need for a diet. Dieting is easier if you don't allow too much excess weight to accumulate. Other times to consider starting a diet are:

1. At the beginning of your vacation. Although this often is difficult to do, you will save money and avoid additional weight gain during a time when everybody has a tendency to overeat.
2. After the November–December holiday season, when temptation is reduced. Or if you are well disciplined, begin during the holiday season.
3. After the "cold and virus" season. The winter months are particularly troublesome due to flu epidemics

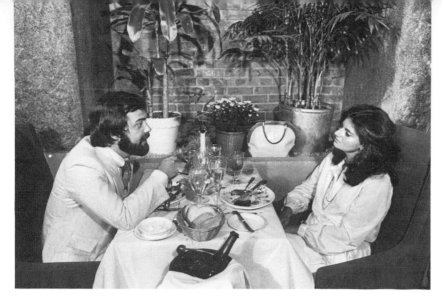

One way to prevent the need for dieting is by planning. When you know you're going to go out for a big meal, eat less before the event.

and colds; avoid adding fuel to the fire with lowered resistance due to dieting.

4. When finances are particularly low in your household. Your chances of eating in a restaurant or stocking "empty" high-calorie treats are minimized.

5. After finishing an organized sport or exercise program. Since the decrease in activity will not be followed by a decrease in appetite, this is a dangerous time when you can't afford to overeat.

Keeping It Off Permanently

Concept: Weight loss that occurs slowly is more likely to be permanent.

A return to an obese or overweight state tends to occur within a period of time proportional to that spent losing a specific amount of weight. Reducing over an extended period of time (minimum of three months) is preferred and generally results in the acquisition of sensible new eating habits, which are more likely to be continued in the future. *Rapid* weight loss, through fasting and other crash programs, can be dangerous and often results in a *rapid* return to old eating habits and an overweight condition. Losing weight over an extended period of time also involves a pleasant personal adjustment to clothes and a new positive self-image so vital to weight control. Controlled weight loss, then, has the advantages of safety and permanency.

Fad Diets and Weight Loss Gimmicks

Concept: Fad diets are an unwise choice for safe, permanent weight loss free from the risk of illness.

There are several reasons why the average diet lasts only five to seven days: boredom, monotony, lack of energy, fatigue, depression, complicated meal planning and purchasing, and failure to lose weight and body fat. These problems are much less likely to occur for individuals on a sound diet. Unfortunately, diet choices are often a direct result of magazine, book, or television publicity that reveals some "secret," easy method of shedding pounds and fat. The gimmick that just might work is often too much for the consumer to resist. Table 8.4 summarizes and evaluates the special claims of many widely publicized diets. Study the table carefully and consult your physician before deciding to try any of these diets.

Table 8.4
SUMMARY AND EVALUATION OF WIDELY PUBLICIZED DIETS

Diet	Special Claims	Allowable Foods	Evaluation
Gimmick Diets			
Pritikin Program	Low-fat and exercise combine to produce weight loss.	Whole grains, vegetables, legumes, fruit; snack on raw vegetables all day and 1 portion from dairy, grain, and fruit groups.	High fiber content causes gas and diarrhea; protein is insufficient; difficult to follow; contains one-quarter normal fat intake; fairly well rounded; devoid of cholesterol, salt, and artificial sweeteners.
Save Your Life Diet	Fiber in foods leads to weight loss which increases by rapid transport of food through the digestive tract.	Vegetable group emphasized, and 1 cup of bran added to six foods; meats and eggs deemphasized.	Side effects may include flatulence; frequent defecation; and soft, bulky stools. Too much fiber binds to some trace minerals and may cause them to pass through the system without being absorbed.
Nibbling Diet	Eating smaller portions will result in fewer calories than eating three meals per day and snacking.	Low carbohydrate, high protein, and nutritious snacking.	With careful calorie counting, weight loss is likely to occur, but difficult to get a balanced diet, and not easy to follow for long periods of time.
Cellulite Diet	Promises removal of the "fat gone wrong" (so-called fat, water, and toxic wastes).	High in fruits and vegetables, low fat and carbohydrate intake; involves kneading the skin, massage under heat lamps to melt the fat away.	No medical condition known as cellulite exists. The fat being described as cellulite cannot be eliminated by a combination of diet and massage (see "Cellulite" section of this chapter).
Cooper's Fabulous Fructose Diet	"Fructose" (sugar from fruit) is used to help lose weight, maintain constant blood-sugar level, keep up energy, and satisfy the sweet tooth.	High protein intake and 1.0 to 1.5 oz fructose supplement.	Weight loss may occur from caloric deficit, not from use of a fructose supplement. Fructose does not help you consume fewer calories and contains the same number of calories as sucrose (4 per gram).
Lecithin, Vinegar, Kelp, and B₆ Diet	Grapefruit and lecithin burn off fat by regulating metabolic rate.	One teaspoon of vinegar with each meal of normal foods.	No one claim (grapefruit or vinegar) can be supported.
The Body Clock Diet	When you eat is nearly twice as important as the number of calories you consume. Lose by eating "breakfast like a king, lunch like a prince, and dinner like a pauper."	Any type of food can be consumed or any diet adapted to the body clock diet.	There is no convincing evidence that eating the big meals early in the day will cause significant weight loss without very close calorie counting. The somewhat hidden implication that calories don't count is inaccurate.
High-Protein Diets			
Women Doctor's Diet for Women New You Diet Doctor's Quick Weight Loss Diet Complete Scarsdale Medical Diet Miracle Diet for Fast Weight Loss	"Specific Dynamic Action" (SDA) is the basis for some high-protein diets: extra calories burned through the process of digesting protein.	Lean meats and poultry, fish, seafood, eggs, and low-fat cheese, no calorie counting.	SDA has no basis. Protein calories are no more or less important than carbohydrate calories. Diets are boring; hard to follow; lacking in vitamins, minerals, and fiber; and can increase blood serum cholesterol levels; dangerous for pregnant women and a poor choice for anyone who wants weight loss to be permanent after a change in eating habits. Ketosis (see Issue) can be dangerous to some people.

High Fat Diets		
Dr. Atkin's Super-Energy Diet Calories Don't Count Diet	In the absence of carbohydrates, stored fat is mobilized and burned for energy. Fat-mobilizing hormone (FMH) is said to be activated to fuel your body with the fat stores.	Unlimited fatty foods: bacon, meat, mayonnaise, rich cream sauces, etc. No calorie counting and avoidance of fruits, vegetables, sugars, starches, bread, and potatoes.	Carbohydrates are needed to oxidize fat completely. If in short supply, fat cannot be used completely and fatigue occurs. Ketone bodies build up in the blood and are excreted in the urine. The existence of a fat-mobilizing hormone has never been substantiated. The diet neglects the four food groups, is dangerous for pregnant women, and is high in cholesterol. Most weight loss is water, which is temporary.
Low Carbohydrate Diets		
Diet of a Desperate Housewife The Drinking Man's Diet No Breakfast Diet Dr. Yudkin's Lose Weight, Feel Great Diet The Brand New Carbohydrate Diet	Claims are similar to those for high-protein diets: a state of ketosis provides a condition conducive to fat loss.	Protein in unlimited amounts with few or no carbohydrates permitted.	Most weight loss is water, and temporary fatigue results from insufficient carbohydrate intake. Ketosis is potentially dangerous over prolonged periods of time. These diets fail to provide adequate foods from the basic four food groups and are difficult to follow.
One Food Diets		
Grapefruit, egg, poultry, melon, banana, steak, beer, fruit, juice, yogurt, rice, etc.	Dieters must concentrate on the food they choose, use a multiple vitamin, and drink plenty of fluid.	Only the one food is permissible.	Impossible to obtain the proper nourishment, even with a vitamin supplement, boring and nearly impossible to follow. Fails to change eating habits, short-term approach. Potentially very dangerous because it is impossible to obtain proper nutrition from the four food groups.
Pill Diets		
Appetite Suppressants: Anorexiants (Amphetamines, Dexedrine, Digitilis)	Appetite is depressed; metabolism is increased.	Medication is designed to restrict total caloric intake. Often used in conjunction with specific diets.	Anorexiants curb appetite and increase metabolic rate. Nervousness, depression, and dependence (physical and mental) are some of the possible side effects.
Metabolic Medication: Thyroid hormone	Increases metabolic rate and energy output to burn more calories. Promotes breakup of lipids.	Used in conjunction with numerous diets.	No evidence is available to support the breakup of lipids. Additional calories are burned as metabolic rate increases. Thyroid hormone induces a state of hyperthyroidism and is dangerous to people with heart disease. It also disrupts the entire endocrine system.
Diuretics: Thiazides	Excess body fluid is lost.	Used in conjunction with numerous diets. Additional potassium is needed to replace that lost through fluid.	Does not increase caloric expenditure. Fluid loss is unrelated to fat and permanent weight loss. Can cause dehydration, nausea, weakness, and drowsiness.
Cathartics (laxatives)	Speeds food through the intestine so nutrients are not absorbed.	Used in conjunction with numerous diets.	May result in bowel difficulty, dehydration, and poor nutrition. Not an effective method of weight loss.

(continued)

Table 8.4 (continued)

Diet	Special Claims	Allowable Foods	Evaluation
Pill Diets (*continued*)			
Nonprescription drugs: Sugar Candy	Curbs appetite when taken prior to meal.	Used in conjunction with numerous diets.	Only mildly effective. Claims of advertisements are not met.
Benzocaine and Methylcellulose	Deadens taste buds to kill hunger and provides a feeling of fullness in stomach.	Used in conjunction with numerous diets.	The amount that can be legally sold is not enough to be effective.
Starvation and Fasting Diets			
The Zip Diet Lockjaw Zen Macrobiotic Diet Liquid Protein Diet	Diets eliminate practically everything but liquids. Jaws wired shut (lockjaw diet) to aid will power. With no calories from chewable foods, weight loss will occur rapidly.	Liquids and some foods.	Extremely dangerous; lacking in vitamins, minerals, roughage. Anemia is likely. The Liquid Protein Diet may have caused over 60 deaths. Weight loss is dramatic at first, then slows considerably, even though you are consuming practically no calories. Quality of weight loss is poor. Too much loss of lean muscle mass, along with fat loss, keeps you flabby.
Vegetarian Diets			
Vegetarian	Reduction in animal fats and cholesterol and less likelihood of excess body fat and heart disease.	Only foods of plant origin, including seeds, grains, nuts, fruits, and vegetables.	Studies in the United States indicate that vegetarians have heart attacks 10 years later in life than meat eaters. An excellent, healthy way to lose weight and keep it off. The diet is safe, providing sufficient protein, iron, calcium, and vitamin B_{12} can be consumed (an iron and B_{12} supplement may be needed). Have your physician confirm that you do not have a peptic ulcer or other inflammation of the digestive tract. On the negative side, the new habits of cooking, purchasing, and eating are not easy to follow at first.
Lacto-vegetarian		Foods of plant origin, plus foods made of milk (yogurt, cheese, and cream).	
Lacto-ovo-vegetarian		All plant foods, plus dairy products and eggs.	

Many of the gimmick approaches to weight loss involve a special apparatus or program. The large majority of them are of dubious value. Vibrating exercise machines result in little caloric expenditure and do not cause weight loss. "Spot-reducing" programs make little sense; research indicates that the greatest weight loss occurs in the area of highest fat deposits, regardless of the body area or part exercised. Steam baths merely remove body fluids; they do not burn calories.

Wearing weights belts throughout the day burns up only a few extra calories; the effect is negligible. The size of the waistline and muscle tone remain about the same, even after prolonged use.

Devices known as "inflatable clothing," or "figure wraps," make the waistline appear smaller because fluids are shifted from one place to another, but only for a short time. By the time you get home and drink a glass or two of water, you'll be back to normal—except for your pocketbook.

Massage is relaxing, can aid muscle tone slightly, and improves circulation, but it burns very few calories and does not cause fluid loss.

WEIGHT CONTROL AND EXERCISE

People who want to lose weight can do so more easily through both diet and exercise. Exercise helps the body burn up excess calories. When the body is both taking in fewer calories and burning all of the calories it takes in, as well as those stored as fat, weight loss occurs. Diet without exercise is a difficult undertaking, although not impossible. Hundreds of weight-reducing clubs provide benefits to thousands of members without exercise. However, without exercise, the dieting person is more likely to have poor muscle tone and conditioning. Also, there is a difference between loss of weight in terms of pounds and loss of fatty tissue in terms of inches. A diet unaccompanied by exercise can lead to a 30 percent loss in fatty tissue and a 70 percent loss in lean muscle. When exercise is added, this ratio can be reversed.

Issues in Health
ARE THE STILLMAN QUICK WEIGHT LOSS DIET AND THE ATKINS HIGH-FAT DIET EFFECTIVE AND SAFE?

Few diets have received such widespread publicity. A tremendous advertising blitz, a best-selling book, and documented examples of actual weight loss are often enough to persuade thousands of people to resort to what appears to be an easy, rapid, and safe approach to weight loss.

Low-carbohydrate diets (such as Stillman's Quick Weight Loss Diet) have been around for a long time. According to the Food and Nutrition Council of the American Medical Association, these diets can be dangerous. Some of the dangers include the possibility of extreme fatigue and a tendency to fainting, headache, nausea, and vomiting. There are also dangers associated with high cholesterol content, the possibility of ketosis, and the possibility of a loss of calcium from the bones with demineralization of the spine.

The low-carbohydrate, high-fat diet described in Atkins' *Diet Revolution* has been under attack since it first appeared. The following statements from the American Medical Association summarize the major concerns:

1. The rationale advanced to justify the diet is, for the most part, without scientific merit. Furthermore, no evidence is advanced that controlled studies were ever carried out to validate the observation that weight can be lost by sedentary subjects who consume a carbohydrate-poor diet providing 5000 kcal/day.

2. The Council is deeply concerned about any diet that advocates an "unlimited" intake of saturated fats and cholesterol-rich foods. In persons who respond to such a diet with an elevation of plasma lipids and an exaggerated alimentary hyperlipemia, the risk of coronary artery disease and

(continued)

Issues in Health (continued)

other clinical manifestations of atherosclerosis may well be increased—particularly if the diet is maintained over a prolonged period.

3. Any grossly unbalanced diet, particularly one which interdicts the 45 percent of calories that is usually consumed as carbohydrates, is likely to induce some anorexia and weight reduction if the subject is willing to persevere in following such a bizarre regimen. However, it is unlikely that such a diet can provide a practical basis for long-term weight reduction or maintenance, i.e., a life-time change in eating and exercise habits.

4. It is unfortunate that no reliable mechanism exists to help the public evaluate and put into proper perspective the great volume of nutritional information and misinformation with which it is constantly being bombarded. The Council believes that, in the absence of such a mechanism, members of the media, and publishers as well as authors of books and articles advising the public on diet and nutrition have a unique responsibility to ensure that such information and advice are based on scientific facts established by responsible research.*

On the positive side, both diets are capable of producing considerable loss of body weight and fat. Although both diets are restrictive and do not provide a balanced diet, a vitamin supplement, it is argued, eliminates the danger of deficiency.

The decision is up to you. ●

*Reprinted, with permission, from Journal of the American Medical Association 224 (10)(June 4, 1973) 1418–1419. Copyright 1973, American Medical Association.

Energy Expenditure

Concept: Even moderate exercise burns many calories and aids weight loss.

Many kinds of exercise can help in weight reduction. To decide what kind of exercise will be most beneficial for them, some dieters consult energy expenditure tables, such as that shown in Table 8.5. These tables are computed for an individual of average height and weight (male: 5 ft 8 in., 150 lbs; female: 5 ft 4 in., 125 lbs) and must be proportionally increased or decreased when there are deviations from this weight norm. Such tables fail to include duration peaks (periods of maximum effort) where the expenditure may reach 1600 to 2000 calories per hour, and they fail to consider the fact that metabolic rate (amount of calories expended at rest) is increased through exercise and remains elevated 40 to 50 calories per hour for as long as six to eight hours after cessation of activity.

According to the chart, a man weighing 200 pounds who has run at a six-minute-mile pace for 30 minutes has expended only 500 calories, or about one-seventh of a pound of fat (3500 calories = 1 lb of fat). But if we adjust this for metabloic rate changes and his extra weight, we find the following:

	Chart (150-lb man)	Actual (200-lb man)
6-minute-mile pace for 30 minutes	500 calories	625 calories
Metabolic rate changes (40–50 calories per hour for 6–8 hours)	—	400
Total	500 calories	1025 calories (almost $\frac{1}{3}$ lb of fat)

The actual energy expenditure in the example above is more than twice that shown in the chart. You can follow the same procedure to estimate the caloric expenditure of your workout. Determine the approximate

Table 8.5
**ENERGY EQUIVALENTS OF FOOD CALORIES EXPRESSED
IN MINUTES OF ACTIVITY**

Food	Calories	Walking	Riding bicycle	Swimming	Running	Reclining
Apple, large	101	19	12	9	5	78
Bacon, 2 strips	96	18	12	9	5	74
Banana, small	88	17	11	8	4	68
Beans, green, 1c	27	5	3	2	1	21
Beer, 1 glass	114	22	14	10	6	88
Bread and butter	78	15	10	7	4	60
Cake, $\frac{1}{12}$, 2-layer	356	68	43	32	18	274
Carbonated beverage, 1 glass	106	20	13	9	5	82
Carrot, raw	42	8	5	4	2	32
Cereal, dry, $\frac{1}{2}$ c, with milk and sugar	200	38	24	18	10	154
Cheese, cottage, 1 tbsp	27	5	3	2	1	21
Cheese, Cheddar, 1 oz	111	21	14	10	6	85
Chicken, fried, $\frac{1}{2}$ breast	232	45	28	21	12	178
Chicken, "TV" dinner	542	104	66	48	28	417
Cookie, plain, 148/lb	15	3	2	1	1	12
Cookie, chocolate chip	51	10	6	5	3	39
Doughnut	151	29	18	13	8	116
Egg, fried	110	21	13	10	6	85
Egg, boiled	77	15	9	7	4	59
French dressing, 1 tbsp	59	11	7	5	3	45
Halibut steak, $\frac{1}{4}$ lb	205	39	25	18	11	158
Ham, 2 slices	167	32	20	15	9	128
Ice cream, $\frac{1}{6}$ qt	193	37	24	17	10	148
Ice cream soda	255	49	31	23	13	196
Ice Milk, $\frac{1}{6}$ qt	144	28	18	13	7	111
Gelatin, with cream	117	23	14	10	6	90
Malted milk shake	502	97	61	45	26	386
Mayonnaise, 1 tbsp	92	18	11	8	5	71
Milk, 1 glass	166	32	10	15	9	128
Milk, skim, 1 glass	81	16	10	7	4	62
Milk shake	421	81	51	38	22	324
Orange, medium	68	13	8	6	4	52
Orange juice, 1 glass	120	23	15	11	6	92
Pancake with sirup	124	24	15	11	6	95
Peach, medium	46	9	6	4	2	35

(continued)

Table 8.5 (continued)

Food	Calories	Walking	Riding bicycle	Swimming	Running	Reclining
				Activity		
Peas, green, ½ c	56	11	7	5	3	43
Pie, apple, ⅙	377	73	46	34	19	290
Pie, raisin, ⅙	437	84	53	39	23	336
Pizza, cheese, ⅛	180	35	22	16	9	138
Pork chop, loin	314	60	38	28	16	242
Potato chips, 1 serving	108	21	13	10	6	83
Sandwiches						
Club	590	113	72	53	30	454
Hamburger	350	67	43	31	18	269
Roast beef with gravy	430	83	52	38	22	331
Tuna fish salad	278	53	34	25	14	214
Sherbet, ⅙ qt	177	34	22	16	9	136
Shrimp, French fried	180	35	22	16	9	138
Spaghetti, 1 serving	396	76	48	35	20	305
Steak, T-bone	235	45	29	21	12	181
Strawberry shortcake	400	77	49	36	21	308

SOURCE: Reprinted by permission from 'Food Energy Equivalents of Various Activities' by Frank Konishi. *J. Am. Dietet. A.* 46:186, 1965. Copyright The American Dietetic Association.

Table 8.6
ACTIVITY RATING CHART

Sport/Activity	Caloric Expenditure	Potential for Heart-Lung Development	Sport/Activity	Caloric Expenditure	Potential for Heart-Lung Development
Apparatus/Tumbling	L	L	Horseshoes	L	L
Archery	L	L	Judo/Karate/Kung Fu	M–H	M
Badminton	M–H	L–M	Running Programs	H	H
Baseball	L	L	Rugby	H	H
Basketball (full court)	H	M–H	Skating	M	M
Bicycling	M–H	M–H	Skiing (cross-country)	H	H
Bowling	L	L	Soccer	H	H
Calisthenics	M	M	Softball	L	L
Canadian Air Force Program	M	M–H	Swimming (competitive)	M–H	M–H
Field Hockey	H	M	Table Tennis	L–M	L–M
Football	H	M	Tennis (singles)	M–H	M
Golf	L–M	L	Volleyball	L	L
Hiking	M	L–M	Wrestling	H	M

Note: L = Low, M = Medium, H = High

calories expended during exercise from Table 8.5 and adjust the calories upward as we did in the example. The importance of exercise as a means of controlling weight can't be overemphasized. The secret is to exercise daily rather than making an occasional effort. A daily expenditure of 1025 calories can result in a loss of two pounds a week, eight pounds a month, and 96 pounds a year.

Which Is The Best Program for You?

Concept: Not all sports and activities expend a high number of calories.

Some sports and activities provide little more than relaxed movement and good fun, but others develop heart and lungs and aid weight loss. Consult Table 8.6 for a rating of various activities according to their potential for caloric expenditure and heart-lung development.

The best type of exercise program for you is one that is enjoyable, expends a high number of calories, develops the heart and lungs, can be continued throughout life, requires no special equipment or facilities, provides the chance for progressive improvement of conditioning, and allows you to start and progress at your present level of fitness.

Girth Control

Concept: Special exercises can help firm the stomach muscles.

Girth control is a common problem in our society. Even though a big stomach is unattractive and unhealthy, both physically and emotionally, too many of us carry one around. This problem can limit mobility; can lead to digestive problems, varicose veins, and hemorrhoids; and can also make breathing more difficult. In addition, those who have large middles have poor stomach muscles, which reduces their ability to protect

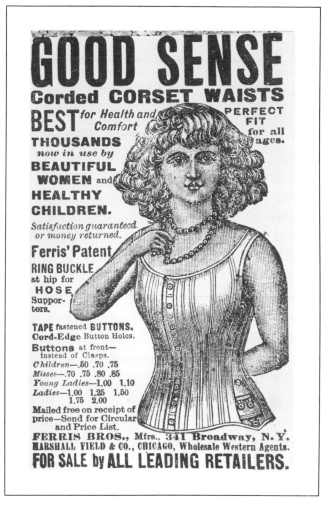

A corset may hide an ample girth, but exercise is the only real way to firm the abdomen.

their backs from strain. Even worse, those who develop fat in the stomach are very likely also accumulating it on the walls of their arteries, which will lead to premature heart attacks, strokes, and poor circulation.

For most people, excess stomach fat is removable, but it requires hard work. The most effective program is dieting combined with calisthenics. The purpose of a calisthenics program directed at firming the stomach is to create what is termed "definition" and to bring out the lines of musculature in the abdominal area by removing fat and increasing the size of the abdominal muscles. The following suggestions will help you begin a program:

1. Measure the waist area carefully before the program starts. Also, use the cut-out fat calipers in Laboratory 1 to take skinfold measures on both sides and in the stomach area. Record these data and compare after several months of exercise.

2. "Definition" can be acquired only through a high number of repetitions. You should attempt to perform a minimum of 100 repetitions daily. For example, if you are doing sit-ups, start with 5 to 25 sit-ups and add between 2 and 5 each day until you can perform 100.

3. Several exercises work the abdominal muscles:
   a) *Sit-ups.* Bend your legs slightly so that you can place a fist between your knees and the floor. Lock your hands behind your neck and sit up slowly, touching opposite elbow to opposite knee. This is a good exercise to assist in eliminating both the spare tire and the "love handles."
   b) *Rowing exercise.* Lying flat on your back, bring your knees up tight against the chest as you sit up.
   c) *Stomach curls.* While lying flat on your back, raise your head and try to touch your chest with your chin. This exercise will help the upper abdominal muscles.
   d) *Side-bender.* While in a standing position, slide your left hand down your leg toward the ankle as far as possible before returning to an upright position. Repeat to the other side.
   e) *Jackknife.* While lying flat on your back, bring both feet into the air as you attempt a sit-up. Touch your feet with both hands.

Remember, it is important to build up to a minimum of 100 repetitions for each exercise. It may be helpful to alternate sit-ups and rowing exercises every other day, and use the side-bender daily. Sit-ups on an incline board are also a useful variation. Finally, don't expect results overnight. Plan to stay with the program for three or four months.

Cellulite

Concept: Lumpy deposits of fat (mistakenly called "cellulite") around the hips, buttocks, and thighs can be prevented.

Weight-reducing salons and some recent diet books define **cellulite** as a gel-like substance made up of fat, water, and wastes trapped in lumpy, immovable pockets beneath the skin. From a medical point of view, there is no such thing as cellulite existing as a particular form of fat. The Federal Trade Commission has stated that cellulite does not exist and that advertised treatments for cellulite are therefore fraudulent.

Regardless of the terminology, lumpy deposits of fat do occur—particularly in women—sometimes at a relatively young age (late teens). Prevention is a lot easier than treatment and centers around regular exercise and weight control. Rapid weight loss and weight gain can contribute to fatty deposits, because these factors tend to reduce skin elasticity. Exercise programs, such as swimming, jogging, bicycling, or rope jumping, performed on a regular basis will help prevent these deposits. The girth control program described in this chapter also offers effective prevention and treatment.

Exercise and Appetite

Concept: Moderate exercise will not significantly increase appetite.

Exercise alone is recommended for those who are trying to lose only a few pounds. Although it is slower than diet, it is a much more reliable method of weight reduction. Research shows that a newly started exercise program does not cause a great increase in appetite. Fat and excess poundage will be reduced by endurance programs, such as distance running (one mile or more), cycling, swimming, and running in place, and by endurance activities, such as basketball, handball, tennis, rugby, soccer, lacrosse, and wrestling, much more rapidly than by any other means. A combination of both endurance running and *mild* dieting (calories should be reduced by no more than 15 to 20 percent when combined with exercise) will produce faster weight loss. An increase in appetite is thus controlled through diet and the caloric expenditure through exercise is *not* offset by increased eating.

Exercise and Carbohydrate Intake

Concept: Exercising when very few carbohydrates are available in the body for energy may aid fat loss.

If the body has no energy-producing foods (carbohydrates) to draw upon for fuel during exercise, it must resort to its fat supply. The result is a reduction in adipose or fatty tissue in the areas of greatest concentration. Obviously, if you exercise in the morning before breakfast and have not eaten since the previous evening, the only available fuel will be fatty tissue. On the other hand, when the body can utilize energy-producing foods for energy, no loss of fatty tissue occurs. If your carbohydrate intake is high, you will burn a greater proportion of carbohydrates with exercise. If your intake is low, you will metabolize a greater amount of fat through exercise.

One disadvantage of performing on an empty stomach is the fact that the blood-sugar level is rather low, and headache and dizziness may occur. A more sound approach, when loss of fatty tissue is desired, is to cut down on carbohydrate intake and increase protein consumption. This will produce similar results without negative side effects.

BEHAVIOR MODIFICATION AND YOU

Factors Influencing Eating Behavior

Concept: Food habits, not hunger pangs, make people fat.

There is a distinct difference between **hunger** and **appetite.** "The difference between human eating, which sees food simultaneously as a symbol, a cultural or religious experience, and a sensual experience, as well as a necessity, and the eating behavior of animals, which is limited to fulfilling survival needs, is the difference between appetite and hunger."[5] Hunger is physiological (inborn), whereas appetite is psychological (a learned response to food). Research shows that obese people seldom feel bodily hunger, nor are they satisfied by what they eat. In fact, obese people do not appear to know when they are hungry or when they are full, suggesting that an empty stomach has little to do with the reason they eat. Such psychological states as boredom, loneliness, and depression have been found to influence eating behavior more than actual hunger. External cues also influence eating behavior. Several theories attempt to explain appetite regulation:

1. The brain monitors blood glucose levels and signals us to eat when glucose is low.
2. Fat cells regulate eating by sending hormonal signals to the brain when they have been fed enough.
3. Centers outside the brain initiate feeding behavior.
4. The feeding behavior switch is always on and must be turned off by a neutral or hormonal switch whenever physiological needs have been met.
5. Appetite is related to both physiological and emotional needs.
6. Obesity is related to a metabolic disorder that increases food intake by affecting hunger-satiety signals transmitted to a "satiety center" or by altering the sensitivity of the satiety center to the signals.

Just which theory or combination of theories is correct remains unclear. Even so, most people can learn to control their eating behavior. To do so, it is important to assess your present eating behavior. For example, you need to know when you eat, what you are doing when you eat (reading, watching TV, studying, etc.), how hungry you are, what portions you eat, and what emotional states or stresses may motivate your over-eating. This assessment is the first step in modifying undesirable eating behavior.

Behaviors Linked to Obesity

Concept: Several specific eating and exercise behaviors linked to obesity can be changed.

Table 8.7 (p. 186) lists eating and exercise behaviors that a jury of experts at Virginia Commonwealth University (health educators, physicians, public school officials, parents, teachers, and students) rated important to weight control. In addition, each behavior was rated from high to low on its potential changeability.

Eating behaviors identified as important to weight control with high potential for behavioral change were: drinking high-calorie drinks instead of water, consuming too much sugar, consuming too many foods high in saturated fats, binge eating, between-meal snacking at school and college on high-calorie foods, overeating

Discovery Activity 8.4
NEGATIVE EATING
BEHAVIORS

Circle those behaviors in Table 8.7 that you feel contribute to your weight problem or to a potential weight problem. Now list each circled behavior on a separate sheet of paper along with some things you might try to lessen the barriers to the behavior, decrease the motivation for the behavior, and eventually avoid or alter the behavior. ●

at lunch and dinner, skipping breakfast, eating a high-calorie breakfast, and failing to preplan snacks.

Exercise behaviors rated important and having the potential to be changed were: no weekend leisure activity, long hours spent watching TV in the afternoons, evenings, and on weekends, and no regular exercise program.

Behavior Modification Techniques

Concept: Changing eating behavior through behavior modification is a slow process, but it can be done.

It is important to recognize that you are in complete control of your own eating behavior. You have the power to alter behaviors that are contributing to obesity or overweight. Now that you have had the opportunity to calculate exactly how many calories you need to consume to reach your desired weight, the next step is to discover what your eating patterns are and what circumstances prompt you to overeat.

Here are fourteen tips to help you modify your eating behavior:

1. Remove temptations by keeping food out of sight, storing a minimum amount of food in kitchen cabinets and pantry, and avoiding the purchase of favorite foods.
2. Keep on hand only those foods that require preparation before they can be eaten.
3. Shop only from a prepared list, and shop after eating.
4. Shop for produce first.
5. Identify and remove the tensions that induce overeating.
6. When you feel you must have that piece of cake, substitute another behavior that prevents eating; for example, go for a walk or chew sugar-free gum.
7. During TV commercials, take a walk but not to the kitchen.
8. Eat only when sitting down.

Discovery Activity 8.5
Identifying Your Eating Patterns

Using the form below, keep accurate records of your eating habits for a seven day period. Copy the form on a separate sheet of paper for each day. Be sure to total your calories on a daily basis.

From your weekly log, identify the cues that seem to prompt you to overeat. List each cue below and devise ways to alter your eating by eliminating or avoiding the cue, substituting for it, or learning to ignore it.

Your eating record will also reveal the number of calories you consume. You will be able to gauge how many calories must be eliminated to reach your desired weight. You may find that eliminating certain types of high-calorie foods; drinking water in lieu of juice, sodas, or beer; or substituting nutritious snacks for high-calorie snacks will eliminate enough calories to reach your weight goal. ●

	Type	Time	Place	Position	With Whom	Assoc. Act.	Mood	Hunger	Food/Drink/Calories
Breakfast									
Lunch									
Dinner									
Snacks									

Type: M—main, S—snack. *Time:* record beginning and ending time. *Place:* K—kitchen, B—bedroom, D—den, A-auto. *Position:* S—sitting, ST—standing, L—lying down. *With whom:* A—alone, W—with others. *Associated activity:* R—reading, T—talking, TV, N—none.

Mood: P—poor, F—fair, E—excellent. *Hunger:* VH—very hungry, MH—moderately hungry, NH—not hungry. *Food/drink/calories:* List foods and drinks consumed and their approximate number of calories.

Eating Cues That Prompt Overeating

1. _____

2. _____

3. _____

4. _____

5. _____

Methods of Controlling the Cue

a. _____

b. _____

a. _____

b. _____

a. _____

b. _____

a. _____

b. _____

a. _____

b. _____

Table 8.7
EATING/EXERCISE BEHAVIORS AND OBESITY

Behavior	Rating	
	Importance	*Changeability*
Eating		
Drinking high-calorie drinks instead of water	high	high
Excessive consumption of simple sugars	high	high
Excessive consumption of foods high in saturated fats	high	high
Excessive consumption of salt	below m.p.	average
Binge eating on weekends	high	high
Binge eating on holidays	average	average
Snacking between meals on high-calorie food/drink in the home	high	above m.p.
Snacking between meals on high-calorie food/drink during school hours	above m.p.	above m.p.
Snacking between meals on high-calorie food/drink on the way home from school	high	high
Overeating at mealtime: breakfast	low	high
Overeating at mealtime: lunch	high	high
Overeating at mealtime: dinner	high	above m.p.
Skipping breakfast	high	high
Eating high-calorie foods at breakfast	high	high
Eating high-calorie foods at lunch	average	average
Eating high-calorie foods at dinner	average	average
Absence of preplanning for snacking	high	average
Exercise		
Absence of exercise program for after school hours	high	average
Absence of weekend exercise program	high	above m.p.
Seeking motorized transportation to and from neighborhood sites within two miles	above m.p.	above m.p.
Watching TV after school	high	average
Watching TV during the evening hours	high	high
Watching TV on weekends	high	high
Absence of a daily exercise program of sports activity for leisure time associated with school	high	average

Each eating and exercise behavior was rated *low, below mid-point, average, above mid-point,* or *high*, depending upon its importance as a contributor to obesity and its changeability (ease with which the behavior can be altered in individuals).

9. Eat only in the kitchen.

10. Do nothing else when you eat.

11. Control the size of the portion you take.

12. Avoid skipping meals, especially breakfast.

13. Eat from a small plate and drink from a small glass, unless you are drinking water.

14. Set your fork down after every other bite.

CONCLUSION

In the final analysis, you are responsible for your own eating and exercise behavior. If you are gaining weight and body fat, you are probably overeating and under-exercising. Once you decide to do something about it, you can apply the information in this chapter to your personal life by evaluating your body weight and fat, by discovering the factors that contribute to your weight problem, and by altering your eating and exercise behavior to eliminate these factors. Weight gain and weight loss are calorie counts. You gain weight by consuming more calories that you expend and lose weight by burning up more calories than you consume. Although it is not easy, you can alter your behavior in several specific areas and slowly reach your weight and fat loss or weight gain objective.

SUMMARY

1. The main cause of overweight and obesity is inactivity combined with overeating.

2. Weight charts serve only as a guide in determining whether you are overweight, obese, underweight, or of normal weight. Skinfold measures (pinching various body parts with calipers), on the other hand, provide an accurate evaluation of both body weight and body fat.

3. Bottle feeding, overeating by the pregnant mother (particularily in the last trimester of pregnancy), and overeating and inactivity the first year of life and during the adolescent growth period result in the production of a high number of permanent fat cells, making it easier for the individual to gain weight throughout life.

4. Calories do count. To lose weight and body fat, and to keep firm, you must burn up, through exercise and daily activity, more calories than you eat. This is best achieved through a combination of diet and exercise.

5. Nutritious snacking on low-calorie, bulky foods is an important part of a weight control program.

6. Six to eight glasses of water should be consumed daily, whether or not you are on a diet.

7. Weight loss should occur slowly, at the rate of no more than 2 to 4 pounds per week. This slow approach is safe and more apt to produce permanent weight loss as eating habits change and remain changed when the diet is discontinued.

8. Extra calories are burned both during exercise and for six to eight hours following the exercise session. These calories are very important to weight and fat loss.

9. Exercise assists in the control of appetite.

10. Hunger and appetite are not the same; hunger is physiological and inborn, whereas appetite is psychological and a learned response to food.

11. Behavior modification programs attempt to place the individual in control of his or her eating habits by discovering the cues that cause overeating and devising ways to substitute, or ignore those cues.

12. Fad diets are potentially dangerous and offer little chance for permanent weight loss.

13. There are no exercise or diet short cuts to permanent, safe weight loss.

REFERENCES

1. American Association for Health, Physical Education and Recreation, *Nutrition for Athletes* (Washington, D.C.: AAHPER, 1971).

2. *American Heart Association Cookbook* (New York: David McKay Co., Inc. 1973).

3. Edwin Bayrd, *The Thin Game* (New York: Newsweek Book, 1978).

4. Theodore Berland, *Rating the Diets* (New York: Beekman House, 1980).

5. *Dietary Goals for the United States.* (Washington, D.C.: Government Printing Office, February 1977).

6. Grace Meynen, "Behavior Therapy with Groups of Obese Female Dieters," Ph.D. Dissertation, Illinois Institute of Technology.

7. Richard Stiller, *Habits: How We Get Them, Why We Keep Them, How We Kick Them* (New York: Thomas Nelson, 1977).

8. Richard B. Stuart and Barbara Davis, *Slim Chance in a Fat World* (Champaign, Ill,: Research Press, 1972).

9. U.S. Department of Agriculture, Science and Education Administration, Human Nutrition Center, Consumer and Food Economics Institute, *Food*, 1981.

Laboratory 1
THE MEASUREMENT OF BODY FAT

Purpose   To determine the percent of body fat through skinfold measures.

Size of Group   Students work in pairs.

Equipment   Scissors and cardboard.

Procedure

Using Fig. 8.2,

1. Trace the skinfold calipers (a) and (b) on a piece of paper.

2. Cut out the traced calipers and paste onto a very stiff piece of cardboard or 1/16 in. plywood backing.

3. Place a brad through the dot in each section of the skinfold calipers, as shown in (c).

4. After measuring a skinfold, place the calipers on the millimeter scale (d).

Figure 8.2
Skinfold calipers and millimeter scale.

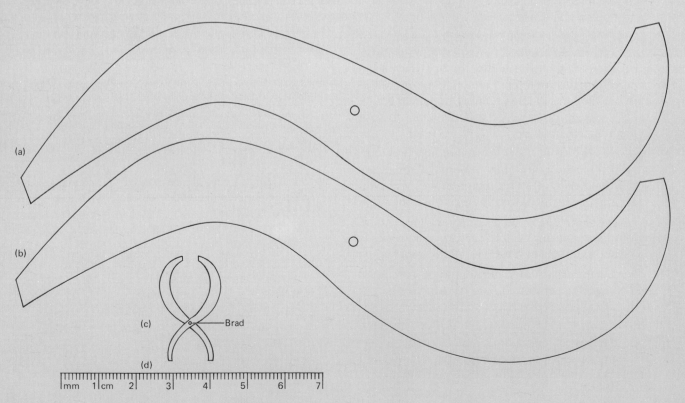

Procedure

1. Working in pairs, practice for ten minutes by taking the measures listed below and described in this chapter. Record the average of three measures on each site.

Men:	Back of the arm (tricep)	_____	mm
	Abdominal	_____	mm
	Chest	_____	mm
Women:	Back of the arm (tricep)	_____	mm
	Iliac crest	_____	mm

Results

1. The back of the arm (tricep) measure can be used as an indicator of obesity in both men and women. Determine whether you can be categorized as obese:

   Obesity in men: a tricep measure greater than 18–20 mm.

   Obesity in women: a tricep measure greater than 25 mm.

2. In the remaining one site for women and two for men, compare your readings with the average values listed here:

AVERAGE SKINFOLD THICKNESS BY AGE AND SEX

	Men		Women	
	23–29	53–57	18–30	46–67
Chest	16.3	27.9		
Abdomen	19.1	26.0		
Iliac crest			22.2	27.1
Tricep	13.7	15.4	21.9	26.9

3. What changes do you feel would be helpful in your diet and exercise routine to reduce body fat?

   Diet changes:

   Exercise changes:

Laboratory 2
CALORIC INTAKE AND EXPENDITURE

Purpose To determine whether a "caloric balance" is in effect for each student. To design a program to reduce calorie intake by 500 calories per day or 3500 calories per week (one pound of fat).

Size of Group Each student works independently in class.

Equipment Scales: In Classroom.
Calorie chart: Approximate from Table 8.2.

Procedure

1. Weigh yourself and record the exact pounds and time of weighing on the chart below (remove shoes).

2. Record all food and drink consumed from the moment of weighing until the next weighing. Include all snacks, approximating portions. Estimate caloric intake from the calorie chart in the appended section of this text.

3. Weigh yourself approximately one week later in class, at the same times as before and under the same conditions (same scales, no shoes).

4. Subtract the difference in the two weights recorded to determine the gain or loss in body weight.

Results

1. *Body Weight Changes*

Body Weight			Difference in calories (Difference in pounds × 3500)
First	Second	Difference (lbs)	

Complete one of the following:

a) Weight gain occurred: A difference of _____ too many calories were consumed.

b) Weight loss occurred: A difference of _____ too few calories were consumed.

c) A caloric balance was attained: Body weight changed less than one pound.

2. *Actual Caloric Intake and Expenditure for One Week.*

	Caloric Intake/Expenditure*							
Day	Breakfast	Lunch	Dinner	Snacks	Total	19 × Wt.	Exercise	Total difference
1								
2								
3								
4								
5								
6								
7								

*Estimate expenditure daily by multiplying 19 calories × each pound of body weight; add additional calories expended through exercise from Table 8.6

a) Add the total *Intake* column for seven days.

b) Add the total *Expenditure* column for seven days.

c) Complete the formula below:

Total caloric intake _____

Less expenditure _____

_____ Caloric balance (intake and expenditure are same)

_____ Positive balance (intake is higher than expenditure and fat gain will occur)

_____ Negative balance (intake is less than expenditure and fat loss will occur)

Remember, it is desirable for growing boys and girls to consume somewhat more calories than they expend.

3. *Removing One Pound of Fat per Week (one pound of fat = 3500 calories)*

a) Describe how you would reduce food intake and/or increase exercise to lose one pound of fat per week. Use calorie table, energy expenditure table, and foods you recorded during the past week.

b) List foods to be eliminated daily.

Food or Drink	Calories
	Total: _____

c) List exercise changes to be added daily.

Exercise	Calories Expended
	Total: _____

drugs and your health

Part four

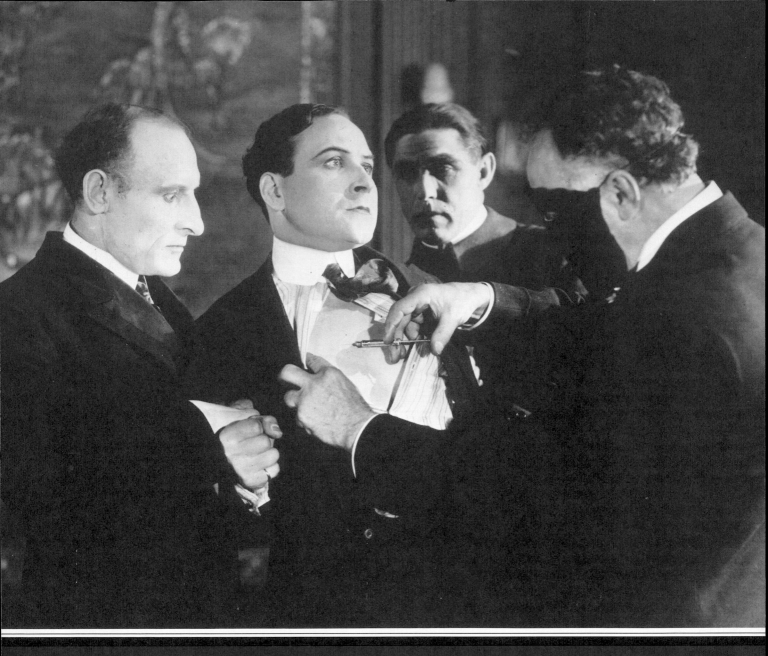

drugs: their use and abuse

- *America: a drug-taking society*
- *drugs: use, misuse, and abuse*
- *taking care of yourself*
- *psychoactive drugs*
- *causes of drug use, misuse, and abuse*

A **drug** is " . . . any substance which by its chemical nature alters structure or function in the living organism."[1] It may include such substances as aspirin or antibiotics, as well as psychoactive drugs that alter mood, thought, and perception. Thus tranquilizers, antidepressants, and marijuana are drugs, as are coffee, tea, alcohol, and nicotine. We discuss alcohol in Chapter 10 and smoking in Chapter 11. Here our focus will be on the other kinds of drugs mentioned above.

Whether drugs have a beneficial or harmful effect is largely determined by how they are used. Just as nuclear power can be used to create energy or wreak destruction, drugs can be used either to enhance or destroy life. In this chapter we will explore a variety of drugs and look at how some of them affect the body and/or the mind. In addition, we will examine some of the reasons people abuse drugs and propose some alternative ways in which people can meet the needs they feel are met by drugs. In light of the information we will present and your own values and needs (discovered in Chapter 2), your task is to decide how or if you will use drugs.

AMERICA: A DRUG-TAKING SOCIETY

Before reading on, can you think of four discoveries of drugs that have revolutionized society? Which four drugs would you list?

1. _____
2. _____
3. _____
4. _____

Perhaps the most important drug discoveries have been the smallpox vaccine and other vaccines (providing protection from many diseases that used to wipe out whole populations), antibiotics (which control many previously fatal bacterial diseases), tranquilizers (a major breakthrough in the treatment of mental illness),

and oral contraceptives (an extremely reliable means of birth control with important social consequences). These discoveries show clearly that drugs have had a significant beneficial impact on our lives.

But for all the good that has come from drugs, many people believe that Americans have become too reliant on medication and mood-altering substances. For many of us, the remedy for anxiety is taking a tranquilizer or smoking a cigarette rather than managing the anxiety ourselves. The remedy for a headache is aspirin. Problems are forgotten with alcohol, and social occasions made more stimulating with cocaine. Americans have access to vast quantities of prescription and nonprescription drugs, as well as psychoactive drugs, and there is no doubt that we use them freely.

Several factors have contributed to this situation. For one thing, we've come to believe that technology is the answer to our problems. Rather than prevent disease from occurring in the first place, for example, we try to find a technological solution to eliminate it once it exists. Consider the vast amounts of money the government and private foundations pour into research to *cure* illness compared to the relatively small amount spent on research concerned with *preventing* illness.

Another factor contributing to the prevalence of drugs in our society is the attitude that life should be entirely free of stress and anxiety. Evidence for this view can be found in the fact that some physicians prescribe tranquilizers when, in many instances, the patient might be better off managing in other ways; or in the barrage of television advertisements for medications that will alleviate "tension" headaches.

Advertising by drug manufacturers exerts a powerful influence. Much of the enormous expenditure on drug advertising is aimed at physicians, who too readily stock and prescribe the products for their patients. Political and economic factors play a role in drug use as well. One need only consider the fact that the government continues to pay subsidies to tobacco farmers, despite the known hazards of smoking, to realize that this is so. Social factors also contribute to the abuse of drugs in our society. We'll look at some of these factors later in the chapter.

DRUGS: USE, MISUSE, AND ABUSE

Concept: Drugs can be used, misused, or abused.

On a separate sheet of paper, list the last ten times you can remember taking a drug. Your list probably includes an occasion when you were ill and took either a drug prescribed by a physician or one available "over the counter." Such remarks, as "I took an aspirin when I had a headache last Tuesday," or "I took some antibiotics that were prescribed by my physician for a urinary tract infection," would fit into this category of drug taking. If used properly (for example, as recommended by a physician), drugs can be helpful. In fact, in some cases physical harm might result if drugs were not used. If you contract pneumonia, for instance, and do not take the drugs prescribed for you, you might die. Drug use of this type is given approval in our society.

Some drugs, however, have useful purposes but are frequently used in ways they were not intended to be used. Aspirin is one of these. Some people swallow aspirin for every headache, muscle tension, pain, or other small discomfort. Prescription drugs are also frequently misused. For example, many people take a larger dosage than is indicated on the principle that if two pills will help, three will really do the trick. We call this practice **drug misuse**.

Defining Drug Abuse

Drug abuse is a more difficult concept than drug misuse. Whether the use of a drug constitutes abuse depends largely on how a society regards the drug at a particular time. In our culture, for example, people who use heroin to achieve a state of euphoria are considered abusers. But in some cultures, use of opium (the naturally occurring drug from which heroin is derived) is regarded as acceptable.

Drug abuse is often defined as use of drugs that are forbidden by law. According to this definition, in most states people who use marijuana or minors who

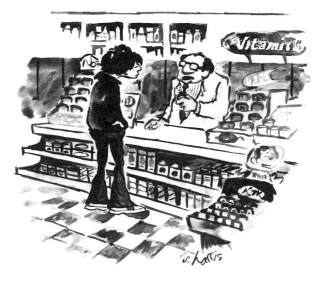

"Shall I wrap it, or do you want to pop them here?"

Reproduced by special permission of
Playboy Magazine; copyright © 1980 by Playboy.

smoke cigarettes would be considered abusers. Whether the use of marijuana for social purposes should be classified as abuse simply because it is illegal is a matter of considerable debate. The important point is that what constitutes drug abuse depends on societal norms and attitudes at a particular time.

Nevertheless, to discuss the problems that can occur with drugs, we must at least try to define drug abuse. For the purposes of this discussion, we will use the following definition: **Drug abuse** occurs when the use of drugs for either medical or recreational purposes results in physiological or psychological harm to the user or to others. Would you define drug abuse differently? If so, how? In what ways do your own values enter into your definition?

Now look again at your list of the last ten times you took drugs. Next to each item on your list write

Table 9.1
TERMS AND SYMPTOMS OF DRUG ABUSE

This chart indicates the most common symptoms of drug abuse. However, all of the signs are not always evident, nor are they the only ones that may occur. Any drug's reaction will usually depend on the person, his mood, his environment, the dosage of the drug, and how the drug interacts with other drugs the abuser has taken or contaminants within the drug.

Drug	Slang terms
Morphine	M, dreamer, white stuff, hard stuff, morpho, Miss Emma, monkey
Heroin	H, snow, junk, horse, dope, smack, skag
Codeine	Schoolboy
Hydromorphone	Dilaudid, Lords
Meperidine	Demerol, Isonipecaine, Dolantol, Pethidine
Methadone	Dolophine, Dollies, dolls, amidone
Exempt preparations	P.G., P.O., blue velvet (Paregoric with antihistamine), red water, bitter, licorice
Cocaine	The leaf, dynamite, gold dust, coke, flake, speedball (when mixed with Heroin)
Marijuana	Smoke, weed, grass, pot, Mary Jane, joint, reefer, tea, hash, roach
Amphetamines	A's, pep pills, bennies, uppers, whites
Methamphetamine	Speed, meth, splash, crystal, methedrine
Other stimulants	Pep pills, uppers
Barbiturates	Yellow jackets, reds, seccy, pink ladies, blues, red and blues, barbs, phennies
Other depressants	Candy, goofballs, sleeping pills
Lysergic acid Diethlamide (LSD)	Acid, cubes, sugar, instant Zen
STP	Serenity, tranquility, peace, DOM, syndicate acid
Phencyclidine (PCP)	PCP, peace pills, synthetic marijuana
Peyote	P, Mescal button, catus, Mesc.
Psilocybin	Sacred mushrooms, mushroom
Dimethltryptamine (DMT)	DMT, 45-minute psychosis, businessman's special

Legend: ○ Symptoms of abuse   ● Symptoms of withdrawal   ▦ Dangers of abuse   ● How taken

SOURCE: Bureau of Narcotics and Dangerous Drugs.

the word that best describes that episode: drug use, drug misuse, or drug abuse.

The symptoms of drug abuse may differ for different drugs. Table 9.1 indicates the most common symptoms that occur with the abuse of drugs.

Drug Dependence

Some drugs cause physical dependence. Sometimes termed addiction, **physical dependence** refers to physiological changes that result in a physical need for the drug. Should this need not be satisfied, the body may experience what we call the **withdrawal syndrome**, a complex of symptoms, including severe discomfort, pain, nausea, vomiting, and convulsions. Sometimes these symptoms even result in death. Withdrawal from barbiturates, for instance, is very dangerous, and the abuser who goes "cold turkey" without being under a physician's care is taking a serious risk.

Other drugs create a **psychological dependence**. Sometimes referred to as a habit, psychological dependence means that in the absence of the drug the person misses it deeply, though no physical symptoms are present. Cocaine, for example, does not result in physical dependence or withdrawal symptoms when it is not available. It does, however, provide a feeling that is so desired by abusers that they rely on it to feel good or to be stimulated. The inability to obtain this drug is a real loss for such persons.

Related to physical and psychological dependence upon drugs is the need to take increasingly large doses. The body builds up a **tolerance** to many kinds of drugs. A heroin addict, for example, might not get the same high feeling ("rush") on the amount of heroin that once provided it; a larger dose is needed. Some drugs seem to work in the opposite manner and are said to develop *reverse tolerance* in the user. Marijuana was thought to be one such drug. It was believed that as an individual smoked more and more marijuana, that person would need less of it to get "high." We know now that marijuana does not result in a reverse tolerance and that the early high by marijuana users has been related to their learning how to get high rather than to the drug's effects on the body. Alcohol, however, does create a reverse tolerance in the latter stages of addiction. In other words, it takes less alcohol for an alcoholic to get drunk in the latter stages of alcoholism than in the early stages.

Factors Related to Drug Effects

Many factors influence the effects of drugs. It is useful to discuss some of these factors, so that you will be aware of them if you consider using particular drugs.

Interaction with other drugs. Two drugs that when used together have opposite effects upon the body are said to be **antagonistic**. An amphetamine abuser taking barbiturates to come down from a high is employing antagonistic drugs.

When two drugs used together have a similar effect upon the body, the psychological effects cannot be easily predicted because of a process called **synergism**. Synergism refers to the fact that the effect on the body of the two drugs taken together is greater than the sum of the effects of the two drugs ingested on separate occasions. For example, barbiturates ingested with alcohol have resulted in coma and death, whereas the separate dosage of either would not have been lethal.

Dosage. Drugs need to be taken in certain amounts (**dosage**) for them to have an effect. Too small a dosage may have no effect; too high a dosage may be harmful. At a particular dosage some drugs may be toxic or poisonous to the body. The dosage required depends on such factors as the user's size, metabolism, and sensitivity to the drug, and the way it is administered.

Potency. A drug's **potency** also influences its effect. Potent drugs require small dosages for the effect sought. Also, two drugs that are initially equal in potency may differ with subsequent use, because one may have chemicals that are maintained within the body, whereas the other's chemicals are excreted from the body. A drug whose chemicals are stored within the body—for example, THC in marijuana—may result in the same effect as another drug but will require a lower dosage.

Solubility. The effects of some drugs may be diluted by the manner in which they are taken. For example, most water-soluble drugs—those that dissolve in water—cannot reach the brain, because their molecules are blocked by what is termed the blood-brain barrier. (Alcohol, however, is an exception.) Fat-soluble drugs, in contrast, can reach the brain, because they can penetrate cell walls, which are composed largely of fat. Most psychoactive drugs are fat-soluble.

Location of action in the body. Some drugs act upon certain sites within the body and other drugs act upon other sites within the body. For example, some antibiotics are termed broad-spectrum—that is, they act throughout the body—whereas other antibiotics act upon only one site.

Individual response. As noted before, the same dosage of a drug can affect different people in different ways, according to weight, height, body fat, and metabolism. In addition, drugs may affect the same person differently depending on the setting in which the drug is taken. For example, drinking with friends at a baseball game may produce a different effect than drinking alone. Further, your mood can affect how you'll react to a drug. A depressed person may become more depressed on a drug, a happy person happier. Finally, psychological set—the expectations you have about a drug based on prior experience—can affect your response.

TAKING CARE OF YOURSELF

Concept: You can medicate yourself safely.

Many common health problems can be taken care of at home with a few basic supplies used wisely (see Table 9.2).

Colds and Coughs

The average American contracts between four and eight colds a year. Though we know colds are caused by viruses, we know little about how to prevent or cure them. All we can do is relieve the symptoms of a cold. Aspirin or acetaminophen relieve fever and aching, and decongestants shrink swollen nasal membranes. Many cold medicines contain alcohol, which causes drowsiness, so be careful to adjust your activities accordingly; for example, don't drive when taking cold medications other than simple aspirin or acetaminophen.

Cough medications can be either expectorants, which liquify and loosen secretions so they can be coughed up, or suppressants, which inhibit coughing. Many of these medications also contain alcohol.

Diarrhea

When diarrhea occurs, switch to a clear liquid diet. You might also want to take Kaopectate, which helps form firmer stools. If diarrhea persists, consult a doctor.

Table 9.2
YOUR HOME PHARMACY

Items in bold print are basic requirements. Other preparations may find use in some households. Keep all medicines out of the reach of children.

Ailment	Medication
Allergy	Antihistamines Nose drops and sprays
Cold and coughs	Cold tablets/cough syrups
Constipation	Milk of magnesia, bulk laxatives
Dental problems (preventive)	Sodium fluoride
Diarrhea	**Kaopectate**, paregoric
Eye irritations	Eye drops and artificial tears
Hemorrhoids	Hemorrhoid preparations
Pain and fever (in children)	**Aspirin, acetaminophen** Liquid acetaminophen,* aspirin rectal suppositories
Poisoning (to induce vomiting)	Syrup of ipecac*
Fungus	Antifungal preparations
Sunburn (preventive)	Sunscreen agents
Sprains	**Elastic bandages**
Stomach, upset	**Antacid, nonabsorbable**
Wounds (minor) (antiseptic) (soaking agent)	**Adhesive tape, bandages** Hydrogen peroxide **Sodium bicarbonate** (baking soda)

*Items are for homes with small children.
SOURCE: Donald M. Vickery and James F. Fries, *Take Care of Yourself: A Consumer's Guide to Medical Care* (Reading, Mass.: Addison-Wesley, 1976), p. 44.

Constipation

Constipation often indicates that you need more fiber in your diet. Exercise may also help. For occasional constipation, milk of magnesia or another mild laxative is helpful, but don't make a habit of using laxatives, because they can be habit-forming and can disrupt your normal bowel patterns.

Hemorrhoids

Over $75 million is spent on hemorrhoid suppositories and ointments each year.[2] There is some disagreement regarding the effectiveness of hemorrhoid preparations. A change in your diet (more fiber) may result in softer stools and fewer problems with hemorrhoids. Anusol is a useful over-the-counter hemorrhoid preparation for occasional problems.

Pain and Fever

Aspirin or acetaminophen (Tylenol) can help control fever and reduce pain. As with other drugs, however, these should be used cautiously. Take aspirin with a full glass of water to reduce the chances of irritating the stomach lining. For infants and small children with fever, it is a good practice to alternate giving aspirin and acetaminophen, because some children have a reaction to aspirin. Reye's syndrome, a potentially fatal disease in children, is suspected of being related to the use of aspirin. If fever or pain persists, consult your doctor.

Poisoning

For the ingestion of certain poisonous materials, the recommended emergency treatment is to induce vomiting with Syrup of Ipecac. However, vomiting should not be induced for poisons that are highly acidic or alkaline. If a household product has been ingested, read the label to find out what the antidote is, and call your local poison control center, or the toll-free poison control hotline (800-682-9211). Appendix B provides more information on first aid for poisoning.

Stomach Upset

It is unclear whether Alka Seltzer and other products that contain sodium bicarbonate actually absorb stomach acid. The nonabsorbable antacids, such as Maalox, are more effective and have no side effects.

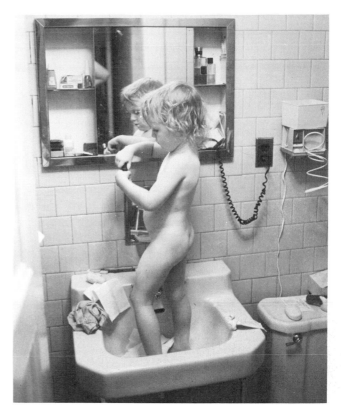

Medications and other dangerous household substances should be placed out of the reach of young children.

Checklist for Correct Drug Use

Before taking drugs, review the following information.

1. Never mix two or more medications without consulting a physician or a pharmacist. Only an expert can evaluate the effects of synergism and antagonistic drugs.

2. Never take prescription drugs unless they are specifically prescribed by a physician for a particular ailment. Drugs prescribed for one illness should not be taken for another without consulting a physician.

3. Make sure you know which medications you are allergic to and keep away from them.

Issues in Health
IS VALIUM OVERUSED?

Valium is a tranquilizing drug that has been the subject of much debate. Some physicians and patients believe Valium is necessary for anxious patients to be able to control their anxiety. They argue that people who are very anxious can't manage other aspects of their lives—for example, family and work responsibilities—much less the situation or stimulus causing anxiety. The Valium is necessary for these patients to function. Proponents argue that Valium has two benefits: (1) it calms the patient to the extent that he or she can profit from psychotherapeutic intervention, and (2) it helps the patient get through the situation, thereby reinforcing his or her perception of being able to manage similar situations on subsequent occasions.

Opponents of Valium argue that it is overused. They believe that Valium prevents users from learning coping techniques. People rely on the calming effect of the drug rather than on their own inner resources, to manage anxiety. Further, they argue, those who use Valium or other tranquilizing drugs in excessive doses over a long period of time develop a tolerance to the drug and psychological and physiological dependence upon it. People have even been known to die from an overdose of Valium or from Valium mixed with alcohol. Therefore, Valium should only be prescribed for the most severe cases of anxiety.

What do you think? ●

Discovery Activity 9.1
YOUR MEDICINE CABINET

List below the medications in your medicine cabinet:

1. _____
2. _____
3. _____
4. _____
5. _____

Have you been following the advice presented above? If not, will you?

Try to recall when you medicated yourself in a manner inconsistent with the advice above. Briefly list these occasions:

1. _____
2. _____
3. _____

In the three instances cited above, how might you have self-medicated in a safer way?

_____
_____
_____
_____ ●

4. Never drink alcoholic beverages while on medication.
5. Keep all your medication out of reach of children and preferably in a locked cabinet.
6. Remember that too much of a good thing might be a bad thing. Know the proper dosage and adhere to it. This will tend to limit any negative side effects.
7. Don't take any medication continually unless it's recommended by a physician.

8. Remember that if you become pregnant stop all medication until you consult a physician. Most drugs will pass through the placenta to the fetus. This can sometimes affect the normal growth and development of the fetus.

9. Ask the pharmacist for the generic rather than the brand name of a drug. The generic drug is the same but is often less expensive.

10. When taking prescription drugs, don't discontinue use when you start feeling better. For example, if you stop using an antibiotic before you've taken the whole dosage, the infection may reappear.

11. Don't use someone else's prescription medication.

12. Ask your doctor or pharmacist about the side effects associated with any drug you are thinking of using.

PSYCHOACTIVE DRUGS

Drugs that affect the central nervous system (the brain and the spinal cord) are called psychoactive drugs. Generally speaking, these drugs can be categorized as **stimulants, depressants, psychedelics,** or **hallucinogens**. These categories will be discussed briefly, in order to give you a general familiarity with them. Consult Tables 9.1 and 9.3 for more information about these drugs.

Stimulants

Three psychoactive drugs that stimulate the central nervous system and thereby speed up body processes are caffeine, amphetamines, and cocaine.

Caffeine. The drug **caffeine** is present in coffee, tea, and cola drinks, as well as in some other soft drinks. For example, a toddler who drinks a six-ounce glass of Sunkist Orange soda is consuming the equivalent, by body weight, of one cup of coffee for an adult. Caffeine is also present in some medications; one dose of Excedrin contains as much caffeine as two cups of instant coffee.[3]

Depending on the amount consumed, caffeine can increase heartbeat, stomach acid, and production of urine. Excessive caffeine consumption (six cups of coffee or a six-pack of cola a day) can lead to disturbed sleep, irritability, nervousness, irritation of the stomach, diarrhea, and headache. However, there is no conclusive evidence that moderate amounts of caffeine are harmful.

Amphetamines. The use of **amphetamines** speed up the body processes so the user feels more energetic, alert, and active. These drugs can also cause irritability, restlessness, anxiety, depression, and high blood pressure. Amphetamines are sometimes prescribed for hyperactive (hyperkinetic) children, but this treatment of hyperkinesis is controversial. Although they curb appetite, amphetamines are no longer used as diet pills because of their potentially harmful side effects.

Cocaine. The drug **cocaine**, which is also called "coke" or "snow," is derived from the coca plant found in Central and South America. Cocaine was once an ingredient in Coca Cola but is no longer legal in the United States, except as a topical anesthetic. In recent years cocaine use has been on the rise, especially among the affluent, because it is relatively expensive. Usually sniffed through the nose but sometimes injected intravenously, its effects are almost immediate, peak within 30 to 60 minutes, and usually disappear within hours.

Cocaine increases respiratory rate, body temperature, heart rate, and blood pressure. Accompanying these physiological effects are the sense of euphoria, restlessness, and excitement. Chronic sniffing of cocaine has been known to harm the tissue of the nose. Possible effects from long-term use include depression and convulsions.

Depressants

Depressants are drugs that depress the central nervous system. Some common psychoactive depressant drugs are barbiturates, tranquilizers, and opiates.

Barbiturates. Taken orally, **barbiturates** are used medically to induce sleep, relieve tension, and control

Table 9.3 SOME SUBSTANCES USED FOR NONPRESCRIBED DRUGGING EFFECTS

Substance	Slang Name	Active Ingredient	Source	Pharmacologic Classification
Morphine	White stuff, M.	Morphine sulphate	Natural (from opium)	Central nervous system depressant
Heroin	H, horse, scat, junk, smack, scag, stuff, Harry	Diacetyl morphine	Semisynthetic (from morphine)	CNS depressant
Codeine	Schoolboy	Methylmorphine	Natural (from opium), semisynthetic (from morphine)	CNS depressant
Oxycodone		14-Hydroxydihydro-codeinone	Semisynthetic (morphine-like)	CNS depressant
Meperidine		Meperidine hydrochloride	Synthetic (morphine-like)	CNS depressant
Methadone	Dolly	Methadone hydrochloride	Synthetic (morphine-like)	CNS depressant
Cocaine	Corrine, coke, flake, snow, gold dust, star dust, Bernice	Methylester of benzoylecgonine	Natural (from coca leaves)	Stimulant, local or topical anesthetic
Marijuana	Pot, grass, tea	Tetrahydrocannabinols	Cannabis sativa	CNS toxin
Hashish	Hash	Tetrahydrocannabinols	Cannabis sativa	CNS toxin
Barbiturates	Barbs, red devils, yellow jackets, phennies, peanuts, blue heavens, candy	Phenobarbital, pentobarbital, secobarbital, amobarbital,	Synthetic	CNS depressant
Amphetamines	Bennies, dexies, hearts, pep pills, speed, lid proppers, wake-ups	Amphetamine, dextroamphetamine, methamphetamine, (desoxyephedrine)	Synthetic	CNS stimulant
Methaqualone	Quads, sopors	2-methl-3-0-tolyl-4 (3H)-quinazolinone	Synthetic	CNS depressant
PCP	Hog, peace pill, angel dust	Phencyclidine	Synthetic	Hallucinogen
LSD	Acid, big D, sugar, trips, cubes	D-lysergic acid diethylamide	Semisynthetic (from ergot alkaloids)	Hallucinogen
DOM	STP, "Serenity, tranquility, peace"	4-methyl-2, 5-dimethoxy alpha methyl phenethylamine	Synthetic	Hallucinogen
THC		Tetrahydrocannabinol	Synthetic	Hallucinogen
Mescaline	Mesc	3,4,5-trimethoxyphenethylamine	Natural (from peyote cactus)	Hallucinogen
Psilocybin		3(2-dimethyl amino) ethylindol 4-oldihydrogen phosphate	Natural (from psilocybe fungus on a type of mushroom)	Hallucinogen
Coffee, tea, colas	Java, coke	Caffeine	Natural	CNS stimulant
Alcohol	Booze, juice, sauce	Ethanol ethyl alcohol	Natural, from fruits, grains	CNS depressant
Tobacco	Fag, coffin nail	Nicotinia tabacum	Natural	CNS toxin (nicotine)
Glue		Aromatic hydrocarbons	Synthetic	CNS depressant

Medical Use	How Taken	Usual Form of Product	Effects Sought
Pain relief	Swallowed or injected	Powder (white) tablet liquid	Euphoria; prevent withdrawal discomfort
None, legally	Injected or sniffed	Powder (white, gray, brown)	Euphoria; prevent withdrawal discomfort
Ease pain & coughing	Swallowed	Tablet, liquid (in cough syrup)	Euphoria; prevent withdrawal discomfort
Pain relief	Swallowed or injected	Tablet	Euphoria; prevent withdrawal discomfort
Pain relief	Swallowed or injected	Tablet, liquid	Euphoria; prevent withdrawal discomfort
Pain relief	Swallowed or injected	Tablet, liquid	P— t withdrawal t
Local or topical anesthesia	Sniffed, injected, or swallowed	Powder (whi⋯⋯	⋯on
Experimental research only	Smoked or swallowed	⋯ucles (dark green or brown)	Euphoria, relaxation, increased perception
Experimental research only	Smoked or swallowed	Solid, brown-to-black, resin	Relaxation, euphoria, increased perception
Sedation, relieve high blood pressure, epilepsy	Swallowed or injected	Tablets or capsules	Anxiety reduction, euphoria
Control appetite, narcolepsy, some childhood behavioral disorders	Swallowed or injected	Tablets, capsules, liquid, powder (white)	Alertness, activeness
Sedation	Swallowed	Tablets	Euphoria, aphrodisiac
Veterinary anesthetic	Smoked or swallowed	Tablets, powder in smoking mixtures	Harsher than LSD
Experimental research only	Swallowed	Tablets, capsules, liquid	Insight, distortion of senses, exhilaration
None	Swallowed	Tablets, capsules, liquid	Stronger than LSD effects
None	Smoked or swallowed	In marijuana or liquid	Stronger than marijuana effects
None	Swallowed	Tablet, capsule	Same as LSD
None	Swallowed	Tablet, capsule	Same as LSD
Mild stimulant	Swallowed	Beverage	Alertness
Solvent, antiseptic, sedative	Swallowed or applied topically	Liquid	Sense alteration, anxiety reduction
Emetic (nicotine)	Smoked, sniffed, chewed	Snuff, pipe, cut particles, cigarettes	Relaxation
None	Inhaled	Plastic cement	Intoxication

(continued)

Table 9.3 (continued)

Substance	Long-Term Possible Effects	Physical Dependence Potential	Psychological Dependence Potential	Organic Damage Potential
Morphine	Addiction, constipation, loss of appetite	Yes	Yes	Yes, indirectly
Heroin	Addiction, constipation, loss of appetite	Yes	Yes	Yes, indirectly
Codeine	Addiction, constipation, loss of appetite	Yes	Yes	Yes, indirectly
Oxycodone	Addiction, constipation, loss of appetite	Yes	Yes	Yes, indirectly
Meperidine	Addiction, constipation, loss of appetite	Yes	Yes	Yes, indirectly
Methadone	Addiction, constipation, loss of appetite	Yes	Yes	Yes, indirectly
Cocaine	Depression, convulsions	No	Yes	Probable
Marijuana	Usually none; bronchitis, conjunctivitis possible	No	Possible	Not determined
Hashish	Usually none, conjunctivitis & psychosis possible	No	Possible	Not determined
Barbiturates	Severe withdrawal symptoms; possible convulsions, toxic psychosis	Yes	Yes	Yes
Amphetamines	Loss of appetite, delusions, hallucinations, toxic psychosis	Possible	Yes	Probable
Methaqualone	Coma, convulsions	Yes	Yes	Yes
PCP	—	No	Possible	Not determined
LSD	May intensify existing psychosis, panic reactions	No	Possible	Not determined
DOM	—	No	Possible	Not determined
THC	—	No	Possible	Not determined
Mescaline	—	No	Possible	Not determined
Psilocybin	—	No	Possible	Not determined
Coffee, tea, colas	May aggravate organic actions	No	Yes	No
Alcohol	Toxic psychosis, addiction, neurologic damage	Yes	Yes	Yes
Tobacco	Loss of appetite, habituation	Possible	Yes	Possible
Glue	Impaired perception, coordination, judgment	No	Yes	Yes

SOURCE: From *Teaching About Drugs: A Curriculum Guide, K–12,* developed and produced by the American School Health Association, Kent, Ohio 44240, and the Pharmaceutical Manufacturers Association, Washington, D.C. 20005. Reprinted by permission.

epileptic seizures. These drugs are fat-soluble and are consequently absorbed into the fatty tissue of the brain. Used on a short-term basis, barbiturates can reduce anxiety and produce euphoria. Over the long-term, however, they are physically addictive. Severe withdrawal symptoms, including convulsion, psychosis, and even death, can occur when the drugs are no longer taken. Consequently, barbiturates can only be legally obtained with a prescription, and those withdrawing from barbiturate dependence are advised to seek medical assistance.

Major and minor tranquilizers. Before tranquilizing drugs were made available in the 1950s, severe forms of mental illness were much more difficult to treat. There was no effective way to calm patients so they could profit from psychotherapeutic counseling. With the availability of **major tranquilizers**, such as chlorpromazine (Thorazine), the management of mental illnesses, such as schizophrenia, became somewhat easier. The **minor tranquilizers**, which include such drugs as diazepam (Valium) and chlordiazepoxide (Librium), are used to treat anxiety and muscle tension. Long-term use of these tranquilizers may produce psychological and physiological dependence and withdrawal symptoms when their use is discontinued. Some experts believe the minor tranquilizers are overprescribed (over 57 million prescriptions for Valium were written in 1977), whereas others believe these drugs are an important precursor to other forms of anxiety treatment (see the accompanying Issue box).

Opiates. The **opiates**, drugs that are synthesized from opium (a derivative of the opium poppy) include morphine, heroin, and codeine. Generally known as **narcotics,** these drugs create both psychological and physiological dependence. The medical use of narcotic drugs has been debated ever since morphine was first synthesized in the early 1800s. Morphine was administered to relieve pain but soon became abused. As a result, the Harrison Narcotic Act of 1914 was passed to prohibit the nonmedical use of narcotics.

Heroin has no medically and legally approved use, although it too was once used for relief of pain. It is derived from morphine and was originally believed to be a nonaddictive pain reliever. However, it soon became known that heroin is addictive, that tolerance is built up, and that discontinuance of heroin use can lead to severe withdrawal symptoms. Heroin can be injected just under the skin ("skin-popping") or intravenously ("mainlining"), smoked, eaten, or sniffed. Use of an unclean hypodermic needle can result in hepatitis. Other effects of heroin are loss of appetite (and the accompanying illnesses and diseases associated with malnutrition), loss of sexual interest, and lethargy. Heroin is very expensive, and many crimes are committed by heroin addicts to support their addiction.

Codeine is a weaker painkiller than either morphine or heroin but can also be psychologically and physiologically addictive. It is medically prescribed on a short-term basis to relieve coughs and sometimes is injected to relieve pain. Most codeine is produced from morphine.

Marijuana

Marijuana is made from the crushed leaves and flowers of the *Cannabis sativa* plant, which grows best in warm, moist climates. The ingredient in marijuana that causes the psychoactive effect is **tetrahydrocannibinol (THC)**. THC can be taken into the body by smoking marijuana or by eating it. Although 43 million Americans have tried marijuana at least once, its use seems to have leveled off in recent years. Among young people it is a very popular recreational drug, whereas adults 35 or older still seem to prefer alcohol. Marijuana is sometimes prescribed for glaucoma patients to relieve pressure on the eyeball and for cancer patients to relieve nausea and vomiting caused by chemotherapy.

Marijuana use results in a relaxed, euphoric feeling with alterations in perception. These changes in perception make it unsafe to drive an automobile while under the influence of marijuana. The effects of long-term, heavy use of marijuana have not been determined conclusively. Some people believe that there are serious psychological effects. For example, they contend that heavy use of marijuana decreases motivation, affects memory and alertness, interferes with the ability to perform complex tasks, and leads ultimately to "dropping out." To date the evidence for these asser-

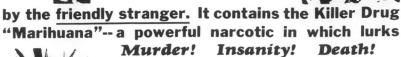

Beware! Young and Old—People in All Walks of Life!

This ▮ may be handed you by the friendly stranger. It contains the Killer Drug "Marihuana"-- a powerful narcotic in which lurks *Murder! Insanity! Death!*

WARNING!

Dope peddlers are shrewd! They may put some of this drug in the 🫖 or in the ᶜᵒᶜᵏᵗᵃⁱˡ or in the tobacco cigarette.

WRITE FOR DETAILED INFORMATION, ENCLOSING 12 CENTS IN POSTAGE — MAILING COST

Address: **THE INTER-STATE NARCOTIC ASSOCIATION**

(Incorporated not for profit)

53 W. Jackson Blvd. **Chicago, Illinois, U. S. A.**

Although the evidence on the long-term effects of marijuana is not all in, it is clear that the drug does not pose the kinds of dangers portrayed in this outdated poster.

tions is not all in. However, it seems likely that the "amotivational syndrome" some have associated with marijuana is probably due more to personal and psychological factors that already existed in the individual than to marijuana use alone.

The physical effects of long-term marijuana use are also the subject of intense debate. It is logical to suppose that regular, heavy use of marijuana may produce respiratory difficulties, such as bronchitis. It also seems possible that heavy users may be more likely to develop lung cancer. However, so far these ideas have not been demonstrated by research.

Even though much is not known about marijuana, some of the popular notions about it have been shown to be unfounded:

1. *Marijuana use leads to heroin use.* Although approximately 85 percent of heroin users previously smoked marijuana, 100 percent previously drank milk and 90 percent previously drank alcohol. No one claims that milk and alcohol lead to heroin addiction. Fewer than 1 percent of marijuana smokers go on to heroin.[4]

2. *Marijuana results in lowered resistance to disease.* Though one study reached this conclusion, subsequent investigations have not verified it.

3. *Marijuana causes chromosomal damage.* This is an early finding that has not subsequently been verified.

4. *Marijuana causes birth defects.* There is no evidence to indicate that in the usual doses this occurs, though in rats tremendously huge doses have resulted in birth defects. Even so, pregnant women should not smoke marijuana.

5. *Marijuana causes impotence.* Though heavy doses of marijuana were found to result in a decreased production of the male hormone testosterone and sperm, this does not mean that impotence occurs. In addition, other investigators have found no decrease in testosterone or sperm production from marijuana use.

One of the reasons that there is so little hard knowledge about marijuana is that research concerning marijuana is difficult to perform and evaluate systematically. Researchers have conducted many informal cross-cultural studies, but their results tend to be unreliable because of numerous methodological shortcomings. Animal studies also tend to be unreliable, and the findings from these studies may not be applicable to human subjects.

With these difficulties in mind, the dilemma confronting legislators reviewing the present marijuana laws (in most states marijuana is still illegal) can be better understood. Knowing that marijuana has not been proved to be the harmful drug it was once reputed to be, yet not knowing much about the effects of its use over a long period of time, lawmakers are faced with a difficult issue. Proponents of legalization argue that marijuana is relatively harmless and should be treated like alcohol and tobacco. They further contend that marijuana laws are not enforced systematically and that as a result there is considerable flouting of the law. In addition, because marijuana is illegal, users are in danger of buying plants that have been sprayed with poisons, such as paraquat. Finally, if marijuana were legalized, the criminal element would be forced out of business and law enforcement agencies would be free to go after more serious crimes.

Those who feel marijuana should not be legalized cite the potential health risks and contend that marijuana is dangerous. Some feel the drug endangers the morals of young people. To legalize marijuana would simply add another problem to the serious problems already posed by alcohol and tobacco. The answer, in their view, is more vigorous enforcement of existing laws.

Currently the states are moving in the direction of "decriminalization"—removing felony penalties for possession of small amounts of the drug. Although it may be some time before marijuana is legalized, it appears that the United States is moving in the direction of greater tolerance of the drug.

Where do you stand on the debate about marijuana? Decide whether you think marijuana should be legal or not. Then list five reasons for the point of view with which you do *not* agree:

1. _____
2. _____
3. _____
4. _____
5. _____

Is there a middle ground? Do you differentiate between using and selling or growing? Do you differentiate between possessing large amounts and small amounts? Would you set a legal age for using marijuana, such as is done now with cigarettes?

Psychedelics and Hallucinogens

Psychedelics and hallucinogens are a broad category that includes LSD and PCP, among others. All psychoactive drugs alter mood and behavior, but psychedelics are more likely than others to produce extreme alterations, such as hallucinations and feelings of paranoia.

LSD. The drug **lysergic acid diethylamide (LSD)** was first synthesized in 1938 by Swiss chemist Albert Hoffman. Use of the drug peaked in the 1960s and 1970s after it was advocated as a means of enlightenment by such gurus as Timothy Leary, at the time a professor at Harvard University. As the "flower children" grew into adulthood and as the potential harmful effects of LSD became known, its use tapered off.

Taken in capsule or liquid form (sometimes poured on sugar cubes), LSD results in excitation; anxiety; euphoria; distortion of perception; and hallucinations involving exotic colors, shapes, and images. The hallucinations have been reported to sometimes be very frightening, and some people experiencing "bad trips" act in a bizarre manner, even jumping out of a window to escape an image. In addition, some users report recurring hallucinations when the drug is no longer being used. This experience is called a **flashback**. Researchers have found that long-term use of LSD is related to chromosomal damage and birth defects, although the evidence is not conclusive. Other dangers include paranoid reactions, psychosis, and serious depression.

PCP. Another psychedelic drug is **phyecyclidine (PCP)**, a white crystalline powder, soluble in water, which is used orally, smoked, injected, or sniffed. It is sold on the streets in tablets, capsules, or powders, or sprinkled on marijuana. PCP is actually a depressant, although in large doses it acts as a psychedelic. It is the active chemical in many street drugs sold as THC (the active chemical in marijuana) and is easily manufactured illicitly. Thus dosage levels and effects vary and are difficult to control.

Originally developed for medical use as an anesthetic (Sernyl), PCP was found to cause agitation, visual disturbances, delirium, increased heart rate, elevated blood pressure, poor speech, lack of muscular coordination, and dizziness. With large doses, convulsion and coma can occur. As a result, it is no longer used for human beings but is instead used as an anesthetic for animals.

Other effects of PCP include disturbances of memory, perception, concentration, and judgment, and, when used in large doses over a period of time, brain and nervous system damage. The drug can result in the development of long-lasting anxiety and depression, as well as psychosis and even death in some cases.

PCP users are often unaware that they have used the drug, because when it is sold on the streets, it is almost always misrepresented, usually as THC. This problem, along with the harmful effects noted above, make PCP an extremely dangerous drug.

CAUSES OF DRUG USE, MISUSE, AND ABUSE

> **Concept:** There are many reasons why people misuse or abuse drugs.

Drugs are often used socially and have sometimes become a part of the culture itself. Wine, for example, is used in certain religious ceremonies. Distilled beverages are consumed at cocktail parties, and beer is consumed at ball parks. These uses are generally accepted in our society.

The *misuse* of drugs is mainly a matter of ignorance. People misuse drugs either because they lack information concerning the drugs or their side effects or because they do not carefully follow instructions concerning their use or dosage. An example of this would be mixing alcohol use and use of a prescription drug because you don't realize this is dangerous.

Discovery Activity 9.2
DRUG CROSSWORD PUZZLE

Before going on, complete the drug crossword puzzle. It will serve to review the discussion so far, as well as provide some new information. The answers appear on p. 212. ●

Reasons for Abuse

The *abuse* of drugs is a different story. Although some drug abusers are ignorant of a drug's side effects, long-term hazards, and legal consequences, many are quite knowledgeable. There is clear evidence that knowledge alone has little effect on drug abuse. People abuse drugs for many and varied reasons. Still, researchers have been able to identify some of the reasons for some people's drug-related behavior.

Discovery Activity 9.3
WHY DO YOU THINK PEOPLE ABUSE DRUGS?

Before reading on, list eight reasons why you think people abuse drugs.

1. _____
2. _____
3. _____
4. _____
5. _____
6. _____
7. _____
8. _____ ●

1	2	3	4	5	6	7		8		9
10	11				12			13	14	15
16			17	18		19	20	21	22	23
24	25	26	27	28	29			30	31	32
33			34	35	36			37		
38	39			40		41		42		
43		44	45	46	47	48	49	50	51	52
53		54		55		56		57		
58				59			60	61	62	
63	64		65		66		67	68	69	
70		71	72	73	74	75				76
77				78			79	80	81	82

ACROSS

1. _____ mixed with barbiturates can cause death
10. Nickname for mother
13. Definite article
17. Abbr. for Police Department
19. A drug made from poppies
24. Abusers of this drug often get hepatitis
30. Abbr. for Marine Military Patrol
34. Abbr. for tender loving care
38. Toward
44. Reaction to the stoppage of an addictive drug
60. Also
63. Negative
67. Name of drug from a fungus on rye
71. Opium is made from the _____ plant
79. A drug-induced departure from reality

DOWN

1. Drug given for weight loss
2. Abbr. for Los Angeles
6. Covering
8. Classification of drugs which cause blood vessels to dilate
9. Common name for the marijuana plant found in India
14. To sing with your mouth closed
17. Slang for marijuana
18. To enlarge or get bigger
29. Abbr. for no charge
41. Poem of praise
44. Pl. of I
59. Abbr. for Constable on Patrol
61. Abbr. for Oh Dear!
65. Opposite of stop
73. Nickname for father
76. Abbr. for the Atlantic and Pacific Co.

SOURCE: Jerrold S. Greenberg, *Student-Centered Health Instruction* (Reading, Mass.: Addison-Wesley, 1978), p. 104.

The literature identifies the following reasons for drug abuse:

1. Alienation. As described in Chapter 2, alienation is comprised of three subfactors: social isolation, powerlessness, and normlessness. People who have no "significant others," who feel unable to control their own destinies, and who have not accepted a set of standards for their behavior have been found to abuse drugs to a greater extent than those not so alienated.[5]

2. Self-esteem. Many drug education programs emphasize the development of a healthy sense of self-esteem rather than knowledge about drugs.[6] The reason for this focus is that those who have a low regard for themselves have been found to abuse drugs to a greater degree than those with positive self-esteem.

3. Lack of confidence. Related to low self-esteem, lack of confidence is one reason for abuse of drugs. People who lack confidence can't relate well

¹A	²L	³C	⁴O	⁵H	⁶O	⁷L		⁸S	⁹H
¹⁰M	¹¹A				¹²N		¹³T	¹⁴H	¹⁵E
¹⁶P			¹⁷P	¹⁸D		¹⁹O	²⁰P	²¹I	²²U ²³M
²⁴H	²⁵E	²⁶R	²⁷O	²⁸I	²⁹N		³⁰M	³¹M	³²P
³³E			³⁴T	³⁵L	³⁶C		³⁷U		
³⁸T	³⁹O			⁴⁰U		⁴¹O		⁴²L	
⁴³A		⁴⁴W	⁴⁵I	⁴⁶T	⁴⁷H	⁴⁸D	⁴⁹R	⁵⁰A	⁵¹W ⁵²N
⁵³M		⁵⁴E		⁵⁵E		⁵⁶E		⁵⁷N	
⁵⁸I					⁵⁹C			⁶⁰T	⁶¹O ⁶²O
⁶³N	⁶⁴O		⁶⁵G		⁶⁶O		⁶⁷L	⁶⁸S	⁶⁹D
⁷⁰E		⁷¹P	⁷²O	⁷³P	⁷⁴P	⁷⁵Y			⁷⁶A
⁷⁷S				⁷⁸A			⁷⁹T	⁸⁰R	⁸¹I ⁸²P

Answers to drug crossword puzzle on page 211.

with others unless they are high. At every party they attend it seems they get high and then, and only then, become the life of the party. Using drugs for confidence is only a temporary solution.

4. Peer pressure. It is reasonable to assume that people who have low self-esteem will not have a great deal of confidence in their own opinions and, consequently, will be unduly influenced by their peers. Many researchers have cited peer pressure as a factor in drug abuse, and it is the objective of some drug education programs to lessen the influence of this pressure in the

decision-making process. The consequence of being excessively influenced by one's peers is that one is less able to be oneself.

4. Adult modeling. We learn adult behavior by observing adults and copying them. Some symbols of adulthood have special meaning to young people who want to feel adult. One of these symbols is having a job and earning money. Another is owning a car and being free to travel. A third is moving out of one's parents' house. Unfortunately, some "adult" behavior is unhealthy, but it too is copied. If children see parents use alcohol, they may imitate this behavior in order to feel adult. If parents misuse or overuse medication, children may also misuse it. Studies have indicated, for instance, that children whose parents smoke cigarettes have a greater tendency to be cigarette smokers than do children whose parents do not smoke.[7]

6. To cope. Coping may take positive forms, such as making friends, getting a job, or acquiring a hobby, or it may take the form of drug abuse. Positive coping focuses on changing the *external* situation. But when drugs are used to cope, the goal is to change the *internal* environment so the situation doesn't seem as bad. However, when the effects of the drug wear off, the situation remains unchanged and the problem unsolved. There are situations in which changing the internal environment may be the only solution. For example, terminally ill people have been given LSD or marijuana to relieve pain or psychological suffering. In most instances, however, the temporary nature of the drug's ability to respond to the situation does not argue for its use. Either more drugs would be needed or the problem would reappear.

7. Mood alteration. Some people abuse drugs for the psychological high they provide. The mellow feeling obtained from some drugs, the excitation from others, and the feeling of invincibility from still others lead some people to seek this experience over and over again. For them, the high is everything.[8]

Did your list of reasons for drug abuse include some of the above? Can you think of other reasons people abuse drugs?

Treating Drug Addiction

Concept: There are many methods for treating drug addicts.

It is very difficult to determine the most effective method of treatment for drug abuse. The circumstances differ widely from one addict to another. Each addict brings to whatever treatment is being considered his or her own level of motivation to get off drugs. Also, addicts differ in background and in situation. Some are fortunate in that they will receive a great deal of family support, others receive none. The financial resources available to treatment programs also vary, and community support services range from generous to nonexistent.

Several approaches to the rehabilitation of drug addicts follow:

1. Therapeutic communities. These communities are designed to house drug addicts trying to kick the habit. They try to meet the addicts' needs (except, of course, drugs) and provide counseling, medical care, and gainful work. They try to instill in the community members a sense of personal and social responsibility. Ex-addicts reside within these communities until they are ready to be eased back into society. Some examples of therapeutic communities are the Delancey Street Family in San Francisco, Phoenix House in New York City and elsewhere, and Daytop Village in New York City.

2. Therapy combined with medical help. For those fortunate enough to be able to afford it or whose

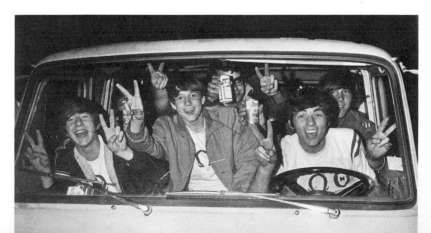

Peer pressure may be an important factor in many young people's decision to use drugs. Teenagers with low self-esteen appear to be especially vulnerable to group influence.

health insurance will cover its cost, psychological counseling, accompanied by medical care, is available. Former First Lady Betty Ford received this sort of help for her dependence upon alcohol and other unspecified drugs on an inpatient basis in a hospital. Outpatient counseling services are also available at many hospitals and have the advantage of allowing the patient to remain with family and friends. Of course, for addicts who are negatively influenced by family and friends, counseling as an inpatient or joining a therapeutic community is recommended.

3. Pharmacological support. Another method of treating addicts is to provide them either with the drug to which they are addicted (for example, heroin maintenance in England), or with a drug that will block the pleasurable effects of the drug to which they are addicted (for example, methadone maintenance or methadone withdrawal). The rationale behind providing drugs to drug addicts is that they will then not have to resort to crime to get the money to support their addiction. Methadone withdrawal programs are designed so that the addict is weaned from a heroin addiction to a methadone addiction. Methadone, a synthetic drug developed during World War II, can then be withdrawn with less difficulty than heroin—at least that was the original thought. Recently, however, drug researchers have begun to question the value of methadone and to look

for other drugs that will act in a similar way but with longer lasting effects. One such promising drug is cyclazocine.

Another method that has been tried is requiring addicts convicted of crimes to join rehabilitation programs. Community drop-in centers and telephone hotlines also have been developed. It appears evident that no one method is a panacea. Rather, what is needed is a multimethod approach, with addicts somehow being directed to the treatment most appropriate for them.

Alternatives to Drugs

There are alternatives to drug abuse that will meet the needs some people seek to meet with drugs. In order to choose one or more of these alternatives, however, you must know yourself.

Recalling how psychosocial factors influence people's health behaviors (Chapter 2), can you now see why people sometimes adopt self-destructive behaviors to alleviate boredom or loneliness, to impress friends, to appear adult, and to feel more self-worth? People who cannot assert their own needs, who feel alienated from society, and who perceive events affecting their lives to be beyond their control may take drugs in spite of the physical harm they know they are risking. As with other health-related behavior, it is not enough for people to *know* about drugs for them to adopt appro-

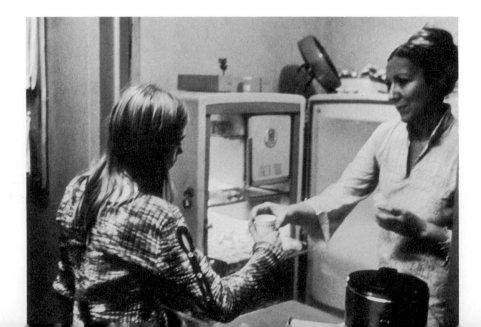

Methadone maintenance as a treatment for heroin addiction has long been controversial. Opponents of this approach contend that the addict simply trades one dependency for another.

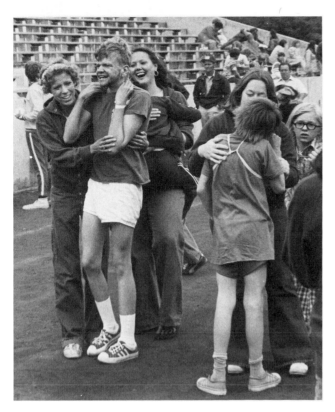

An active involvement in life and a concern for other people can provide a fulfillment not possible with drugs. Here teenage volunteers aid participants in the Special Olympics program for retarded youngsters.

priate drug behavior. Certainly this knowledge is necessary and important. However, the psychosocial influences upon us are so pervasive and so strong that, in addition to the knowledge about drugs, we must have knowledge about ourselves—about our needs and motivations, our perceptions and philosophies, and our goals and desires. Only self-knowledge will allow us to make decisions that are right for us.

Such activities as meditation, exercise, yoga, sky diving, hang gliding, kiting, participation in religion, and social service are alternative ways to feel the "high" or "rush" that drugs provide—only in a health-enhancing manner. Some people get so involved in the Special Olympics, for example, that when they see the thrill on the faces of the young competitors, they feel

Issues in Health
HOW SHOULD SOCIETY DEAL WITH DRUG ADDICTS?

Some states (New York, for one) have decided that drug dealers must be shown that they will be dealt with sternly. Consequently, laws in these states concerning the possession, sale, and manufacture of drugs require jail sentences for those found guilty, with little leeway for plea bargaining. The idea behind these stern laws is to discourage drug activities through the fear of long jail sentences and to prevent lenient judges from circumventing the intent of the laws by making jail sentences mandatory. In many instances, however, those arrested for drug-related offenses are themselves addicted. What should be done with these addicts? Consider the following questions:

1. Should convicted addicts be placed in therapeutic programs of one kind or another, or should they be jailed? Who should decide this?

2. Should any differentiation be made between those just possessing drugs and those selling them?

3. Should either the age of the seller or the age of the purchaser be a consideration?

4. What should be done with the addict caught in a crime such as burglary or prostitution if the crime is designed to support the addiction? Should the addict be arrested and jailed or placed in a program of therapy? ●

high. Others find their work so absorbing that they feel a rush when they've accomplished a job-related goal. Still others report that the experience of learning a new skill or acquiring new knowledge is akin to a drug-induced state.

There are many alternatives to drugs that will hold appeal for you. The trick is to match one of these alternatives to your personality and needs. Only you can do that for you.

CONCLUSION

This chapter has presented information about types of drug-related behavior (use, misuse, and abuse), classification of drugs and their physiological effects, and reasons for the abuse of drugs. Whether or not to use drugs is not the question. Each of us probably ingests drugs, applies drugs to our skin, or has drugs injected into our bodies at one time or another. The question you must answer for yourself is: Considering the presentation made in this chapter and all that you have learned elsewhere, and considering the validity of these sources, how and when will you use drugs? This question is of profound importance, should be given most serious consideration, and should be reconsidered periodically as health scientists learn more about drugs and their effects upon human beings.

Why not take some time *now* to contemplate your drug-related behavior? If you wait until you're confronted with a situation necessitating a decision related to drugs, you may have to make a hasty decision, and a decision made hastily is more likely to be wrong for you than one well thought out.

SUMMARY

1. A drug is any substance whose chemical nature alters structure or function in the living organism.

2. Americans tend to rely on drugs to relieve their anxious feelings, make them happier, and help them to relax.

3. Drug use is the use of a legal drug as recommended by a physician or approved by society. Drug abuse is the use of a chemical substance so as to cause the user serious physiological or psychological harm.

4. The effect of a drug depends on such factors as its interaction with other drugs, the dosage taken, its solubility, and its location of action within the body, and on such individual user characteristics as weight, height, body fat, and personality. In addition, the user's frame of mind and the setting in which the drug is taken affect its action.

5. People can learn to take care of minor health problems at home with a few basic supplies used wisely. The conditions for which self-care are appropriate include colds, coughs, diarrhea, constipation, hemorrhoids, pain, fever, poisoning, and stomach upset. Follow-up care is recommended for some of these conditions, but initially self-care is appropriate.

6. People can become dependent on drugs—psychologically, physiologically, or both. Physical dependence occurs as the user builds up a tolerance to the drug and needs increasingly large dosages to obtain a drug effect. When the drug is discontinued, withdrawal from physiological dependence may be marked by shaking, sweating, and convulsion, and may even lead to coma or death.

7. Psychoactive drugs can be classified as stimulants, depressants, or hallucinogens. Caffeine, amphetamines, and cocaine are examples of stimulant drugs. Barbiturates, tranquilizers, and the opiates are examples of depressant drugs. Marijuana, LSD, and PCP are examples of hallucinogenic drugs.

8. Drug abuse can be caused by alienation, poor self-esteem, lack of confidence, peer pressure, adult modeling, an attempt at coping, or a desire to seek mood alteration.

9. Drug abuse is treated in residential therapeutic communities, in nonresidential therapy programs combined with medical help, by providing pharmacological support (for example, methadone

maintenance), or through a combination of these treatments.

10. Alternatives to getting high on drugs are involvement in family, religion, community service, hang gliding, sky diving, meditation, or some other means appropriate to the individual's personality and needs.

REFERENCES

1. Walter Mondale, "Mass Drug Catastrophes and the Role of Science and Technology," *Science* 21 (1967): 346.

2. Joe Graedon, *The People's Pharmacy-2* (New York: Avon Books, 1980), p. 36.

3. Consumers Union of the United States, Inc., "Caffeine: What It Does," *Consumers Report* 46 (October, 1981): 595–596.

4. Dorothy V. Whipple and Dodi Shultz, "Answers to the Most Controversial Questions About Drugs," *Today's Health* 50 (1972): 16–20, 60, 61.

5. Eileen M. Harris, "A Measurement of Alienation in College Student Marijuana Users and Non-Users," *The Journal of School Health* 41 (1971): 133.

6. Jerrold S. Greenberg, Testimony presented before the New York State Assembly Subcommittee on Drug Control, October 24, 1973.

7. Richard Lannes, Franklin Banks, and Martin Keller, "Smoking Behavior in a Teenage Population: A Multivariate Conceptual Approach," *American Journal of Public Health* 62 (1972): 808.

8. Dorothy Dusek and Daniel A. Girdano, *Drugs: A Factual Account*, 3rd ed. (Reading: Mass.: Addison-Wesley, 1980), p. 9.

Laboratory 1
ATTITUDES TOWARD MARIJUANA*

Purpose   To determine attitudes toward marijuana.

Size of Group   Group of nine students.

Equipment   None.

Procedure

Circle the numbers of *each* of the statements below with which you agree. Make no marks next to those statements with which you disagree.

4.9 149 Smoking marijuana is a requirement for successful living.

4.7 147 Smoking marijuana is necessary if one is to achieve his or her potential.

4.5 145 Smoking marijuana is an excellent way to increase one's understanding of the world about him.

4.3 143 Smoking marijuana is too good a thing to be given up.

4.1 141 Smoking marijuana can be a helpful way of adjusting to the world around us.

3.9 139 A person should be allowed to smoke marijuana if he or she wants to.

3.7 137 Smoking marijuana can be justified.

3.5 135 Smoking marijuana is all right in some cases.

3.3 133 The benefits of smoking marijuana depend entirely upon the individual.

3.1 131 Smoking marijuana is not necessarily wrong.

2.9 129 Smoking marijuana is one way of trying to be different.

2.7 127 Smoking marijuana isn't absolutely bad but it isn't good either.

2.5 125 I question whether or not it is morally right to smoke marijuana.

2.3 123 Smoking marijuana is not a necessary part of life.

2.1 121 Smoking marijuana is an emotional "crutch."

1.9 119 Smoking marijuana is a foolish thing to do.

1.7 117 Smoking marijuana is wrong.

1.5 115 Smoking marijuana is bad.

1.3 113 Smoking marijuana is a foolish way to try to escape reality.

1.1 111 Smoking marijuana shows an utter lack of self-respect.

Now score your responses by figuring out the middle scale value of those statements whose numbers you circled. For example, if you circled numbers 141, 133, 129, 123, 121, your middle scale value would be 2.9 (the scale value next to 129). The statement next to 2.9 would best represent your attitude toward marijuana. If an even number of numbers have been circled, your attitude would best be represented by both the middle statements. This attitude scale runs from a high of 4.9 (highly favorable toward marijuana) to a low of 1.1 (extremely opposed to marijuana). Any scale value between 2.1 and 2.9 is right in the middle of the scale and represents a fairly neutral attitude toward marijuana.

After doing this individually, compute a small-group scale value by averaging all the individual members' scale values.

Next compute a total class scale value by averaging the small-group values.

*Scale derived from Raymond J. Vincent, "A Scale to Measure Attitude Toward Smoking Marijuana," *Journal of School Health* 40 (1970): 454–456. Copyright 1970, American School Health Association, Kent, Ohio 44240.

Results

	Me	My Group	The Class
Lowest scale value			
Highest scale value			
Scale value			

How different is your attitude toward marijuana from that of your group and your class?

Is one's attitude toward marijuana determined *prior to* smoking it or used as a *rationalization* either for smoking or not smoking it?

What do you think the scale values would be for:

Police officers _____

College professors _____

Your best friend _____

Your parents _____ _____

A ten-year-old _____

The authors of this textbook _____

Discuss the above.

Laboratory 2
PEER PRESSURE

Purpose To demonstrate the effect of peer pressure on behavior.

Size of Group Total class.

Equipment None.

Procedure

Have five of your classmates volunteer to bring a friend to class. Tell these five visitors that you want outsiders' opinions regarding drug abuse. The real reason you want them in class, however, is to observe their reaction to the following:

Arrange in advance for the instructor to give a signal (e.g., pulling on his or her earlobe) five minutes after the class has begun that will result in everyone in the class sitting on their desks and facing the back of the room. (If there are no desks, everyone can stand and face the back of the room.) Allow several minutes, as the instructor continues to lecture, for the visitors to react. Probably some of the visitors will eventually do the same as everyone else, while others will stay seated.

Results

1. Number of visitors facing back of room _____

2. Number of visitors staying seated _____

Discuss:

1. Ask the visitors who faced the back of the room why they did so.

2. Ask the visitors who remained seated why they did not face the back of the room.

3. How does this activity pertain to peer pressure and to drug abuse?

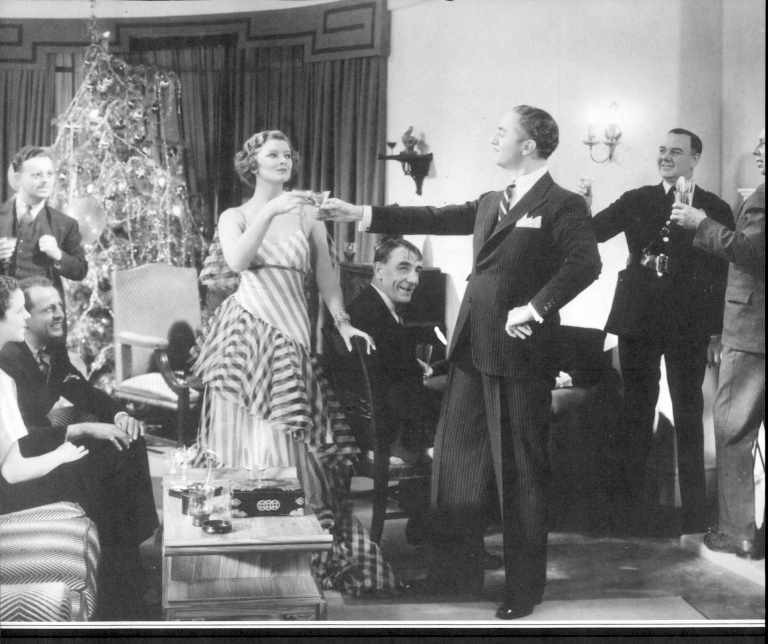

chapter *10*

alcohol and health

- *alcohol in American society*
- *physiological effects of alcohol*
- *alcoholism*

This chapter was written by Dr. Lawrence A. Cappiello, Department of Health Education Professions, State University of New York at Buffalo.

Even though much information is available concerning alcohol and health—both in textbooks and through the mass media—various public and private agencies report that more and more people have problems that are linked with drinking alcohol and that alcoholism is the third leading health problem in this country. Why is alcohol such a widespread problem? What do you need to know in order to avoid the problems associated with alcohol? In this chapter we will attempt to answer these questions and provide information that is essential for you in deciding, first, whether, when, and how you will use alcoholic beverages; and second, what your attitude will be toward those who use alcoholic beverages compulsively—alcoholics.

ALCOHOL IN AMERICAN SOCIETY

One way of outlining the patterns of alcohol consumption in American society and the consequences of alcohol abuse is to consider the findings of a 1981 special report to Congress from the National Institute on Alcohol Abuse and Alcoholism. Among the findings of the report were the following:

- During the 1970s, the nation's apparent consumption of ethanol continued to rise, but the rate of increase slowed considerably. By 1978, apparent consumption had risen to more than 2.7 gallons per year of ethanol per person 14 years of age and older.

- Beer accounts for 49 percent of the ethanol consumed by Americans; wine accounts for 12 percent; and distilled spirits for 39 percent.

- In the heavier drinking category, males (14 percent) outnumber females (4 percent). While 25 percent of males reported abstaining from alcohol, 40 percent of females reported abstaining.

- Heavier drinking appears to peak at age 21–34 for males (19 percent) at age 35–49 for females (8 percent), and to decline thereafter for both sexes.

- While the frequency and quantity of adolescent drinking does not appear to have changed much since the 1974 national survey, the proportion of 10th–12th graders who reported ever having consumed alcohol is very high—87 percent.

- In terms of volume of drinking, in the year prior to the 1978 survey, 25 percent of 10th–12th graders reported abstention, 7.6 reported infrequent drinking and 18.8 percent reported light drinking. Heavier drinkers constituted approximately 15 percent of the sample surveyed.

- Larger number of adolescent females reported abstention while larger numbers of adolescent males reported heavier drinking.[1]

In addition, the report summarizes some of the social implications of alcohol use and abuse:

- In the United States, 10 percent of all deaths are alcohol related, and 10 percent of American adults who drink are either problem drinkers or alcoholics.

- In the United States, traffic accidents are the major cause of violent death. Between 35 and 64 percent of the drivers in fatal accidents had been drinking prior to the accident. Between 45 and 60 percent of all fatal crashes involving a young driver are alcohol related.

- Approximately one-half of adult fire deaths involve alcohol. Alcoholics were found to be 10 times more likely to die in fires compared with the general populations.

- Alcohol plays a significant role in drownings. One study reported that 68 percent of drowning victims had been drinking and another study reported that 50 percent of such victims had been drinking.

- The relationship of alcohol to criminal behavior is complex. However, problem drinkers seem more likely than other offenders to have been drinking prior to or during, the commission of a crime.

- Alcoholics are at particularly high risk of committing suicide. Between 15 and 64 percent of suicide attempters and up to 80 percent of suicides had been drinking at the time of the event. The risk of suicide for alcoholics is as much as 30 times greater than that for the general population.

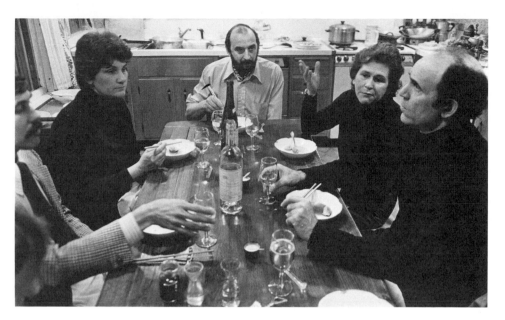

Maturity and personal stability are significant factors contributing to responsible alcohol use.

- Alcohol is related to spouse abuse. Studies of women seeking services for spouse abuse indicate that alcohol consumption by abusing husbands is clearly involved in this subpopulation.

- Problem drinking among adolescents appears to be associated with pessimism, unhappiness, boredom, aggressiveness, frustration, impulsiveness, distrust, cynicism, irresponsibility, inflexibility, and dissatisfaction. Correlations exist between adolescent problem drinking and antisocial or delinquent behavior. Heavier consumption has been linked to precocious sexual behavior, poor school performance, problem behavior in the classroom, number of classes cut from school, problems within the family, other drug use, and higher dropout rates.

- The economic costs of alcoholism and alcohol misuse to the individual and to society are difficult to estimate. In terms of lost production, health care expenditures, motor vehicle accidents, violent crimes, fire losses, and social responses, alcoholism and alcohol misuse have been estimated to cost $42 billion a year.[2]

Societal Factors in Alcohol Use

Concept: Decisions about using alcoholic beverages are subject to multiple influences.

It might sometimes appear as though some of the decisions that we are called on to make have already been made for us, at least in part. In this country when we pull our car into a drive-in for a bite of lunch, we are programmed to expect a flat portion of ground meat placed between two ovals of soft bread. We are further programmed to lift one of those pieces of bread and place a bright red and/or yellow sauce on top of the meat. Our programming goes on, and we find ourselves ordering a flavored, bubbling fluid to drink. We have been programmed by our society to make a meal of the hamburger and soft drink. What this means is that a nutritional decision has been made for us by the tastes and customs of our peers.

In a similar way, society influences our individual decisions concerning the use of alcoholic beverages. Your own first encounter with alcohol probably did not even take the form of an active decision. For many of us, our first drink containing alcohol was handed to us at a social gathering, or we were confronted with a situation where, if we wanted to quench our thirst, the only beverages available were alcoholic drinks. Others were introduced to alcoholic beverages in an even more deeply cultural manner: through rituals associated with ethnic eating habits or religious ceremonies, such as a communion rite or a Bar Mitzvah.

Much has been said about the possible influences of mass advertising on our individual decisions as consumers. Certainly that cannot be downplayed in the case of alcohol. We are constantly exposed to advertising portraying people who drink as young, "with it," popular, and attractive. Many people find this image hard to resist.

We recognize that many people do not drink alcoholic beverages and were just as programmed to that decision as were those who do drink. In both cases, one's parents, church, experiences, and peers have influenced the decision.

Children commonly are first exposed to alcohol within their own family.

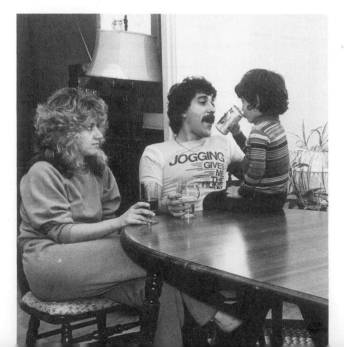

Discovery Activity 10.1
YOUR FIRST DRINK

Can you remember your first alcoholic drink? _____

What was the setting? _____

How old were you? _____

Were you frightened? _____

Were you with your family? _____

Were you sneaky about it?* _____

Were you afraid your folks would find out?* _____

Were you pressured into it?* _____

Were you alone? _____

Most of you have already decided whether or not to drink alcoholic beverages. If you have decided not to:

Have you been embarrassed by that decision? _____

Do you have trouble defending it? _____

Has it restricted your social life? _____

If you classify yourself as a social drinker:

Do you very often not order an alcoholic beverage when the others you are with do? _____

Do you have trouble refusing a drink? _____

If you do have trouble, can you analyze why? _____

Do you ever feel that you really *need* a drink? _____

Do you ever become aware that you change your behavior patterns after a drink or two? _____

As you can see, our alcohol-related behavior (drinking or abstinence) is a function of various influences; and the consequences of that behavior can necessitate coping skills. For example, you must manage the peer pressure either to join others who are drinking or to abstain from drinking. ●

*Note that peer pressure and experimentation are implied here.

PHYSIOLOGICAL EFFECTS OF ALCOHOL

Concept: The part of the drink that affects your behavior is the alcohol.

Determining Alcohol Content in the Body

How often have you heard people say something like, "How can you drink vodka? That stuff really hits me hard." We have probably all known people who claim that one type of drink is, for them, more or less potent than another. Many teenage drinkers prefer beer to other types of alcohol not only because of the price, but also because of the misconception that beer is less likely to cause intoxication than hard liquor. For some reason, the concept we are about to discuss is difficult for people to accept. Maybe if we begin with some simple mathematics it will be helpful.

The most common size bottle or can of beer is 12 fluid ounces. Most beer brewed in the United States is roughly 5 percent alcohol. If we multiply the 12 fluid ounces by the 5 percent alcohol, we find that the amount of alcohol in beer is 0.60 fluid ounces.

The standard wine glass for most restaurants and drinking establishments holds 5 fluid ounces of wine. The alcohol content of wine is determined by the sugar in the grapes and by the fermentation process, with the natural limit at about 12 percent. If we multiply 5 fluid ounces by 12 percent, we find that the amount of alcohol in a glass of wine is 0.60 fluid ounces.

Repeating the procedure for hard liquors (gin, vodka, scotch, bourbon, rye, etc.), we multiply the contents of a standard "shot" (1.5 fluid ounces) by the percentage of alcohol in the drink (one-half its proof, as stated on the label). Thus, one shot of an 80 proof bourbon whiskey translates to 1.5 × 0.40, or 0.60 fluid ounces of alcohol.

These calculations show that we are only fooling ourselves if we think that one type of drink is less potent than the others; each contains roughly the same amount of alcohol. Obviously, if you drink an 8-ounce rather than a 12-ounce beer, or a small glass of wine, or a whiskey of lower proof, you will reduce the amount of alcohol ingested. However, the fact is that anyone who drinks beer or wine as a protection against intoxication is making a decision based on misconception. It is the alcohol that intoxicates, and we ingest just about the same amount, whichever of the three drinks we choose.

Some information concerning the so-called light beers is called for here. These beers are characterized by reduced calorie content; some have only half or fewer than half the calories of the regular product of the same brewer. The advertising strongly implies that because it has fewer calories, light beer can be consumed in greater quantity than regular beer. You should keep in mind that although the calories have been reduced significantly, the alcohol content has not. People who drink a greater quantity of light beer may not get as fat, but they get just as drunk.

Another problem with drinking beer and ale as a means of reducing the alcohol one consumes is that the consumer has no way of knowing the actual alcohol content of the product, except in those few states allowed to sell "3.2 beer" (beer containing no more than 3.2 percent alcohol). The brewer is prohibited by federal regulations from stating the alcohol content of the product, and although there is a tax on the alcohol, that tax is levied on a per-barrel basis. Nevertheless, most experts agree that beer is in the 4 to 5 percent alcohol range.

Absorption and Metabolism

Concept: The roles of absorption and metabolism control the intoxication process.

Alcohol is absorbed directly into the bloodstream through the walls of the stomach and the small intestine. Once in the bloodstream, between 80 and 90 percent of the alcohol is metabolized (broken down chemically) by the liver. What is not metabolized may travel to the brain before it is eventually eliminated from the body.

It is true that you can slow down the absorption of alcohol by eating immediately before and/or while

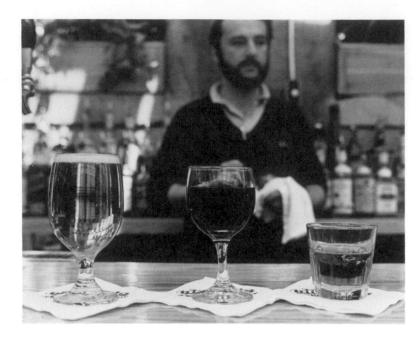

A twelve ounce glass of beer, a five ounce glass of wine, and a shot glass of distilled liquor: which drink is most potent? (See text.)

drinking. The problem, however, is that only a small percentage of alcohol is absorbed through the stomach wall; the major portion is absorbed through the wall of the small intestine. In any event, the alcohol does not disappear; it merely takes a bit longer to be absorbed.

It is important to understand the relationship between the liver's rate of metabolizing alcohol and the amount of alcohol in the bloodstream. Unlike many drugs, alcohol is metabolized at a relatively slow, constant rate, regardless of the amount consumed. Thus, drinking coffee, running around the block, taking a cold shower, and other efforts people use to "sober up" have no effect on the rate of alcohol metabolism.

The most important factor in determining what effect alcohol will have on a person's behavior is **blood alcohol level (BAL)**. This refers to the concentration of alcohol in the blood that is carried to the brain. If the alcohol is absorbed more rapidly than it is metabolized, intoxication will occur. These symptoms of intoxication will not begin to disappear until the intake of alcohol stops and the liver has time to metabolize the alcohol

remaining in the bloodstream and in all other water-bearing parts of the body. Thus, *time* is the essential ingredient in the sobering-up process.

Effects of Different Blood Alcohol Concentrations

Concept: Small differences in blood alcohol concentrations make big differences in our reactions.

These effects can be illustrated by a discussion of drinking and driving.

A blood alcohol concentration of .10 percent is evidence of driving while intoxicated in all but two states (Utah and Idaho, where it is 0.08 percent). "The alcohol in two 12-ounce beers consumed in an hour or less can slow a driver's reaction time by two-fifths of a second. An automobile going 60 miles per hour travels 34 feet in two-fifths of a second—possibly the difference between a near miss and a crash."[4] Furthermore, "When BAL (blood alcohol level) reaches 0.06 percent the probability of causing an accident is twice that of alcohol-free drivers, at 0.10 the probability is 6 times greater; at 0.15 the probability has risen to 25 times; and at 0.18 percent the driver is 60 times more likely to be responsible for a fatal accident than if he had not been drinking at all."[5]

Carlson[6] and Waller[7] have shown that age and experience are important factors in drinking and au-tomobile accidents. They point out that young drivers have accidents when they have relatively low concentrations of blood alcohol. Both researchers attribute this finding to young people's inexperience as drivers and as drinkers. A general description of the effects of alcohol can be found in Table 10.1. Depending on the amount of alcohol consumed, there may be no overt effects, a sense of relaxation, slower reaction to stimuli, decreased muscular coordination, blurred vision, slurred

Table 10.1

PSYCHOLOGICAL AND PHYSICAL EFFECTS OF VARIOUS BLOOD ALCOHOL CONCENTRATION LEVELS[a]

Number of Drinks per Hour[b]	Blood Alcohol Concentration (%)	Psychological and Physical Effects
1	0.02–0.03	No overt effects, slight feeling of muscle relaxation, slight mood elevation.
2	0.05–0.06	No intoxication, but feeling of relaxation, warmth. Slight increase in reaction time, slight decrease in fine muscle coordination.
3	0.08–0.09	Balance, speech, vision, and hearing slightly impaired. Feelings of euphoria. Increased loss of motor coordination.
4	0.11–0.12	Coordination and balance becoming difficult. Distinct impairment of mental facilities, judgment, etc.
5	0.14–0.15	Major impairment of mental and physical control. Slurred speech, blurred vision, lack of motor skill. Legal intoxication in all states (0.15%).
7	0.20	Loss of motor control—must have assistance in moving about. Mental confusion.
10	0.30	Severe intoxication. Minimum conscious control of mind and body.
14	0.40	Unconsciousness, threshold of coma.
17	0.50	Deep coma.
20	0.60	Death from respiratory failure.

[a]For each one-hour time lapse, 0.015% blood alcohol concentration, or approximately one drink.
[b]The typical drink—three-fourths of an ounce of alcohol—is provided by:

- a shot of spirits (1.5 oz of 50-percent alcohol—100-proof whiskey or vodka);
- a glass of fortified wine (3.5 oz of 20-percent alcohol);
- a larger glass of table wine (5 oz of 14-percent alcohol);
- a pint of beer (16 oz of 4.5-percent alcohol).

SOURCE: Dorothy Dusek and Daniel A. Girdano, *Drugs: A Factual Account*, 3rd ed. (Reading, Mass.: Addison-Wesley, 1980), p. 49.

speech, lack of balance, impaired judgment, and lack of motor skills. Extremely high levels of blood alcohol can result in loss of motor control, mental confusion, unconsciousness, coma, or even death.

Alcohol and Drugs

The relationship between the use of small amounts of alcohol and certain gastrointestinal conditions is well known. The same is true for certain cardiovascular conditions. For example, ulcers can be aggravated by alcohol. Although some research indicates that consumption of one ounce of alcohol a day is more common among those without coronary heart disease than among those with it, excessive alcohol consumption is harmful to individuals with poor hearts and/or circulatory problems.

Fetal Alcohol Syndrome

Physicians have recently drawn attention to the **fetal alcohol syndrome**, a condition found in babies born to women who are heavy users of alcohol. Babies born with fetal alcohol syndrome have low birth weight, stunted growth, and various anatomical defects; some are mentally retarded.

A recent study at the University of Washington suggests that not only heavy but moderate drinking creates a dangerous environment for the unborn child. The study was concerned with daily consumption rates of as little as one ounce of absolute alcohol, which, according to our earlier calculations, can be translated to as few as two drinks per day. According to the findings of this study, ". . . daily consumption of one ounce of absolute alcohol before pregnancy is associated with a decrease in birth weight of 91 grams. One ounce consumed in late pregnancy is associated with a decrease in birth weight of 160 grams."[8]

Earlier studies of the fetal alcohol syndrome viewed the nutritional status of the mother as a possible factor; the Washington study points the finger directly at alcohol consumption. Important questions are now being raised concerning blood alcohol content at the time of conception and during the first trimester of pregnancy. The safest course of action for pregnant women is to abstain from alcohol during pregnancy.

Using Alcohol Responsibly

In our discussion of the physiological effects of alcohol, we pointed out that responsible drinking requires that you learn how much alcohol you can drink without reaching a high blood alcohol level. Using alcoholic beverages responsibly also involves deciding when it is appropriate to drink, drinking in moderation, and showing concern for the health and safety of others who are with you. The following list provides some guidelines that you may find useful when you are serving alcohol in your own home and when you are attending a party or other activity where alcoholic beverages are being served.

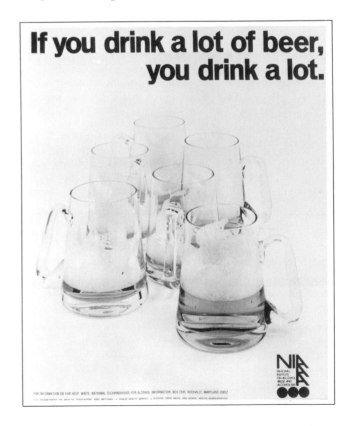

If you drink a lot of beer, you drink a lot.

1. Use alcohol as an adjunct to an activity rather than the primary purpose.
2. Set a limit as to the number of drinks you are going to drink.
3. Know your limit and stick to it.
4. Respect a person who chooses not to drink.
5. Provide alternative beverages at your party.
6. Serve food with alcoholic beverages.
7. Show displeasure to someone who has drunk too much.
8. Do not be insistent about refilling or refreshing someone's drink.
9. Make sure alcohol is used carefully in connection with other drugs.
10. Take a taxi, ask for a ride, or stay over at a friend's if you are in no condition to drive, and insist that others for whom you are responsible do the same.

ALCOHOLISM

> **Concept:** Alcoholics are persons whose use of alcohol creates physical, personality, and/ or social problems in their lives.

Those individuals who do not, or cannot, exercise control over their drinking behavior become problem drinkers. They may ultimately become **alcoholics** if their drinking interferes with or disrupts major areas of their life on a continuing basis. Each of us, as we read this, probably has someone we know well in mind. Before you read on, respond to the categories in the activity.

Factors Contributing to Alcoholism

Alcoholism has always been regarded as a serious problem in our society, but only in recent decades have attitudes begun to change regarding the factors contributing to alcoholism. During the nineteenth and early

Discovery Activity 10.2
WHO IS MOST LIKELY TO BE AN ALCOHOLIC?

What is your perception of the person who is likely to have alcohol-related problems? Fill in the blanks below based only on your personal opinion.

Age: _____

Sex: _____

Ethnic background: _____

Marital status: _____

Employment status: _____

Educational status: _____

Socioeconomic status: _____

Wine drinker: _____

Beer drinker: _____

Hard liquor drinker: _____

Residence (urban, rural): _____

Later in the chapter you'll find a table that profiles persons who are and are not most likely to have alcohol-related problems. Compare the table with your responses above. ●

twentieth centuries, most people who opposed alcohol use believed that alcoholics were morally weak. It was this perception that helped give rise to the prohibition of the sale of alcoholic beverages from 1919 to 1933. Today there is much greater awareness of the complexity of this disorder:

> We now know that alcoholism involves an interplay of biological, behavioral, and cultural components within the individuals who are afflicted. We have come to understand that alcoholism involves biological factors, either as etiological indicators or as biomedical consequences, and that psychological and

sociocultural factors enter in as well. The interaction of these components, varying as they do from individual to individual, further deepens the complexity of this disease and makes it quite unlike any other.[9]

Let's take a look at some of the factors that contribute to alcohol-related problems.

Personality disturbance.   "The common description of the alcoholic given by those who work in the rehabilitation process is a frustrated, fearful, self-punishing, immature person. *Incidentally*, that person also uses alcohol to excess."[10] The position held by many psychiatrists is that alcohol abuse is a symptom of personality disorder; it is the person's way of seeking relief. "He seeks relief in drinking as opposed to other symptoms of acting out. As he becomes increasingly dependent upon it he becomes addicted to it, so that he has a physiologic, as well as psychological, need for drink."[11]

The personality factors identified as typical of the problem drinker are also characteristics that would cause an individual to come under stress in a social or cultural situation. The conflict between societal and personal goals and expectations, cultural differences that may tend to place a person apart from the immediate population, or attitudes toward the act of drinking may bring about the stressful situations from which relief is sought.

Physiological factors.   Among current studies of the possible physiological determinants of various types of addiction, including alcohol addiction, research concerning the possibility of inherited differences and differences in the functioning of the endocrine system bears watching. This research focuses on the ability of the body to produce the enzyme necessary for alcohol metabolism. It is well documented that children of alcoholics are more likely to become alcoholics themselves than are children of nonalcoholics. One possible cause of this relationship is a physiologically inherited trait in alcoholism. However, some experts contend that alcoholism runs in families because of the family environment and that therefore alcoholism is sociologically rather than physiologically determined.

Sociocultural correlates.   Certain factors in alcoholism are referred to in the literature as sociocultural correlates. The National Institute on Alcohol Abuse and Alcoholism (NIAAA) states that, "Among such factors are sex, age, ethnic background, religious affiliation, education, socioeconomic status, occupation, and area of residence and degree of urbanization."[12] These factors alone or in combination, and the psychological factors already mentioned, may lead to problem drinking and alcoholism. Some of the sociocultural correlates are described below.

1. *Sex.* Surveys representative of the total population of men and women in the United States, from abstainers to heavy drinkers, have found that men are three times more likely to become heavy drinkers than women are. "The highest proportion of heavier drinkers occurred among men aged 18 to 20 and 35 to 39. Women aged 21 to 29 had the highest proportion of heavier drinkers."[13] However, the NIAAA reports that more and more adult women are now drinking and that this number has been steadily increasing since World War II.

Some years ago, it was generally accepted that one in five alcoholics would be female. Today, those who work in the rehabilitation field are revising this estimate. They believe that the number of female alcoholics is rapidly approaching the number of male alcoholics, and some say that there will soon be statistical parity.

In the 1981 special report to the Congress[14] the NIAAA cited several research studies that point to changing sex roles as a key factor in alcoholism among women. These studies found that employed women and employed married women had higher rates of problem drinking than women who were homemakers with no outside employment or who were single and employed. Perhaps the stress encountered in the work place, combined with responsibilities at home, creates intense pressures on many women, who seek solace in alcohol. Some women may also drink out of loneliness or feelings of inferiority caused by the lower status of women in our society.

2. *Age.* NIAAA also cites surveys showing that the greatest number of drinkers are in their early twenties;

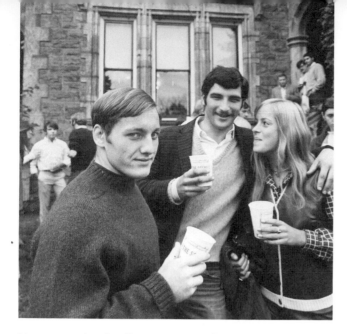

Young people of college age report high levels of drinking. What factors do you think influence them to use alcohol?

moreover, "18 to 20-year-olds reported the highest levels of frequent consumption of five or six drinks at an occasion."[15]

NIAAA states that the greatest percentage of male drinkers were in the 18–20 age group, whereas the highest percentage of female drinkers were in the 21–23 age group, with a relatively steady decline in drinking as age increased.[16]

As a class exercise, you might discuss the possible reasons that young people in these age ranges apparently consume more alcohol. We suggest that socialization and recreational drinking are two probable causes; that is, people in early adulthood drink in social situations, such as at dating bars and discos, and there is considerable peer pressure to drink among this age group. As these young people grow older, perhaps they grow more independent and may not perceive drinking as such an important part of being accepted by others.

3. *Ethnic background.* Many years ago, researchers in alcoholism noted that there were rather dramatic differences in rates of alcoholism among certain white ethnic groups. It was commonly reported that the rate of alcoholism among men of Irish extraction was many times greater than the rate among men from countries

Issues in Health
SHOULD WE BRING BACK PROHIBITION?

It has been suggested that the number of people who have problems associated with alcohol is rising dramatically, and recent studies suggest that even moderate use of alcohol can be dangerous to our health. Therefore, it may be time again to institute a national prohibition against the manufacture and use of alcoholic beverages.

Advocates of this view cite statistics concerning employment difficulties, domestic relations, child and other abuse, accidents, the number of alcoholics, and the decreasing age at which problem drinking begins as proof that we are unable to be responsible in our use of alcoholic beverages.

Others state that when one analyzes the statistics concerning alcohol-related problems against all those who use alcoholic beverages, it becomes clear that only a very small percentage of those who drink ever have trouble. The many should not be inconvenienced for the benefit of the few. In addition, our present experience with laws concerning drug abuse and our past experience with prohibition prove that such laws are unrealistic.

What do you think? ●

bordering the Mediterranean Sea, and alcoholism was almost unknown among Jews. "Alcoholism and problem-drinking rates tend to be low among those groups whose drinking habits are well integrated with the rest of their culture. It is, therefore, not surprising that ethnic background and generational status are important determinants of drinking patterns in the United States."[17]

The introduction of the act of drinking alcohol as a family-centered activity, or as part of a religious observance or ceremony seems to be very important. The degree to which the family group and the societal circle accept or reject recreational drinking and intoxication evidently affects people's attitudes. A society sends a message to its children by the way it uses alcohol and by its tolerance of intoxication.

Among ethnic groups, Native Americans appear to have the highest prevalence of drinking problems. The NIAAA found that for this group, five of the ten major causes of death are alcohol-related: accidents, cirrhosis of the liver, alcoholism, suicide, and homicide. The major factor implicated in serious alcohol problems among Native Americans seems to be the displacement from tradition and culture that they have suffered throughout American history.

Regarding racial differences in drinking patterns, the NIAAA found that blacks of both sexes reported relatively high rates of abstention from alcohol. Among black adults who drink, the proportion of self-reported heavy drinkers was similar to the proportions among other groups.[18] The higher rate of abstention among blacks seems to be associated with several sociological variables, including lower average economic status, lower average educational level, lower average occupation, and higher proportion of membership in conservative Protestant churches.[19]

4. *Education and economic level.* The NIAAA has also reported that educational and socioeconomic levels are important factors in drinking behavior. The higher a group is on those scales, the heavier the drinking.[20] This relationship may be explained by stress and opportunity. More highly educated individuals tend to have jobs involving substantial responsibility and therefore high levels of stress. In addition, they have money to support heavy drinking, as well as many job-related social opportunities to drink. High income itself can be stressful in that the more money one earns, the more painful the thought of losing that income.

Now that you have read about some of the major factors in alcohol abuse, take a moment to study Table 10.2, which gives profiles of those persons most and least likely to have alcohol-related problems. Does your description written in Activity 10.2 fit the description of the problem drinker in Table 10.2? What stereotypes of the alcoholic have you found that you hold? Use the discrepancy, if there is any, between your description and Table 10.2 to uncover these stereotypes.

Table 10.2
PROFILES OF POTENTIAL PROBLEM AND NONPROBLEM DRINKERS

Profile of Persons with High Rates of Alcohol-Related Problems

Males at low socioeconomic levels

Separated, single, and divorced persons

Persons with no religious affiliation, followed by Catholics and liberal Protestants

Those with childhood disjunctions

Beer drinkers, as opposed to hard liquor drinkers

Persons who believe that drunkenness is not a sign of irresponsibility

Residents of large cities

Profile of Those Most Likely Not to Have Alcohol-Related Problems

Persons over 50

Widowed or married

Jewish religious affiliation

Rural residents

Residents of southern states

Wine drinkers

Persons with postgraduate education

SOURCE: U.S. Department of Health, Education, and Welfare, National Institute of Mental Health, *Alcohol and Health* (Washington, D.C.: Government Printing Office, 1978).

Stages in the Development of Alcoholism

Concept: There are recognizable stages in the development of problem drinking and alcoholism.

The vast majority of individuals who have trouble handling alcohol arrived at their present stage of drinking behavior after a long period of drinking. Alcoholism is not the type of condition that happens today because of a decision someone did or did not make yesterday, last week, last month, or even last year. It is a gradual process that begins with social drinking and culminates—sometimes decades later—in an addictive drinking pattern that eventually controls most aspects of the individual's life.

As outlined by Dusek and Girdano, alcoholism generally develops in four phases: the prealcoholic phase, the early alcoholic phase, the true alcoholic phase, and complete alcoholic dependence.[21] During the first three phases the drinker's tolerance to alcohol steadily increases, whereas it dramatically decreases in stage four.

The prealcoholic phase is characterized by social drinking (controlled drinking in social situations, such as parties and eating out). The pattern evolves into drinking occasionally to escape from tensions and eventually into using alcohol more and more frequently as an escape from tension and frustration.

During the early alcoholic phase, drinking itself becomes a more and more important event. The very act of drinking—going to places where drinking takes place rather than to places where one knows it will not, socializing with people who drink rather than with those who do not, planning for the drinking part of a social or recreational event rather than the event itself—becomes a pattern to the point where the drinker is uncomfortable in nondrinking situations and will seek out a drinking situation as a substitute.

One of the most important signs of the early alcoholic phase is **blackout**, that is, the loss of memory of what occurred in a drinking situation. This loss of memory may or may not be associated with intoxication. The individual may have difficulty remembering who the drinking partners were, where the drinking took place, what events occurred while drinking, who drove, etc. These blackouts may be of short or long duration.

Problem drinkers and alcoholics who undergo treatment commonly state that blackouts occurred very early in their drinking careers, often during their earliest contacts with alcohol. For this reason we have come to look on the blackout in alcoholism as one would look at a lump in breast cancer or shortness of breath in heart disease. It is a sign that should be taken very seriously. In relation to alcoholism, it is the sign that tells one to learn to live without the use of alcohol.

During the true alcoholic phase, alcohol comes to dominate the drinker's life. Family relationships begin to deteriorate because of the drinking, and family members may try to reorganize their lives to avoid confrontations with the alcoholic and isolate him or her from the family. As a result, the alcoholic is likely to feel self-pity and turn to alcohol for consolation. At this point the alcoholic generally cannot stop after one drink. It is this element of need or compulsion that separates the alcoholic from other heavy drinkers. The alcoholic feels that drinking is essential, that it is the most important part of life.

The final stage, complete alcoholic dependence, is characterized by physiological addiction such that if the drinker does not have alcohol he or she is likely to experience severe withdrawal symptoms. The alcoholic at this stage is physically in danger from poor nutrition and possible liver and brain tissue damage. Without medical and psychological help, the alcoholic may die prematurely.

We must reiterate that these stages take several years to unfold, and that in most cases they represent such a gradual evolution that they do not spell trouble to the individual, friends, or family. Of course, like everything else in the human dimension, these stages do not apply to every case of alcoholism. Some problem drinkers exhibit the symptoms of later stages in the earliest part of their drinking careers.

Discovery Activity 10.3
SIGNS OF ALCOHOLISM*

1. Do you occasionally drink heavily after a disappointment, a quarrel, or when the boss gives you a hard time? _____

2. When you have trouble or feel under pressure, do you always drink more heavily than usual? _____

3. Have you noticed that you are able to handle more liquor than you did when you were first drinking? _____

4. Did you ever wake up the "morning after" and discover that you could not remember part of the evening before, even though your friends tell you that you did not "pass out"? _____

5. When drinking with other people, do you try to have a few extra drinks when others will not know it? _____

6. Are there certain occasions when you feel uncomfortable if alcohol is not available? _____

7. Have you recently noticed that when you begin drinking you are in more of a hurry to get the first drink than you used to be? _____

8. Do you sometimes feel a little guilty about your drinking? _____

9. Are you secretly irritated when your family or friends discuss your drinking? _____

10. Have you recently noticed an increase in the frequency of your memory blackouts? _____

11. Do you often find that you wish to continue drinking after your friends say that they have had enough? _____

12. Do you usually have a reason for drinking heavily on certain occasions? _____

*©1982 by the National Council on Alcoholism, Inc. Reproduced by written permission only.

13. When you are sober, do you often regret things you have done or said while drinking? _____

14. Have you tried switching brands or following different plans for controlling your drinking? _____

15. Have you often failed to keep the promises you have made to yourself about controlling or cutting down on your drinking? _____

16. Have you ever tried to control your drinking by changing jobs or moving to a new location? _____

17. Do you try to avoid family or close friends while you are drinking? _____

18. Are you having an increasing number of financial and work problems? _____

19. Do more people seem to be treating you unfairly without good reason? _____

20. Do you eat very little or irregularly when you are drinking? _____

21. Do you sometimes have the "shakes" in the morning and find that it helps to have a small drink? _____

22. Have you recently noticed that you cannot drink as much as you once did? _____

23. Do you sometimes stay drunk for several days at a time? _____

24. Do you sometimes feel very depressed and wonder whether life is worth living? _____

25. After periods of drinking, do you sometimes see or hear things that aren't there? _____

26. Do you get terribly frightened after you have been drinking heavily? _____

Those who answer "yes" to *any* questions may have some symptoms of alcoholism. "Yes" answers to *several* of the questions indicate these stages of alcoholism:

Questions 1–8: early alcoholic phase,

Questions 9–21: true alcoholic phase,

Questions 22–26: complete dependence phase. ●

If you recognize these signs in yourself or in others, you have arrived at a point where you have to make a health decision. If it is your own drinking behavior that is in question, you will have to seek help. If it is another person's drinking behavior you are concerned about, you will have to consider what role you will play in giving help. There are agencies in your community to provide help. In addition to **Alcoholics Anonymous**, a fellowship of recovering alcoholics dedicated to helping others recover, your local telephone book will lead you to various mental health and other agencies that will work with you. Not the least among these will be your own physician or health care facility.

This discussion of the progression of alcoholism should help those of you who have no problem with alcohol to see that those who do are ill and that they need understanding and help with their illness. For you it is a decision of attitude; for those who have the problem it is a decision of action.

Alcoholism and the Family

Concept: Alcoholism is a family disease.

You may have firsthand knowledge of the disruption to a family unit in which one member is an alcoholic. Whether the family unit consists only of husband and wife or includes children or other relatives as well, the disruption and resulting problems are so great that some authors refer to such units as **co-alcoholic**.[22] The family members are so intertwined with the alcoholic that they are unable to escape and feel trapped and helpless.

Family members typically experience feelings of guilt, alternately blaming the alcoholic, for disrupting the family, and themselves, individually or collectively ("What have I done that caused this to happen?").

The question of cause and effect is a difficult one. Is the stress of family responsibility or the inability to

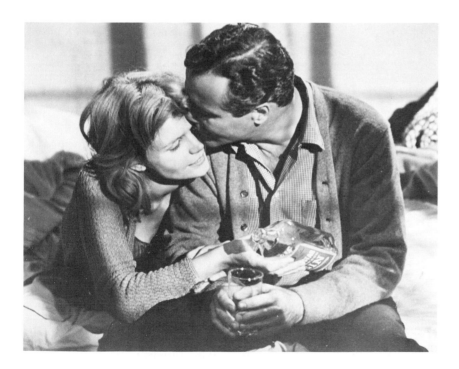

The film "Days of Wine and Roses" poignantly depicts the disintegration of a loving marriage because of alcoholism.

SHOULD DRUNK DRIVERS BE DEALT WITH MORE SEVERELY?

National citizens groups have been established to reform laws and court practices relating to driving while intoxicated. RID (Remove Intoxicated Drivers) and MADD (Mothers Against Drunk Drivers)* were formed as a reaction to the many deaths and injuries caused by drunken drivers on parole, awaiting trial, or recently imprisoned for a similar offense. Advocates of more severe penalties for drunk drivers cite the statistic that half of all driving accidents involve a person who is under the influence of alcohol. The only way to prevent these accidents—and the death and injury they cause—is to lock up drunk drivers so that they cannot cause other accidents. Certainly, they argue, repeat offenders ought to be treated in this manner.

Opponents of more severe treatment for drunk drivers believe alcoholism is an illness that requires treatment, not imprisonment. Better methods of referring drunk drivers to treatment programs and more effective means of treating alcoholism are the answers, they continue, not jail sentences. Further, drunk drivers have families as well as do their victims. What of the consequences to the alcoholic's family when deprived of his or her economic support, love, and presence? Opponents of stricter penalties for drunk drivers argue that the best way to prevent subsequent drunk driving is to treat the alcoholic with the help and support of the family rather than separating them by jailing the drunk driver.

What do you think? ●

*RID, P.O. Box 520, Schenectady, New York 12301. MADD, California 95628.

cope with family life actually the cause of the drinking problem? Or did the problem exist already and became associated with family life simply by virtue of the progressive nature of the disease? No matter which position one takes, it is now common practice to include the immediate family in therapy; that is, to see the alcoholic as a member of a family unit that both affects and is affected by the alcoholic. The reason for this is suggested in the following passage:

> The fact that alcoholics live with, or in some important way are in contact with significant others is only one dimension of the rationale for looking to family therapy for help in treating alcoholism. Along more functional dimensions, all aspects of family life are compromised when a member of the family is abusing alcohol. The marital relationships, parents and often the development of the children suffer.[23]

Separation and divorce are very common in marriages in which one partner is an alcoholic. The result may be difficult for children, especially if the parent who retains custody of the children is the alcoholic.[24,25]

Are children of alcoholic parents likely to become alcoholic? Although there is no hard evidence for genetic factors in alcoholism, some researchers believe heredity might contribute to the disease. What the experts do agree on is that in many cases it is very difficult for a child to develop normally in an alcoholic home. Children who face aggression, abuse, or rejection from the alcoholic parent and overprotection from the nonalcoholic parent may have trouble developing the self-esteem necessary to lead a happy and productive life. For these reasons, experts commonly refer to the children of alcoholics as being *predisposed* to alcoholism.

Treatment of Alcoholism

Alcoholism is a complex problem requiring careful analysis of its development in each individual. Standard treatment regimes can relieve the physical (physiological) problems that are associated with or may accompany the illness. They relieve the symptoms, but they do not eliminate the disease.

Modern treatment programs make a step-by-step analysis of the factors contributing to alcoholism (personality, physiology, and sociocultural correlates) with the aim of helping the alcoholic readjust his or her life to control the need for alcohol. For example, **antabuse**—a drug that causes nausea when alcohol is subsequently ingested—has been used in attempting to control drinking behavior. Individual and group counseling programs and family therapy programs can sometimes offer effective treatment. Programs of inpatient hospital care offer a combination of treatments.

We have already mentioned Alcoholics Anonymous, a self-help organization for alcoholics. Since its founding in the late 1930s, this organization—along with groups subsequently patterned on it, Alanon for the family and friends of alcoholics and Alateen for children of alcoholics—has been the single most important factor in the recovery of thousands of alcoholics. The twelve steps of AA describe the approach that is used:

1. We admitted we were powerless over alcohol—that our lives had become unmanageable.

2. Came to believe that a Power greater than ourselves could restore us to sanity.

3. Made a decision to turn our will and our lives over to the care of God *as we understood Him*.

4. Made a searching and fearless moral inventory of ourselves.

5. Admitted to God, to ourselves and to another human being the exact nature of our wrongs.

6. Were entirely ready to have God remove all these defects of character.

7. Humbly asked Him to remove our shortcomings.

8. Made a list of all persons we had harmed, and became willing to make amends to them all.

9. Made direct amends to such people wherever possible, except when to do so would injure them or others.

10. Continued to take personal inventory and when we were wrong promptly admitted it.

11. Sought through prayer and meditation to improve our conscious contact with God, *as we under-stood Him*, praying only for knowledge of His will for us and the power to carry that out.

12. Having had a spiritual awakening as the result of these steps, we tried to carry this message to alcoholics, and to practice these principles in all our affairs.

One very important factor to keep in mind: It is generally accepted by those involved in alcoholism therapy that alcoholics do not truly recover from their illness; that is, they can never expect to return to social drinking. Their recovery is dependent on total and continuing abstinence from alcohol.

CONCLUSION

In the final analysis, we have to think about what kind of family members we are or are going to be. We have to take a close look at how we treat other people, how we respond to the needs of others for security, friendship, and understanding. The important question is not how much, or even when and how a person drinks, but *why* a person drinks. We have discussed some of these reasons, or at least some of the factors that may lie behind those reasons. By regulating our attitudes and relations to others, each of us may be able to promote those conditions that help people to cope better with their lives and to develop a sound base for growth and development.

SUMMARY

1. By 1978, annual consumption of ethanol had risen to more than 2.7 gallons per person 14 years of age or older.

2. Beer accounts for 49 percent of the ethanol consumed by Americans, wine accounts for 12 percent, and distilled spirits for 39 percent.

3. Between 35 and 64 percent of the drivers in fatal automobile accidents had been drinking prior to the accident.

4. The media and advertising, social gatherings, cultural rituals, and peer pressure influence drinking behavior.

5. Beer and wine are no less likely to cause intoxication than hard liquor. It is the alcohol that intoxicates, and the alcohol content in a 12-ounce bottle of beer is equivalent to that in one shot (1.5 fluid ounces) of an 80-proof whiskey.

6. Once in the bloodstream, between 80 and 90 percent of the alcohol is metabolized by the liver. What is not metabolized may travel to the brain before it is eventually eliminated from the body.

7. Depending on the amount of alcohol consumed, its effects on the body can range from no overt effects to a sense of relaxation, slower reaction time, impaired judgment, blurred vision, poor motor coordination, coma, and even death.

8. Those *most* likely to have problems with their consumption of alcohol include males, unmarried individuals, those with no religious affiliation, and residents of large cities.

9. Those *least* likely to have problems with consumption of alcohol include people over 50 years of age, those who are widowed or married, those of Jewish religious affiliation, rural residents, and those with a postgraduate education.

10. Alcoholism generally develops in four phases: the prealcoholic phase, the early alcoholic phase, the true alcoholic phase, and complete alcoholic dependency.

REFERENCES

1. U.S. Department of Health and Human Services, *Fourth Special Report to the United States Congress on Alcohol and Health*, DHHS Pub. No. (ADM) 81–1080 (Washington, D.C.: Government Printing Office, 1981), p. 1.

2. Ibid.

3. Ibid., p. ix.

4. James L. Malfetti, Esther A. McGrath, and Angelo G. DeMeo, *Instructor's Manual-DWI Mini-Course for High School Driver Education Programs* (New York Teachers College Press, Columbia University, 1976), p. 41.

5. Ibid., p. 44.

6. William L. Carlson, "Age, Exposure, and Alcohol Involvement in Night Crashes," *Journal of Safety Research* 5(4) (1973): 247–259.

7. Julian A. Waller, "Factors Associated with Alcohol Responsibility for Fatal Highway Crashes," *Quarterly Journal of Studies on Alcohol* 33 (1) (1972): 160–170.

8. Ruth E. Little, "Moderate Alcohol Use During Pregnancy and Decreased Infant Birth Weight," *American Journal of Public Health* 67 (12) (1977): 1154–1156.

9. U.S. Department of Health and Human Services, *Fourth Special Report to the United States Congress on Alcohol and Health*.

10. Lawrence A. Cappiello, "Prevention of Alcoholism—A Teaching Strategy," *Journal of Drug Education* 7 (4) (1977): 311–316.

11. J. R. Ewalt and D. J. Farnsworth, *Textbook of Psychiatry* (New York: McGraw-Hill, 1963), pp. 137–138.

12. U.S. Department of Health and Human Services, *Second Special Report to the United States Congress on Alcohol and Health* DHEW Pub. No. (ADM) 74–124 (Washington, D.C.: Government Printing Office, 1974).

13. Ibid., p. 12.

14. U.S. Department of Health and Human Services, *Fourth Special Report to the United States Congress on Alcohol and Health*.

15. Ibid., p. 15.

16. Ibid., p. 20.

17. U.S. Department of Health and Human Services, *Second Special Report to the United States Congress on Alcohol and Health*, p. 15.

18. U.S. Department of Health, Education and Welfare, *First Special Report to the U.S. Congress on Alcohol and Health*, DHEW Pub. No. (HSM) 72–9099 (Washington, D.C.: Government Printing Office, 1971).

19. Ibid., pp. 24–25.

20. U.S. Department of Health and Human Services, *Second Special Report to the United States Congress on Alcohol and Health*, pp. 16–18.

21. Dorothy Dusek and Daniel A. Girdano, *Drugs: A Factual Account*, 3rd ed. (Reading, Mass.: Addison-Wesley, 1980).

22. Stephanie A. Leary, "The Co-Alcoholic: Hostage in the Home?" *Alcoholism* 1 (1) (1980): 9–10.

23. William E. Fann *et al.*, *Phenomenology and Treatment of Alcoholism* (New York: SP Medical and Scientific Books, 1980), p. 112.

24. Jim Orford and Griffith Edwards, *Alcoholism*, (Maudsley Monographs, No. 26) (New York: Oxford University Press, 1977).

25. Vasanti Burtle, ed., *Women Who Drink* (Springfield, Ill.: Charles C. Thomas, 1979).

Laboratory 1
PROFILING DRINKING BEHAVIOR

Purpose   To draw a profile of the drinking behavior of the class.

Size of Group   The class.

Equipment   The survey instrument.

Procedure

1. Place a check mark ($\sqrt{}$) in the box most descriptive of your own behavior for each of the questions.

Profile of the Drinking Behavior of the Class

a) Where do you drink?
   (1) your own home ☐   (3) bar ☐
   (2) someone else's ☐   (4) restaurant ☐
       home

b) With whom to you drink?
   (1) alone ☐   (3) strangers ☐
   (2) close friends ☐   (4) the gang ☐

c) Time of day?
   (1) 9 A.M.–12 ☐   (4) 6 P.M.–9 ☐
       P.M.   P.M.
   (2) 12 P.M.–3 ☐   (5) 9 P.M.–12 ☐
       P.M.   A.M.
   (3) 3 P.M.–6 ☐   (6) 12 A.M.–3 ☐
       P.M.   A.M.

d) Day of week?
   (1) every day ☐   (5) Wednesday ☐
   (2) Sunday ☐   (6) Thursday ☐
   (3) Monday ☐   (7) Friday ☐
   (4) Tuesday ☐   (8) Saturday ☐

e) Why?
   (1) something to do ☐ (4) to get high ☐
   (2) companionship ☐   (5) don't know ☐
   (3) because others ☐
       are drinking

f) How much in one day?
   (1) 1–3 ounces ☐   (4) 10–12 ☐
   (2) 4–6 ☐   (5) more ☐
   (3) 7–9 ☐

g) Average consecutive time spent in drinking activity (hours)?
   (1) 1 ☐   (3) 3–4 ☐
   (2) 2–3 ☐   (4) 4–5 ☐

h) How often have you been intoxicated?
   (1) never ☐   (4) 2–5 times in ☐
                              past year
   (2) once in my life ☐ (5) 6 or more ☐
                              times in past
                              year
   (3) once in past ☐   (6) whenever I ☐
       year   drink

i) What do you drink?
   (1) beer ☐   (3) liquor ☐
   (2) wine ☐   (4) mixed drinks ☐

2. Transfer individual *anonymous* responses to a class master-response form.

3. Work out frequency responses for each test item.

Result

The class members will see their own profile in relation to those of their peers.

Laboratory 2
ALCOHOL AND VALUES

Purpose   To demonstrate how values affect drinking behavior.

Size of Group   Four students per group.

Equipment   None.

Procedure

1. Rank order each of the following sets by placing a "1" next to the most important to you, a "2" next to the second most important, and a "3" next to the least important.

   _____ a. friends   _____ a. feeling good

   _____ b. money   _____ b. being healthy

   _____ c. respect   _____ c. acting smart

   _____ a. be responsible   _____ a. to think well of
                                        yourself

   _____ b. have fun   _____ b. to be thought
                                        well of by
                                        friends

   _____ c. feel un-   _____ c. to be thought
           restricted   well of by
                                        adults

2. Place yourself on the following continuum as it pertains to alcohol:

1	1	1	1	1
Always high	Often high	High on weekends	Seldom drink alcohol	Never drink alcohol

3. Complete the following sentences:

   a. Alcohol _____

   b. Being high _____

   c. My friends _____

   d. I drink alcohol when _____

   e. The pressure to drink alcohol _____

   _____

4. Now form groups with four students in each and discuss the responses to the above. In particular, answer the question "How do my values influence my drinking behavior?"

Results

Write a paragraph starting with "In this activity, I learned that . . . "

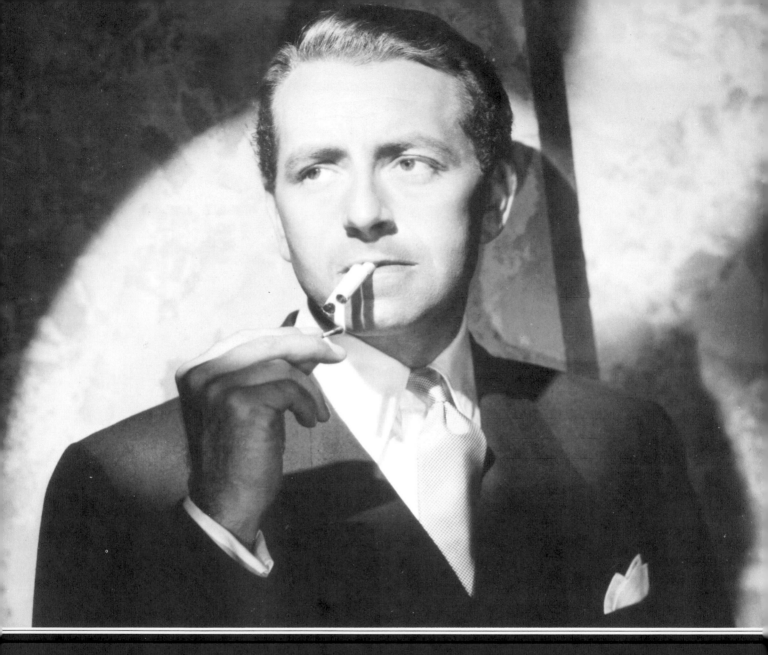

chapter *11*

smoking and health

- *physiological effects of smoking*
- *why people smoke*
- *nonsmokers*
- *kicking the tobacco habit*

In ancient Greece the tobacco plant (*Solanaceae*) was prescribed for medicinal purposes. The same plant, now referred to as *Nicotiana*, was brought to western Europe sometime after the expeditions of Columbus. Almost everywhere it was introduced, it was popularly used for smoking, in the face of claims that it could cure numerous diseases and ailments. Its early use was associated with cultural ceremony and the demonstration of good faith and peaceful intentions; later, social use for pleasure became popular. Increased mechanization in the nineteenth century, invention of the cigarette-manufacturing machine for large-scale production, and advances in mass communication in the twentieth century led to an estimated domestic consumption of more than 600 billion cigarettes annually in the 1970s. Advertising receives the greater share of the credit (or blame) for increased sales and a steadily increasing number of habitual smokers of all ages.

During the early nineteenth century, there was considerable opposition to public smoking, with religious groups branding the practice as immoral, unhealthy, and improper for respectable people. Protective laws were introduced prohibiting minors and women from smoking. Taxation was imposed to curb the practice. Today, however, only the law forbidding the sale of tobacco to minors remains on the books. Smoking among women and youth is widespread, and taxation exists only for the sake of producing revenue. Today smoking is one of the major health problems in the United States.

PHYSIOLOGICAL EFFECTS OF SMOKING

If you are a smoker, complete and score Discovery Activity 11.1: *What Do You Think the Effects of Smoking Are?* Analyze your score and rate your present knowledge in this area.

Concept: Tobacco use in any form is harmful to health.

Concern for the health of the smoker has developed slowly over recent decades. The medical profession started to become concerned over the effects of smoking in the 1930s, and public concern began in the 1950s, when statistics were published showing the rise in the number of cases of lung cancer and other ailments and the higher death rates among smokers (see Fig. 11.1). The now-famous Surgeon General's Report, released in 1964, substantiated the public's worst fears: "Cigarette smoking is a health hazard of sufficient importance in the United States to warrant appropriate remedial action." Shortly after the report was published, millions of people stopped smoking. Unfortunately, the impact was short-lived, and ten years later, in 1974, 42.2 percent of men over 21 and 30.5 percent of women over 21 were still smoking. Although the percentage of adult smokers (particularly men) has declined in the past ten years, the actual number of cigarettes smoked per year has increased.

Researchers have produced overwhelming and highly conclusive evidence demonstrating that cigarette smoking is a severe health hazard. Although propaganda and ongoing research by the tobacco industry continue to attempt to cast doubt, evidence of physical harm is increasing. In the following sections we'll consider some of the major findings.

Components of Tobacco Smoke

Concept: Cigarettes contain several harmful substances.

Tobacco smoke is a combination of gases, vapors, and small particles. It is these components that have harmful effects on the body.

Nicotine is a colorless, oily compound that produces physical dependence or addiction. Smokers who inhale

Discovery Activity 11.1
WHAT DO YOU THINK THE
EFFECTS OF SMOKING ARE?*

For each statement, circle the number that shows how you feel about it. Do you strongly agree, mildly agree, mildly disagree, or strongly disagree?

Important: Answer every question.

	Strongly Agree	Mildly Agree	Mildly Disagree	Strongly Disagree
A. Cigarette smoking is not as dangerous as many other health hazards.	1	2	3	4
B. I don't smoke enough to get any of the diseases that cigarette smoking is supposed to cause.	1	2	3	4
C. If a person has already smoked for many years, it probably won't do him much good to stop.	1	2	3	4
D. It would be hard for me to give up smoking cigarettes.	1	2	3	4
E. Cigarette smoking is enough of a health hazard for something to be done about it.	4	3	2	1
F. The kind of cigarette I smoke is much less likely than other kinds to give me any of the diseases that smoking is supposed to cause.	1	2	3	4
G. As soon as a person quits smoking cigarettes he begins to recover from much of the damage that smoking has caused.	4	3	2	1
H. It would be hard for me to cut down to half the number of cigarettes I now smoke.	1	2	3	4
I. The whole problem of cigarette smoking and health is a minor one.	1	2	3	4
J. I haven't smoked long enough to worry about the diseases that cigarette smoking is supposed to cause.	1	2	3	4
K. Quitting smoking helps a person to live longer.	4	3	2	1
L. It would be difficult for me to make any substantial change in my smoking habits.	1	2	3	4

How to score:

1. Enter the numbers you have circled to the test questions in the spaces below, putting the number you have circled to question A over line A, to question B over line B, and so on.

2. Total the three scores across on each line to get your totals. For example, the sum of your scores over lines A, E, and I gives you your score on *Importance*—lines B, F, and J give the score on *Personal relevance;* and so on.

Totals

_____ + _____ + _____ = _____ 6 or below indicates you may shrug off evidence available.
  A   E   I   Importance

__*1*__ + _____ + __*2*__ = _____ 6 or below may indicate the "it-can't-happen-to-me" attitude.
  B   F   J   Personal relevance

_____ + _____ + _____ = _____ 6 or below suggests an unawareness of health benefits occurring when
  C   G   K   Value of stopping   you quit.

_____ + _____ + _____ = _____ 6 or below suggests you feel stopping would be difficult.
  D   H   L   Capability for stopping

Scores can vary from 3 to 12. Any score 9 and above is *high;* any score 6 and below is *low.*

*SOURCE: National Clearinghouse for Smoking and Health (USPHS), Bethesda, Md., 1974.

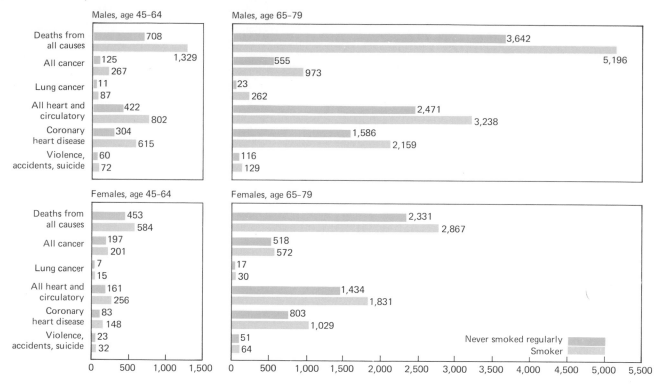

Figure 11.1
Death rates of smokers versus nonsmokers per 100,000 population.

SOURCE: U.S. Department of Health, Education and Welfare, Chart Book on Smoking, Tobacco and Health, p. 11.

absorb about 90 percent of the nicotine into the body; noninhalers absorb 25 to 30 percent. Nicotine first acts as a stimulant, then as a tranquilizer. It is a powerful drug that stimulates the cerebral cortex (the outer layer of the brain controlling complex behavior and mental activity) and the adrenal glands. The resulting bodily changes include increased blood pressure and heart rate, constriction of blood vessels, depression of hunger contractions, interference with the production of urine, and dulling of taste buds. Nicotine is also linked to heart and respiratory disease.

Tar is a dark, thick, sticky by-product of burned tobacco containing hundreds of different chemicals, both poisonous and carcinogenic. These chemicals lodge in the forks of the bronchial tubes in the lungs to produce precancerous changes. Tar also damages the mucus and the cilia in the bronchial tubes, thereby decreasing their ability to remove foreign matter from the lungs.

Carbon monoxide is another by-product of burned tobacco, which displaces oxygen in the blood and produces shortness of breath. Smoking can result in levels of carbon monoxide in the blood as much as 400 times the safety limit specified by industrial hygienists.

Smoking-Related Diseases

Lung cancer. Research findings in several countries agree that cigarette smoking is the cause of the modern lung cancer epidemic. Pipes, cigars, and general air pollution play a relatively small part in lung cancer. Most studies have identified a clear, quantitative relationship between the number of cigarettes smoked, the number of years of smoking, and the incidence of lung cancer (see Fig. 11.2). In addition, heavy inhalation increases the lungs' exposure to smoke and increases the risk of cancer (see Fig. 11.3). The risk can be slightly reduced by smoking filtered cigarettes. However, no cigarette is completely safe, not even the low-tar brands. Although not all smokers develop lung cancer, due to differences in smoking patterns, family history, and environmental and genetic differences, all suffer from lung damage. The only solution is the complete cessation of smoking. Research has demonstrated that smokers who quit permanently rapidly reduce their risk of developing lung cancer over the next ten years.

Figure 11.2
Death rates of smokers by age when smoking began per 100,000 population.
SOURCE: U.S. Department of Health, Education and Welfare, Chart Book on Smoking, Tobacco and Health, p. 13.

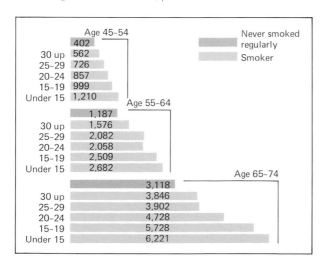

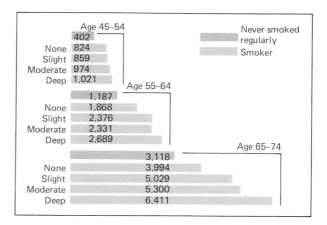

Figure 11.3
Death rates of smokers by degree of inhalation per 100,000 population.
SOURCE: U.S. Department of Health, Education and Welfare, Chart Book on Smoking, Tobacco and Health, p. 13.

Oral problems. Most people are aware that constant cigarette, cigar, or pipe smoking causes bad breath and stained teeth. Unfortunately, several more serious oral problems also occur more frequently among smokers, including (1) edentulism, or loss of teeth; (2) formation of white patches on the mucous membranes in the mouth, with patches becoming malignant in some individuals; (3) delayed healing of tooth sockets after extraction; (4) lip and tongue cancer (among pipe smokers) and cancer of the mouth, pharynx, larynx, and esophagus (among cigarette smokers); (5) periodontal disease (pyorrhea), a disease of the gums spreading to the sockets containing teeth and resulting in destruction of the supportive structure of the teeth; and (6) gingivitis a gum inflammation resulting in bleeding gums, pain, and foul odor.

Chronic bronchitis and emphysema. Cigarette smoking is the most important predisposing cause of both **chronic bronchitis** and **emphysema.**[1] Constant coughing and expectorating of mucus, particularly upon rising in the morning, are common symptoms of chronic bronchitis. While other causative factors may exist, cigarette smoking is the most common cause of inflammation of the bronchial tubes and their subdivisions and of the production of excessive mucus.

Emphysema is 13 times more prevalent among cigarette smokers than among nonsmokers. The irritants in cigarette smoke reduce the lung's effectiveness as an oxygenating organ, making it more susceptible to disease.

With cessation of smoking, mild bronchitis will improve, although severe damage to the lungs (emphysema) cannot be repaired. Figure 11.4 shows an emphysema victim making an unsuccessful attempt to

Figure 11.4
An emphysema victim making an unsuccessful attempt to summon enough air to blow out a match.
Courtesy American Cancer Society.

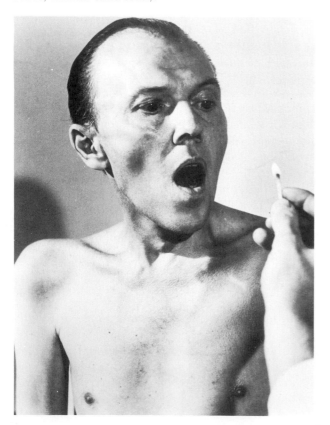

generate enough air to blow out a match. Take a moment to test your own ability to summon air to blow out a match held six inches from the mouth. Open your mouth and generate the air without puckering your lips as you normally would to blow out candles on a birthday cake. This is not a difficult task for the normal individual. Avoidance of cigarette smoking and keeping fit through regular aerobic exercise (see Chapter 6) offer the best protection against chronic bronchitis and emphysema.

Coronary artery disease, heart attacks, and stroke. Cigarette smoking is a major factor in the high death rate from circulatory diseases, heart attacks, and strokes. It contributes to an estimated 188,000 deaths each year in the United States alone. Between the ages of 45 and 54, the death rate for male smokers from coronary heart disease is three times higher than the rate for nonsmoking males and two times higher than the rate for nonsmoking females. Research findings link nonfatal heart attacks to cigarette smoking independently of any other causative factors. Experimental evidence has also demonstrated the damaging effects of smoking on the heart and coronary arteries. Moderate to advanced thickening of the coronary arteries is more common in heavy smokers. Numerous autopsy studies show increased atherosclerosis in the coronary arteries of smokers. In addition, strokes and arterial disease of the leg are related to cigarette smoking.

Cessation of smoking at any age sharply decreases the risk of heart attacks, strokes, and other circulatory diseases within one year. After ten years of abstinence, the risk is nearly as low as for an individual who has never smoked.

Effects of Smoking During Pregnancy

Smoking during pregnancy poses dangers to both the mother and the fetus. Smoking results in the absorption of carbon monoxide and reduction in the supply of oxygen to the mother and unborn baby. Smoking one pack of cigarettes per day can reduce oxygen supply to the unborn fetus by 20 percent or more. In addition,

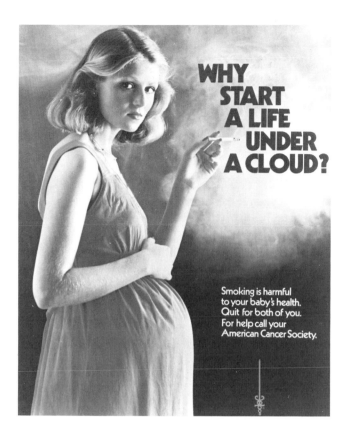

WHY START A LIFE UNDER A CLOUD?

Smoking is harmful to your baby's health. Quit for both of you. For help call your American Cancer Society.

smoking elevates fetal heart rate and blood pressure, constricts blood vessels, and impairs breathing.

While no direct cause-and-effect relationship has been established, it has been found that women who smoke during pregnancy have more stillbirths and spontaneous abortions than nonsmoking pregnant women. Their infants have a higher mortality rate during the first month of life, and twice as many of them are premature. Traces of nicotine have been found in the milk of mothers, which will affect the nursing infant.

Some studies indicate a trend toward a reduction of smoking during pregnancy.[2] In one study 36 percent of the pregnant women surveyed felt that women should stop smoking completely (22 percent actually did), and 36 percent felt that they should reduce the number of cigarettes smoked (37 percent did). According to this study, women continued to smoke during pregnancy

Issues in Health
DOES OCCASIONAL CIGARETTE SMOKING DECREASE PERFORMANCE IN RECREATIONAL ACTIVITIES AND EXERCISE PROGRAMS?

Light, low-tar smokers (less than a pack per day) assume that the health hazards of smoking do not pertain to them and that light smoking has no adverse physiological effect on their bodies. After all, what effect can a few cigarettes have if research indicates that it takes two packs or more per day for 20 years to induce cancer in animals? Light smokers who exercise frequently report no noticeable effects, such as breathlessness or early fatigue, either during or immediately following exercise. Regular exercise, they argue, negates the potential harmful effects of cigarette smoking and keeps their lungs clear and pink, like those of the nonsmoker. Light smokers also point out that several professional and high-caliber amateur athletes smoke moderately. If smoking is harmful, how can these athletes perform so efficiently? Very little evidence exists to show that smoking a few cigarettes daily will decrease performance in physical activity.

Opponents of smoking feel that a definition of "occasional smoking" is needed. If occasional means two to three cigarettes per day, perhaps the risk of decreased performance in exercise programs is only slight. However, smoking one-half to one pack per day may produce quite different results.

Research does show that smoking one-half pack per day produces some physiological changes in the human body that potentially could reduce physical performance: (1) the oxygen-carrying capacity of the blood is reduced as a result of carbon monoxide absorption, (2) the efficiency of the lungs to take in and use oxygen is reduced, (3) heart rate and blood

(continued)

Issues in Health (continued)

pressure are elevated, (4) skin temperature drops, (5) small arteries that carry blood to the lung's surface for oxygenation are damaged, (6) the nervous system is irritated, and (7) the ability to perform coordinated motor movements is decreased. The type of cigarette, degree of inhalation, and how far down each cigarette is smoked all alter the degree to which these physical changes occur.

By smoking several cigarettes daily, inhaling only lightly, and discarding each cigarette when it is half gone, it may be possible to maintain performance in recreational activities or exercise programs. On the other hand, one could perhaps be more physically efficient by not smoking any cigarettes. Evidence is lacking on both the hazards of very light smoking and its effect on performance.

What do you think? ●

in spite of their knowledge of the evidence for one of two reasons: They did not accept the evidence or they did not receive adequate social support. This demonstrates again that knowledge does not necessarily lead to a change in behavior.

Other Health Problems

Tobacco is capable of harming practically every organ and system in the body. Cancer of the bladder, esophagus, and pancreas has been linked to smoking. Gastric and duodenal ulcers, pulmonary tuberculosis, lower body weight, and decreased physical fitness are a few additional consequences of tobacco smoking. Heavy cigarette smoking has even been correlated with deep wrinkling in the face, most noticeable at the corner of each eye. There is evidence suggesting that smoking heavily can result in a facial appearance that is 10 to 15 years beyond one's chronological age. Finally, a long-term study of thousands of women in California found that the use of birth control pills in conjunction with smoking increases the risk of heart disease, hypertension, and blood clot formation.

WHY PEOPLE SMOKE

If you are a smoker, before reading this section, complete and score the test in Discovery Activity 11.2. Analyze your scores carefully to determine the basic reasons for your smoking behavior and the best approaches to quitting. Then read this section and compare your reasons for smoking with those given by other smokers in the United States.

Smoking Trends in the United States

Concept: Understanding why you smoke can be helpful in breaking the habit.

A study by the U.S. Department of Health, Education and Welfare,[3] involving a representative sample of 3009 households, provides insight into current trends in

Discovery Activity 11.2
WHY DO YOU SMOKE?*

Here are some statements made by people to describe what they get out of smoking cigarettes. How *often* do you feel this way when smoking them? Circle one number for each statement.

Important: Answer every question.

		Always	Frequently	Occasionally	Seldom	Never
A.	I smoke cigarettes in order to keep myself from slowing down.	5	4	3	2	1
B.	Handling a cigarette is part of the enjoyment of smoking it.	5	4	3	2	1
C.	Smoking cigarettes is pleasant and relaxing.	5	4	3	2	1
D.	I light up a cigarette when I feel angry about something.	5	4	3	2	1
E.	When I have run out of cigarettes I find it almost unbearable until I can get them.	5	4	3	2	1
F.	I smoke cigarettes automatically without even being aware of it.	5	4	3	2	1
G.	I smoke cigarettes to stimulate me, to perk myself up.	5	4	3	2	1
H.	Part of the enjoyment of smoking a cigarette comes from the steps I take to light up.	5	4	3	2	1
I.	I find cigarettes pleasurable.	5	4	3	2	1
J.	When I feel uncomfortable or upset about something, I light up a cigarette.	5	4	3	2	1
K.	I am very much aware of the fact when I am not smoking a cigarette.	5	4	3	2	1
L.	I light up a cigarette without realizing I still have one burning in the ashtray.	5	4	3	2	1
M.	I smoke cigarettes to give me a "lift."	5	4	3	2	1
N.	When I smoke a cigarette, part of the enjoyment is watching the smoke as I exhale it.	5	4	3	2	1
O.	I want a cigarette most when I am comfortable and relaxed.	5	4	3	2	1
P.	When I feel "blue" or want to take my mind off cares and worries, I smoke cigarettes.	5	4	3	2	1
Q.	I get a real gnawing hunger for a cigarette when I haven't smoked for a while.	5	4	3	2	1
R.	I've found a cigarette in my mouth and didn't remember putting it there.	5	4	3	2	1

*SOURCE: National Clearinghouse for Smoking and Health (USPHS), Bethesda, Md., 1974.

(continued)

Discovery Activity 11.2 (continued)

How to score:

1. Enter the numbers you have circled to the Test questions in the spaces below, putting the number you have circled to question A over line A, to question B over line B, and so on.

2. Total the three scores on each line to get your totals. For example, the sum of your scores over lines A, G, and M gives you your score on *Stimulation*—lines B, H, and N give the score on *Handling,* etc.

Totals

_____ + _____ + _____ = _____
  A   G   M   Stimulation

11 or above suggests you are stimulated by the cigarette to get going and keep going. To stop smoking, try a brisk walk or exercise when the smoking urge is present.

_____ + _____ + _____ = _____
  B   H   N   Handling

11 or above suggests satisfaction from handling the cigarette. Substituting a pencil or paper clip, or doodling may aid in breaking the habit.

_____ + __2__ + _____ = _____
  C   I   O   Pleasurable relaxation

11 or above suggests you receive pleasure from smoking. For this type of smoker, substitution of other pleasant habits (eating, drinking, social activities, exercise) may aid in eliminating smoking.

__3__ + __2__ + __2__ = _____
  D   J   P   Crutch: tension reduction

11 or above suggests you use cigarettes to handle moments of stress or discomfort. Substitution of social activities, eating, drinking, or handling other objects may aid in stopping.

_____ + _____ + _____ = _____
  E   K   Q   Craving: psychological addiction

11 or above suggests an almost continuous psychological craving for a cigarette. "Cold turkey" may be your best method of breaking the smoking habit.

_____ + _____ + _____ = _____
  F   L   R   Habit

11 or above suggests you smoke out of mere habit and may acquire little satisfaction from the process. Gradually reducing the number of cigarettes smoked may be effective in helping you stop.

Scores can vary from 3 to 15. Any score 11 or above is *high;* any score 7 and below is *low.*

●

smoking behavior in the United States and some reasons for these trends. A summary of the findings follows:

1. Although smoking among the adult population has dropped significantly, the nation's youth, particularly teenage girls and young women, are smoking in greater numbers and smoking more cigarettes per person than in the past.

2. This rise has occurred in spite of the fact that the antismoking message has reached the public. The majority of individuals surveyed were aware of the harmful effects to people of all ages, that it is not safe to smoke low-tar cigarettes, and that smoking during pregnancy can harm the fetus. However, their belief that "everybody smokes" and the fact that people they admire smoke counterbalance the knowledge of the harmful effects of smoking.

3. The individuals shown in cigarette advertising are almost always attractive, well dressed, sexy, young, and healthy. Teenage girls seem to be influenced by this image of sophistication.

4. Moral norms have changed drastically among teenage girls and young women. With teenage boys, smoking has long been related to social rebellion. Rebellion against adult society is now a factor in smoking among adolescent girls and represents a drastic change for that group.

5. Most young men and women who smoke have parents who smoke now or did in the past. Many of the parents do not object to their children smoking. The number of high school smokers is twice as high if one or both parents also smoke.

6. Curiosity, impressing others, and conformity are also factors in smoking among adolescents.

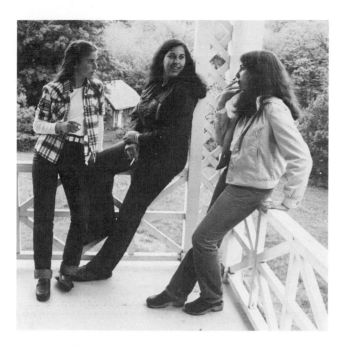

Surveys indicate that more teenage girls and young women are smoking despite signs of reduced smoking among the adult population as a whole. What factors do you think account for this trend?

Table 11.1
THE BALANCE SHEET: TEENAGERS AND YOUNG WOMEN

The Plus Side	The Minus Side
Smoking is a minority phenomenon	The increase in smoking
Teenage girl smokers do not consider smoking to be a social asset	The all-pervasive smoking environment
Smoking is not a necessary social prop—at least for the girls	The "everybody smokes" theory
The "evils" of smoking are known	Health hazards are seen as exaggerated for teenagers
The militant nonsmoker—a new form of peer pressure	Relaxation of restrictions at home
Most smokers want to quit	Boys still smoke to express their masculinity
Most young smokers are not yet committed	Smoking rooms in schools
The New Values: emphasis on self, self-control, self-fulfillment	Cutback in television anti-smoking advertising
Importance of physical appearance and fitness	Peer pressure; smokers come in pairs and groups
The example of former smokers	Parents who smoke
Pregnancy and smoking	The advertised image of the smoker
Children as allies	Doctors don't speak up
Fear of gaining weight is not an inhibiting factor	"The new values": anti-authority, emphasis on the emotional rather than the rational
The readiness for antismoking regulation	Belief that smoking is addictive makes quitting harder
	The problems of being a housewife encourage young women to smoke
	"The cure is just around the corner" crutch for smokers

SOURCE: United States Department of Health, Education and Welfare, *Cigarette Smoking among Teenagers and Young Women,* 1976.

Table 11.1 summarizes both the factors that inhibit teenagers and young women from smoking and the factors that encourage them to smoke.

Young adult smokers have a rationale of their own for their behavior. They are very much aware of the harmful effects of smoking but feel that these dangers are exaggerated, that there is an overemphasis on things that are bad for you these days (such as saccharin, food additives, auto fumes, and other so-called carcinogens), and that air pollution is as much a cause of lung cancer as cigarettes are. Unfortunately studies have revealed that air pollution plays only a minor role in lung cancer and deserves little or none of the blame for the modern-day epidemic of that disease.

Characteristics of Smokers

Surveys reveal that the majority of smokers give several social or psychological reasons for their smoking habit, such as stimulation, pleasure, alleviation of anxiety, relief from tension or anger, relief of a craving for smoke, or merely because it is a habit.[4] Other studies reveal two broad groups of smokers: those motivated by inner needs (moods, hunger, or solitude) and those motivated by social factors (smoking in a group to gain confidence). Social factors were more common among adolescents.

The Influence of Advertising

Concept: Advertising has a significant influence on smoking, especially among young people.

The purpose of cigarette advertising is to sell cigarettes, not to provide people with accurate information for use in decision making. Over $300 million is spent for cigarette advertising each year. This constant barrage of procigarette propaganda rather successfully undermines antismoking efforts. Although the elimination of cigarette advertising on television was an important step in stemming the tide, the cigarette industry has diverted its vast resources to magazines, newspapers, and billboards.

Cigarette advertisments relate smoking to sexual attractiveness, athletic prowess, youth, femininity and masculinity, popularity, and health. Teenagers are particularly susceptible to these messages because they are concerned with appearing mature, sexy, and sophisticated. In addition, it is difficult for teenagers to understand that smoking now could shorten their lives as adults, because they generally don't think far ahead into the future.

Factors That Encourage Smoking

Numerous political, social, and economic forces almost guarantee the continuance of tobacco smoking in the United States. It is unlikely that anyone sent to Congress from a tobacco-growing state will work toward the abolishment of cigarettes, or that any state or the federal government receiving several billion cigarette tax dollars annually will lobby to eliminate smoking. An example of the dilemma is that the Department of Health and Human Services is charged with eliminating cigarette smoking while it and a number of other federal agencies are funded from the $2 billion or more received in cigarette taxes each year. Money is provided in the form of agricultural subsidies to tobacco growers, and cigarette tax dollars are used by federal agencies, yet, at the same time, large sums of money are spent searching for cures for lung cancer when a preventive approach through strong legislation offers an immediate solution. Economically, the picture is even more gloomy, with tremendous expenditure and profits for advertising, manufacturing, shipping, and distributing involved. The power of the tobacco industry cannot be underestimated. Their insistence that there is no link between smoking and health is evidence of their utter defiance based on vested interest and economic pressures.

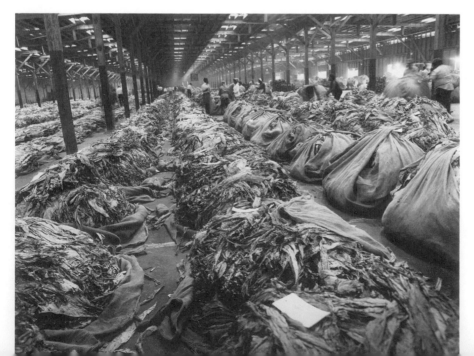

One of the most powerful forces that encourage the continuance of smoking in our society is the tobacco industry, which wields enormous economic and political influence.

What Can Be Done?

The American Cancer Society continues its battle to eliminate tobacco smoking and has reaffirmed its decision to intensify and expand the fight along the following lines:

1. The Society supports federal action to reduce tar and nicotine content of cigarettes; to require disclosure of tar and nicotine content on cigarette packages and in advertising; to require a stronger warning label.

2. Since the Society sees no reason why the major cause of lung cancer should be advertised, we seek the elimination of cigarette advertising in all media. It is hoped that this can be achieved by voluntary self-regulation and that governmental action will not be necessary.

3. Since 1971, when explicit advertising of cigarettes on television became illegal, cigarette companies have made indirect reentry to television through sponsorship of sports events with huge television audiences. The Society opposes such sponsorship and will work to persuade managers of these events to reject it.

4. The Society urges TV personalities and entertainers to refrain from smoking during their broadcasts, because of their influence on the smoking habits of the young.

5. The American Cancer Society supports restriction on smoking in places of public assembly such as theaters, restaurants, offices, hospitals; and in places of transport such as elevators, buses, trains, airplanes, because (a) it helps to discourage the smoker from smoking, and (b) it protects the nonsmoker from the noxious effects of other people's smoke.

6. Units should increase their sponsorship of group cessation activities, particularly in industry, hospitals, health centers, schools, and colleges, and should help others to organize similar programs. The goal is a minimum of one ongoing cessation program in each community. Company incentive programs against cigarette smoking should be encouraged.

7. The Society should maintain its support of research on: the health hazards of smoking; the carcinogenic components of cigarette smoke; the development of less hazardous cigarettes; the nature of addiction to cigarettes and the motivations for smoking; the most effective methods for persuading and helping people to stop smoking, including smoking cessation clinics; the effects of cigarette smoke on the nonsmoker.

8. Since the lung cancer death rate for women has doubled in the past ten years, and since smoking by teenage girls is increasing at an alarming rate, the American Cancer Society has designated women's smoking as a special problem requiring special program emphasis at all organizational levels.

9. Health professionals are persuasive and effective examples. Special efforts must be made to involve practicing physicians, dentists, and nurses in local programs and to persuade them to urge patients not to smoke.

10. Face-to-face education is the most powerful force in persuading smokers to give up the habit. Educational programs for students in primary and secondary schools should be expanded, with new emphasis on teacher involvement and teachers as examples. The Society takes the position that smoking areas should not be provided on school grounds or in school buildings.

11. The Society should expand its antismoking information program through films, television and radio spots, magazine and newspaper articles, posters and brochures.

12. To counteract the reduction of antismoking television messages resulting from the ban on TV advertising of cigarettes, national and local efforts should be intensified for increased use of these messages.

13. In winning acceptance for the antismoking message, nonsmokers are far more convincing than smokers. First educational targets should be health professionals who smoke, antismoking activists who smoke, and any of the Society's staff and volunteers who smoke.[5]

NONSMOKERS

Characteristics of Nonsmokers

Concept: Nonsmokers possess unique characteristics of their own.

While not all nonsmokers can be grouped into a single category, several characteristics are common to this group. Some nonsmokers are very religious, respectful of authority, and turned off by the new moral values discussed previously. Others share many of the same values as smokers but feel by not smoking they will be more in control of their own lives. Nonsmokers are likely to be concerned about nicotine addiction and to emphasize physical fitness and health. In recent years nonsmokers have been increasingly vocal about insisting on certain rights they believe are essential to preserving the health, comfort, and safety of everyone. Figure 11.5, the Nonsmoker's Bill of Rights, outlines these rights.

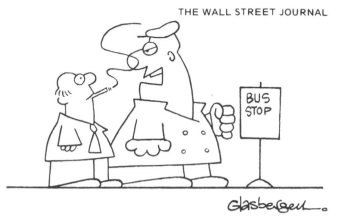

"Warning: Bernie Bronski has determined that smoking near Bernie Bronski may be hazardous to your face."

From The Wall Street Journal,
Permission-Cartoon Features Syndicate.

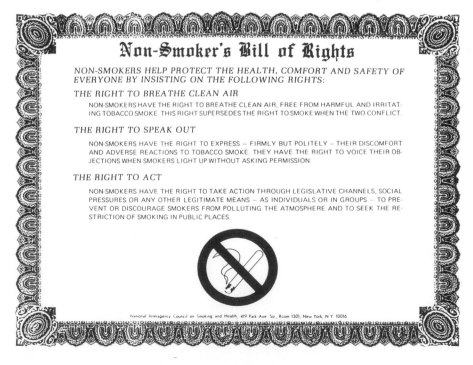

Non-Smoker's Bill of Rights

NON-SMOKERS HELP PROTECT THE HEALTH, COMFORT AND SAFETY OF EVERYONE BY INSISTING ON THE FOLLOWING RIGHTS:

THE RIGHT TO BREATHE CLEAN AIR

NON-SMOKERS HAVE THE RIGHT TO BREATHE CLEAN AIR, FREE FROM HARMFUL AND IRRITATING TOBACCO SMOKE. THIS RIGHT SUPERSEDES THE RIGHT TO SMOKE WHEN THE TWO CONFLICT.

THE RIGHT TO SPEAK OUT

NON-SMOKERS HAVE THE RIGHT TO EXPRESS — FIRMLY BUT POLITELY — THEIR DISCOMFORT AND ADVERSE REACTIONS TO TOBACCO SMOKE. THEY HAVE THE RIGHT TO VOICE THEIR OBJECTIONS WHEN SMOKERS LIGHT UP WITHOUT ASKING PERMISSION.

THE RIGHT TO ACT

NON-SMOKERS HAVE THE RIGHT TO TAKE ACTION THROUGH LEGISLATIVE CHANNELS, SOCIAL PRESSURES OR ANY OTHER LEGITIMATE MEANS — AS INDIVIDUALS OR IN GROUPS — TO PREVENT OR DISCOURAGE SMOKERS FROM POLLUTING THE ATMOSPHERE AND TO SEEK THE RESTRICTION OF SMOKING IN PUBLIC PLACES.

National Interagency Council on Smoking and Health, 419 Park Ave. So., Room 1301, New York, N.Y. 10016

Figure 11.5
Nonsmoker's Bill of Rights.

Discovery Activity 11.3
SMOKING AND
HEART RATE

The next time you are in an automobile, sit quietly for five to ten minutes before taking your radial pulse. To take your pulse, place the index and middle fingers of your right hand in the small hollow just below your left thumb. Count the beats for 30 seconds and record that number for future reference. Repeat the above procedure in an automobile immediately after someone has smoked one cigarette. Compare the two heart rates. What did you find? ●

Benefits for
the Nonsmoker

The obvious benefits of not smoking are improved health and vitality, reduced risk of the chronic and degenerative diseases discussed early in this chapter, healthier offspring, improved performance in exercise, and a longer life. There are additional advantages. For example, there is strong speculation that smoking and sexual performance are related. It is known that carbon monoxide reduces the blood oxygen level and impairs hormone production. There is also evidence that nicotine constricts blood vessels and may inhibit sexual excitement and, in men, the physiological capability for a full erection. For some individuals, a low level of fitness due to sedentary living, obesity, and smoking can reduce stamina and the ability to continue intercourse for as long as they'd like. Whether discolored teeth and smoking breath make one less sexually attractive or desirable depends upon the partner. They are apparently much less offensive when both partners are smokers.

Another advantage to the nonsmoker is cost. For the heavy smoker or a family with two or more smokers, the habit can be quite expensive. In addition, a number of life, accident, and disability insurance companies provide discount rates for nonsmokers. Studies clearly demonstrate that nonsmokers live longer, have fewer automobile accidents, and are less likely to become disabled. Depending upon the state, the nonsmoker may pay 5 to 20 percent less in insurance premiums.

Issues in Health
SHOULD SMOKERS BE
REQUIRED BY LAW TO
SMOKE IN PRIVACY?

Advocates of nonsmokers' rights argue that smoking directly affects the lives of others. Some people are offended by smoke due to eye, nose, and throat sensitivity; some by odor or sight; and some on moral or religious grounds. "Secondhand (exhaled) smoke" is dangerous to the nonsmoker who has not developed a tolerance for smoke. It causes a number of physiological changes in the nonsmoker in a closed, poorly ventilated room or vehicle, including an increase in heart rate and blood pressure, and a rise in carbon monoxide levels in the blood. In addition, the system takes in by-product poisons, such as cadmium (related to high blood pressure, bronchitis, and emphysema), and these poisons are actually higher in the exhaled smoke and burn off than in the smoke inhaled by the smoker. Smoke from an idling cigarette gives off more tar and nicotine than a smoker consumes from inhaling. The level of carbon monoxide in the nonsmoker's blood can double depending upon room ventilation. In addition, approximately 34 million people are sensitive to smoke and about 2 million of them suffer smoke-induced asthma attacks. Lung illness among the children of parents who smoke is twice that found in nonsmoking families. All these health hazards, it is argued, make smoking a violation of the human rights of the nonsmoker.

Legislation concerning nonsmokers' rights has been passed in numerous cities and states and is pending in others. Smokers argue that such legislation is unconstitutional and undemocratic. In a free society people have the right to make their own decision about smoking. Also, they claim that the effects of secondhand smoke are greatly exaggerated and that most people complain only because it is fashionable to do so in this temporary period of antismoking hysteria. If nonsmokers are offended (physically or emotionally) by smoke, they should leave the area.

What do you think? ●

KICKING THE TOBACCO HABIT

The single most important factor in eliminating any habit is motivation. If you are a smoker, complete and score Discovery Activity 11.4, *Do You Want to Change Your Smoking Habits?* Surveys indicate that most young smokers want to quit, and only a minority are actually committed to smoking. From your scores on the test, determine whether you are committed to smoking or whether a sufficient amount of evidence suggests you may want to quit.

Concept: To stop smoking involves terminating the dependence on nicotine.

According to the American Cancer Society, 21 million people in the United States (one in five adult men) have kicked the smoking habit. The four most common reasons for giving up cigarette smoking are: (1) concern over the effects on health; (2) desire to set an example; (3) esthetics, or the unpleasant aspects of smoking; and (4) the desire for self-control. The success rate is higher among light smokers (less than one pack per day). Cessation programs are based on eliminating dependence on nicotine. Breaking the dependence may involve supportive social or psychological measures or a pharmacological approach aimed toward changing the smoker's behavior.

Studies in which nicotine has been administered intravenously, orally, or by inhalation have identified nicotine as the main dependence-producing substance in tobacco smoke. This dependence can be acquired after less than one month of regular smoking. The person who has a dependence on nicotine and decides to kick the habit may experience what is known as the abstinence syndrome. This involves depression; aggression; vertigo; craving for sweets; hunger; drowsiness; and a lowering of blood pressure, pulse rate, and cortisol plasma rate. The syndrome is most severe after three days and generally wears off after 14 days. The syndrome may be severe and quitting difficult even if the dependence is only mild. Terminating a strong dependence is difficult regardless of the intensity of the

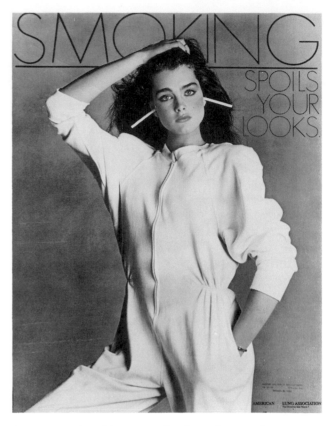

A recent antismoking campaign featuring popular actress Brooke Shields is focused on countering the perception held by many teenage girls that smoking will make them look attractive and sophisticated.

abstinence syndrome.[6] It can be done, however, regardless of how much and how long you have been smoking.

Health Education Programs

Although it would seem logical to assume that a smoker, when presented with the medical facts, would change his or her smoking behavior, this rarely occurs. The high failure rate of traditional educational programs aimed at helping people stop smoking is explained by the following:

Discovery Activity 11.4
DO YOU WANT TO CHANGE
YOUR SMOKING HABITS?*

For each statement, circle the number that most accurately indicates how you feel. For example, if you completely agree with the statement, circle 4, if you agree somewhat, circle 3, and so on.
Important: Answer every question.

		Completely Agree	Somewhat Agree	Somewhat Disagree	Completely Disagree
A.	Cigarette smoking might give me a serious illness.	4	3	2	1
B.	My cigarette smoking sets a bad example for others.	4	3	2	1
C.	I find cigarette smoking to be a messy kind of habit.	4	3	2	1
D.	Controlling my cigarette smoking is a challenge to me.	4	3	2	1
E.	Smoking causes shortness of breath.	4	3	2	1
F.	If I quit smoking cigarettes it might influence others to stop.	4	3	2	1
G.	Cigarettes cause damage to clothing and other personal property.	4	3	2	1
H.	Quitting smoking would show that I have willpower.	4	3	2	1
I.	My cigarette smoking will have a harmful effect on my health.	4	3	2	1
J.	My cigarette smoking influences others close to me to take up or continue smoking.	4	3	2	1
K.	If I quit smoking, my sense of taste or smell would improve.	4	3	2	1
L.	I do not like the idea of feeling dependent on smoking.	4	3	2	1

How to score:

1. Enter the numbers you have circled to the test questions in the spaces below, putting the number you have circled to question A over line A, to question B over line B, and so on.

2. Total the three scores across on each line to get your totals. For example, the sum of your scores over lines A, E, and I gives you your score on *Health*—lines B, F, and J give the score on *Example,* and so on.

Totals

```
_____  +  _____  +  _____  =  _____        9 or above suggests the harmful effects of smoking may be enough
    A           E           I            Health      for you to want to quit smoking.

_____  +  _____  +  _____  =  _____        6 or less indicates you are probably not interested in giving up
    B           F           J            Example     cigarettes to set an example for others.

_____  +  _____  +  _____  =  _____        9 or above suggests you are disturbed enough by some of the un-
    C           G           K            Esthetics   pleasantness of smoking to give up the habit.

_____  +  _____  +  _____  =  _____        9 or above suggests you are aware that you are not controlling
    D           H           L            Mastery     your desire to smoke and may want to challenge your self-control
                                                     and give up smoking.
```

Scores can vary from 3 to 12. Any score 9 and above is *high;* any score 6 and below is *low.*

*SOURCE: National Clearinghouse for Smoking and Health (USPHS), Bethesda, Md., 1974.   ●

1. Nicotine dependence can be very intense and can counter one's desire to quit smoking.

2. Peer pressure can negate educational efforts.

3. A link between the message (harmful effects of smoking, benefits of stopping) and the personal well-being of the smoker must be established. The smoker must associate the information with *his or her* life and health. The concept that cessation of smoking now will allow an individual to live until age 72 instead of age 65 is meaningless to a 16-year-old.

4. Experiencing the physical, social, emotional, and psychological changes that result from several weeks of abstinence from smoking would be much more effective than merely hearing what it would be like. A program in which smokers volunteer to give up the habit for a few weeks would have a higher success rate than a traditional educational program.

In spite of these limitations, some programs do work. A "group spirit and peer pressure program," for example, produced a 45 percent success rate, with 99 of 222 volunteers still not smoking after one year.[7] The names of those who remained in the program were published monthly in a local newspaper. Social pressure appears to have been the strong motivator for program continuance.

Education probably contributes best to the overall effort to quit smoking by providing continuous information for abstaining to aid against relapses, prevent experimenters from becoming regular smokers, and discourage new smokers.

Pharmacological Programs

Programs employing nicotine substitutes (which do not produce dependence); drugs having drying effects on the mucous membranes, sedatives to manage psychological withdrawal problems; and metallic salts, which produce an unpleasant taste during tobacco inhalation, have been relatively ineffective. However, programs using a combination of nicotine substitutes (adminstered both orally and by injection), sedation, group therapy (including positive suggestion therapy), and aversion therapy have had a higher success rate.

Nicotine chewing gum and other substances containing nicotine have been only about 25 percent effective in helping smokers to quit, because relapse tends to occur when the supply of nicotine is cut off. These substances should not be given to children, because they are likely to produce nicotine dependence in youngsters who do not use tobacco and may turn to it later. Programs attempting to replace smoking-induced nicotine with chewing gum, snuff, or chewing tobacco all have one serious limitation—nicotine dependence is left untreated.

Smoking Low-Tar and Low-Nicotine Cigarettes

The cigarette industry's response to public awareness of the harmful effects of smoking has been a vigorous promotion of low-tar and low-nicotine brands of cigarettes. The industry maintains that a less hazardous cigarette with reduced tar and nicotine is not harmful to health. However, research does not fully support this theory. Several carefully conducted studies reveal that the amount of nicotine directly affects cigarette consumption and the degree of inhalation. Subjects, unaware of the brand they are smoking, automatically increase the number of cigarettes smoked when using a brand with low nicotine. Conversely, consumption decreases among subjects smoking a brand high in nicotine. Those smoking nicotine-free brands tend to "cheat" and substitute their own brand. Synthetic tobacco substitutes, although lower in carcinogen content, tend to rank higher in carbon monoxide, have an objectionable taste, and are poor sellers. In fact, low-poison-content cigarettes account for less than 0.5 percent of sales, in spite of elaborate advertising campaigns.

Adding to the problem is the knowledge that nicotine consumption from any cigarette varies by a factor of as much as 100 depending on the depth of inhalation. A mild increase in the depth of inhalation will compensate for the decreased nicotine content of a cigarette. Evidence also suggests that telling a smoker not to inhale is useless since many are not even aware that they do inhale.

While partial measures, such as use of low-poison-content cigarettes, inhaling less, and smoking each cigarette only halfway, appear to be steps in the right direction, such actions do not guarantee the smoker protection from lung cancer. It has been demonstrated that 20 percent of all lung cancer patients are light smokers who have smoked 1 to 20 cigarettes daily for 10 years or more. The only answer to improved health and reduced risk of lung cancer is complete abstinence.

Cold Turkey

"Cold turkey," or quitting all at once, is effective for some smokers and not for others. It may be the best approach for the heavily addicted, whereas gradual withdrawal may be less painful and more effective for those only mildly addicted. Some authorities, such as Dr. Robert Felix, psychiatrist and Director of the National Institute of Mental Health, believe that cold turkey is the only way: "There's no magic formula. I wish there were, I'd make a fortune. . . . The only way to quit is to quit—all at once."

The 5-Day Plan

Seventh-Day Adventist medical doctors and ministers have been successful in helping people give up smoking through their "5-Day Plan." Five consecutive two-hour sessions, using proven principles to overcome the craving for nicotine, are scheduled. Plans are held wherever there is a Seventh-Day Adventist medical institution or a Seventh-Day Adventist church of sufficient size. About 85 percent of smokers remaining with the program for the entire five days are likely to break the habit. For information on such a program in your area, write: 5-Day Plan, Hinsdale Sanitarium and Hospital, 120 North Oak Street, Hinsdale, Illinois, 60521.

Other Programs

Pacifiers (noncombustible plastic cigarettes) to keep the mouth and fingers occupied, mild electroshock to the hands (to create a negative association), hypnosis, and various behavior modification programs have been tried. The success rate has been rather low for all these approaches.

Preparing to Quit

Concept: Preparing for Q-day (Quit day) requires careful planning.

As we noted, for some people, willpower alone may be enough to break the smoking habit. For others, willpower must be combined with careful preparation for the target Q-day, learning new behavior in order to break the habit permanently. Many smokers fail in their first, second, and even third attempts before finally succeeding. One important behavioral change that is necessary is to stop thinking of quitting. This is very difficult because smoking is perceived as rewarding. A useful approach is to substitute another reward to make up for the loss of smoking as a reward. We will describe some substitute rewards in the next section.

The American Cancer Society suggests some basic steps in preparing for and carrying out the Q-day approach:[8]

1. Set an exact date (one to four weeks in advance) for Q-day, the day you will stop smoking completely.
2. As Q-day approaches, gradually reduce the number of cigarettes smoked day by day or week by week.
3. Use whatever suggestions below work for you.
   a) Smoke only one cigarette per hour.
   b) Avoid smoking between 9 and 10 A.M., 11 and 12 P.M., and/or 3 and 4 P.M., extending the nonsmoking time by a half hour, an hour, two hours.

c) Smoke exactly half as many cigarettes the first week and half this amount again each week until Q-day arrives.

d) Inhale less and with less vigor, avoiding deep inhalation.

e) Smoke each cigarette only halfway before discarding.

f) Remove the cigarette from your mouth between puffs.

g) Smoke slowly.

h) Smoke brands with low nicotine and tar content.

i) Make it difficult to locate a cigarette by leaving yours at home, not carrying pocket change, etc.

j) Place unlighted cigarettes in your mouth when you have the urge to smoke.

k) Switch to a brand you dislike.

4. Maintain a daily record of your smoking habit, using the chart shown in Table 11.2. As you slowly withdraw, attempt to eliminate those cigarettes you rate 1, 2, or 3, or take the opposite approach and eliminate the least needed cigarettes first. Use the log to uncover data about yourself. Are you mainly a social smoker (at parties, in groups); an automatic smoker, who doesn't even realize it's happening; a positive effect smoker, who lights up for a stimulant, pleasure, relaxant, or something at the end of the meal; a negative effect smoker, lighting up to reduce fear, shame, disappointment, or distress; or an addictive smoker who is always aware of not smoking, with the absence of a cigarette in hand causing need, desire, or discomfort?

Making It Permanent

Many people are able to stop smoking temporarily. A much harder task is to stay off cigarettes permanently. After Q-day, when you have an impulse to smoke, try some of these suggestions:

1. Drink a lot of water, nibble fruit and roughage, suck candy, chew gum.

2. Chew bits of fresh ginger or bite a clove, enjoying the aroma.

3. Start an exercise program—jogging, cycling, walking, or any other activity you enjoy. Exercise can give you a naturally "high" feeling.

Table 11.2
RECORD OF SMOKING HABITS

Copy this record sheet seven times for seven days. Make a check for each cigarette you smoke, hour by hour, and indicate how much you need it: a mark in the box opposite 1 shows low need; a mark opposite 6, high need, opposite 4, moderate need; etc. Then decide which cigarette you wish to eliminate.

Need	Morning Hours (A.M.)							Afternoon, Evening Hours (P.M.)												
	6	7	8	9	10	11	12	1	2	3	4	5	6	7	8	9	10	11	12	1
1																				
2																				
3																				
4																				
5																				
6																				

4. Spend time in places where smoking is prohibited, such as libraries and movie theaters.

5. Avoid friends who smoke the first several weeks after Q-day.

6. After a meal or coffee, when the urge for a cigarette is strong, use a pleasant-tasting mouth wash. Alter your pattern of behavior after dinner. If you usually have a cigarette then, substitute another reward or activity.

7. Reward yourself with a pleasant food or drink. Although some people gain weight when they stop smoking, this is usually only a temporary problem.

8. Remind yourself frequently why you quit smoking.

Not all tips will be helpful to everyone. Try numerous suggestions and resort to those that work for you. The agony of giving up cigarettes is much the same as that of dieting. It passes quickly after the first three or four days. Unfortunately, most dieters and would-be exsmokers give up during this initial period.

CONCLUSION

The decision to smoke is generally made during the early teens. In spite of the evidence, 40 percent of the adult population continue to subject their bodies to the harmful effects of tobacco smoke. The sidestream smoke (secondhand smoke) that can be inhaled by those in close proximity to the smoker also poses health hazards to the nonsmoker. A controversy has arisen over an individual's right to smoke and the nonsmoker's right to breath clean air. If you smoke, you can decide to give up the habit at any time. Depending upon your level of addiction, the habit can be stopped by inner motivation and willpower alone or through one of the smoking cessation programs discussed in this chapter. After several weeks of abstinence from cigarettes, you will discover some pleasant changes in your body.

SUMMARY

1. Cigarette smoke contains several substances that are harmful to both the smoker and the nonsmoker.

2. Cigarette smoking is associated with lung cancer; oral disease; chronic bronchitis and emphysema; coronary artery disease; heart attack; stroke; damage to an unborn fetus; pulmonary tuberculosis; facial skin wrinkling; and cancer of the bladder, esophagus, and pancreas.

3. Smoking has declined among the adult population and increased among the nation's youth, particularly among teenage girls and young women.

4. Adolescent smoking behavior is encouraged more by peer influence, rebellion, curiosity, and advertising than by inner motivation.

5. Nonsmokers tend to be more health conscious and feel more in control of their lives than do smokers.

6. Nonsmokers have the right to breathe uncontaminated air in public places.

7. Many young smokers want to terminate their dependence on nicotine.

8. Approaches to help people quit smoking include health education programs, pharmacological programs, cold turkey, the 5-Day Plan, mild electroshock, hypnosis, and behavior modification programs.

REFERENCES

1. Royal College of Physicians, *Smoking and Health Now* (Great Britain: Staples Printers, Ltd., 1976), pp. 1–17.

2. Baric et al., "A Study of Health Aspects of Smoking Education in Pregnancy," *Supplement to International Journal of Health Education* 19 (April/June 1976).

3. U.S. Department of Health, Education and Welfare, Public Health Service, NIH, National Cancer Institute, *Cigarette Smoking among Teen-agers and Young Women,* 1976.

4. American Cancer Society Journal, World Smoking and Health 2 (1) Summer 1977.

5. American Cancer Society, *A Statement on Cigarette Smoking: A 13-Point Program to Reduce Cigarette Smoking,* 1974. Reprinted by permission.

6. Jonas Hartelius and Lita Tibbling, "Nicotine Dependence and Smoking Cessation Programs: A Review," *World Smoking and Health* 2 (1) Summer 1977:4–10. An American Cancer Society Journal.

7. Ibid.

8. American Cancer Society, *If You Want to Give Up Cigarette Smoking,* 1970. Reprinted by permission.

Laboratory 1
CIGARETTE SMOKING AND HEART RATE

Purpose   To determine the effects of smoking upon resting heart rate. To compare the resting heart rate of smokers and nonsmokers.

Size of Group   Group I: All nonsmokers.
Group II: All smokers.

Equipment   One pack of each of the following types of cigarettes: filtered, regular or unfiltered, and low tar.
Wristwatch.

Procedure

1. Smokers and nonsmokers are seated in separate halves of the room, as far apart as possible. Both groups remain in their seats for a minimum of 15 minutes without rising. During this period, students practice self-administering the carotid pulse check; using the tips of the three middle fingers, gently press up under the rear portion of the jaw bone until a pulse is felt. Avoid exerting hard pressure.

2. After the 15-minute rest period, each student determines his or her carotid pulse rate for 30 seconds before doubling that count. A recorder lists the resting pulse rates separately for each group.

3. During the next 15 minutes of class time, each member of the smoking group (Group IIa: filtered; Group IIb: unfiltered; Group IIc: low tar) may light up and smoke at his or her normal rate until the time limit expires. No one is permitted to stand or walk around the room. Nonsmokers should be as far away as possible to reduce the effects of secondhand smoke.

4. After the 15-minute smoking period, both smokers and nonsmokers again take and record their carotid pulse.

Results

1. Compare the carotid pulse rates of smokers (regardless of the type of cigarette used) and nonsmokers, using only the initial count (prior to the smoking period). What is the average pulse rate of:

Smoking men _____
Nonsmoking men _____
Difference _____
Smoking women _____
Nonsmoking women _____
Difference _____

2. Compare the initial pulse rate with the second pulse rate for the smoking group and record below:

Average pulse rate (initial pulse) _____
for all smokers
Average pulse rate (second test) _____
for all smokers
Difference _____
Average pulse rate (initial test)— _____
unfiltered
Average pulse rate (initial test)—filtered _____
Average pulse rate (initial test)—low tar _____
Average pulse rate (second test)— _____
unfiltered
Average pulse rate (second test)—filtered _____
Average pulse rate (second test)—low tar _____

a) What effect did smoking (regardless of the type of cigarette) have on heart rate?

b) Using 70 cc of blood per beat (approximate volume pumped per beat), calculate how much extra blood the heart must pump because of smoking to carry out the same function and maintain sitting posture in a chair.

c) How effective were the low-tar and filtered cigarettes in reducing the poison content (based on heart rate changes)?

3. Compare the initial pulse rate with the second pulse rate for the nonsmoking group and record below:

Average pulse rate (initial test)   _____

Average pulse rate (second test)   _____

a) Did changes in heart rate occur for the non-smoker?

b) Could secondhand smoke have affected the nonsmoking group? Was the room large, small, well ventilated, hot, cool?

4. Discuss how other factors may have affected the heart rates of students, such as coffee consumed prior to class, time of day, mood and tone of the instructor, activity during the smoking period, emotional anxiety created by others smoking, etc.

5. What conclusions can be drawn from this study?

Laboratory 2
SMOKE BY-PRODUCTS COLLECTED BY THE LUNGS

Purpose   To demonstrate the amount of smoke by products retained in the lungs by inhaling cigarette smoke. To determine the effectiveness of filters in removing tobacco poisons.

Size of Group   Four or five in each of three groups—only smokers.

Equipment   One pack of each of the following types of cigarettes: filtered, regular or unfiltered, and low tar.

Procedure

Tar and nicotine retained in the lungs:

Group 1:   Using a regular unfiltered cigarette, a smoker draws cigarette smoke into the mouth (without inhaling) and exhales the smoke through a clean portion of a handkerchief or clean tissue. A total of three puffs are taken, one at a time, and exhaled through the same portion.

The above process is now repeated; however, this time the smoker inhales deeply before exhaling the smoke through an adjacent clean portion of the tissue.

The darkness of the two spots is now compared.

Group II: The above steps are performed using filtered cigarettes

Group III: The above steps are performed using low-tar cigarettes

All Groups: A spokesperson is appointed from each group to come to the front of the room and display the tissue, labeled according to the type of cigarette and whether inhaled or not.

Results

1.   Were there differences in the darkness of the soiled handkerchief when smoke was not inhaled? Why? Did the lungs absorb the difference?

2.   Even without inhaling, do you think some poisons enter and remain in the lungs?

3.   Compare the spots made by different types of cigarettes. Do the low-tar and filtered cigarettes result in less accumulation on the tissue than the unfiltered cigarette?

4.   What conclusions can be drawn from this study?

Note: Another method of checking the effectiveness of filters and comparing filtered, regular, and low-tar cigarettes is to place the tissue cloth over the smoked end of the cigarette before taking several deep draws. The spots left on the tissue should be less dark with low-tar and filtered cigarettes.

sex and family life

Part Five

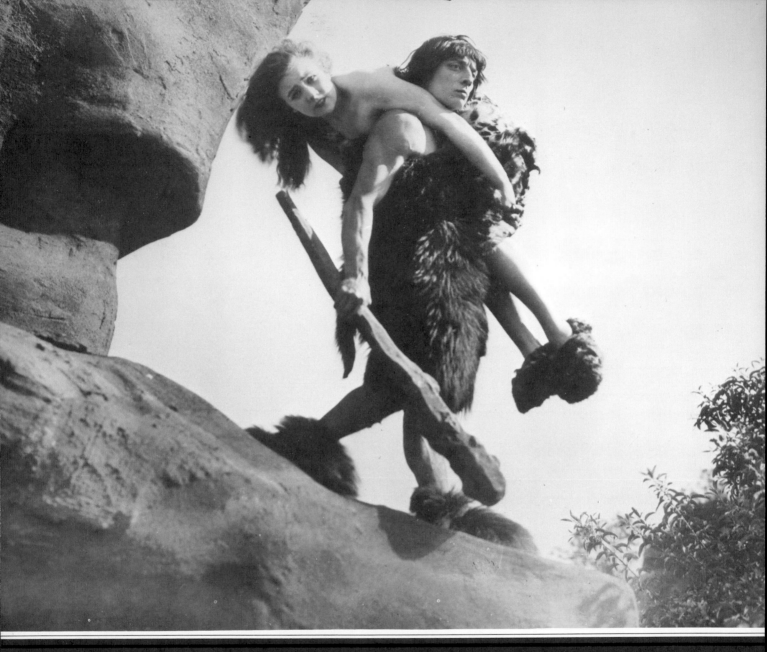

chapter *12*

male/female:
masculine/feminine

- *the reproductive systems*
- *the influence of hormones*
- *sex roles*

An important part of your life is your sexuality. Sexuality is what you are. It includes your reproductive anatomy, the roles you play, and the societal expectations you adopt. Sex, on the other hand, is something you do: kissing, petting, having intercourse, and the like. We might say that sexuality is at your essence, your being, you, whereas sex is concerned only with sexual behavior. Sexuality is an implicit theme of this chapter. The next chapter will deal with sexual behavior and response from both the physiological and social viewpoints.

If you were called a car mechanic or police officer, you would know how to dress, what you would be responsible for, and what was beyond your capabilities. Maleness and femaleness, however, cannot be so clearly defined. Even in biological terms, there are many similarities. On a separate piece of paper, write a paragraph defining what it means to be a male and another paragraph defining what it means to be a female. Don't forget to include social and psychological characteristics, as well as physical ones. Now write a third paragraph describing the differences between females and males. As you read this chapter, refer back to your definitions and periodically revise them as you learn new information.

THE REPRODUCTIVE SYSTEMS

The Male Reproductive System

Figure 12.1 depicts the male reproductive system. The external male reproductive structures include the scrotum, penis, and urethra. The **scrotum** is a baglike structure containing the two **testes,** which produce **sperm** and the male sex hormone. Each testis consists of several parts. The sperm is produced by cells in the **seminiferous** tubules. Each testis contains approximately 1000 seminiferous tubules, and some 50,000 sperm

Discovery Activity 12.1
THE MALE REPRODUCTIVE SYSTEM

To test your understanding of the male reproductive system, see if you can match the following numbered items with the lettered items that most pertain to them. ●

Correct Letter	Numbered Item		Lettered Item
c	1. Ampulla	a.	Stores testes
a	2. Scrotum	b.	Surrounded by the bulbocavernosa muscle
f	3. Corpora cavernosa	c.	Stores sperm
	4. Epididymis	d.	Stores sperm and contracts during ejaculation
b	5. Corpora spongiosa	e.	Produces sperm
g	6. Seminiferous tubles	f.	Its engorgement with blood results in erect penis
h	7. Vas efferentia	g.	Carries sperm to the epididymis
e	8. Vas deferens	h.	Transports sperm from epididymis to ampulla
i	9. Testes	i.	Secretes substance to make sperm live longer
j	10. Prostate	j.	Secretes preejaculatory fluid
	11. Cowper's gland	k.	Produces testosterone

cells are produced each minute (150 million daily). Once produced, the sperm are carried through the **vasa efferentia,** out of the testes to the **epididymis,** where the sperm are stored and nourished. Some of the sperm then proceed to the **ampulla,** by way of the **vas deferens,** and are stored there. **Seminal vesicles** located nearby provide nutrients for the sperms' further maturation. When **ejaculation** (forceful exit of **semen** during **orgasm**) is about to occur, the seminal vesicles empty into the ejaculatory duct, and the sperm pass through this duct into the **urethra.** As shown in Fig. 12.1, the urethra passes through the **prostate,** which secretes a substance that helps increase sperm life. Next, the sperm pass through the urethra, which has been lubricated by the secretion of the **Cowper's gland.** This secretion neutralizes any acidity remaining in the urethra from urine. Any preejaculation fluid that may be noticed is really secretion from the Cowper's gland, but it may also contain some sperm. The sperm next pass into the penis, which has become erect due to sexual stimulation, causing the arterioles leading to the **corpora**

cavernosa to dilate. This dilation results in the corpora cavernosa becoming engorged with blood and thereby erect.

Ejaculation is the result of contractions of muscles in the glands and ducts of the male reproductive system. The ampulla and seminal vesicles contract, as does the **bulbocavernosa muscle,** which surrounds the **corpora spongiosa** of the penis. The semen, or ejaculate, consists of fluids from the seminal vesicles, prostate, and Cowper's gland, as well as sperm. Each ejaculate contains, on the average, 300 million sperm.

Male hormone production in the male reproductive system is accomplished by the interstitial cells, which lie between the seminiferous tubules.

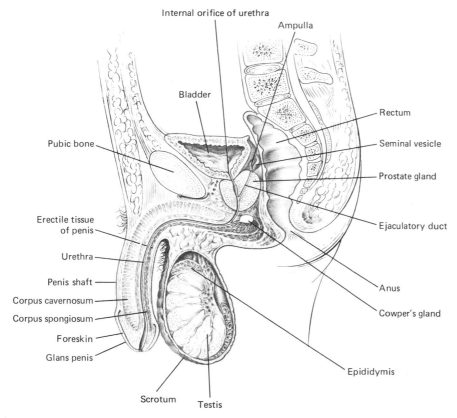

Internal orifice of urethra
Ampulla
Bladder
Rectum
Pubic bone
Seminal vesicle
Prostate gland
Ejaculatory duct
Erectile tissue of penis
Urethra
Penis shaft
Corpus cavernosum
Corpus spongiosum
Anus
Foreskin
Cowper's gland
Glans penis
Epididymis
Scrotum
Testis

Figure 12.1
Cross-section of the male penis.
SOURCE: Eric T. Pengelley, *Sex and Human Life* (Reading, Mass.: Addison-Wesley, 1974).

The Female Reproductive System

The external structures of the female reproductive system (known collectively as the **vulva**) are the labia majora, labia minora, clitoris, hymen, and vestibule. The internal structures are the vagina, uterus, Fallopian tubes, and ovaries. Figure 12.2 depicts the relationship of these organs to one another and their structure. The two large outer folds surrounding the total external structure of the female reproductive system are the **labia majora.** Usually providing protection for the vulva, the labia majora become engorged with blood and expand during sexual stimulation, thereby opening the vulva.

The two thin folds of tissue that lie just inside the labia majora are called the **labia minora.** Loaded with blood vessels and nerve receptors, the labia minora are very sensitive to stimulation. During sexual excitement,

Discovery Activity 12.2
THE FEMALE REPRODUCTIVE SYSTEM

To test your understanding of the female reproductive system, see if you can match the following numbered items with the lettered items that most pertain to them. ●

Correct Letter	Numbered Item		Lettered Item
C	1. Labia majora	a.	Labia majora, labia minora, clitoris, hymen, and vestibule
A	2. Vulva	b.	Two thin folds of tissue loaded with blood vessels and nerve receptors
B	3. Labia minora	c.	Two large folds of tissue surrounding the external genitalia
G	4. Clitoris	d.	A thin connective tissue
F	5. Vestibule	e.	The birth canal
D	6. Hymen	f.	Contains the vaginal and urethral openings
	7. Vagina	g.	Homologous to the penis
	8. Uterus	h.	Where ovum are stored prior to being discharged
H	9. Ovary	i.	Where the egg is usually fertilized
I	10. Fallopian tubes	j.	Where the fertilized egg is implanted and nourished

the blood vessels fill with blood, spreading the labia minora and revealing the **vagina.** The hood of the **clitoris** is composed of the upper part of the labia minora.

The clitoris in the female is similar (homologous) to the penis in the male. The clitoris contains a large number of nerve cells and is the most sensitive structure in the female body. The clitoris includes a corpora cavernosa (as does the male penis) but no corpora cavernosa spongiosa. During sexual stimulation, the corpora cavernosa becomes engorged with blood and erect (as does the penis). When the labia minora are separated, the area that is visible and that contains the vaginal and urethral openings is called the **vestibule.**

The last external structure is the **hymen,** a thin connective tissue with a relatively large number of blood vessels, which separates the vestibule from the vagina. Although its function is uncertain, the hymen may protect the vagina from infection early in life. It is usually ruptured during the first coitus, unless previously ruptured by accident or during exercise. In some cases a physician may have to remove the hymen surgically if the tissue is very thick.

As depicted in Fig. 12.3, the vagina is an elastic organ that can stretch during sexual arousal to accommodate any size penis. Menstrual flow leaves the body through the vaginal canal, and it is also the usual route of exit for the newborn. The vaginal walls contain muscular membranes, which make the vagina capable of expanding so that a baby can pass through it. The tis-

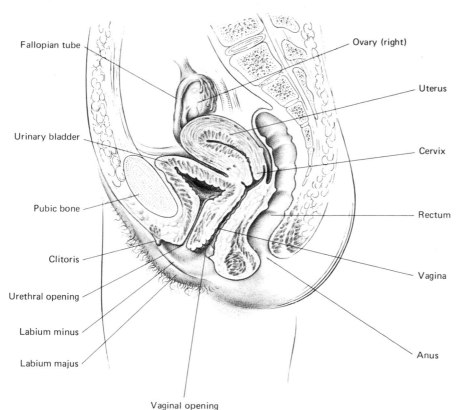

Fallopian tube

Urinary bladder

Pubic bone

Clitoris

Urethral opening

Labium minus

Labium majus

Vaginal opening

Ovary (right)

Uterus

Cervix

Rectum

Vagina

Anus

Figure 12.2
Cross-section of female pelvis.
SOURCE: Eric T. Pengelley, *Sex
and Human Life* (Reading, Mass.:
Addison-Wesley, 1974).

Figure 12.3
External genitalia of the human female.
SOURCE: Gilbert D. Nass, *Marriage and
the Family* (Reading, Mass.: Addison-
Wesley, 1978).

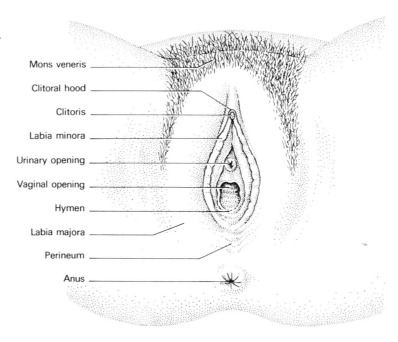

Mons veneris

Clitoral hood

Clitoris

Labia minora

Urinary opening

Vaginal opening

Hymen

Labia majora

Perineum

Anus

sues surrounding the vagina secrete a lubricant when the female is sexually stimulated; the presence of this lubricant is the first physical sign of female sexual arousal.

The vagina leads to the **uterus,** a thick-walled muscular organ the size and shape of a pear. The mouth of the uterus, termed the **cervix,** extends into the vagina. The other end of the uterus is termed the **fundus.** It consists of three layers. The outermost layer is the **perimetrium,** which is very elastic and allows the uterus to expand during pregnancy. The middle layer, the **myometrium,** is muscular (smooth muscle) and can contract to push the newborn out through the cervix and into the birth canal (vagina). The inner layer is the **endometrium,** which is abundant in blood vessels and is partly discharged during menstruation. It is in the uterus that the fertilized egg, or **ovum,** is implanted and develops into an **embryo** (to 12 weeks) and then a **fetus** (after 12 weeks).

Leading from the uterus back toward the ovaries are the **Fallopian tubes,** which are hollow and have muscular walls. The sperm usually fertilizes the ovum in one tube or the other. Once fertilized, the ovum passes down the Fallopian tube toward the uterus (see Fig. 12.4).

The egg is originally deposited by the ovary and eventually works its way through the Fallopian tube. The ovary contains approximately 400,000 ova at birth and at puberty begins releasing one each month. When released, the ovum is caught by one of the **fimbria,** the fingerlike projections that jut out from the end of the Fallopian tubes (ampulla). The ovary is also responsible for female hormone production.

THE INFLUENCE OF HORMONES

How Sex Hormones Work

Concept: Hormones are responsible for the development of secondary sexual characteristics, and they trigger the reproductive functions.

Hormones are chemical substances produced by the **endocrine** (ductless) glands. They affect the functioning

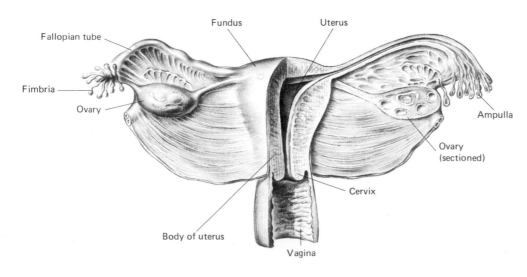

Figure 12.4
Uterus and ovaries
(front view).
SOURCE: Eric T. Pengelley, *Sex and Human Life* (Reading, Mass.: Addison-Wesley, 1974).

Fallopian tube
Fundus
Uterus
Fimbria
Ovary
Ampulla
Ovary (sectioned)
Cervix
Body of uterus
Vagina

of various organs throughout the body. Hormones also play an important role in sexual development and sexual behavior throughout our lives. For example, during prenatal development, hormonal secretions are released at just the right time so that the embryo develops sexual organs appropriate to its sex.

Two hormones produced by the **pituitary gland** are of particular importance, because they stimulate the production of sex hormones. In females the **follicle-stimulating hormone (FSH)** and the **luteinizing hormone (LH)** stimulate the manufacture and secretion of the female sex hormones, **estrogen** and **progesterone.** In males the luteinizing hormone is called **interstitial-cell-stimulating hormone (ICSH)** because it stimulates the interstitial cells of the testes to manufacture and secrete the male hormone, **testosterone.** FSH and LH (ICSH) are called **gonadotrophins.**

During puberty, sex hormones are responsible for the development of secondary sexual characteristics. In females estrogen triggers the development of pubic hair, breasts, and fat deposits. In males testosterone triggers the growth of pubic, facial, and chest hair; deepening of the voice; and muscle enlargement. The sex hormones also stimulate menstruation and ovulation in females and sperm production in males.

The Menstrual Cycle

Concept: Hormonal secretions control the menstrual cycle.

Menstruation is a word derived from the Latin *menis,* meaning month. Though considered to occur monthly, the **menses** (period) may be quite unpredictable. Beginning at **menarche** (from 9 to 14 or 15 years of age) and ceasing at **menopause** (between 45 and 55 years of age), menstruation is a normal physiological response to hormonal changes occurring in the female.

The hormones involved in menstruation are the estrogens. The menstrual cycle begins when the anterior portion of the pituitary gland secretes FSH, signaling the ovary to ripen one egg. The anterior portion of the pituitary gland also secretes LH, which aids in **ovulation** (the release of one egg by the ovary). Once the egg is released by the ovary, the area from which it was released (**Graafian follicle**) converts into a yellow body called the **corpus luteum.** The Graafian follicle secretes estrogen, and the corpus luteum secretes progesterone. Progesterone causes the endometrium of the uterus to thicken and store nutrients in preparation

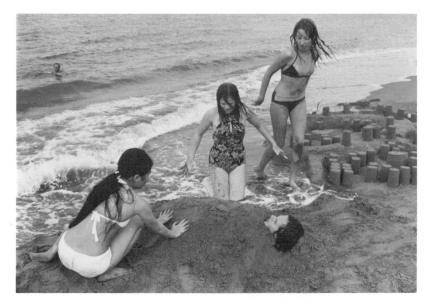

Hormones play a central role in the development of secondary sexual characteristics during puberty.

Discovery Activity 12.3
MENSTRUATION

To test your understanding of the menstrual cycle fill in the blanks in the following sentences:

1. The gonadotrophic hormones produced by the pituitary gland are _____ and _____.

2. FSH stimulates the production of the _____ _____ from which the egg is released.

3. LH stimulates the development of the _____ _____.

4. The place from which the egg is released from the ovary (answer to question 2 above) secretes the hormone _____. This hormone tells the pi-

tuitary gland to increase production of the hormone _____.

5. After 14 days of a 28-day menstrual cycle, the place from which the egg was released from the ovary secretes the hormone _____. This hormone tells the pituitary gland to slow down production of the hormone _____ if the egg is not fertilized by a sperm.

6. During a 28-day menstrual cycle, ovulation occurs around day _____.

7. The menstrual flow continues for about _____ days during a 28-day cycle.

Consult Fig. 12.5 *only* after filling in the blanks above, if you are unsure of your answers. ●

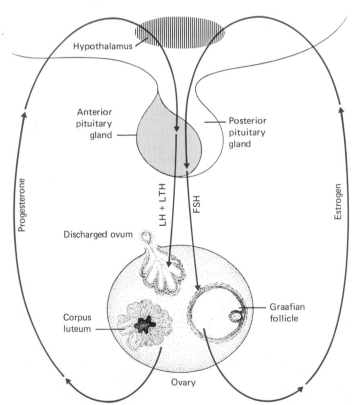

Figure 12.5
The menstrual cycle. During a 28-day cycle, ovulation will occur on day 14, with secretion of progesterone from then until day 25. Estrogen is produced throughout the 28 days, though in varying degrees. Menstruation will occur during days 1–5 of a 28-day cycle.

to receive, implant, and nourish a fertilized egg. If the egg is not fertilized, the corpus luteum degenerates and is no longer able to secrete progesterone. The lack of progesterone is a signal to expel the unneeded nutrient-full endometrium, and menstruation begins. The cycle is then ready to begin anew. Figure 12.5 depicts the phases of the menstrual cycle.

Menopause

Between the ages of 45 and 55 women usually begin **menopause.** Menopause is the end of monthly expulsion of the nourished endometrium. Menopause is the result of hormonal changes. Immediately preceding menopause, there is an increase in the secretion of gonadotrophic hormones (FSH and LH).[1] As a consequence, the feedback mechanism of estrogen and progesterone production upon the pituitary gland is disturbed, resulting in the cessation of both ovulation and menstrual flow. Several physiological changes take place during menopause: thinning of the vaginal walls, narrowing and shortening of the vagina, and shrinking of the labia majora. In addition, there is less vaginal lubrication during sexual arousal, and uterine contractions during orgasm become stronger. These changes may make intercourse painful for a small number of women. The most commonly experienced menopausal symptom is "hot flashes," a sensation of heat caused by irregular dilation of the blood vessels, often in the face.

Some physicians view menopause as a deficiency condition caused by insufficient amounts of estrogen. As a result, many women take prescription estrogen pills aimed at restoring the appropriate hormonal balance and thereby relieving symptoms. However, **estrogen replacement therapy (ERT)** is a controversial treatment, because studies have linked it to uterine cancer. Women taking estrogen pills were found to be six times more likely to develop cancer of the endometrium than women not taking estrogen. Consequently, ERT should be prescribed only in cases of severe symptoms and in the smallest possible dosages. Most menopausal symptoms can be treated with relatively safe medications, such as aspirin, tranquilizers, and antidepressants. Although most menopausal women do experience some discomfort, only about one-quarter have symptoms that prompt them to seek medical help.[2]

Contrary to the notion that menopause is a major life trauma, most women make the transition smoothly. Many report increased interest in and enjoyment of sexual intercourse, because the fear of pregnancy has been eliminated.[3] These findings run contrary to the myth that postmenopausal women can no longer enjoy sex.

Do you know someone going through menopause? If you do, it might be useful to discuss with this person the changes she is experiencing. Too often menopause is considered inappropriate for discussion, and consequently some menopausal women who might need support from family and friends do not get it. Such support can be enormously useful in helping a woman cope with this life change.

Research has shown that, contrary to popular myth, many post-menopausal women experience greater enjoyment of sexual relations because they no longer need be concerned about pregnancy.

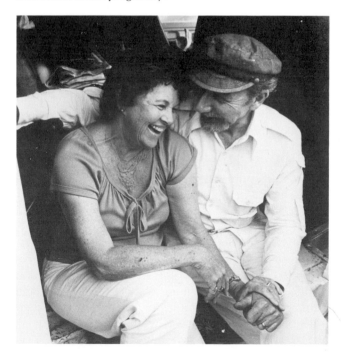

The Male Climacteric

There is evidence that men experience some physiological changes related to their reproductive system, but these changes are not as obvious and rapid as the changes that occur in women. There is a gradual decline in production of testosterone, which causes a decrease in the frequency of erection, amount of ejaculate, and force of ejaculation. The testicles decrease slightly in size and the prostate gland enlarges. Some middle-aged men find that they require longer to achieve an erection than they did in their younger years. However, many men remain fertile throughout life.

Some men report physical symptoms related to the male climacteric, including impotence, frequent urination, headaches, and even hot flashes. Changes in hormone levels may be related to some of these symptoms, but certain common aspects of middle age, such as stress at work and reevaluation of life goals, also seem to play a large role.

SEX ROLES

Sex Differences: Myth and Fact

A great many assumptions are made about differences in the abilities and traits of men and women, purely on the basis of gender. Table 12.1 shows the results of recent studies of gender differences. Some of the findings may not surprise you. For example, males tend to be physically stronger, more aggressive, and more active; and females tend to have better verbal skills and to be more nurturant and more sociable. However, some stereotypes simply are not supported by the research. For example, no differences have been established between the sexes on intelligence, creativity, assertiveness, competitiveness, achievement orientation, or emotionality. What stereotypes did you possess before looking at Table 12.1? Which were supported by the literature and which were not? How do you think you developed your views of the abilities and traits of men versus those of women?

Sex Roles

Concept: Males and females are stereotyped by sex roles.

He is playing masculine. She is playing feminine. She is playing feminine *because* he is playing masculine. He is playing masculine *because* she is playing feminine. He is playing the kind of man that he thinks the kind of woman she is playing ought to admire. She is playing the kind of woman that she thinks the kind of man he is playing ought to desire.

If he were not playing masculine, he might well be more feminine than she is—except when she is playing very feminine. If she were not playing feminine, she might well be more masculine than he—except when he is playing very masculine.

So he plays harder. And she plays—softer.

He wants to make sure that she could never be more masculine than he. She wants to make sure that he could never be more feminine than she. He therefore seeks to destroy the femininity in himself. She therefore seeks to destroy the masculinity in herself.

She is supposed to admire him for the masculinity in him that she fears in herself. He is supposed to desire her for the femininity in her that he despises in himself.

He desires her for her femininity which is *his* femininity, but which he can never lay claim to. She admires him for his masculinity which is her masculinity, but which she can never lay claim to. Since he may only love his own femininity in her, he envies her her femininity. Since she may only love her own masculinity in him, she envies him his masculinity.

The envy poisons their love.

He, coveting her unattainable femininity, decides to punish her. She, coveting his unattainable masculinity, decides to punish him. He denigrates her femininity—which he is supposed to desire and which he really envies—and becomes more aggressively masculine. She feigns disgust at his masculinity—which she is supposed to admire and which she really envies—and becomes more fastidiously feminine. He is becoming less and less what he wants to be. She is becoming less and less what she wants to be. But now he is more manly than ever, and she is more womanly than ever.

Her femininity, growing more dependently supine, becomes contemptible. His masculinity, growing more oppressively domineering, becomes intolerable. At last she loathes what she has helped his masculinity to become. At last he loathes what he has helped her femininity to become.

So far, it has all been very symmetrical. But we have left one thing out.

The reward for what his masculinity has become is power. The reward for what her femininity has become is only security which his power can bestow upon her. If he were to yield to what her femininity

Table 12.1
GENDER-LINKED DIFFERENCES IN ABILITIES AND IN PHYSICAL AND PSYCHOLOGICAL TRAITS

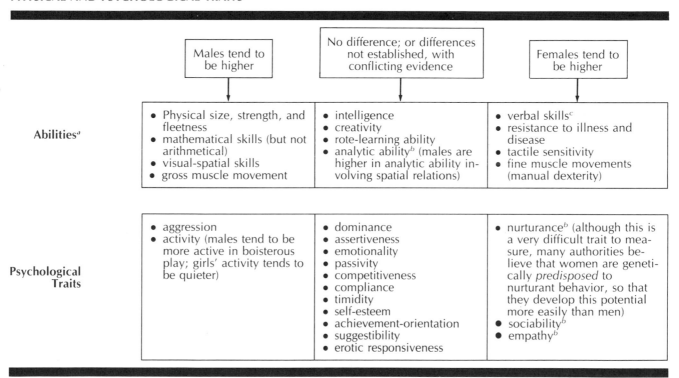

	Males tend to be higher	No difference; or differences not established, with conflicting evidence	Females tend to be higher
Abilities[a]	• Physical size, strength, and fleetness • mathematical skills (but not arithmetical) • visual-spatial skills • gross muscle movement	• intelligence • creativity • rote-learning ability • analytic ability[b] (males are higher in analytic ability involving spatial relations)	• verbal skills[c] • resistance to illness and disease • tactile sensitivity • fine muscle movements (manual dexterity)
Psychological Traits	• aggression • activity (males tend to be more active in boisterous play; girls' activity tends to be quieter)	• dominance • assertiveness • emotionality • passivity • competitiveness • compliance • timidity • self-esteem • achievement-orientation • suggestibility • erotic responsiveness	• nurturance[b] (although this is a very difficult trait to measure, many authorities believe that women are genetically *predisposed* to nurturant behavior, so that they develop this potential more easily than men) • sociability[b] • empathy[b]

[a]Gender-linked abilities not indicated here are the four biological imperatives (gestation, lactation, and menstruation in the female, and sperm production in the male).

[b]These abilities and traits are especially controversial. Men tend to be superior in analyzing problems that have to do with manipulating objects in space; some authorities find that more women than men are predisposed to being nurturant by their genetic programming; some authorities find that women are superior in personal relations, empathy, or sociability—judging emotions and expressions better than men.

[c]It is curious that although most writers, orators, and newscasters are men, girls score higher on tests of verbal ability, and remedial reading and writing programs enroll far more boys than girls. Either verbal ability in children is not related to later professional verbal skills, or cultural factors (opportunity and expectation) must explain this phenomenon.

SOURCE: Lloyd Saxton, *The Individual, Marriage and the Family.* (Belmont, Calif.: Wadsworth Publishing Company, 1980), p. 47. Reprinted by permission.

has become, he would be yielding to contemptible incompetence. If she were to acquire what his masculinity has become, she would participate in intolerable coerciveness.

She is stifling under the triviality of her femininity. The world is groaning beneath the terrors of his masculinity.

He is playing masculine. She is playing feminine.

How do we call off the game?[4]

The passage above describes how males and females are victimized by sex role stereotyping. **Sex roles** refer to the behaviors and tasks that our society expects of men and women by virtue of their sex. Traditional attributes fostered in males are dominance, aggression, rational decision making, and the like. Females traditionally have been expected to display nurturant, passive, and emotional qualities. In terms of roles, men have traditionally been expected to be breadwinners and women to be homemakers and mothers. As the excerpt shows, expectations of masculinity and femininity often have a profound effect on people's lives, forcing both sexes to play roles that may stifle them and put them at odds.

Sex role perceptions greatly influence the decisions men and women make about occupation, the opportunities they are afforded in society, and the roles they assume in marriage and family relationships. The rapid rate of change in today's society, difficult economic conditions, changing views of the roles of men and women, and more effective means of birth control are among the factors that have prompted many people to question traditional role expectations. Today more people want to be able to define their own roles rather than accept sex-based definitions that may not suit their individual needs. You can decide whether the roles and tasks you have assumed to this point because of your sex are the most suitable for you, or whether you wish to change them. To make this decision, however, it is useful to have a basic understanding of how your perceptions of yourself as masculine or feminine developed.

Sex Role Development

Sex role development is a complex process that begins at birth and continues throughout an individual's formative years. The differing expectations our society has of the roles of males and females appear to result from a complex combination of biological and learning factors. There is still great debate over how these factors operate, however, and over whether biology or learning is more important. Hutt states that "the effects of

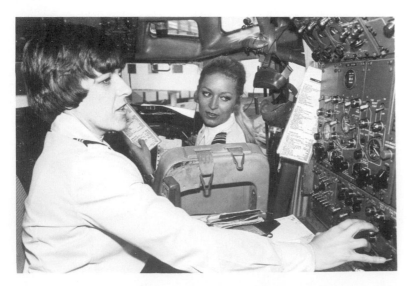

Some women today are entering vocations that were once considered the traditional reserve of men. For these female airline pilots, the sky is apparently no limit.

Discovery Activity 12.4
ABILITIES AND APTITUDES DESIRABLE FOR MEN AND WOMEN

For each trait listed below, indicate whether you feel it is more desirable in males (M), more desirable in females (F), or equally desirable in both sexes (B).

1. Athletic ability
2. Social ability
3. Mechanical ability
4. Interpersonal understanding
5. Leadership
6. Art appreciation
7. Intellectual ability
8. Creative ability
9. Scientific understanding
10. Moral and spiritual understanding
11. Theoretical ability
12. Domestic ability
13. Economic ability
14. Affectional ability
15. Observational ability
16. Fashion sense
17. Common sense
18. Physical attractiveness
19. Achievement and mastery
20. Occupational ability ●

In one study college students of both sexes were asked which abilities and aptitudes were desirable for males and females. They cited the odd-numbered items on your list and item 20 as desirable for males and the even numbered items (except item 20) as desirable for females.¹ How do your responses compare? Why do you think the results turned out as they did?

Issues in Health
IS SEX ROLE STEREOTYPING BAD?

Some people believe that sex role stereotyping serves a useful purpose and should be maintained. They argue that clearly defined sex roles provide guidance to young people—boys and girls—regarding the training they should acquire. Girls should develop nurturance by baby-sitting, learn how to cook by helping their mothers, and prepare for a career that will also allow them to do their homemaking and mothering chores, (for example, teaching). Marriages are breaking up because sexual roles are not clearly defined, they contend. A man and a woman enter a marriage expecting certain things from each other. If the roles aren't well defined, these expectations are likely to go unmet, resulting in marital dissatisfaction and divorce. Further, schools should teach children to accept traditional sex roles, because the purpose of schooling is to help young people fit into society. Otherwise, schools create citizens who are ill prepared to contribute to a stable society and who will be social malcontents.

Others believe sex role stereotyping is too limiting; that is, it prohibits a free choice of lifestyle. Why shouldn't people be free to choose those roles they want rather than having certain ones forced upon them? People cannot be self-actualized unless they are able to choose a career suited to them, can develop a family style consistent with their needs, or develop abilities and characteristics natural to them. These opponents of sex role stereotyping believe schools should develop citizens with inquiring minds who can examine their society and identify ways to improve it. Teaching young people to fit into the society, with no questions asked, rather than help it to evolve, would defeat this purpose.

What do you think? ●

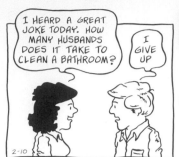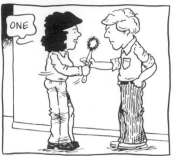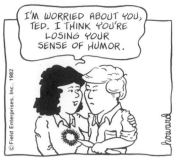

Sally Forth by Greg Howard. © 1982 Field Enterprises, Inc. Courtesy of Field Newspaper Syndicate.

the male and female sex hormones determine that physiologically the sexes function very differently.''[6] Hutt believes that due to early hormonal secretions, and therefore physiological differentiation between males and females, societal influences affect them differently and determine their sex roles.[7]

Learning plays a vital role in shaping masculine and feminine behavior. Parents, teachers, peers, toys, books, and other media are all influential in teaching children the conduct and qualities deemed appropriate for their sex. Boys and girls are treated differently even from birth, when boys are wrapped in blue blankets and girls in pink blankets. There is evidence that parents perceive boy babies as larger, sturdier, and more active and girl babies as smaller, more delicate, and weaker.

The toys and books parents give their children tend to foster different qualities in boys and girls. Boys' toys, such as guns, space toys, and trucks, encourage aggressive, active, and dominant behaviors, whereas girls' toys, such as dolls and kitchen equipment, promote nurturant, passive behaviors.

Children learn many behaviors, including appropriate behavior for their sex, by imitating their parents. Girls imitate the nurturant behavior of their mothers and are rewarded for adopting these ''feminine'' behaviors. It has been suggested that boys, in contrast,

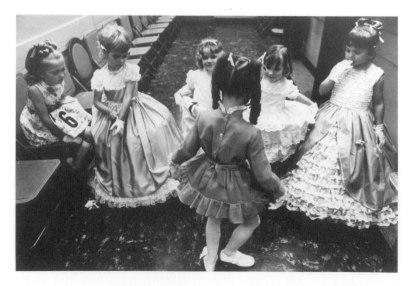

Little girls often learn that being pretty and ladylike are what counts most.

learn their roles through more negative processes; that is, they are more often told what behaviors *not* to express, such as crying, showing dependency, or playing with dolls. Thus, boys may actually have a more limited range of acceptable behaviors than girls. If a girl enjoys "boys'" activities, she's called a "tomboy," but a boy who displays feminine characteristics and interests is labeled a "sissy." One author has even concluded that, as a result of sex role stereotyping, males "have fewer role options than females."[8]

Because formal schooling involves a great deal of one's time, particularly during the formative years, its influence in determining sex roles is important to consider. Educational materials and personnel have been studied to determine the extent to which they foster sex role stereotyping, and the results of these studies have not been encouraging. For example, textbooks for elementary school children have many more male than female characters. Boys are portrayed as aggressive, active, and problem solvers, whereas girls are shown as engaged in fantasy and carrying out behaviors directed by others.[9]

Even educational tests tend to be biased regarding sex roles. When educational test batteries were studied, it was found that the test items referred more often to males and their worlds. Boys described in these test items tended to be active and girls passive; and boys were involved outside the home, girls predominantly in it.[10]

Other aspects of schooling also show evidence of sex role stereotyping. For instance, girls' athletic programs have long been treated as second cousins to boys' programs. Coaches of female interscholastic sports teams traditionally receive lower salaries than coaches of male teams.[11] In addition, vocational education programs have often provided more slots for boys than girls, have provided a greater variety of courses for boys than girls, and have labeled certain vocational options as more appropriate for one sex than another.[12] Title IX of the Education Amendments Act of 1972 directed toward the elimination of sex bias in schools, and as a result of this legislation, many of these practices have been or are being corrected. Nevertheless, their efforts will probably long be with us.

Issues in Health
SHOULD EMPLOYERS BE REQUIRED TO HIRE MORE WOMEN?

Some people believe it is unfair to expect a business to hire more women. Given two qualified candidates, one male and one female, the logical choice is the male. Many jobs require costly and time-consuming training programs, they contend, and men are better candidates because they cannot become pregnant and are unlikely to have to move due to their spouse's job requiring such a move. Why train women who may not make use of the training long enough? In addition, pregnant employees draw on the company's health insurance benefits, thereby increasing the premiums the company must pay the insurance carrier. Lastly, opponents of equal job access to women believe that, in most cases, the woman is not the breadwinner, is less likely to take her job as seriously, and will probably be absent from work when her children are ill.

Advocates of equal job access for women take issue with all these points. Most households must have two earners. Women are working not just to bring in extra money but to help the family meet its expenses. Furthermore, many women are careerminded and have educational backgrounds comparable to their male counterparts. Such women are unlikely to leave a job after undergoing costly training, and if they do become pregnant, they are likely to return to the job within a short period of time. Although some women may occasionally have to be absent from work because their children are ill, this is not a typical occurrence and results from the fact that we have no system of national day care. In addition, there is no evidence that women do not take their jobs as seriously as men. Finally, job discrimination on the basis of sex is against the law, and employers should be forced to comply with laws that protect the rights of citizens.

What do you think? ●

Discovery Activity 12.5
SEX ROLE STEREOTYPING AND YOU

How does sex role stereotyping relate to you? List below those tasks, traits, and expectations associated with your sex that you would like to give up.

1. _____ 4. _____
2. _____ 5. _____
3. _____ 6. _____

Next list those tasks, traits, and expectations associated with the opposite sex that you would like to adopt.

1. _____ 4. _____
2. _____ 5. _____
3. _____ 6. _____

Why are the tasks, traits, or expectations that you first listed associated with your sex? Why would you like to give them up? Why are the tasks, traits, or expectations you listed second associated with the opposite sex? Why would you like to adopt them? •

Changing Attitudes and Expectations

Since the mid-1970s there has been a significant change in the roles expected of men and women. It has become almost fashionable for men to admit to sensitivity and for women to pursue a career aggressively, for example. Although some of the rhetoric is just that, there has been an increasing acceptance of freedom of choice in career patterns, family lifestyles, and sexual behavior. The two-earner family has become common, while at the same time homemaking has regained its status as a vital and worthwhile occupation. The media periodically describes the life of a "househusband," making that option more acceptable. More women are becoming active in sports and other physical activities, and more men are helping with housework.

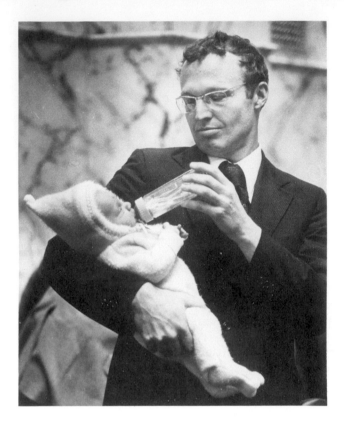

The key to this change lies in changing attitudes, which have made available a greater number of options for men and women. The result of this better "fit" might well be improved psychological health for the individual and improved sociological health for the community. This movement toward a blending of masculine and feminine characteristics in one person—called **androgyny**—is one of the most exciting and promising trends in today's society.

CONCLUSION

Although there are differences between males and females, there are also many similarities. Males and females differ anatomically but are complementary in the reproductive function. Males and females differ in the site of action of hormones but are similar in the hormones secreted. Both males and females suffer from sex role stereotyping. The importance of the consideration of sex roles was summarized by Rosen and Rosen:[13] ". . . sexuality is a way of relating to our fellow human beings, and many of the greatest rewards—and disappointments—of human sexuality arise from the nature of our sexual relationships and life styles."

SUMMARY

1. The male reproductive system consists of external structures—the scrotum, penis, and urethra—and internal structures—the testes, vas deferens, seminal vesicle, prostate and Cowper's glands, and the ampulla.

2. The female reproductive system consists of external structures—the labia majora, labia minora, and clitoris—and internal structures—the vagina, uterus, Fallopian tubes, and ovaries.

3. Hormones are chemical substances produced by endocrine glands and affecting organs throughout the body. The hormones that affect sexual development are estrogen and progesterone in females and testosterone in males.

4. The menstrual cycle is governed by the hormones FSH, LH, estrogen, and progesterone.

5. There is some evidence supporting the existence of a male menopause; for example, testosterone levels diminish over time. However, the changes in males are not as dramatic as those in females, and some men remain fertile throughout life.

6. The stereotypes of male and female abilities and traits do not necessarily hold up under investigation. Traits such as physical strength and aggressiveness have been found to be more prevalent in males, and sociability and verbal skills have been found to be more prevalent in females. However, no difference has been demonstrated between the sexes with regard to such traits as intelligence, creativeness, and emotionality.

7. Learning plays a vital role in shaping masculine and feminine behavior. Parents, teachers, peers, toys, books, and other media are all influential in teaching children the conduct and qualities deemed appropriate for their sex.

8. There is a trend toward androgyny—a blending of masculine and feminine characteristics in one person—in today's society. In addition, a greater choice of lifestyles is available today than ever before for men, as well as for women.

REFERENCES

1. Robert Kaplan, *Aspects of Human Sexuality* (Dubuque, Iowa: Wm. C. Brown, 1973), p. 53.

2. James Leslie McCary, *Human Sexuality: A Brief Edition* (New York: D. Van Nostrand, 1973), p. 51.

3. William H. Masters and Virginia E. Johnson, *Human Sexual Response* (Boston: Little, Brown, 1966).

4. Betty Roszak and Theodore Roszak, *Masculine/Feminine: Readings in Sexual Mythology and the Liberation of Women* (New York: Harper & Row, 1969), pp. vii–viii. Reprinted with permission.

5. R. Centers, "Evaluating the Loved One," *Journal of Personality* 39 (1971):311.

6. Corinne Hutt, *Males and Females* (Baltimore: Penguin Books, 1972), p. 17.

7. Ibid., p. 18.

8. David F. Shope, *Interpersonal Sexuality* (Philadelphia: W. B. Saunders, 1975), p. 95.

9. Terry N. Saario, Carol Nagy Jacklin, and Carol Kehr Tittle, "Sex Role Stereotyping in the Public Schools," in *What Do You Expect: An Inquiry into Self-Fulfilling Prophecies,* Paul M. Insel and Lenore F. Jacobson, eds. (Menlo Park, Calif.: Cummings, 1975), pp. 144–146.

10. Ibid., p. 153.

11. National Education Association, *Salary Schedule Supplements for Extra Duties, 1971–72.* Research Memo. Washington, D.C., April 1972.

12. New York City Board of Education, *Public High School, New York City 1970–1971* (New York: Bureau of Educational and Vocational Guidance, 1972).

13. Raymond Rosen and Linda Reich Rosen, *Human Sexuality* (New York: Alfred A. Knopf, 1981), p. 79.

Laboratory 1
THE SEXY COLLAGE

Purpose   To define masculinity and femininity.

Size of Group   Two groups: one all males and one all females.

Equipment   Each group will need:
magazines brought to class by the students
newsprint pad

Procedure

1. The two groups meet separately and develop two collages from pictures and words cut out of the magazines. One collage will depict how you *would like* the opposite sex to view your sex. The other collage will represent how you think the opposite sex *actually does* view your sex.

2. When all the collages are completed, show your group's collages to the other group and explain the rationale behind them. Listen while the other group does the same.

Results

Organize into two concentric circles: an inside circle of females and an outside circle of males. The inside circles of females should face outward toward the circle of males.

In this concentric circle formation, discuss the meaning that can be gleaned from the collages. Questions such as the following can serve as a basis for discussion:

1. What stereotypes did each sex believe characterized the other sex? Are these stereotypes actually true of the other sex?

2. Were the ways in which each group wished to be perceived by the opposite sex possible? What could each sex do to be perceived in the way they prefer.

3. How have these stereotypes developed?

4. Which stereotypes are accurate descriptions and which are inaccurate?

5. How does each sex behave toward the other based upon their stereotypic beliefs?

Laboratory 2
GENDER AND EROTICISM

Purpose   To discuss the differences between males' and females' views of eroticism and whether these differences are innate or learned.

Size of Group   Originally the total class; then divided by sex.

Equipment   None.

Procedure

1. As homework, each student is to write his or her conception of an erotic adventure on one side of one sheet of paper. On the other side of the paper, write the letter *F* if the erotic adventure was written by a female and the letter *M* if written by a male.

2. A box should be placed in front of the room for the erotic adventures to be deposited in when students enter class.

3. The erotic adventures should then be spread out, face up, on a table in front of the room. Each student should take one, read it, and guess whether it was written by a female or a male prior to turning it over to check for an *F* or *M*. When one paper has been read, it should be replaced and another taken, with the same procedure applying. This should continue for 20 minutes.

4. Next the males should meet in one room and the females in another. They should discuss any generalities they can identify about what females find erotic, what males find erotic, and the similarities and differences between the two. Specifically, they should discuss:

   a. The setting of the fantasy and its accoutrements (for example, candlelight or the sound of ocean surf),

   b. Who's passive and who's active in the fantasy,

   c. How many sexual partners are involved and of what sex,

   d. If there is any relationship other than sexual between the people in the fantasy.

Results

The class should reconvene to present the conclusions drawn by each group and express agreements and disagreements with each group's conclusions. The causes (learned behavior, hormonal, or genetic) of differences and similarities between male and female conceptions of eroticism should be discussed.

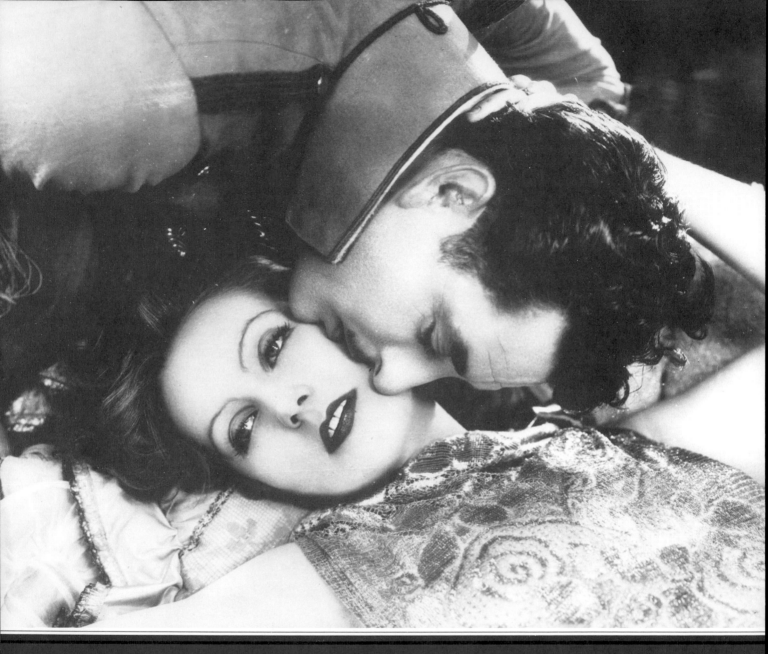

chapter *13*

sexual behavior and response

- *sexual response*
- *purposes of sexual behavior*
- *forms of sexual expression*
- *sexual dysfunction*
- *sexual diversity*
- *sex-related crimes*
- *sexual behavior: deciding for yourself*

Sexual behavior is a subject about which people have strong feelings and many misconceptions. The information presented in this chapter is intended to help you understand sexual response and the sources of sexual difficulties. It should also give you a basis for assessing your own attitudes toward varieties of sexual behavior and such controversial issues as rape and incest.

SEXUAL RESPONSE

Concept: The human sexual response can be described.

The Sexual Response Cycle

The most significant research in the area of human sexual response was conducted by William Masters and Virginia Johnson.[1] They found that the human sexual response could be divided into four distinct phases:

1. **Excitement phase.** This phase begins with sexual stimulation of some sort, whether physical, psychological (thoughts), or both. Sexual arousal in males is indicated by erection of the penis and in females by vaginal lubrication.

2. **Plateau phase.** If the excitement phase is not interrupted, sexual tension is intensified. In the male preejaculatory fluid is emitted at this point, and in the female the clitoris retracts under its hood.

3. **Orgasmic phase.** This phase consists of an involuntary muscular contraction concentrated in the clitoris, vagina, and uterus in the female and in the penis, prostate, and seminal vesicles in the male. It is in this phase that the male ejaculates.

4. **Resolution phase.** After orgasm, sexual tension is dissipated and the person returns to the preexcitement state. Although the female can return to the orgasmic phase if sexually stimulated during resolution, the male enters a refractory period during which sexual stimulation cannot produce another full erection. In other words, females are capable of multiple orgasms, or orgasms close in time to one another, whereas males are not.

The sexual response cycle in males and in females is detailed in Tables 13.1 through 13.4.

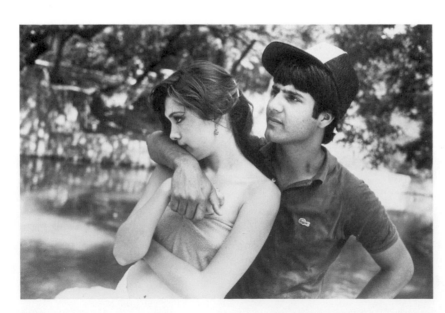

Table 13.1
**SEXUAL RESPONSE CYCLE OF THE HUMAN FEMALE—
EXTRAGENITAL REACTIONS**

	I. Excitement Phase	II. Plateau Phase	III. Orgasmic Phase	IV. Resolution Phase
Breasts	Nipple erection; increased definition and extension of venous patterning; increase in breast size; tumescence of areolae	Turgidity of nipples; further increase in breast size; marked areolar engorgement	No observed changes	Rapid detumescence of areolae and involution of nipple erection; slower decrease in breast volume and return to normal venous patterning
Sex flush	Appearance of maculopapular rash late in phase, first over epigastrium, spreading rapidly over breasts	Well-developed flush; may have widespread body distribution late in phase	Degree of flush parallels intensity of orgasmic experience (est. 75 percent incidence)	Rapid disappearance of flush in reverse order of its appearance
Myotonia	Voluntary-muscle tension; some evidence of involuntary activity (vaginal-wall expansion, tensing of abdominal and intercostal musculature)	Further increase in voluntary and involuntary tension; semispastic contractions of facial, abdominal and intercostal musculature	Loss of voluntary control; involuntary contractions and spasm of muscle groups	Myotonia rarely carried more than 5 min. into phase but not lost as rapidly as many evidences of vasocongestion
Rectum	No observed reaction	Voluntary contraction of rectal sphincter as stimulative technique (inconsistent)	Involuntary contractions of rectal sphincter occurring simultaneously with contractions of orgasmic platform	No observed changes
Hyperventilation	No observed reaction	Appearance of reaction occurs late in phase	Respiratory rates as high as 40 per min.; intensity and duration indicative of degree of sexual tension	Resolves early in phase
Tachycardia	Heart rate increases in direct parallel to rising tension regardless of technique of stimulation	Recorded rates average from 100 to 175 beats per min.	Recorded rates range from 110 to 180+ beats per min.; higher heart rates reflect more variation in orgasmic intensity for female than for male	Return to normal
Blood pressure	Elevation occurs in direct parallel to rising tension regardless of technique of stimulation	Elevation in systolic pressure of 20–60 mm Hg, diastolic 10–20 mm Hg	Elevations in systolic pressure of 30–80 mm Hg, diastolic 20–40 mm Hg	Return to normal
Perspiratory reaction	No observed reaction	No observed reaction	No observed reaction	Appearance of widespread film of perspiration, not related to degree of physical activity

From *Human Sexual Response* by W. H. Masters and V. E. Johnson, published in 1966 by Little, Brown and Company, Boston, pp. 286–287. Drs. Masters and Johnson are currently at the Masters & Johnson Institute, St. Louis, Missouri.

Table 13.2

SEXUAL RESPONSE CYCLE OF THE HUMAN FEMALE—GENITAL REACTIONS

	I. Excitement Phase	II. Plateau Phase	III. Orgasmic Phase	IV. Resolution Phase
Clitoris	Tumescent reaction of clitoral glans; vaso-congestive increase in diameter of clitoral shaft; shaft elongation	Withdrawl of clitoral body (shaft and glans) from normal pudendal-overhang positioning and retraction against anterior body of symphysis	No observed changes	Return to normal positioning within 5 to 10 sec. after cessation of orgasmic-platform contractions; slower detumescence and loss of vasocongestion
Vagina	Appearance of vaginal lubrication 10–30 sec. after initiation of sexual stimulation; expansion and distention of vaginal barrel; vaginal wall color alteration from normal purplish-red to darker, purplish hue of vasocongestion	Development of orgasmic platform at outer third of vagina; further increase in width and depth of vaginal barrel	Contractions of orgasmic platform starting at 0.8-sec. intervals and recurring 5–12 times; after first 3 to 6 contractions, intercontractile intervals lengthen and contractile intensity diminishes	Rapid detumescence of orgasmic platform; relaxation of vaginal walls; return to normal coloring (may take as long as 10–15 min.)
Uterus	Partial elevation of anteriorly placed uterus; development of corpus irritability	Full uterine elevation into false pelvis; cervical elevation produces tenting effect in midvaginal plane; increasing corpus irritability	Corpus contractions beginning in fundus, progressing through midzone, and expiring in lower uterine segment; contractile excursion parallels intensity of orgasmic experience; multipara, est. 50 percent size increase	Gaping of external cervical of which continues 20–30 min.; return of elevated uterus to unstimulated resting position in true pelvis; cervical descent into seminal basin
Labia majora	Nullipara: flattening, separation and antero-lateral elevation of labia away from vaginal outlet	Nullipara: labia may become severely engorged with venous blood during prolonged phase	Nullipara: no observed reaction	Nullipara: return to normal thickness and midline positioning
	Multipara: vasocongestive increase in diameter; slight lateral movement away from midline	Multipara: further vasocongestive swelling depending upon degree of varicosity involvement	Multipara: no observed reaction	Multipara: involution of labial vasocongestion
Labia minora	Minor labial thickening and expansion extending vaginal barrel approximately 1 cm	Vivid color change ranging from bright red to deep wine color; this sex-skin reaction pathognomonic of impending orgasm	No observed reaction	Color change from deep or bright red to light pink within 10–15 sec.; loss of vasocongestive size increase
Bartholin's glands	No observed changes	Secretion of drop or two of mucoid material aiding in lubrication of vaginal outlet during long-maintained coitus	No observed changes	No observed changes

From *Human Sexual Response* by W. H. Masters and V. E. Johnson, published in 1966 by Little, Brown and Company, pp. 288–289. Drs. Masters and Johnson are currently at the Masters & Johnson Institute, St. Louis, Missouri.

Table 13.3
SEXUAL RESPONSE CYCLE OF THE HUMAN MALE—EXTRAGENITAL REACTIONS

	I. Excitement Phase	II. Plateau Phase	III. Orgasmic Phase	IV. Resolution Phase
Breasts	Nipple erection (inconsistent and may be delayed until plateau phase)	Nipple erection and turgidity (inconsistent)	No observed changes	Involution of nipple erection (may be prolonged)
Sex flush	No observed reaction	Appearance of maculo-papular rash late in phase (inconsistent); originates over epigastrium and spreads to anterior chest wall, neck, face, forehead, and occasionally to shoulders and forearms	Well-developed flush; degree parallels intensity of orgasm (est. 25 percent incidence)	Rapid disappearance of flush in reverse order of appearance
Myotonia	Voluntary-muscle tension; some evidence of involuntary activity (partial testicular elevation, tensing of abdominal and intercostal musculature)	Further increase in voluntary and involuntary tension; semispastic contractions of facial, abdominal, and intercostal musculature	Loss of voluntary control; involuntary contractions and spasm of muscle groups	Myotonia rarely carried more than 5 min. into phase but not lost as rapidly as many evidences of vasocongestion
Rectum	No observed reaction	Voluntary contraction of rectal sphincter as stimulative technique (inconsistent)	Involuntary contractions of rectal sphincter at 0.8-sec. intervals	No observed changes
Hyperventilation	No observed reaction	Appearance of reaction occurs late in phase	Respiratory rates as high as 40 per min.; intensity and duration indicative of degree of sexual tension	Resolves during refractory period
Tachycardia	Heart rate increases in direct parallel to rising tension regardless of technique of stimulation	Recorded rates average from 100 to 175 beats per min.	Recorded rates range from 110 to 180 beats per min.	Return to normal
Blood pressure	Elevation occurs in direct parallel to rising tension regardless of technique of stimulation	Elevations in systolic pressure of 20–80 mm Hg, diastolic 10–40 mm Hg	Elevations in systolic pressure of 40–100 mm Hg, diastolic 20–50 mm Hg	Return to normal
Perspiratory reaction	No observed reaction	No observed reaction	No observed reaction	Involuntary sweating reaction (inconsistent), usually confined to soles of feet and palms of hands

From *Human Sexual Response* by W. H. Masters and V. E. Johnson, published in 1966 by Little, Brown and Company, Boston, pp. 290–291. Drs. Masters and Johnson are currently at the Masters & Johnson Institute, St. Louis, Missouri.

Table 13.4
SEXUAL RESPONSE CYCLE OF THE HUMAN MALE–GENITAL REACTIONS

	I. Excitement Phase	II. Plateau Phase	III. Orgasmic Phase	IV. Resolution Phase
Penis	Rapid occurrence of erection which may be partially lost and subsequently regained during a prolonged phase, or may be easily impaired by the introduction of asexual stimuli	Increase in penile circumference at coronal ridge; color change in coronal area (inconsistent)	Expulsive contractions of entire length of penile urethra; contractions start at 0.8-sec. intervals and after the first three or four are reduced in frequency and in expulsive force; minor contractions continue for several seconds	Detumescence occurs in two stages: (1) rapid loss of vasocongestion until penis is from 1 to 1½ times enlarged; (2) slower involution to normal state, usually extended process
Scrotum	Tensing and thickening of scrotal integument; flattening and elevation of scrotal sac	No specific reactions	No specific reactions	Rapid loss of congested, tense appearance of scrotum and early reappearance of integumental folding; sometimes delayed process
Testes	Partial elevation of both testes toward perineum accomplished by shortening of spermatic cords	Enlargement of testes to a 50 percent increase over their unstimulated noncongested state; elevation to a position of close apposition to perineum; full testicular elevation pathognomonic of impending ejaculation	No recorded reaction	Loss of vasocongestive increase in testicular size and full descent of testes into relaxed scrotum; may occur rapidly or slowly depending upon length of plateau phase
Secondary organs	No observed changes	No observed changes	Contractions of secondary organs which develop sensation of ejaculatory inevitability and initiate ejaculatory process	No observed changes
Cowper's glands	No observed changes	Have been suggested as source of preejaculatory emission of two or three drops of mucoid fluid; timing is essentially same as that of secretory activity of Bartholin's glands in female; active spermatozoa have been observed in this fluid	No observed changes	No observed changes

From *Human Sexual Response* by W. H. Masters and V. E. Johnson, published in 1966 by Little, Brown and Company, Boston, pp. 292–293. Drs. Masters and Johnson are currently at the Masters and Johnson Institute, St. Louis, Missouri.

Similarities in Male and Female Response

Concept: Males and females have many similarities in their sexual physiological responses.

Masters and Johnson found a number of similarities in the sexual response of males and females.

1. *Nipples.* Erection of the nipples is evident in both sexes. In an early study, Masters and Johnson found nipple erection in 30 percent of men; however they later upgraded that figure to 50 to 60 percent on the basis of further research. Not only do the nipples become erect in both sexes, they also increase in diameter.

2. *Sex flush.* During high levels of sexual tension, due to **vasocongestion** (a lot of blood accumulating in an area), both sexes experience a darkening of the skin. This sex flush occurs on the neck, face, and forehead of both males and females, as well as on the chest.

3. *Muscle tension.* Medically termed **myotonia,** muscle tension in both sexes first develops during the plateau phase and involves the legs, arms, abdomen, neck, and face. In addition, both sexes contract the gluteal (buttocks) muscles prior to orgasm. During orgasm both sexes contract the muscles of the abdomen, chest, and face. Finally, muscle tension is released by both sexes during the resolution phase. "No difference has been observed between the sexes in rapidity of muscle tension release."[2]

4. *Deep and rapid breathing.* Termed **hyperventilation,** deep and rapid breathing occurs in both sexes.

5. *Increased heart rate.* Both sexes experience **tachycardia** (increased heart rate). During the orgasmic phase, Masters and Johnson found heart rates to increase up to 180+ beats per minute.

6. *Increased blood pressure.* Blood pressure is elevated significantly in both males and females during sexual excitement.

7. *Perspiration.* Approximately 33 percent of both sexes will develop involuntary sweating immediately following orgasm.

8. *Vasocongestion.* Increased blood flow to the pelvic area occurs in both sexes, causing penile erection in the male and vaginal lubrication in the female. In addition, vasocongestion results in elevation of the male scrotal sac, and elevation of the major labia in females who have never given birth and a thickening and separation of the labia in females who have borne children.

Differences in Male and Female Response

Concept: Males and females have many differences in their sexual physiological responses

The differences between males and females in their physiological and anatomical sexual responses include the following:

1. *Nipples.* Though both sexes experience nipple erection during sexual stimulation, the female more often experiences this erection during the excitement phase. Males also experience nipple erection during the excitement phase but are more apt to have it delayed until the plateau phase than are females. In addition, female nipple erection disappears rapidly after orgasm, whereas male nipple erection may be prolonged after ejaculation.

2. *Sex flush.* Though both exhibit a sex flush, the female experiences it late in the excitement phase or early in the plateau phase, whereas the male sex flush occurs only in the plateau phase. The neck, face, forehead, and chest of both sexes become flushed, but the flush is also evident on the lower abdomen, thighs, lower back, and buttocks of females only.

3. *Muscle tension.* Myotonia results in an increase in the length of the vagina and expansion of the di-

ameter of the cervix in females. In males elevation of the testes occurs.

4. *Deep and rapid breathing.* Both sexes experience hyperventilation prior to orgasm. Once orgasm has occurred, the male must wait for hyperventilation to subside during the resolution phase before he can be orgasmic again. However, the female can move from one orgasm to the next (multiorgasmic) without waiting for hyperventilation to subside.

5. *Blood pressure.* Whereas blood pressure increases for both sexes, the range of increase differs. For males the range is 40 to 100 mm Hg systolic pres-

sure and 20 to 50 mm Hg diastolic. For females the range is 30 to 80 mm Hg systolic and 20 to 40 mm Hg diastolic.

6. *Perspiration.* In males sweating after orgasm is predominantly confined to the soles of the feet and the palms of the hands. In females it is more likely to occur on the back, thighs, and chest, and sometimes on the trunk, head, and neck.

7. *Patterns of response and orgasm.* As shown in Fig. 13.1(a), males have an orgasm with a refractory period as part of their response cycle. Fig. 13.1(b) shows that the female sexual response

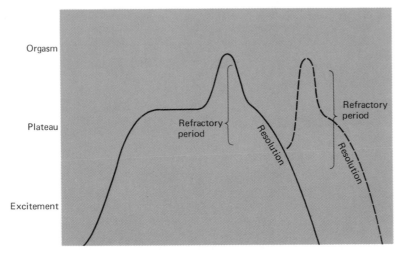

Figure 13.1(a)
The male sexual response cycle.
SOURCE: Masters and Johnson, *Human Sexual Response* (Boston: Little, Brown and Company, 1966), p. 5. Reprinted by permission.

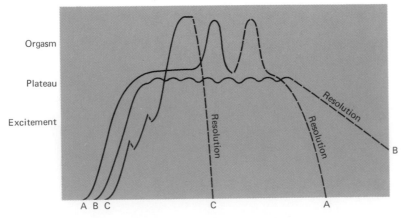

Figure 13.1(b)
The female sexual response cycle.
SOURCE: Masters and Johnson, *Human Sexual Response* (Boston: Little, Brown and Company, 1966), p. 5. Reprinted by permission.

and orgasm can take several forms. Pattern A most closely resembles the male pattern, except that it shows the potential of the female for additional orgasms without the refractory period necessary for males. In Pattern B the woman reaches the plateau level but does not have an orgasm, and in Pattern C she experiences a rapid rise to orgasm followed by a quick resolution. Another important difference, as noted previously, is that multiple orgasms are within the capacity of most women, whereas men always experience a refractory period after orgasm. The fact that not nearly as many women actually have multiple orgasms as are capable of them may be related to the source of stimulation used to achieve orgasm. Masters and Johnson found that repeated orgasms are more often possible through manual, oral, or mechanical stimulation than through penile thrusting.

PURPOSES OF SEXUAL BEHAVIOR

Concept: Sex is engaged in for many reasons.

People engage in sexual activity for many reasons, some of which are more acceptable in our society than others. For example, sex for having babies or as an expression of intimacy and love tends to be more acceptable than sex for fun or as a remedy for loneliness. Each individual evaluates sexual behavior according to his or her own values and morals. Thus it is difficult to decide objectively which expressions of sexual activity and which purposes are "right" and which are "wrong."

How do you use sexual behavior? You have probably used sex for many reasons: perhaps to show your love, to relieve boredom, for excitement, or because it was expected of you. To analyze how you use sexual behavior, complete the accompanying Discovery Activity 13.1. Afterward, spend some time determining which of these purposes you want to eliminate and which you want to emphasize in your life. In this manner you will be making more sense out of your sexual lifestyle.

Discovery Activity 13.1
THE USES OF SEX

People use sex for many reasons. How do you use it? Read the list below, and place a check mark next to those phrases that represent how you sometimes use sex.

_____ Sex as purely playful activity.

_____ Sex as a way to have babies.

_____ Sex as fun.

_____ Sex as an expression of hostility.

_____ Sex as punishment.

_____ Sex as a mechanical duty.

_____ Sex as an outlet from physiological or psychological tension.

_____ Sex as a protection against alienation.

_____ Sex as a way of overcoming separateness or loneliness.

_____ Sex as a way to communicate deep involvement in the welfare of others.

_____ Sex as a form of "togetherness."

_____ Sex as a reward.

_____ Sex as a revenge.

_____ Sex as an act of rebellion.

_____ Sex as an experiment.

_____ Sex as an adventure.

_____ Sex as a deceit.

_____ Sex as a form of self-enhancement.

_____ Sex as an exploitation for personal gain.

_____ Sex as proof.*

Now go back over this list and circle those uses you checked with which you are not happy. How will you try to change your behavior as a result of this activity? ●

*Adapted from J. L. Malfetti and E. M. Eidlitz, *Perspectives on Sexuality* (New York: Holt, Rinehart and Winston, 1972). Reprinted by permission.

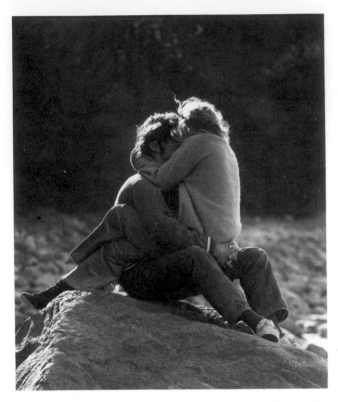

Most people believe that sexual behavior should be used for positive purposes such as to express intimacy and caring. When sex is used for negative purposes, the individual is probably experiencing an adjustment or emotional problem.

FORMS OF SEXUAL EXPRESSION

Concept: Sexual expression can take a number of different forms.

Until recently, our society imposed many restrictions on the forms of sexual expression that were considered appropriate. Today, however, a much wider range of behaviors is regarded as acceptable. Sexual intercourse is only one of many sexual choices. Indeed, people may choose different forms of sexual expression under different circumstances or at different times in their lives. Our sexual attitudes and behavior are influenced by what we think others regard as appropriate. As you read the following sections, consider to what degree your own sexual behavior has been influenced by what your peers are doing.

The most extensive study of human sexual behavior was conducted by Kinsey *et al.*[4,5] These researchers interviewed thousands of people of varied socioeconomic status, educational attainment, marital status, and sex education experiences. Although published in 1948 (*Male Sexual Behavior*) and 1953 (*Female Sexual Behavior*) their studies are still considered the landmark research in American sexual behavior. In our discussion of forms of sexual expression, we will refer to some of the Kinsey findings, as well as to more recent studies.

Masturbation

Masturbation refers to erotic self-stimulation, usually to the point of orgasm. It has been practiced in all societies since ancient times. Even infants explore their genitals and receive pleasure from touching them. Often self-stimulation continues throughout life, whether or not the individual is a partner in a permanent intimate relationship.

Gender apparently has a substantial effect on the practice of masturbation, with males more likely to masturbate than females. This is probably the result of different socialization of males and females. A 1972 study of the masturbatory behavior of college students found that 80 percent of freshman males but only 33 percent of freshman females had engaged in masturbation (see Table 13.5). However, the incidence for both males and females in their senior year was nearly the same (about 75 percent).[6]

Even though masturbation is quite widespread, most men and women still feel somewhat ashamed of the practice. This is probably a carryover from their upbringing and from folklore that stamped masturbation as sinful, evil, and even physically and mentally harmful. Such ideas are entirely false, and today sex therapists and other experts believe that masturbation can be beneficial. It serves as a sexual outlet, a way to become more comfortable with one's own body in heterosexual lovemaking, and an alternative form of sexual expression when no partner is available.

Table 13.5
COLLEGE STUDENTS' SEXUAL BEHAVIOR

Independent Variable	Number	Incidence of Masturbation (%)	Frequency of Masturbation*	Incidence of Sexual Intercourse (%)
1. Sex				
male	52	84.62	6.73	76.93
female	75	52.00	1.82	69.33
2. Marital status				
married	21	61.90	2.81	100.00
not married	106	66.04	4.04	72.45
3. Class in school				
freshman				
male		80.00		
female		33.33		
total	27	51.85	4.07	51.85
sophomore				
male		100.00		
female		50.00		
total	29	55.17	1.62	72.41
junior				
male		90.48		
female		57.14		
total	42	73.81	3.86	76.19
senior				
male		75.00		
female		76.92		
total	29	75.86	5.79	86.21
4. Race				
Negro	7	33.33	0.57	55.56
Caucasian	111	76.24	4.17	80.20
other	9	42.86	2.22	85.71

*Number of times per month.
SOURCE: Jerrold S. Greenberg, "The Masturbatory Behavior of College Students," *Psychology in the Schools* 9(1972): 427–432. Reprinted with permission.

Petting and Oral Sex

Heterosexual **petting** is defined as erotic stimulation of a person by a sexual partner. It can include kisses, genital caresses, and oral-genital contact, and may culminate in orgasm. During adolescence petting is often a way for young people to experience intense sexual excitement without actually engaging in intercourse. Petting is carried over into adult sexual relationships as foreplay or for sexual variety.

Oral-genital stimulation takes two basic forms. **Cunnilingus** is oral stimulation of the vulva, and **fellatio** is oral stimulation of the penis and scrotum. Until recently, oral sex was viewed negatively by many people in the United States. Some have objected for religious reasons (because oral sex does not lead to procreation), others for sanitary reasons, and others because they feel uncomfortable about engaging in it. In Kinsey's surveys only 15 percent of high school–educated married men reported engaging in cunnilingus. However,

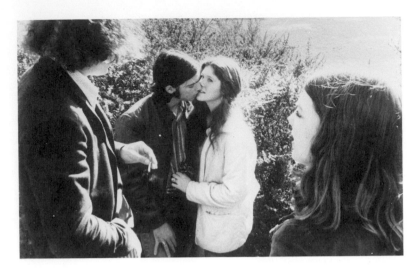

Teenagers today are engaging in sexual experimentation at earlier ages than in the past. Young women, particularly, seem to be "catching up" to young men in terms of their sexual experience.

more recent surveys suggest that oral-genital sex is becoming increasingly widespread. In a study conducted by Hunt in the 1970s, a majority of both male and female respondents under the age of 25 reported engaging in cunnilingus and fellatio.[7]

Sexual Intercourse

Sexual intercourse, or **coitus,** is penile-vaginal intercourse. It usually begins with petting, and when the partners are sufficiently aroused, the penis is guided into the vagina. Almost all men have an orgasm with every intercourse, but this is not true of all women. A survey of 26,000 people conducted by *Redbook Magazine* in 1980 found that 60 percent of women had an orgasm every time or almost every time they had intercourse.[8] A major reason that women do not have as high a rate of orgasm during intercourse is that intercourse alone may not provide sufficient clitoral stimulation. For many women, manual stimulation of the clitoris during intercourse and/or choosing a position that permits effective stimulation of the clitoris are effective means of reaching climax.

The incidence of young people engaging in sexual intercourse has been rising in recent years. In a study of college students conducted by Parcel, 40 percent of freshmen, 55 percent of sophomores, 73 percent of

juniors, and 85 percent of seniors reported having sexual intercourse.[9] The most profound change in incidence has occurred among women. Only 33 percent of Kinsey's sample of female subjects under 25 years of age reported engaging in sexual intercourse, compared to 75 percent of Hunt's sample. The incidence for males has not increased significantly since Kinsey's study, so it appears that women are now "catching up" to men in terms of their sexual experience. Recent studies have also shown that both males and females are having their first experience of intercourse at an earlier age, many by age 14 or 15.

SEXUAL DYSFUNCTION

Concept: Both males and females can experience sexual dysfunction.

Although occasionally an individual may not be able to function sexually, for example, after drinking a lot of alcohol these infrequent occurrences need not cause alarm. But if such occasions are the rule rather than the exception, there may be a problem requiring expert attention.

Sexual Problems in Males

Premature ejaculation.   The two most frequent sexual problems occurring in males are premature ejaculation and impotence. **Premature ejaculation** is defined as the inability of the male to "control his ejaculatory process for a sufficient length of time during intravaginal containment to satisfy his partner in at least 50 percent of their coital connections."[10] Other than the rare cases caused by surgery, trauma, or disease, premature ejaculation is a function of the psyche; that is, the mind is not able to control the body's need to ejaculate. Though not related to frequent masturbation, there does seem to be a relationship between premature ejaculation and "a long history of heavy petting which progresses into withdrawl as a method of contraception."[11] In addition, it has been hypothesized, though not as yet tested, that the dwindling use of condoms has led to larger numbers of premature ejaculators. Pierson and D'Antonio argue that the condom results in less stimulation than skin-to-skin contact, thereby causing inexperienced males to be able to control ejaculation.[12] As the use of the condom decreases, more and more males are not learning to control ejaculation and are subsequently experiencing premature ejaculation. Other explanations for the increasing number of men experiencing premature ejaculation are (1) that the women's movement is causing women to become more sexually assertive and demanding, and (2) that more is being said about this dysfunction, so that men who experience it are better able to recognize that the problem exists and less apt to want to hide it.

Fortunately, there is an effective treatment for premature ejaculation. Developed by Masters and Johnson and described in detail in their book, *Human Sexual Inadequacy*, the "squeeze" technique is easily applied, effective, and well publicized so that sexual counselors and therapists are aware of it. The technique entails a squeezing of the penis by the man's partner when ejaculation is approaching.

Impotence.   **Impotence** is the "inability of a man to attain or maintain an erection long enough to have sexual intercourse."[13] Masters and Johnson distinguish between primary and secondary impotence. Primary impotence is never having been able to achieve or maintain an erection long enough to have sexual intercourse. Secondary impotence occurs when a male is only infrequently able to achieve or maintain an erection long enough to have sexual intercourse but has previously been coitally effective.[14] Impotence can be caused by various factors: neurological or anatom-

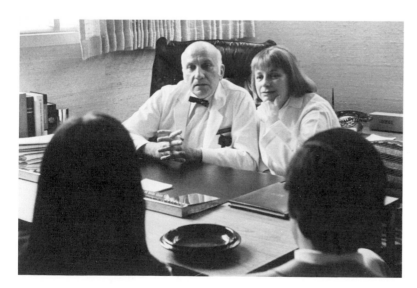

The research of William H. Masters and Virginia E. Johnson on the physiology of human sexual response laid the foundation on which a useful treatment for sexual problems could be based.

ical damage to the reproductive system, drug or alcohol abuse, hormonal deficiency, circulatory problems, aging, or physical exertion. The most prevalent cause, however is psychological. "Performance anxiety" refers to a fear of not performing well during sexual intercourse. This fear may serve as a self-fulfilling prophecy; that is, the fear of not performing well leads to poor performance. Other psychological factors that may lead to impotence include guilt over masturbation (not masturbation itself), guilt over sexual relations, feelings of inferiority, and a view of sex as dirty.[15]

Sexual Problems in Females

Orgasmic dysfunction. The most common causes of sexual dysfunction in females are orgasmic dysfunction, sexual anesthesia, dyspareunia, and vaginismus. Although they may enjoy sexual intercourse, some females cannot, or can at best rarely, achieve an orgasm. **Orgasmic dysfuntion** may be caused by such psychological factors as anger, guilt, fear, embarrassment concerning one's body, or hostility. It may also be caused by factors external to the woman; for example, an inexperienced partner, inappropriate setting (such as an uncomfortable back seat of a car), or alcohol. Lack of orgasm in young women is usually caused by one of these external factors.

Other causes of orgasmic dysfunction are anatomical defects in the female reproductive system, hormonal deficiency or imbalance, disorders of the nervous system, drugs, and alcohol. Note the similarity between this list and the causes of male impotence.

Therapy for orgasmic dysfunction that is psychological in nature usually involves both partners, because communication between the partners is often at the core of the problem and/or the solution. "A knowledgeable, understanding, and aware male sexual partner is an important part of the therapy for orgasmic dysfunction."[16]

Sexual anesthesia. This disorder used to be called frigidity, but therapists have dropped this value-laden term. **Sexual anesthesia** is defined as the inability to experience erotic pleasure from sexual contact. Some

women with this problem are difficult to treat because they show evidence of personality disorders.[17] Unhealthy socialization may contribute to attitudes regarding sex as sinful, men as exploiters, or sexual excitement as dirty. Contrary to popular belief, however, rape does not seem to be a cause of this sexual dysfunction, although women who are raped may temporarily not want to engage in sexual relations.[18]

Discovery Activity 13.2
SEX KNOWLEDGE INVENTORY

Circle the correct answer for each statement.

	True	*False*
1. The most satisfying position is with the male on top of the female.	T	F
2. Sex during menstruation is unclean and harmful.	T	F
3. Sex should be avoided during pregnancy.	T	F
4. A small penis is less satisfying to a woman than a large one.	T	F
5. Prostitutes are either frigid or homosexual or both.	T	F
6. Anal intercourse is perverted and dangerous.	T	F
7. It's good to sublimate the sex drive for long periods.	T	F
8. An excessively amorous woman is a nymphomaniac.	T	F
9. Advancing age means the end of sex.	T	F
10. Any man who can't have sexual relations with a woman is suffering from severe psychiatric problems.	T	F

These statements are all untrue. Here are the correct answers:

1. The most satisfying position for sexual partners varies with the individuals and the situation.

2. Coitus during menstruation is safe and healthy and depends only upon the personal preferences of the individuals involved.

3. Sex during pregnancy is safe except for women who have a history of miscarriage or other serious difficulties in their pregnancies.

4. The vagina expands to the size of the penis and contracts around it; therefore the size of the penis is not related to either partner's satisfaction during coitus.

5. Women become prostitutes for many reasons. Their private sexual lives are often similar to other people's sexual lives.

6. Anal intercourse is a matter of personal preference, and is not dangerous if health precautions are taken (a lubricant such as K-Y Jelly, and a condom to protect against infection).

7. There is no benefit in sublimating the sex drive for long periods of time since the only result will be frustration.

8. An "excessively" amorous woman may be just that—amorous. There is no reason to believe that women who enjoy a lot of sexual activity are abnormal.

9. Old age requires some adjustments to sexual activity—for example, lubrication of the vagina with jelly may be necessary and penile erection may take longer—but not its end.

10. Although the predominant causes of sexual dysfunction are psychological, there are other reasons for sexual dysfunction, for example, a medical condition. ●

Dyspareunia. The condition known as **dyspareunia,** or painful intercourse, can stem from psychological or physical causes. Painful intercourse might result from irritation of the vaginal barrel by the glans of the penis or insufficient lubrication of the vagina resulting from physical causes. Dyspareunia can also result from too frequent intercourse or from insufficient vaginal lubrication due to insufficient sexual stimulation. Although much more common in females, males may also experience painful intercourse. In males the cause is usually irritation from contraceptives (the same ones as in the female), blisters or a rash on the glans of the penis, or a nonretracting foreskin. Because dyspareunia makes sexual intercourse unenjoyable, medical examination should be sought immediately.

Vaginismus. In **vaginismus,** the muscles in the vagina involuntarily tighten so that the penis either cannot enter or causes a good deal of pain when it does enter. This condition is primarily psychological in origin; therefore the treatment is psychological in nature. Conditions found related to vaginismus include a sexual relationship with an impotent man, religious guilt, a traumatic sexual experience, or dyspareunia.

It should be emphasized that a temporary sexual dysfunction upon occasion is not unusual, but a frequently recurring or permanent dysfunction should be of concern. There are effective means of helping both males and females to overcome these problems. If you feel you have a sexual problem, you should seek counseling. Perhaps the first place to start is with your own physician. If your physician determines that no physical problem exists, he or she can refer you to a reputable sexual and/or psychological counselor.[19]

SEXUAL DIVERSITY

Homosexuality

Although most people are sexually attracted to people of the opposite sex, a minority are attracted to members of their own sex. **Lesbianism** in women and **homosexuality** in men (both herein termed "homosexuality") refer to a sexual preference for persons of the same sex. One need not be homosexual to have had a homosexual experience. For instance, 37 percent of the males and 13 percent of the females studied by Kinsey *et al.* reported at least some overt homosexual experience to the point of orgasm.

There are many reasons for homosexual behavior. Some people are isolated from people of the opposite sex (for example, those in prisons, all-male or all-female schools, or the military), and their only opportunity for human sexual activity (other than masturbation) is with someone of the same sex. These situational homosexuals usually are heterosexual when given the choice. Others experiment with homosexual behavior during adolescence but soon behave exclusively heterosexually. A small percentage of people are **ambi-**

Issues in Health
SHOULD HOMOSEXUALS BE EMPLOYED AS SCHOOL TEACHERS?

Some people believe that homosexuals should not be employed as school teachers. They argue that because children are in their formative years, they are impressionable and are likely to be influenced to be homosexual. Even if they don't become homosexuals per se, these children may be influenced to experiment with homosexual activities that are illegal or are viewed as immoral. Because adults in positions of authority serve as role models for children, these people argue that homosexuals should be denied employment in jobs where they are in charge of children or youth.

Others find these arguments absurd. They contend that there is no evidence that a teacher's sexual preference has any impact on students. Most homosexual teachers are not likely to make their sexual preferences known, because a person's sexuality is not an appropriate topic for classroom discussion. Further, there have always been homosexual teachers; they simply didn't make this fact known. Most sex researchers believe that an individual's sexual orientation is developed by age four or five. Therefore, children are in no danger from well-adjusted teachers of either sexual persuasion. Only teachers with psychological problems might have an adverse effect.

What do you think? ●

sexual; that is, they engage in sexual behavior with males on some occasions and females on others. It has been estimated that 4 percent of males and 2 percent of females are exclusively homosexual.

Myths about homosexuality.   Many myths have been perpetuated about homosexuality. Perhaps one reason for this is that most of the early researchers who studied homosexuality used the only sample available to them—homosexuals who sought psychological counseling or therapy, or homosexuals in psychiatric institutions. Encouraged by the current trend toward acceptance of the homosexual lifestyle, and aided by the political activities of homosexuals themselves, many homosexuals who function well and are productive members of society have "come out of the closet"—that is, they no longer hide their sexual preference. Research using this new sample of homosexuals suggests that many of the earlier findings were inaccurate. Here are some of the popular myths that have been dispelled by research:

1. *Homosexuals are more promiscuous than heterosexuals.* Some are and some aren't. Homosexual relationships are similar to heterosexual ones. Some homosexuals maintain a single longterm relationship, whereas others seek out sexual variety. This is equally true of heterosexuals.

2. *Homosexuals are likely to seduce young children.* The data just does not support this myth.

3. *Homosexuality is abnormal.* The term "abnormal" is a relative one. What is abnormal in one society or culture may be normal behavior in another. Homosexuality has been acceptable in many cultures throughout history.

4. *It is easy to recognize homosexuals by how they walk or talk.* Only a small percentage of homosexuals walk with a "swish" or talk in an effeminate or [in the case of lesbians] "butch" manner. Most are indistinguishable from heterosexuals

5. *Homosexuals can be "cured" by having sexual relationships with the "right" persons of the opposite sex.* There is no known, effective, and agreed upon manner to change one's sexual preference. How our sexual preference develops remains unclear and, therefore, how to change it is also unclear.

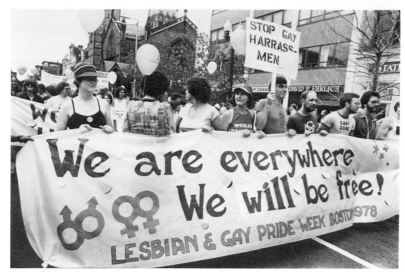

Political activism by gay rights groups has probably helped to alleviate some of the traditional prejudice against homosexuals.

6. *There are more female homosexuals than male homosexuals.* As we've stated earlier, there are double the number of male homosexuals as female homosexuals.

7. *Homosexuals have more psychological problems than heterosexuals.* Several studies have found that there is no difference between the mental health of homosexuals and heterosexuals.[20]

Homosexuality and society.   Until recently, homosexuality was considered a psychiatric illness. In 1973, however, the American Psychiatric Association reclassified homosexuality so that it is no longer considered a mental disorder. In the past, homosexuals were considered poor security risks, were sometimes treated as criminals, and were generally rejected by American society. More recently, homosexuals have become a powerful, organized political force. For example, it is said that a person who does not have the support of homosexuals cannot be elected mayor of San Francisco, where the homosexual population is large and well organized.

With research findings showing that most homosexuals are mentally healthy, are productive members of society, and have many similarities in their sexual lifestyles with heterosexual couples, homosexuality is becoming more acceptable and homosexuals are experiencing less prejudice.

Sexual Deviations

Sexual deviations refer to a category of behavior characterized by sexual interest in objects rather than people or by coitus performed under bizarre circumstances. People who engage in deviant behaviors are assumed to have a personality disorder. The following behaviors are among the sexual deviations that usually come to the attention of psychiatrists and psychologists:

1. *Fetishism.* A compulsion in which sexual arousal is brought about by a specific object (for example, articles of clothing), or some part of the body but not the whole (for example, a foot).

2. *Exhibitionism.* Exposure of one's genitals to involuntary observers.

3. *Necrophilia.* Sexual relations with a dead body.

4. *Bestiality.* Sexual relations with animals.

5. *Voyeurism.* Watching others engage in sexual behaviors as one's primary means of sexual arousal. A voyeur is a "Peeping Tom."

6. *Transvestism.* Gender identification with the opposite sex; usually males who dress as females.

7. *Pedophilia.* Sexual molestation of a child for gratification of the adult.

People with these characteristics can be treated psychotherapeutically and should be referred for help.

SEX-RELATED CRIMES

In recent years sex-related crimes—particularly rape and incest—have been the subject of growing concern.

Rape

Rape is the fastest-growing violent crime in our society. During 1977, 63,020 rapes were reported to the FBI, a figure twice the number reported 10 years earlier. The actual incidence of rape is undoubtedly much higher, because a great many women do not report being raped. It is believed that for every rape that is reported, 3 to 10 other rapes go unreported.[21]

Rape is defined as sexual penetration of an individual (usually female) against her will. **Statutory rape** is a special category referring to unlawful sexual intercourse with a female minor. The "age of consent" varies from 12 to 21 years, depending on the state one lives in. If a male participates in sexual intercourse with a minor, he is committing statutory rape in spite of the female's willingness, assistance, or initiation of the intercourse. In 1981 the Supreme Court upheld the constitutionality of the statutory rape laws, stating that because female minors are in jeopardy of pregnancy, they should be uniquely protected by such laws.

Many popular misconceptions contribute to the problems of women who are raped. For example, many people still believe that rape victims "ask for it" or that women secretly enjoy being raped. Until recently, it was permissible to reveal a rape victim's past sexual history at a rape trial as a means of discrediting her testimony. As a result of pressure from women's advocates, many states now prohibit this practice. Even so, much needs to be done to erase the myths surrounding rape.

What do we know about rape? Although many people believe that the rapist and victim are usually of different races, in fact in 90 to 95 percent of cases, they are of the same race. According to the Uniform Crime Reports, over half of those arrested for rape were under 25 years of age, and half the victims were under 21. Although young women may be more frequent victims, females of all ages, from children to elderly, have been rape victims. In about 60 percent of cases reported to the FBI, the rapist and victim were strangers; in the remaining 40 percent, they were acquainted.

Most rapists are never caught, and those who are are unlikely to be convicted. According to the National Institute of Law Enforcement and Criminal Justice, only 5 percent of reported rapes result in the capture of a suspect, and only 3 percent result in a conviction.[22]

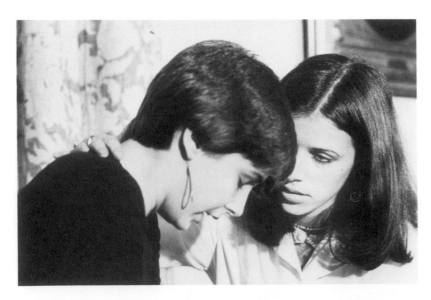

Supportive, sympathetic counseling can help rape victims deal with the trauma they have experienced.

There are two main theories about why men commit rape. One hypothesis connects rape with personality disturbance, such as the inability to control impulsive behaviors. The other hypothesis is that rapists are more likely than nonrapists to accept the unsupported myths about rape that are prevalent in our society. For example, they may be more likely to believe that women unconsciously wish to be raped, that women who are raped are sexually provocative, or that women enjoy violent sex. The research on these theories has not yet yielded clear results, and more study is needed.

Rape on college campuses has recently become a problem, and many colleges are now taking precautions against rape. These include better lighting, security gates, locking of dormitories after a certain hour, escort services during evening hours, rape counseling and education programs, campus police patrolling the most likely rape locations, and even the distribution of rape whistles. What is your campus doing in this regard? How could you help?

Figure 13.2 illustrates self-defense techniques that can be employed against a potential rapist. Although

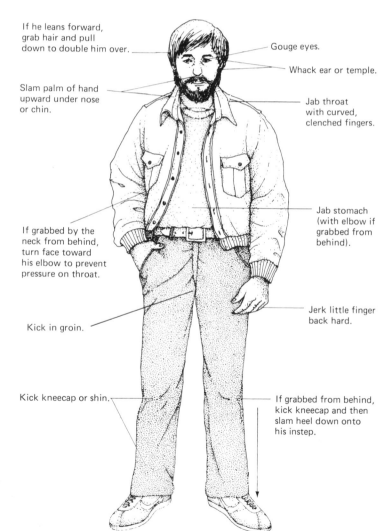

If he leans forward, grab hair and pull down to double him over.

Gouge eyes.

Whack ear or temple.

Slam palm of hand upward under nose or chin.

Jab throat with curved, clenched fingers.

If grabbed by the neck from behind, turn face toward his elbow to prevent pressure on throat.

Jab stomach (with elbow if grabbed from behind).

Kick in groin.

Jerk little finger back hard.

Kick kneecap or shin.

If grabbed from behind, kick kneecap and then slam heel down onto his instep.

Figure 13.2
Self-defense tactics for women. Some women learn "dirty street fighting" tactics like these in hopes of warding off a sexual assault. If a woman chooses to use such tactics when she is attacked, speed, vigor, and the feeling of being in control of the situation are crucial to her ability to escape. If she struggles unsuccessfully, her attacker may become more violent.

SOURCE: From G. D. Nass, R. W. Libby, and M. P. Fisher, *Sexual Choices*, p. 397. Copyright © 1981 by Wadsworth, Inc. Reprinted by permission of the publisher, Wadsworth Health Sciences Division, Monterey, California.

there is still controversy about whether a rape victim should resist her attacker, most experts believe that if you can resist without risking serious harm, you should do so; however, if the attacker has a gun, knife, or other lethal weapon, the best course of action may be to submit and then seek an opportunity to escape.

Incest

> **Concept:** Incest is a coercive sexual behavior within a family setting, often having profound psychological consequences.

Incest technically refers to sexual intercourse between close blood relatives. However, many therapists and researchers now define incest as any form of coercive sexual contact (not only intercourse) between a child and a relative, including stepparents and adoptive parents. Incest often engenders feelings of helplessness, guilt, shame, and anger in both parties. People (teachers, pediatricians) whose occupations bring them in contact with children are often the ones who report these incestuous relationships once the child opens up to them.

From 1 to 2 million cases of incest are reported each year.[23] The most common form of reported incest is between father and daughter. The incestuous father is typically aggressive and domineering and may be a heavy drinker. In many cases the mother is passive or submissive and frequently suffers from such problems as depression, alcoholism, or major illness. Because the mother's disabilities interfere with her maternal responsibilities, most tasks are shifted to the oldest daughter, to whom the father turns for emotional and sexual satisfaction.

Treatment programs for both parents and children have been developed to deal with incest and the problems it entails. These programs are usually based upon the following principles:[24]

1. The complaint of sexual abuse is always believed, false reports of incest are rare.

2. Sexual abuse is always reported to the proper authorities (for example, the police or a social worker).

In this manner the professional is implicitly siding with the child rather than with the offending parent. Reporting sexual abuse to the proper authorities is required by law.

3. The relationship between the mother and daughter must be strengthened. The child should be assured that she is not to blame for what has happened, and the mother should receive medical or psychiatric help so that she can become a more assertive parent.

4. The offender is treated under court orders. A useful approach is group therapy with other abusive fathers, which combines a supportive approach with direct confrontation of the problem.

SEXUAL BEHAVIOR: DECIDING FOR YOURSELF

> **Concept:** Campus life presents special considerations in terms of sexual behavior.

Though sexual behavior is important throughout one's life, it seems expecially important during the college years. We have already noted one study in which it was found that 52 percent of freshmen had experienced sexual intercourse, and by the time they were seniors, 86 percent had. Another study found that 40 percent of freshmen and 85 percent of seniors had experienced sexual intercourse. It seems obvious that, at least concerning sexual intercourse, colleges truly are institutions for learning. This is understandable when several factors are considered. First, many students are away from home for the first time and are experimenting with a new-found freedom. This experimentation is manifested in their sexual behavior as well as in other areas of their lives. Related to this is the need to find new friends and achieve a new status among peers on the campus, a process that took years to accomplish back home. Sexual behavior might seem to be an easy solution. A female might think about how popular she could be if she were more sexually active. A male might want to become a bigshot by bragging about "sexual conquests." Some students do use sex this way.

Some people cite the availability of contraception as another reason for increased sexual activity during the college years. Students reach legal age during college and are offered sexual counseling and/or health services on campus. Thus contraceptives are more available to college students than ever before. This is another reason why sexual behavior during the college years deserves special consideration.

Obviously sexual decision making is also necessary beyond the college years. Married couples must decide how often they should engage in sexual relations and in what form, that is, which sexual activities are acceptable to them and which are not. They must also decide whether to limit their sexual activity to their mate or engage in extramarital sex (see the accompanying Issue). Single adults must decide how sexually active to be. Whether single or married, adults who work outside the home must often decide whether a sexual advance comprises sexual harassment—sexual advances made by someone of power or authority who threatens firing, lack of promotion, or some other sanction if sex is declined—and if so what to do about it.

Sexual decision making is a part of living. It is inescapable. The best we can do for ourselves is to make these decisions as logically and rationally as we can after we have gathered the pertinent information.

CONCLUSION

It is not our intention to suggest that you adopt any particular lifestyle. But we do strongly urge that you consider your sexual behavior as seriously as you consider any other important aspect of your life. Make decisions regarding your sexual behavior after consideration of your values, needs, desires, alternative choices, the consequences of these choices, and the realization that your choice need not be etched in stone. If you are unhappy with your sexual behavior after considering these factors, a change of behavior may be in order. That change requires some careful thought as well.

Issues in Health
IS EXTRAMARITAL SEX HEALTHY BEHAVIOR?

Albert Ellis believes that it is possible for a person to have extramarital sexual relationships for healthy reasons. Although he refers to "adultery," we prefer the term extramarital sex, because it is less judgmental.

1. The healthy adulterer is nondemanding and noncompulsive. He prefers but does not need extramarital affairs. He believes that he can live better with than without them, and therefore he tries to arrange to have them from time to time. But he is also able to have a happy general and marital life if no such affairs are practicable.

2. The undisturbed adulterer usually manages to carry on his extramarital affairs without unduly disturbing his marriage and family relationships or his general existence. He is sufficiently discreet about his adultery, on the one hand, and appropriately frank and honest about it with his close associates, on the other hand, so that most people he intimately knows are able to tolerate his affairs and not get too upset about them.

3. He fully accepts his own extramarital desires and acts and never condemns himself or punishes himself because of them, even though he may sometimes decide that they are unwise and may make specific attempts to bring them to a halt.

4. He faces his specific problems with his wife and family as well as his general life difficulties and does not use his adulterous relationships as a means of avoiding any of his serious problems.

5. He is usually tolerant of himself when he acts poorly or makes errors; he is minimally hostile when his wife and family members behave in a less than desirable manner; and he fully accepts the fact that the world is rough and life is often grim, but that there is no reason why it *must* be otherwise and that he can live happily even when

(continued)

Issues in Health (continued)

conditions around him are not great. Consequently, he does not drive himself to adultery because of self-deprecation, self-pity, or hostility to others.

6. He is sexually adequate with his spouse as well as with others and therefore has extramarital affairs out of sex interest rather than for sex therapy.

Although the adulterer who lives up to these criteria may have still other emotional disturbances and may be having extramarital affairs for various neurotic reasons other than those outlined in this paper, there is also a good chance that this is not true. The good Judeo-Christian moralists may never believe it, but it would appear that healthy adultery, even in our supposedly monogamous society, is possible.*

What do you think? How will you behave if and when you get married? ●

*Reproduced by permission from *Encounter with Family Realities* by Powers and Lees, copyright © 1977, West Publishing Company. All rights reserved.

SUMMARY

1. Sexuality is what you are: the roles you play, the societal expectations you adopt. Sex, on the other hand, is something you do: kissing, petting, having intercourse.

2. The human sexual response cycle consists of four phases: the excitement phase, the plateau phase, the orgasmic phase, and the resolution phase.

3. In some respects, females and males are similar in their sexual responses. For example, when sexually aroused, they both experience nipple erection, sex flush, muscle tension, deep and rapid breathing, and increases in the heart rate and blood pressure.

4. In other respects, females and males differ in their sexual responses. For example, when sexually aroused, male blood pressure increases more, female perspiration is more widespread, and females can be multiorgasmic, whereas males experience a refractory period.

5. People engage in sexual activity for many reasons, including to express intimacy, for fun, to relieve loneliness or boredom, as a reward or punishment, and to have babies.

6. Homosexuals have become more politically active and better organized in recent years. Consequently, homosexuality is accepted more by society as an alternative lifestyle.

7. Sexual expression takes many forms. Masturbation—experienced by about 75 percent of college seniors—is one form of sexual expression; others are petting, oral sex, and intercourse.

8. Cunnilingus is the oral stimulation of the vulva, and fellatio is the oral stimulation of the penis and scrotum. Oral-genital sexual behavior is more prevalent today than it was when Kinsey conducted his landmark studies.

9. Male sexual dysfunctions include premature ejaculation and impotence. Female sexual dysfunctions include orgasmic dysfunction, sexual anesthesia (previously termed frigidity), dyspareunia, and vaginismus.

10. Some of the more common forms of sexual deviation are fetishism, exhibitionism, necrophilia, bestiality, voyeurism, transvestism, and pedophilia.

11. Rape and incest are two sex-related crimes that have received increased attention in recent years. Rape is the fastest-growing violent crime in America. Counseling programs for victims of rape and incest have been developed to respond to the victims' needs.

REFERENCES

1. William H. Masters and Virginia Johnson, *Human Sexual Response* (Boston: Little, Brown, 1966).

2. Ibid., p. 277.

3. Jerrold S. Greenberg, *Student-Centered Health Instruction: A Humanistic Approach* (Reading, Mass.: Addison-Wesley, 1978), p. 134.

4. Alfred C. Kinsey et al., *Sexual Behavior in the Human Female* (Philadelphia: W. B. Saunders, 1953).

5. Alfred C. Kinsey et al., *Sexual Behavior in the Human Male* (Philadelphia: W. B. Saunders, 1948).

6. Jerrold S. Greenberg, "The Masturbatory Behavior of College Students," *Psychology in the Schools* 9 (1972): 427–432

7. Morton Hunt, *Sexual Behavior in the 1970s* (Chicago: Playboy Press, 1974).

8. Philip Sarrel and Lorna Sarrel, "The Redbook Report on Sexual Relationships," *Redbook* (October 1980):73–80.

9. Guy S. Parcel, "A Study of the Relationship Between Contraceptive Attitudes and Behavior in a Group of Unmarried University Students," doctoral dissertation, Pennsylvania State University, 1974.

10. William H. Masters and Virginia Johnson, *Human Sexual Inadequacy* (Boston: Little, Brown, 1970), p. 92.

11. Elaine C. Pierson and William V. D'Antonio, *Female and Male: Dimensions of Human Sexuality* (Philadelphia: J. B. Lippincott, 1974), p. 52.

12. Ibid., p. 52

13. Michael S. Haro et al., *Explorations in Personal Health* (Boston: Houghton Mifflin, 1977), p. 147.

14. Masters and Johnson, *Human Sexual Inadequacy.*

15. Donald A. Read, *The Concept of Health*, 3d ed. (Boston: Holbrook Press, 1978), p. 168.

16. Haro et al., *Explorations in Personal Health*, p. 147.

17. J. P. Brady, "Frigidity," *Medical Aspects of Human Sexuality* (November 1967):42.

18. J. P. Brady et al., "Roundtable: Frigidity," *Medical Aspects of Human Sexuality* (February 1968):26.

19. For a discussion on the qualifications of certified sex counselors and therapists, see Clint E. Bruess and Jerrold S. Greenberg, *Sex Education: Theory and Practice* (Belmont, Calif.: Wadsworth, 1981), pp. 232–233.

20. Alan P. Bell and Martin S. Weinberg, *Homosexualities: A Study of Diversity among Men and Women* (New York: Simon and Schuster, 1978).

21. *Uniform Crime Reports* (Washington, D.C.: Federal Bureau of Investigation, 1978).

22. National Institute of Law Enforcement and Criminal Justice, *Forcible Rape Final Project Report* (Washington, D.C.: Government Printing Office, March 1978).

23. Karen C. Mieselman, *Incest* (San Francisco: Jossey-Bass, 1979).

24. "Incest," *The Harvard Medical School Health Letter* (March 1981):4.

Laboratory 1
SEXUAL BEHAVIOR EMPATHIZING

Purpose   To understand viewpoints regarding sexual behavior that are contrary to your own.

Size of Group   Total class.

Equipment   None.

Procedure

Divide the class into two groups: one that favors legalizing prostitution, and one opposed to legalizing prostitution.

The groups should meet separately and brainstorm a list of arguments that support their position.

Placing the lists aside for the meantime, one group stands on one side of the room and the other group on the other side. The groups face each other and verbally debate the legalization of prostitution. However, the groups must assume the viewpoint opposed to their own. In other words, the group favoring legalization of prostitution must argue *against* legalization; the group opposed to legalization of prostitution must argue *for* legalization.

At the conclusion of the argument, the groups meet separately and develop a list of reasons supporting the position for which they verbally argued. The result should be that each group has a list of reasons for and a list of reasons against legalizing prostitution.

Results

Each group should briefly discuss their two lists among themselves. The groups should then come together to discuss what they have learned from this experience.

Note: Other topics that can be similarly considered are:

1. Premarital sexual intercourse
2. Extramarital sexual intercourse
3. Homosexuality
4. Transvestism
5. Transsexualism
6. Statutory rape

Laboratory 2
SEXUAL SENTENCE COMPLETIONS

Purpose To provide a structured format for discussions of sexual behaviors.

Size of Group Small groups of five members each. Students who feel most comfortable with each other should be allowed to form their own groups. The nature of this activity requires a feeling of openness and trust.

Equipment None.

Procedure

Each student should complete the following sentences:

1. Sexual intercourse _____

2. Fellatio _____

3. Cunnilingus _____

4. Homosexuality _____

5. Petting _____

6. Orgasm _____

7. Sex and love _____

8. Masturbation _____

9. Sexual experience _____

10. Virginity _____

Once all group members have completed these sentences, a group discussion should commence, concentrating on each person's sentence topic by topic. In other words, each student presents his or her sentence for "sexual intercourse," then each student presents his or her sentence for "fellatio," etc. When discussing the sentence completions, each student should describe the *reasons* for completing the sentences as he or she did.

Results

A general group discussion, once all the specific sentence completions have been presented, should include consideration of the following:

1. How did thoughts, feelings, and opinions differ among the group members?
2. How did religious beliefs affect responses?
3. How did past experience affect responses?
4. How honest do you think the group members were?
5. How do you think your parents would have completed these sentences? Why?

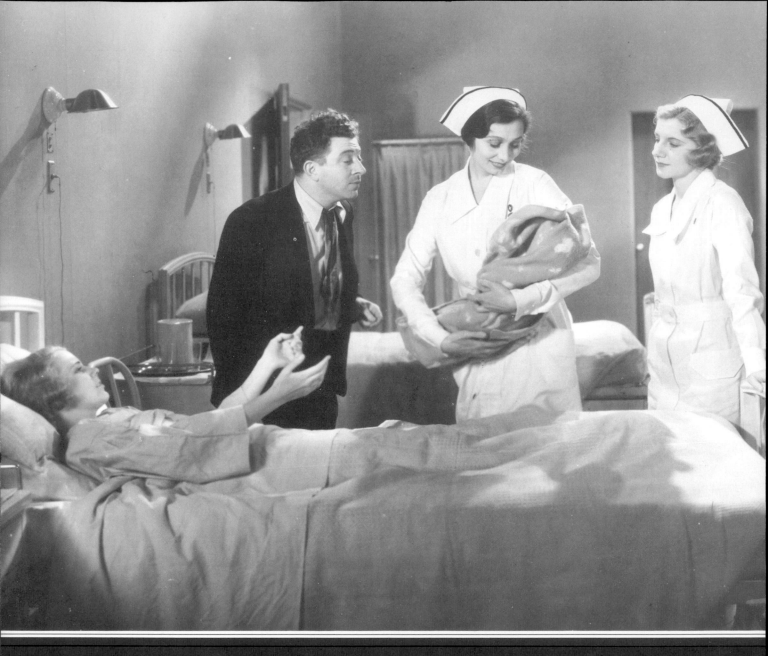

conception control, pregnancy, and birth

- *conception control*
- *abortion*
- *pregnancy*
- *childbirth*
- *infertility and its treatment*

There are several sexual crossroads at which many people periodically find themselves. If you are sexually active, you must decide whether to use birth control and, if so, what method you want to use. If you decide to conceive a child, you must decide whether to drink alcohol or take other drugs, and what to eat, because all of these factors can affect the fetus. Prior to the birth process you also have to make decisions: the method of delivery, the place of delivery, whether to use pain relievers, and the nature of the postdelivery phase.

Decisions about contraception and pregnancy are obviously very personal and are related to religious beliefs, value systems, and societal attitudes. These decisions can have an enormous impact on both physical and mental health, as well as on intimate relationships. This chapter offers some basic information about contraception, pregnancy, and birth so that you will be better prepared to make the right decisions for you in these areas of your life.

CONCEPTION CONTROL

Reasons Why People Don't Use Contraception

Concept: A variety of social factors may influence a person against using contraception.

In recent years there have been great strides in contraceptive technology. Information on birth control is widely available. Such organizations as Planned Parenthood/World Population offer advice and information, as well as contraceptive devices, regardless of age or marital status.

Nevertheless, the rate of adolescent pregnancy has increased dramatically in recent years. Research indicates that one out of every 10 women in the United States now becomes pregnant by age 17. Obviously these young people either are not using contraception or are using it sporadically or incorrectly. What are

some of the factors that may influence people against using contraception? Before reading on, complete Discovery Activity 14.1, which asks you to consider the answer to this question.

The most obvious reasons are religious. Catholics, for example, have been taught that natural family planning is the only permissible contraceptive method. Nevertheless, a recent poll indicates that nearly the same percentage of Catholics are using other contraception as are non-Catholics. Because rhythm is not as effective as some other means of contraception, Catholics who want to adhere to their religious beliefs and want to limit the size of their families at the same time face a real dilemma. Some choose rhythm, whereas others opt for more effective methods.

Parcel conducted a study of college students to determine the methods of contraception used and the reasons for sometimes not using any method. The stu-

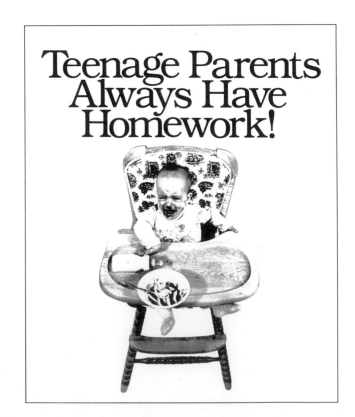

Teenage Parents Always Have Homework!

Discovery Activity 14.1
REASONS FOR
NOT USING
CONTRACEPTION

List all the reasons you can think of to explain why many people don't use contraception, based either on your own experience or that of others whom you know.

1. _____
2. _____
3. _____
4. _____
5. _____
6. _____
7. _____
8. _____
9. _____
10. _____ ●

dents studied were unmarried and enrolled in a large, state-supported university in the eastern United States. It was found that for the first intercourse, the majority of the students used no contraception, and for their last intercourse experience over 23 percent used no method of contraception. Asked why they sometimes used no contraception, almost 58 percent of the students said that it was because they "didn't plan ahead of time."[1] Almost 13 percent said they didn't use a contraceptive because they left it up to their partner.

Some of the reasons most frequently given for not using contraception are reflected in the following statements:

1. It (pregnancy) couldn't happen to me.
2. I feel guilty (immoral) if I plan in advance.
3. I'm too embarrassed to buy contraceptives.
4. Someone (for instance, parents) may find out I'm using contraceptives.

5. If I start using contraceptives, I won't be able to stop myself from participating more.
6. It wasn't a planned experience.
7. It hasn't happened yet (pregnancy or sexual intercourse), so it won't.
8. It's not natural to use contraceptives.
9. It ruins the fun.
10. I'm too lazy.
11. I could not imagine myself having a child (it's beyond my comprehension).
12. I have intercourse too infrequently to be concerned with contraception.

Did you list some of the reasons given above? Did you think of other reasons in addition to these?

One implication of points 1, 7, 11, and 12 is that many people (especially teenagers) don't seem to understand how conception takes place and believe they are somehow immune to becoming pregnant. There is evidence that low self-esteem is a factor in teenage pregnancy. The idea that sexual activity isn't something to be planned is also especially influential among adolescent women. These youngsters believe that if they don't use contraception, they can pretend that they aren't really sexually active and therefore are still "good girls." Finally, lack of maturity is a significant factor in nonuse of contraception. Adolescents who don't use contraception seem to be less able than their peers to exercise self-control and foresee the consequences of their behavior.

Evaluating Contraceptive Effectiveness

Concept: Methods of birth control can be evaluated according to their effectiveness in preventing pregnancy.

One of the things you need to know before deciding on a birth control method is how well they work. The effectiveness of contraceptives is measured in terms of how successfully they work to prevent pregnancy during one year in 100 sexually active women. When

Table 14.1
CONTRACEPTIVE EFFECTIVENESS

Method	Theoretical Effectiveness %	Actual User Effectiveness %
Abstinence	100	?
Withdrawal	91	75–80
Rhythm	87	60–86
Ovulation Method	98	75
Condoms	97	90
Diaphragm (with spermicide)	97	83
Cervical Cap	97	83
IUD	97–99	95
Spermicidal Foam	97	78
Spermicidal Suppositories	97	75–80
Oral Contraceptives	99.7	96
Douching	?	60

discussing effectiveness rates for methods of contraception, a differentiation is made between theoretical effectiveness and actual user effectiveness. **Theoretical effectiveness** refers to how effective the method is if used perfectly—the maxium possible effectiveness. **Actual user effectiveness** is always lower, because people do not use contraceptives perfectly. Table 14.1 lists the rates of theoretical and actual user effectiveness for the methods we'll discuss. Our intent is not to influence you toward any particular method but rather to provide you with the necessary information you might need to make an informed decision if you are sexually active and plan to use contraception.

Methods of Contraception

Abstinence. One way to prevent conception is to abstain from sexual intercourse. Obviously, if the penis does not come near or enter the vagina, there is no chance of pregnancy.

People abstain from sexual intercourse for various reasons. Among unmarried couples, a common reason

is a religious or moral objection to nonmarital sexual intercourse. Another factor for many unmarried people is their concern about contracting one of the sexually transmitted diseases. We know, however, that approximately two-thirds of all unmarried men and women are sexually active by age 19. Abstinence, then, is clearly not for most people. Those who are sexually active and do not want to become pregnant or (in the case of men) cause a pregnancy, need some effective means of preventing conception. Let's consider the methods that are available.

Withdrawal. Also called **coitus interruptus,** this method requires the male to withdraw his penis from the female's vagina prior to ejaculating. In theory it makes sense that withdrawal will prevent sperm from entering the female. However, in practice coitus interruptus isn't very effective, because it requires considerable self-control. Often the male is not able to identify the imminence of ejaculation quickly enough. The first drops of the ejaculate contain a higher concentration of sperm than later ones;[2] therefore not withdrawing soon enough can lead to pregnancy. Moreover, pre-ejaculatory fluid contains some sperm and can lead to impregnation. Consequently, a penis near or in a vagina can deposit sperm even prior to ejaculating.

Withdrawal is not a popular method of birth control among married couples in the United States. However, among teeneagers it is widespread.

Rhythm method. Fertility control by the **rhythm method** is based upon an understanding of the female menstrual cycle. As described in Chapter 12, an egg is released by a female approximately once a month. The object is not to have a sperm meet that egg while it is still viable. Though an egg begins to degenerate 24 hours after ovulation if not fertilized, sperm and the egg can remain alive up to 72 hours. The task, then, is to identify the day of ovulation and abstain from intercourse 72 hours before (so that no sperm will remain alive in the female) and after the day of ovulation. However, during a 28-day menstrual cycle, ovulation may occur anywhere from the seventeenth to the thirteenth day before the next menstruation begins. As a result, to employ the rhythm method, abstinence should be practiced from day 10 through day 17 of a 28-day cycle.

The rhythm method requires considerable commitment and presents some difficulties. Many women have irregular menstrual cycles, making it difficult for them to pinpoint the time of ovulation. It is recommended that women keep exact records of the length of their menstrual cycles for one year.

The most common way to determine the time of ovulation is to identify a shift in basal body temperature (BBT): a decrease of approximately 0.3 degree just before ovulation and an increase of approximately 0.5 to 0.6 degree during ovulation.[3] To be effective in identifying time of ovulation, BBT readings should be taken each morning before getting out of bed. A BBT thermometer can be purchased in a drugstore.

If the BBT reading is usually 97.9 (it is usually lower in the morning than during the day), it will decrease to 97.6 just prior to ovulation, increase to 98.4 or 98.5 during ovulation, and remain there for three days after ovulation (the time it takes the egg to disintegrate). After the three days of a 0.5 to 0.6 degrees rise in BBT, the safe days begin.

One problem with this means of identifying ovulation is that illness or activity may change the BBT. To diminish the chance of incorrectly identifying the time of ovulation, it is recommended that the thermometer and calendar be used hand in hand, the calendar helping to identify shifts in BBT resulting from sources other than ovulation, and the thermometer helping to identify an early or late ovulation.

Couples using the rhythm method of fertility were found to be more effective in preventing conception if they viewed their successes or failures as a result of their own behavior (internal locus of control) than if they possessed an external locus of control.[4] Despite the fact that the rhythm method is somewhat difficult, it has the advantage of permitting a couple to *plan* as well as prevent a pregnancy, and it is acceptable to the Roman Catholic church.

Ovulation method. Use of the **ovulation method** entails identifying the onset of ovulation by interpreting the woman's cervical mucus pattern. Developed by Dr.

John Billings, the ovulation method requires keeping records of the days on which mucus is secreted through the vagina and recognizing the characteristics of this mucus. When the woman is not fertile, the mucus is thinner, more elastic, clear, and lubricative. This method has several advantages. It is relatively easy to teach a woman how to "read" her cervical mucus pattern, and this method is more reliable than basal body temperature. Like rhythm, the ovulation method has no side effects, is acceptable to those religions advocating the rhythm method, and can be used to plan a pregnancy as well as prevent one.

One disadvantage of the ovulation method is the possibility of misinterpreting the mucus discharge. About 30 percent of women do not have a recognizable mucus pattern. In addition, this method requires abstinence during the woman's fertile period of each menstrual cycle.

Condoms. Also called "rubbers," **condoms** are sheaths of rubber placed on the erect penis to prevent sperm from entering the vagina. Condoms come in various shapes and colors, and are about 7.5 inches long when unrolled (see Fig. 14.1, page 322).

The condom is most effective if the male removes the penis from the vagina shortly after ejaculation to avoid the possibility of semen leakage into the vagina. Breakage of the condom is rare but possible. Condoms should never be reused and should not be kept in a wallet near the body, because they can deteriorate with heat. Lubricating jelly will also deteriorate rubber condoms and should not be used with them. Though the condom has been critized by some couples because it requires an interruption in foreplay to put on, other couples have used the placing of the condom on the male penis as a part of foreplay. An advantage of the condom is that it does not have the side effects that accompany some of the other techniques. In addition, condoms are inexpensive and easily obtained in drugstores, by mail, and from some public bathroom vending machines. No prescription is needed to purchase them, and they are very effective if used correctly. Another important advantage of the condom is the protection it provides from sexually transmitted diseases and infection.

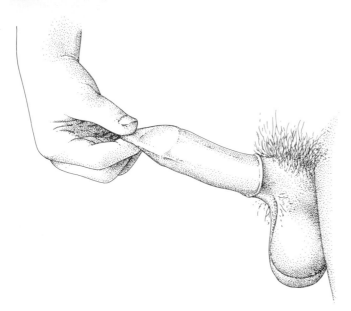

Figure 14.1
Placing the condom on the penis. The condom should be rolled on the penis only after it has been slightly unrolled to allow for a space, once the condom is on, between the tip of the penis and the condom. This space will serve as the deposit for the ejaculate. Without this space, it is likely that the ejaculate will overflow the condom and enter the vagina.

Diaphragm.   Another means of preventing conception is to create a barrier that sperm cannot penetrate. The **diaphragm,** a rubber cap around a collapsible metal ring, is designed to cover the cervix and prevent sperm from traveling through the uterus and up the Fallopian tubes, where the egg might be fertilized. To perform its function well, the diaphragm must be fitted by a physician and should be refitted after a pregnancy or weight gain or loss of 10 pounds or more. To further assure that live sperm will not enter the uterus, the diaphragm is lubricated with a spermicidal cream or jelly that will kill sperm on contact. The cream is placed around the edge and inside the cup of the diaphragm prior to putting it in place. Figure 14.2 shows the diaphragm in place.

The diaphragm can be inserted any time prior to intercourse but must be left in place at least six hours afterward. Additional cream or jelly must be applied before each act of intercourse. It is recommended that the diaphragm not be left in place more than 24 hours. The disadvantages to the use of a diaphragm include the need to plan prior to intercourse and the possibility of improper insertion.

Cared for, the diaphragm can be used effectively and comfortably for several years. Couples report that its presence does not hinder sexual enjoyment for either the male or the female.

It is recommended that the diaphragm be washed with warm water and mild soap, rinsed, and air dried.

Figure 14.2
Cross-section of the female pelvis showing diaphragm in position. Generally used in conjunction with a jelly or cream, the diaphragm blocks sperm from entry into the uterus and thus prevents conception.
SOURCE: Eric T. Pengelley, *Sex and Human Life* (Reading, Mass.: Addison-Wesley, 1974).

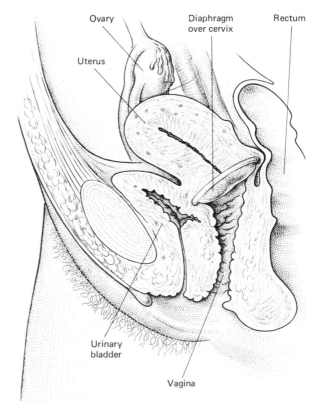

It should be dusted with cornstarch (scented talcs or petroleum jelly will weaken the rubber). Periodically check the diaphragm for wear, looking for thin spots or holes.

Cervical cap. The device known as the **cervical cap** is a rubber, plastic, or metal cap covering the cervix. Like the diaphragm it creates a barrier to the sperm. It is more popular in Europe than in the United States. However, with concern over side effects of other methods of contraception, the cervical cap is gaining popularity in this country as well. As of this writing, the Food and Drug Administration is conducting studies in order to determine the effectiveness of the cap, how long it can be worn safely, and to identify any side effects not presently known. The cervical cap appears to be both safe and effective when fitted properly and when the user inserts it correctly. Its failure rate is about the same as for the diaphragm. In addition, the cervical cap can be left in place for days or weeks. It is more difficult to insert properly than the diaphragm.

The Pill. Some form of **birth control pill** is used by 10 to 15 million women in the United States. To understand how the Pill functions as a contraceptive, you must understand the hormonal involvement in the menstrual cycle, described in Chapter 12. Estrogen in the Pill works on the hypothalamus of the brain to prevent the pituitary gland from producing FSH and LH. The result of this action is the prevention of ovulation, and with no egg to fertilize, pregnancy can't occur. In simple terms, the body is fooled into believing it is pregnant, thereby not having to ovulate any longer. The progestins in the Pill serve to prepare the endometrium for implantation and to maintain pregnancy. When provided prior to ovulation, however, progestins are thought to inhibit implantation. Progestin also creates a cervical mucus that results in decreased sperm transport and penetration.

The Pill is really many pills. Some contain estrogen and progestin in combination, some only estrogen, some only progestin. In addition, the amount of the hormone or hormones contained in the Pill varies greatly from one brand to the next. A physician is the person best qualified to recommend which pill to take, but it is

Issues in Health
HAS THE RESEARCH ON CONTRACEPTION BEEN SEXIST?

Some people wonder why contraceptive research has concentrated almost exclusively on the female reproductive system. Past research has focused upon preventing ovulation or on placing mechanical barriers in the female, and current research is still aimed primarily at contraceptives for women. These observers accuse the predominantly male group of contraceptive researchers of being sexist. They argue that we would have pills today designed to prevent sperm production if more attention had been directed toward males rather than toward experimentation with females. Male researchers are willing to experiment with the female reproductive system, but they don't want to ask men to accept the same risks of side effects that women already accept. Before all the recent research, males were responsible for contraception anyway. More research should be directed at males now, so that men and women can truly share responsibility for contraception.

Others argue that it is only logical that research has concentrated on females, because it is females who become pregnant, and more is known about the female reproductive system. They also point to the current work on a male pill. This research has tested the use of synthetic hormones to stop sperm production. Unfortunately researchers have been unable to reduce the sperm count to zero, and these pills have led to lowered sexual interest, signs of feminization, and toxic effects upon the liver. Further, research funds are limited, because drug companies have focused upon improving available and proven contraceptives rather than on conducting extensive research on new methods. Those viewing contraceptive research as balanced argue that the dramatic increase in condom sales since 1975 shows that men are willing to share responsibility for contraception. Thus there is no pressing need to develop more contraceptives for men.

What do you think? ●

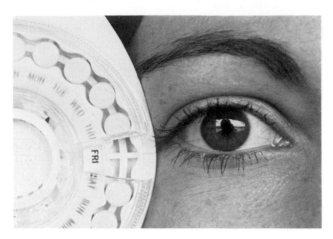

Although birth control pills are very effective, women who wish to use them need to become fully informed about potential side effects.

suggested that a woman starting on the Pill take one with 50 mcg or less of estrogen to minimize the possibility of blood-clotting complications.[5]

Some varieties of the Pill are taken each day for 21 days and then not taken for the next 7 days to allow for menstruation. Others are taken every day. It is suggested that during the first month on the Pill another means of contraception (such as a condom) be used to allow time for the Pill to become effective.

One type of pill is the "minipill," which is taken every day (even during menstruation) and contains only progestin. The advantage of this pill is that it is thought to cause fewer side effects than pills containing estrogen. A disadvantage is that it is slightly less effective than combined pills, although about as effective as the IUD.

The Pill is extremely effective in preventing pregnancy. Other advantages of the Pill are that it doesn't require an interruption of lovemaking and, unlike the IUD, it serves to regulate the menstrual period.

The main disadvantage of the Pill is its side effects. About 40 percent of users of the Pill experience side effects ranging from nausea, weight gain, headaches, and yeast infections to gallbladder disease, hypertension, and blood clots.

You should not take the Pill if you are over 35 years old, are pregnant or nursing, are a smoker, or have any of the following conditions:*

Thromboembolic disorders (for example, blood clots)

Cerebrovascular accident (stroke, coronary disease)

Impaired liver function

Malignancy of breast or reproductive system

Migraine headaches

Hypertension

Diabetes or strong family history of diabetes

Full-term gestation terminated within past two weeks

Gallbladder disease

Active or postcholecystectomy (surgical removal of the gallbladder)

History of cholestatis (jaundice) during pregnancy

Acute phase of mononucleosis

Sickle-cell disease

Undiagnosed abnormal vaginal bleeding

Surgery planned in next four weeks

Long leg cast or injury to lower leg

Cardiac or kidney disease

Uterine fibromyomata

Fibrocystic breast disease or breast fibrodenomas

Epilepsy

Depression

Any woman who takes the Pill should be alert to the development of any of the above conditions. See your physician immediately if any of these are present, or if you experience headaches, blurred vision, leg pain, chest pain, or abdominal pain.

Intrauterine device. The **intrauterine device (IUD)** is a small plastic object that is inserted by a physician into the uterus to prevent pregnancy. IUDs come in a variety of designs (see Fig. 14.3). Some contain cop-

---

*From Robert A. Hatcher et al., *Contraceptive Technology 1976–1977* (New York: Irvington Publishers, 1980). Used with permission.

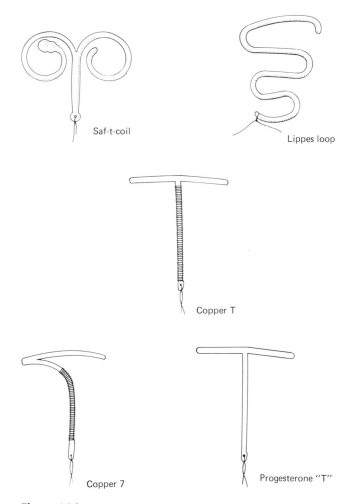

Saf-t-coil

Lippes loop

Copper T

Copper 7

Progesterone "T"

Figure 14.3
IUDs.

3. In the case of copper-treated devices, alter the chemical environment needed or the hormonal secretions necessary for the development of the fertilized ovum.

Severe complications from using IUDs have been reported, including pelvic infection and uterine perforation. Another complication associated with IUD usage is the possibility of expulsion without the user's knowledge. When this happens, the woman is unprotected and pregnancy may result. For this reason, women wearing IUDs should check often to see that they are still in place by feeling for the string that leads from the IUD through the cervix into the vagina. Figure 14.4 depicts the IUD in place with its descending string.

Figure 14.4
Lippes loop in position in the uterus. The thread
projecting from the cervix enables the woman to
check at intervals to ensure that the IUD has not
been ejected from the uterus.
SOURCE: Eric T. Pengelley, *Sex and Human Life* (Reading, Mass.: Addison-Wesley, 1974).

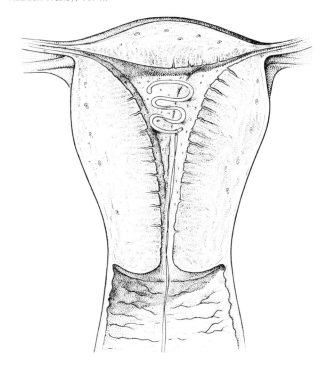

per, and some contain the hormone progesterone. Although it is not known for sure how IUDs work, they are believed to do one of several things to prevent pregnancy.

1. Prevent the fertilized ovum from implanting itself on the endometrium of the uterus so that it cannot be nourished,

2. Immobilize the sperm,

Other complications can arise if pregnancy occurs while the IUD is in the uterus. If the IUD is removed during pregnancy, there is a 25 percent chance of spontaneous abortion, whereas if it is kept in place, infection, blood poisoning, bleeding, or premature labor may result.[6] Finally, IUDs may lead to heavier than usual menstrual bleeding and a more painful menstrual period, particularly for three months or so after first being inserted.

The advantages of IUD usage relate to its effectiveness and its constantly being in place. Couples not wanting to interrupt intercourse to insert a diaphragm or use a condom, for example, may find the IUD appealing.

Spermicides. Spermicidal preparations offer another form of contraception. The **spermicide** is applied so as to be placed against the cervix (see Fig. 14.5).

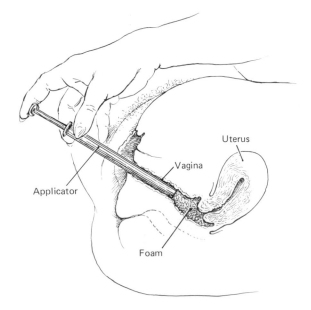

Figure 14.5
Application of a spermicidal foam.
SOURCE: Wayne Middendorf and Bruce Middendorf, *A Sperm and Egg Handbook* (Buffalo: University Press, 1971), p. 15.

Applicator

Uterus

Vagina

Foam

The spermicide blocks the sperm from entering the cervix, as well as immobilizing and killing them. Spermicidal jellies and creams are not very effective unless used with a diaphragm. Spermicidal foam offers much better protection because it is more evenly distributed. To be effective, the foam must be inserted just before intercourse, and a new application is required with each act of intercourse. The effectiveness of foam is greatly increased when used in combination with a condom. Spermicides are available without a prescription.

Spermicidial suppositories are also available. When inserted in the vagina, the moisture and warmth effervesces or dissolves the suppository into a sperm-killing barrier. The suppository should be inserted at least 10 to 15 minutes before intercourse, and it remains effective for approximately one hour. A new suppository should be inserted for each act of intercourse.

Spermicidal suppositories are free of serious side effects. However, they are less effective than spermicidal foam, because they do not distribute the spermicide as evenly.

Douching. **Douching** refers to squirting a special solution into the vagina after sexual intercourse in an effort to flush all of the semen out of the vagina. This method is extremely ineffective, because sperm can reach the cervical canal as quickly as 90 seconds after ejaculation. Some experts contend that douching may actually facilitate the passage of sperm to the cervical opening, because the douche is squirted under pressure. In addition, frequent douching may irritate the tissues of the vagina. Although some women douche for sanitary reasons, there is no evidence that this practice is necessary or beneficial.

Sterilization. **Sterilization** is usually a permanent form of birth control that can be applied to either the male or the female. In the case of the male, the vas deferens is cut and tied by a physician so that the sperm cannot be transported out of the penis. Termed a **vasectomy,** this procedure is performed on an outpatient basis, and the patient can return home shortly after the procedure. Only a small incision in each side of the

Vasectomy

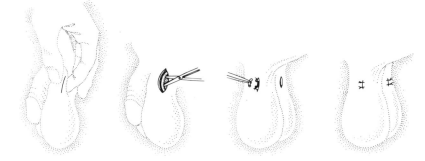

Figure 14.6
Vasectomy. These drawings show the incision in the testicles and the removal of a small portion of the vas deferens on each side.

scrotum, to reach the vas, is necessary (see Fig. 14.6). At present the procedure is generally considered irreversible, although use of microsurgery has become increasingly effective in reversing vasectomies. Research is now being conducted with a new sterilization technique for males that does not require surgery. This new procedure involves an injection of ethanol and formaldehyde into the vas deferens. The result is scarring in the vas, which prevents the sperm from moving through it.

The female sterilization procedure is termed **tubal ligation.** In this procedure the Fallopian tubes are cut and tied to prevent the sperm and egg from meeting (see Fig. 14.7). One or two small incisions are made in the abdomen through the navel, and a viewing instrument, known as a laparoscope, is inserted so that the physician can locate the tubes. This procedure is termed a **laparoscopy** and can usually be done under local anesthesia. This method is the least complicated and easiest for the woman. Other means of cutting or cauterizing the Fallopian tubes require a larger abdominal incision (laparotomy) or approach the Fallopian tubes through the vagina (culpotomy). The preferred method, however, is usually laparoscopy.

A nonsurgical sterilization procedure for females is now being studied. This procedure plugs up the Fallopian tubes with injections of silicone, which becomes a rubberlike solid, preventing the egg from reaching the uterus and the sperm from reaching the egg. Each

silicone plug can be removed and fertility restored. Testing of this procedure on human subjects is already under way.

Table 14.2 summarizes the methods of contraception we have discussed.

Figure 14.7
Tubal ligation. This is a relatively safe surgical procedure, which is generally irreversible. In sterilization the procedure is performed on both tubes.

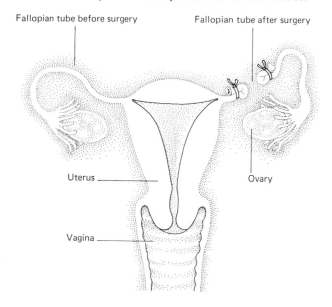

Fallopian tube before surgery

Fallopian tube after surgery

Uterus

Ovary

Vagina

Table 14.2
COMPARATIVE SUMMARY OF CONTRACEPTIVE METHODS

	The Pill	Minipills	Intrauterine device (IUD)	Diaphragm with Spermicidal Jelly or Cream
	Pills with two hormones, an estrogen and progestin, similar to the hormones a woman makes in her own ovaries.	Pills with just one type of hormone: a progestin, similar to a hormone a woman makes in her own ovaries.	A small piece of plastic with nylon threads attached. Some have copper wire wrapped around them. One IUD gives off a hormone, progesterone.	A shallow rubber cup used with a sperm-killing jelly or cream.
How does it work?	Prevents egg's release from woman's ovaries, makes cervical mucus thicker and changes lining of the uterus.	It may prevent egg's release from woman's ovaries, makes cervical mucus thicker and changes lining of uterus, making it harder for a fertilized egg to start growing there.	The IUD is inserted into the uterus. It is not known exactly how the IUD prevents pregnancy.	Fits inside the vagina. The rubber cup forms a barrier between the uterus and the sperm. The jelly or cream kills the sperm.
How would I use it?	Either of two ways: 1. A pill a day for 3 weeks, stop for one week, then start a new pack. 2. A pill every single day with no stopping between packs.	Take one pill every single day as long as you want to avoid pregnancy.	Check string at least once a month right after the period ends to make sure your IUD is still properly in place.	Insert the diaphragm and jelly (or cream) before intercourse. Can be inserted up to 6 hours before intercourse. Must stay in at least 6 hours after intercourse.
Are there problems with it?	Must be prescribed by a doctor. All women should have a medical exam before taking the Pill, and some women should not take it.	Must be prescribed by a doctor. All women should have a medical exam first.	Must be inserted by a doctor after a pelvic examination. Cannot be used by all women. Sometimes the uterus "pushes" it out.	Must be fitted by a doctor after a pelvic exam. Some women find it difficult to insert, inconvenient, or messy.
What are the side effects or complications?	Nausea, weight gain, headaches, missed periods, darkened skin on the face, or depression may occur. More serious and more rare problems are blood clots in the legs, the lung, or the brain, and heart attacks.	Irregular periods, missed periods, and spotting may occur and are more common problems with minipills than with the regular birth control pills.	May cause cramps, bleeding, or spotting; infections of the uterus or of the oviducts (tubes) may be serious. See a doctor for pain, bleeding, fever, or a bad discharge.	Some women find that the jelly or cream irritates the vagina. Try changing brands if this happens.
What are the advantages?	Convenient, extremely effective, does not interfere with sex, and may diminish menstrual cramps.	Convenient, effective, does not interfere with sex, and less serious side effects than with regular birth control pills.	Effective, always there when needed, and usually not felt by either partner.	Effective and safe.

Spermicidal Foam, Jelly or Cream	Condom ("Rubber")	Condom and Foam Used Together	Periodic Abstinence (Natural Family Planning)	Sterilization
Cream and jelly come in tubes; foam comes in aerosol cans or individual applicators and is placed into the vagina.	A sheath of rubber shaped to fit snugly over the erect penis.		Ways of finding out days each month when you are most likely to get pregnant. Intercourse is avoided at that time.	Vasectomy (male). Tubal ligation (female). Ducts carrying sperm or the egg are tied and cut surgically.
Foam, jelly and cream contain a chemical that kills sperm and acts as a physical barrier between sperm and the uterus.	Prevents sperm from getting inside a woman's vagina during intercourse.	Prevents sperm from getting inside the uterus by killing sperm and by preventing sperm from getting out into the vagina.	Techniques include maintaining chart of basal body temperature, checking vaginal secretions, and keeping calendar of menstrual periods.	Closing of tubes in male prevents sperm from reaching egg; closing tubes in female prevents egg from reaching sperm.
Put foam, jelly or cream into your vagina each time you have intercourse, not more than 30 minutes beforehand.	The condom should be placed on the erect penis before the penis ever comes into contact with the vagina. After ejaculation, the penis should be removed from the vagina immediately.	Foam must be inserted within 30 minutes before intercourse and condom must be placed onto erect penis prior to contact with vagina.	Careful records must be maintained of several factors: basal body temperature, vaginal secretions and onset of menstrual bleeding.	After the decision to have no more children has been well thought through, a brief surgical procedure is performed on the man or the woman.
Must be inserted just before intercourse. Some find it inconvenient or messy.	Objectionable to some men and women. Interrupts intercourse. May be messy. Condom may break.	Requires more effort than some couples like. May be messy or inconvenient. Interrupts intercourse.	Difficult to use method if menstrual cycle is irregular. Sexual intercourse must be avoided for a significant part of each cycle.	Surgical operation has some risk but serious complications are rare. Sterilizations should not be done unless no more children are desired.
Some women find that the foam, cream or jelly irritates the vagina. May irritate the man's penis. Try changing brands if this happens.	Rarely, individuals are allergic to rubber. If this is a problem, condoms called "skins" which are not made out of rubber are available.	No serious complications.	No complications.	All surgical operations have some risk but serious complications are uncommon. Some pain may last for several days. Rarely, the wrong structure is tied off or the tube grows back together.
Effective, safe, a good lubricant and can be purchased at a drugstore.	Effective, safe, can be purchased at a drugstore; excellent protection against sexually transmitted infections.	Extremely effective, safe, and both methods may be purchased at a drugstore without a doctor's prescription. Excellent protection against sexually transmitted infections.	Safe, effective if followed carefully; little if any religious objection to method. Teaches women about their menstrual cycles.	The most effective method; low rate of complications; many feel that removing fear of pregnancy improves sexual relations.

SOURCE: *Family Planning Methods of Contraception,* U.S. Public Health Service, 1980.

Discovery Activity 14.2
CONTRACEPTIVE DECISION MAKING

If you are thinking about using contraception or changing the method you use, the following questions are intended to help you decide what method might be suitable for you.

1. How important are each of the following to you in a birth control method? Effectiveness, safety, spontaneity, religious acceptability, ease of use.

2. Are you concerned about the possible side effects of chemical means of contraception, in particular the pill?

3. Are you concerned about the possibility of contracting a sexually transmitted disease?

4. How often do you plan to have sexual intercourse? Frequently? Infrequently?

5. For how long a period of time do you plan to use contraceptives? Short term? Long term?

6. Do you have specific health or behavior patterns or problems that make some forms of contraception less advisable?

7. Who in a relationship do you feel should take responsibility for birth control?

8. How important is it to you to avoid becoming pregnant or causing a pregnancy at this point in your life?

After you've thought about these questions, study Table 14.2 to help you decide which methods might be suitable. It's also a good idea to talk to your doctor or visit a Planned Parenthood office. ●

ABORTION

Abortion is the termination of a pregnancy. If the pregnancy is not terminated purposefully, the abortion is said to be spontaneous. If the abortion is purposeful, it is said to be induced. There are several methods of induced abortion, with the stage of the pregnancy usually determining which method is used. During the first trimester of pregnancy, either **dilation and curettage (D and C)** or **suction curettage** is the method of choice. In dilation and curettage the cervix is opened (dilation) and an instrument inserted to scrape out the products of conception. Suction curettage uses a vacuum to suck out the products of conception.

During the second trimester, the growth of the fetus is such that other methods are dictated. One method, **evacuation and curettage,** requires scraping the products of conception prior to vacuuming, because the conceptus is too large to fit through the vacuum otherwise. Another method which is used only rarely, is **hysterotomy:** removal of the products of conception through an abdominal incision. One of the most frequently used methods of abortion during the second trimester is **induced labor,** in which a saline solution is injected into the amniotic fluid surrounding the fetus to induce labor and discharge the fetus. Sometimes prostaglandins are injected instead of saline solution.

We should also mention the use of **diethylstilbestrol (DES),** a synthetic estrogen administered in a massive dose. Sometimes called the "morning-after pill," DES is prescribed only in emergency cases, such as rape or incest, because this drug has been associated with a significant risk of cancer of the cervix or vagina.

The Abortion Controversy

During the past decade abortion has been the subject of considerable controversy in the United States. Even though abortion was legalized in 1973, highly vocal antiabortion groups have sought to overturn the Supreme Court decision and make abortion a crime. These "Right-to-Life" advocates argue that personhood begins at conception and that therefore abortion is murder. "Pro-Choice" advocates, on the other hand, contend that it is impossible to determine when life begins and that it is the right of a woman to choose whether or not to bear a child. According to a 1979 Gallup poll, the great majority of Americans favor permitting therapeutic abortion during at least the first trimester of pregnancy. Only 17 percent of the people surveyed opposed abortion under all circumstances. Discovery Activity 14.3 gives you an opportunity to express your views on abortion.

Discovery Activity 14.3
SHOULD ABORTIONS BE PERMITTED?

1. Should abortions ever be allowed?

   yes   no

2. If yes, under what circumstances?

   a) Only if conception is a result of rape or incest

      yes   no

   b) If the pregnancy will cause economic hardship

      yes   no

   c) If the pregnancy will harm the woman's physical health

      yes   no

   d) If the pregnancy will harm the woman's mental health

      yes   no

   e) Only during the first trimester

      yes   no

   f) During the first and second trimesters

      yes   no

   g) If the woman is unmarried

      yes   no

   h) If the woman is a teenager

      yes   no

   i) If the woman is over 40

      yes   no

   j) If amniocentesis determines that the fetus is defective

      yes   no

   k) Only if the woman undergoes counseling first

      yes   no

3. Should government funds be used for abortions for poor women?

   yes   no

4. Should the father's agreement be required before an abortion can be performed?

   yes   no

5. Should the father be held financially responsible for the cost of the abortion?

   yes   no

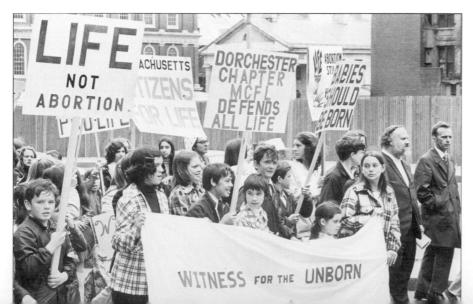

The right-to-life movement is extremely active in its campaign against abortion. Nevertheless, polls have consistently indicated that the great majority of Americans favor permitting abortion under some circumstances.

SHOULD THE GOVERNMENT PAY FOR ABORTION?

Those who believe life begins at conception consider abortion murder. The government, they argue, should not be party to murder. In 1977 the efforts of the antiabortion forces resulted in passage of legislation that permits the states to deny payment to physicians or hospitals from Medicaid funds for abortion services. Though the individual states can still use state funds to pay for abortion services, and many do, passage of this legislation has provided encouragement for those advocating a ban on all abortions. These "Right-to-Lifers" are lobbying for a Constitutional amendment outlawing abortion.

Another group of opponents of federally funded abortions views abortion as genocide. Dr. Mildred Jefferson, a black surgeon from Boston and a chairperson of the national Right to Life organization, believes that a federally funded abortion program is aimed at eliminating the poor, black population in the United States. She contends that "abortion is accomplishing what 200 years of slavery and 300 years of lynching didn't,"[7] and points out that 30 percent of all Medicaid-funded abortions were performed on black women.

Proponents of federally funded abortion argue that although wealthy women will have the money and be able to find a physician for abortions, poor women will not. Without government assistance, poor women are likely to obtain inferior abortion services or even attempt to abort themselves. The dangers of quack abortionists and self-induced abortion were demonstrated vividly in the years prior to legalization of abortions. Many women suffered serious complications or even died. The "Pro-Choice" groups argue further that women throughout history have terminated unwanted pregnancies and will continue to do so. Poor women need government assistance to obtain safe, reputable care.

What do you think? ●

PREGNANCY

Determining Pregnancy

Although pregnancy may be indicated by such symptoms as morning sickness, swollen breasts, and frequent urination, these can all be signs of other bodily processes. Even a missed mentrual period is not a sure sign of pregnancy, because many women do not ovulate every month during their menstruating life.

Pregnancy can be determined most accurately by examination of the urine. The most frequently used urine test looks for the presence of the hormone **human chorionic gonadotropin,** a hormone produced by the uterus once the fertilized ovum is implanted in it. This test for pregnancy is highly accurate when the menstrual period is two weeks overdue. Because early identification of pregnancy is necessary for proper prenatal care, it is wise not to postpone diagnosis by a physician or medical laboratory. If six weeks have passed since your last menstrual period and you have participated in sexual intercourse, you should have a pregnancy test. Results can be obtained about two minutes after the urine is analyzed.

You may have seen **early pregnancy tests (EPTs)** sold at a neighborhood drugstore. These do-it-yourself kits test for the presence of a human chorionic gonadotropin (HCG) hormone in the urine. If HCG is present, the antibodies in the pregnancy test kits, which are added to the urine contains HCG; therefore the brown ring indicates a positive result.

Consumers Union reports these tests to be very accurate when the result is positive.[8] However, up to 25 percent of women receiving negative results may be pregnant. These are termed "false negatives." In fact, the earlier in the pregnancy the kit is used, the more likely a false negative will occur. Since the kits are usually used prior to consulting a physician and obtaining a laboratory test, Consumers Union recommends having only one test, the laboratory test. If a self-test is made, it is suggested it be done no sooner than 14 days after a missed period, and if the result is negative, a second self-test should be administered a few days later.

Our advice: save your money and peace of mind by having the test done at a physician's office, a clinic (for example, Planned Parenthood), or a county or state health department office.

Prenatal Care

Concept: Prenatal care is essential to ensuring the health of the fetus.

The **embryo** (conceptus prior to 12 weeks) and **fetus** (conceptus after 12 weeks) are nourished through the blood of the mother. The blood carries nutrients and oxygen necessary for the baby's development in the uterus and is passed to the baby through the **placenta.** The placental membrane prevents certain substances or organisms from passing from the mother to the fetus. Other substances, however, some harmful, can pass through this placental barrier. For this reason, it is highly important that a pregnant woman obtain prenatal care as soon as she knows she is pregnant. The most crucial phase of development in utero is the first three months. This is the time when what the mother does is most important. What she eats, whether or not she smokes or drinks alcohol—all of these decisions should be made with medical assistance. At the very least, medication, alcohol, and cigarettes should be discontinued until medical advice is obtained.

The need for early medical advice cannot be over-emphasized. Lower-birth-weight babies are statistically related to late prenatal care and tend to have more birth defects of all kinds than do babies of greater birth weight. Genetic disorders are discussed in Chapter 17.

To help make wise decisions, pregnant women should be aware of the following findings:

1. Although past practice had suggested that pregnant women limit their weight gain to 20 pounds, a woman of average weight is now usually advised to gain between 24 and 30 pounds during pregnancy.

2. Smoking during pregnancy is associated with lower birth weight, shorter gestation period, higher rates of spontaneous abortion, more frequent complications of pregnancy and delivery, and higher rates of infant mortality.

3. Research with monkeys demonstrates that tetra-hydrocannabinol (THC), the primary psychoactive agent in marijuana, can pass through the placental barrier and concentrate in the fatty tissue of the fetus.

4. Even moderate consumption of alcohol while pregnant is related to central nervous system dysfunction and growth deficiency in babies. **Fetal alcohol syndrome** is the name given to the physical and psychological characteristics present in babies of mothers who drank heavily when pregnant.

5. Aspirin taken by the mother is suspected of being associated with physical defects, blood-clotting problems, and central nervous system dysfunction in the baby.

6. Mothers addicted to heroin will give birth to babies addicted to heroin. The newborn must then go through withdrawal. Other narcotic drugs will lead to similar addictions.

7. Pregnant women need to eat foods that are high in protein to aid fetal tissue growth and high in calcium to aid bone growth.

8. Several complications of pregnancy can occur and should be recognized. **Toxemia** is pregnancy-induced hypertension, with swelling caused by fluid retention and the possibility of coma or convulsion. At the first signs of these symptoms a physician should be consulted.

9. Some pregnant women have an Rh negative blood factor that destroys the baby's Rh positive red blood cells. This combination is usually dangerous in second and subsequent pregnancies, where, if untreated, the baby could die. The method of treatment is to give the newborn a transfusion with Rh negative blood. In time, the baby will replace this Rh negative blood with the Rh positive blood it produces.

Gestation

Gestation is the period of time from conception to birth. The term of pregnancy is usually divided into three time periods, called **trimesters,** each of which is three months long.

The first trimester. At the end of the first month of pregnancy the embryo is approximately 0.25 inch long. During this month, three cell layers are formed: the **ectoderm,** or outer layer, from which the skin, sense organs, and nervous system will form; the **mesoderm,** or middle layer, from which the muscular, circulatory, and excretory systems will form; and the **endoderm,** or inner layer, from which the digestive and glandular systems and the lungs will form.

At the conclusion of the second month, the embryo is approximately 1.25 inches long and weighs 1/30th of an ounce. At this point the embryo slightly resembles a small human, although its head is half its bulk and the forehead is very large. Also noticeable at this stage of development are the eyes, ears, nose, lips, and tongue.

At the end of the first trimester the fetus is 3 inches long and weighs 1 ounce. The fetus can move now but this movement is not noticeable or felt by the mother. At this stage, nails have grown on the fingers and toes, and the genitalia can be identified as male or female.

The second trimester. The fourth month is characterized by great growth. The fetus grows to 6 inches in length, with the head now only one-third the body length. The fetus demonstrates an ability to suck. Usually by the end of this month the fetal movements can be felt by the mother. This movement is called **quickening.**

The conclusion of the fifth month finds the fetus 12 inches long and weighing 1 pound. The fetus now has all its essential structures.

At the end of the sixth month the fetus is about 14 inches long and weighs about 2 pounds. The eyes have formed, and the fetus is sensitive to light. The fetus can also hear uterine sounds.

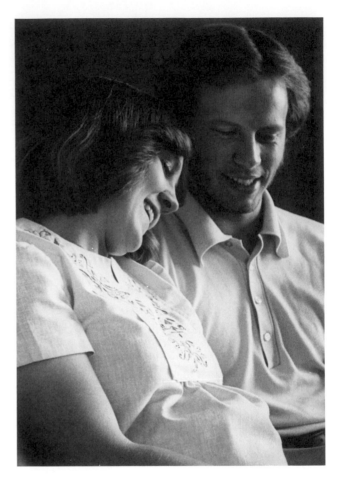

During a first pregnancy, fetal movement—called quickening—can usually be felt by the end of the fourth month.

The third trimester. During the last trimester the fetus develops a layer of fat, making it appear more babylike. By the seventh month the fetus generally has a good chance of survival if born prematurely. By the end of the eighth month the fetus weights about 5 pounds, 4 ounces, and is 20 inches long. During the last month of pregnancy the baby's head moves into position in the pelvis. Figure 14.8 shows the development of the fetus at several stages.

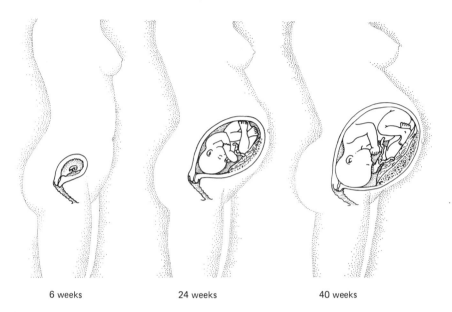

6 weeks   24 weeks   40 weeks

Figure 14.8
Development of the fetus at 6 weeks, 24 weeks, and term. The relationship
between changes in the fetus and changes in the mother is shown.

CHILDBIRTH

The Birth Process

Concept: The birth process occurs in three stages.

The birth process begins with rhythmic contraction of the uterine muscles. This first stage of **labor** lasts an average of 10.5 hours for the first pregnancy and 6.5 hours for subsequent pregnancies. The task of the first stage of labor is to open the neck of the cervix wide enough (10 centimeters) for the fetus to exit.

The second stage of labor, consisting of pushing by the abdominal muscles, lasts about one-half to two hours. As the head of the fetus appears in the vaginal opening, an incision, known as an **episiotomy,** may be made by the physician to prevent the vaginal tissue from tearing. Episiotomies used to be common practice; now they are often deemed unnecessary.

The third stage of labor results in the discharge of the placenta and occurs from two to 20 minutes after birth. When the umbilical cord stops pulsating, it is clamped and then cut. The baby is then checked for vital body functions and drops are deposited in its eyes to prevent gonorrheal infection.

Of course, this routine birth process can vary. If the fetus is positioned in the uterus with the buttocks rather than the head first (**breech birth**), or if the pressure on the head of the fetus becomes too great, thereby decreasing its oxygen supply, other procedures are employed. The fetus may be delivered with the aid of forceps to pull it out gently or removed through an incision in the woman's abdomen. Figure 14.9 portrays the birth process.

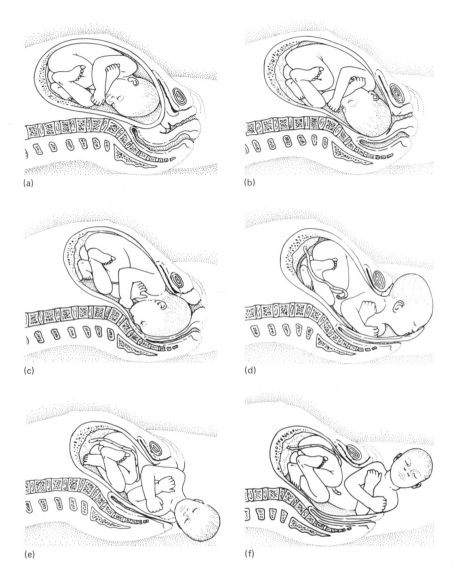

Figure 14.9
The birth process. (A) The baby floats in the amniotic fluid before labor begins. (B) Rhythmic contractions force the baby's head against the cervix. (C) Descent through the birth canal begins, with the head gradually rotating and extending. (D) The head crowns and the baby begins to emerge from the birth canal. (E) and (F) Again the baby rotates, as first one shoulder and then the other is delivered.

Cesarian section. Delivery of the fetus by incision through the abdominal wall into the uterus is called a **cesarian section** (C-section). This procedure is performed when a delivery through the vagina would be a risk to the mother or baby. The baby's head may be too large, labor may be prolonged, or labor contractions may not be strong enough for a vaginal delivery.

The number of C-sections has been increasing at a very high rate in the past decade (from 6 to 18 percent of births). One reason for this increase may be the use of the electronic fetal monitor, which checks uterine contractions and fetal heart beat during labor and can reveal problems physicians might otherwise miss. However, some physicians may misinterpret a labor variation as "fetal distress" and overreact by performing a C-section. Consequently, it has been suggested that the fetal monitor be used only in cases where there is a special need to watch the fetus.

Making Decisions about Birthing

Concept: Couples can now choose from several approaches to managing the birth process.

As a result of the increasing evidence that drugs used to decrease pain during childbirth remain in the baby's system long after birth, many women are choosing to give birth without drugs. Prepared childbirth consists of classes that teach the prospective parents what to expect and how to behave during delivery. Women are taught to relax through breathing exercises. Men are taught to coach. An important decision regarding birth, then, is whether to give birth without drugs.

Another decision being made more frequently in recent years is to deliver in the home rather than in the

Home birth is becoming a popular alternative among couples who want to experience birthing within a family setting.

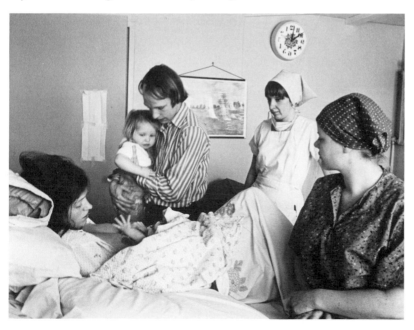

hospital. Nass and McDonald summarize the pros and cons of home birth as follows:[9]

> Home birth offers a number of advantages, including the familiar surroundings, the presence and often the active participation of family and friends, the ability to make decisions about delivery with a doctor who is sympathetic to the couple's particular needs, the reduced expense, and the assurance that the couple will not be separated from their newborn for any length of time. The major drawback is the lack of immediate emergency equipment should complications arise.
>
> Home births require careful planning. Couples are screened for possible risks, they generally attend classes designed especially for those planning home births, and they often employ the services of a midwife who monitors the course of the pregnancy and is present at the birth along with a doctor. Women who are under 20 or over 30 and are giving birth for the first time are considered at higher risk and are usually discouraged from home birth. And women who experience problems during a first pregnancy or have a history of pregnancy-related problems are advised to give birth in a hospital.

Another decision relates to the ideas of French obstetrician Frederick Leboyer. Leboyer believes that birth is traumatic for the baby and should be made as comfortable as possible. He argues that the delivery room should be dimly lit, quiet, and warm. Further, the baby should not be turned upside down and spanked to encourage breathing but rather placed gently on the mother's abdomen and permitted to begin breathing gradually. Next the baby should be placed in water warmed to body temperature. Some physicians worry that babies will not begin to breathe properly if handled as recommended by Leboyer; others see no special advantage in the Leboyer method.

Still another decision in hospital births is whether to have the baby kept in the mother's room (**rooming-in**) or in a nursery area of the hospital, from which it is brought periodically to the mother for feeding and attention. Though the mother obtains valuable rest when the baby is kept in the nursery, there is evidence to suggest that mothers of first children who choose rooming-in feel more confident in themselves as mothers than those who do not choose rooming-in.[10]

Bonding

There is evidence that **bonding,** or attachment between mother and newborn, develops quickly and can be delayed by extended separation just after birth. The initial contact between mother and child—fondling, holding, gazing, talking—somehow seems to enhance attachment of the mother to the newborn. Studies have shown a higher incidence of child abuse and a greater number of deaths in infants separated from their mothers at birth, compared to infants not separated from their mothers at birth. Premature infants are often separated from their parents, and the greater attention they require may cause stress for the parents.

The importance of bonding between father and child should also be recognized. Father–child attachment can be enhanced through home birth or natural childbirth, because in both types of birth the father is present and involved during the birth process.

Breast and Bottle Feeding

During pregnancy, secretions of estrogen, progesterone, and lactogen lead to an increase in breast tissue and glandular ducts. After delivery, a pituitary hormone named **prolactin** activates the mammary glands to produce milk. For three to four days after delivery, a thin, yellowish liquid called **colostrum** is secreted; mature milk production begins four to seven days after delivery.

Breast milk has several advantages over infant formula and is therefore recommended by the American Academy of Pediatrics. It contains antibodies that provide the infant with immunity to several diseases. In addition, the psychological attachment between mother and baby is enhanced by breast feeding.

Not all women are able to breast feed, and many prefer the convenience of bottle feeding. Although infant formula cannot supply the antibodies breast milk does, it provides all the nourishment a baby needs in

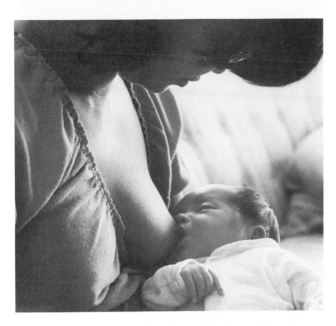

One advantage of breast feeding is that it provides the infant with antibodies from the mother to protect it against disease.

order to thrive. Some couples prefer bottle feeding because it enables the father to participate in feeding the baby. Breast feeding for some meals and bottle feeding for others is another way of ensuring that the father is able to enjoy this aspect of baby care.

INFERTILITY AND ITS TREATMENT

Infertility is generally defined as the inability to conceive after a year or more of sexual relations without contraception. About 10 to 15 percent of American couples who want a child are infertile. In about 30 percent of cases both partners have a fertility problem; in the remaining 70 percent about half of the problems can be traced to the woman and half to the man.

In men infertility usually results from insufficient production of sperm or low **motility** (ability of the sperm

to swim). Infertility in women can be caused by pelvic infection, blockage of the Fallopian tubes, **endometriosis** (a condition in which tissue that normally grows in the uterus grows on various other abdominal structures), or several other factors.

The success rate of treatment for infertility has been rising in recent years, and it is estimated that 50 to 70 percent of all childless couples are eventually able to have a baby. In cases where the male is infertile, many couples choose to have **artificial insemination,** in which sperm from an anonymous donor is introduced into the woman's vagina with a syringe. Over 14,000 American babies are conceived each year by this method.

Perhaps the most widely publicized new treatment for infertility is **in vitro fertilization.** This procedure was developed to enable women who have blocked Fallopian tubes to conceive. The mature ovum is removed from the ovary and mixed with the male partner's sperm. Once it has divided into eight or 16 cells, the fertilized ovum is reimplanted into the uterus. The success rate for in vitro fertilization is quite low; however, successful births have taken place (most recently in the United States) and the technique appears to be quite promising.

CONCLUSION

Many decisions must be made about contraception, pregnancy, and birth. Unmarried people must decide whether to participate in sexual intercourse; if so, whether to use contraceptives; if pregnancy occurs, whether to abort or deliver the unborn; and if the latter, whether to raise the baby, give it up for adoption, or abandon the child. Married people make similar decisions.

Additional decisions that must be made concern where to give birth, what method of delivery to use, and whether to breast feed.

The information and issues discussed in this chapter should help you make informed decisions about contraception, pregnancy, and birth.

SUMMARY

1. There are many reasons why people choose not to use conception control even though they do not wish to conceive a child: they believe pregnancy couldn't happen to them, they feel guilty or immoral planning for coitus in advance, they're too embarrassed to purchase contraceptives, or they believe they experience coitus too infrequently to be concerned with contraception.

2. Contraceptive effectiveness is evaluated in terms of failure rates. Theoretical or ideal failure rate refers to how effective the method is when used perfectly; actual user failure rate refers to how effective the method is when used by people outside of controlled laboratory situations.

3. Conception control can be obtained in several ways: abstinence, withdrawal, rhythm, natural family planning, condoms, diaphragm, cervical cap, intrauterine devices, spermicides, the Pill, and sterilization.

4. Abortion is termination of a pregnancy. Abortions that do not occur purposefully are called spontaneous. Abortions performed purposefully are called induced. Methods of abortion include dilation and currettage, evacuation and curettage, hysterotomy, and induced labor by injection of saline solution. The choice of method depends on the stage of pregnancy.

5. Pregnancy is usually determined by a laboratory test for the hormone human chorionic gonadotropin in the urine. Results can be obtained about two minutes after the urine is analyzed.

6. Prenatal care is recommended as soon as pregnancy is determined. Good prenatal care and nutrition are related to fewer birth defects and lower infant mortality.

7. Cigarette smoking, use of drugs, consumption of alcoholic beverages, and poor nutrition are related to spontaneous abortion, birth defects, and infant mortality. Therefore pregnant women should adjust their behavior in these respects during the gestation period.

8. Childbirth consists of three stages of labor. In the first stage the neck of the cervix opens wide enough for the fetus to exit, in the second stage the baby is delivered, and in the third stage the placenta is discharged.

9. Among the decisions regarding childbirth are where to have the delivery, whether to use drugs or deliver without medication, whether to have rooming-in, and whether to subsequently breast feed.

10. Infertility is a problem for some 10 to 15 percent of couples in the United States who want a child. The success rate for treatment of infertility has been rising in recent years. When the male is infertile, many couples choose artifical insemination, in which sperm from an anonymous donor is introduced into the vagina of the female partner with a syringe.

REFERENCES

1. Guy S. Parcel, "A Study of the Relationship between Contraceptive Attitudes and Behavior in a Group of Unmarried University Students," doctoral dissertation, Pennsylvania State University, 1974.

2. Kenneth L. Jones, Louis W. Shainberg, and Curtis O. Byer, *Sex* (New York: Harper & Row, 1969), p. 71.

3. E. James Lieberman and Ellen Peck, *Sex and Birth Control: A Guide for the Young* (New York: Schocken Books, 1973), p. 53.

4. Alexander Tolar, Frank J. Rice, and Claude A. Lanctot, "Characteristics of Couples Practicing the Temperature-Rhythm Method of Birth Control," *Proceedings of the 81st Annual Convention of the American Psychological Association* 8 (1973): 353–354.

5. Robert A. Hatcher, *Contraceptive Technology, 1980–81* (New York: Irvington, 1980), p. 29.

6. Robert A. Hatcher, *Contraceptive Technology, 1980–81*, p. 4.

7. "Doctor Attacks Abortion Plan as 'Class War,'" *Buffalo Evening News,* October 3, 1977, p. 7.

8. "Test Yourself for Pregnancy?" *Consumer Reports* (November 1978):644–645.

9. Gilbert D. Nass and G. W. McDonald, *Marriage and the Family,* 2nd ed. (Reading, Mass.: Addison-Wesley, 1982), pp. 321–322.

10. M. Greenberg, I. Rosenberg, and J. Lind, "First Mothers Rooming-in with Their Newborns: Its Impact upon the Mother," *American Journal of Orthopsychiatry* 43 (1973): 783–788.

Laborabory 1
CONTRACEPTIVE SURVEYING

Purpose   To learn why sexually active college students either use or do not use contraceptives.

Size of Group   Four students per group.

Equipment   Access to duplicating equipment (a mimeo or copying machine).

Procedure

1. Identify where large groups of students congregate, for example, the library, dining halls, cafeteria, student union, or dormitories.

2. Assign a group to each place so that the whole class can cover as many places as possible.

3. The group then goes to these places and asks students to complete the form below *confidentially* and deposit their completed forms in a centrally located box. The form should ask:

    a. Are you sexually active?

        yes _____   no _____

    b. Do you use a method of birth control?

        yes _____   no _____

        If yes, which method do you use?

        _____

    c. Why do you use this method? (check as many reasons below as pertain to *your* choice of birth control.)

        _____ It's convenient.

        _____ It's effective.

        _____ It doesn't interrupt sex act.

_____ It's accepted by my religion.

_____ It has very few or no side effects.

_____ It's inexpensive.

_____ It's not embarrassing to obtain.

_____ It's not messy.

_____ It prevents sexually transmitted diseases.

_____ It's not my responsibility but rather my partner's.

_____ I've never thought about other options.

    d. Now rank order the reasons you checked. Which is first in importance, second, etc.?

4. Once each group has obtained approximately 25 completed forms *from students who use some means of birth control,* they should bring these forms together and tally the results.

Results

The total class should discuss the results in terms of the following questions:

1. Which method of contraception is most often used?

2. Why is that method chosen?

3. Is that method the safest one?

4. Is that method effective? Are there more effective means of birth control?

The discussion should conclude with a statement about the specific needs of the student body regarding education about contraception.

Laboratory 2
RESPONSIBLE SEXUAL BEHAVIOR

Purpose To practice regarding responsible sexual behavior.

Size of Group Initially the total class.
Later, students pair up.

Equipment None.

Procedure

1. Form a large circle with everyone in the class. Have one male and one female volunteer role play, in the middle of the circle, the following situation:

   John and Mary are on a date. John has taken Mary to a movie and then over to his apartment. He holds Mary, and they kiss and hug for awhile. He next attempts to have sexual intercourse with Mary. Mary inquires as to whether John has any contraceptives (such as a condom). John says no, so Mary says no. The role-playing situation begins with John trying to talk Mary into having sexual intercourse with him then and there, and Mary trying to refuse because of fear of pregnancy and a desire to exhibit responsible sexual behavior.

   Only the actors speak. No one in the outside circle may say anything.

2. After 15 minutes of role playing, and without analyzing the situation just acted out, pair up (one male, one female) and act out the same situation. This time, however, incorporate into your arguments anything heard in the role playing you observed, or add to what you've heard.

Results

Form one large group of the total class after sufficient time has been provided for step 2 above (approximately 15 minutes), and discuss the following:

1. What did you add to the arguments offered by John and Mary? Why?

2. What did you delete from the arguments offered by John and Mary? Why?

3. What does "responsible sexual behavior" mean?

4. In the situation you acted out, someone might argue that John was sexually irresponsible for wanting to engage in intercourse without using any method of contraception, whereas others might argue that Mary was irresponsible for disregarding John's sexual needs. What do you think?

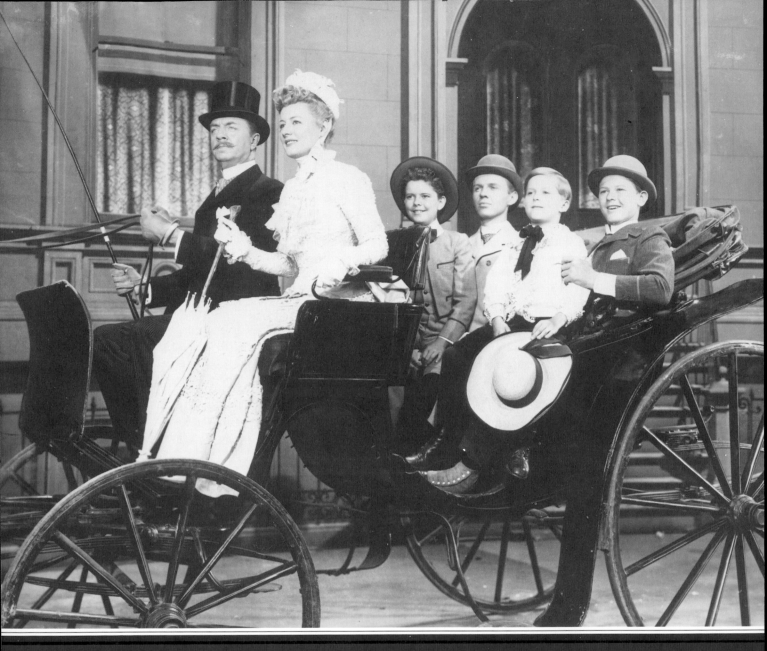

chapter *15*

intimate relationships: dating, marriage, and the family

- *intimacy: a learned process*
- *marriage*
- *parenthood*
- *alternatives to marriage*

The need for intimate relationships is central to most people's lives. Loving and being loved provide a sense of belonging, security, and well-being. We generally think of people who do not have the emotional support of relatives, friends, lovers, or spouses as being sad or isolated. In our society most people still regard marriage as the ultimate intimate relationship, achieved through a sequential progression beginning with dating and culminating in the formation of a new family unit. Although many people experience a smooth progression, many others find the route to intimacy a difficult one. The high incidence of divorce in our society and the large number of single-parent families are testimony to this fact. In this chapter we will focus on intimate relationships, how they form, and why they often fail. We'll also examine alternative routes to intimacy, such as cohabitation and single-hood. Finally, we'll consider some of the issues surrounding parenthood and family life. Your task will be to see how you can use what you learn in this chapter to build satisfying intimate relationships in your own life.

INTIMACY: A LEARNED PROCESS

The ability to form an intimate relationship that might lead to marriage does not come naturally; it is learned. Much of our early learning about close relationships comes from our family background. You have evolved into the person you are through inherited traits and interaction with your environment. You have inherited a physical appearance and an intellectual potential. You come from a certain socioeconomic background. You had many experiences as a boy or girl that shaped your perceptions of life. You had parents or other caretakers whom you observed interacting, perhaps brothers and sisters to model, and friends with whom you shared important aspects of your life. The interaction between your heredity and your environment has led you to become the person you are. If your family background and early experiences were happy, if you were loved and cherished, it is likely that you will develop the ability to love and cherish others. If your experiences were unhappy, the process may be more difficult. But many people who have had an unhappy family background are also able to develop into warm, nurturing individuals, although they may need more help along the way.

The Challenge of Intimacy

Intimacy doesn't just happen; it requires work. To be intimate with another person we must be willing to be vulnerable and to reveal ourselves to that person. Some people are afraid to reveal what they are to others because they fear rejection. Others are afraid that if they become too close to others they might lose their individuality. Building a healthy relationship means being willing to take these risks and to find a way to balance self-revelation and closeness with the need to be one's own person. A crucial element in your ability to do this is your self-esteem. As we saw in Chapter 2, people with low self-esteem are more anxious and insecure than people with positive self-esteem. They see themselves as inadequate and lack confidence in their own ideas. People with high self-esteem, in contrast, believe in themselves and accept their own feelings. They are more likely to be able to risk rejection in a relationship, because their overall perception of themselves is positive. When a relationship doesn't work out, they may be unhappy about it, but they aren't likely to retreat into themselves and never try again. Before you can expect to be happy with another person, then, you have to be happy with yourself.

Another vital component in achieving a healthy intimate relationship is communication, as we will see later in the chapter. Can you think of some other factors that contribute to building healthy relationships?

Dating

Our first intimate relationships, of course, are with our parents and siblings. As children we also form friendships with playmates and schoolmates. At some point in adolescence, most people begin to focus their need

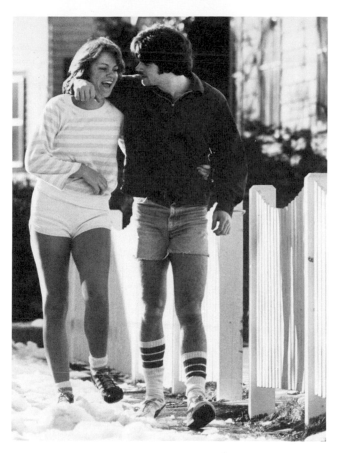

Dating gives the individual a chance to try out and evaluate behavior that may be relevant to future interpersonal relationships, including marriage.

for intimacy outside their immediate family. As they grow more independent and mature sexually, young people become increasingly interested in forming relationships with members of the opposite sex. "Dating" used to be the popular term to describe young people going out together. Today, however, many people talk about "getting together." This phrase seems to imply a more informal process of social interaction at work.

The purpose of dating, or getting together, may initially be companionship or recreation, rather than for courtship, but it nevertheless serves as a training ground for future intimate relationships, including marriage. It affords people the opportunity to try out behaviors and observe how others react to them and to experience a degree of intimacy. Eventually, over a

period of time, it helps people decide what qualities appeal to them in an intimate partner and what kinds of relationships they want to avoid.

Factors in date selection. Three factors appear to be related to the selection of dating partners: prestige considerations, physical attractiveness, and personality characteristics. *Prestige considerations* are based on our understanding that when we obtain things valued by our peers, we gain status in their eyes. Similarly, when we date someone who has characteristics valued by our peers, we gain prestige. If going out with the captain of the football team or the head cheerleader is valued by our friends, we might seek to date these people so as to improve our status with our friends. Dating a pre-med student may be more prestigious than dating a forestry major and, if so, would improve our status with our peers. Because prestige considerations relate to the values of a specific reference group—for example, our friends—they are not objective; that is, prestige considerations may vary according to sex, age, and region of the country. What is valued by your reference group? How does that affect your dating decisions?

The second factor related to the selection of dating partners is *physical attractiveness.* Facial attractiveness, physique, grooming, and dress all enter into the physical attractiveness equation. Although researchers have found physical attractiveness to be more important to males than it is to females, it is a factor in dating for both sexes. Of course, there is no concrete ideal against which all dates are measured. Some men and women find a tall date attractive, whereas others do not. Some men and women like plump dates, whereas others do not. Beauty *is* in the eye of the holder.

The last factor related to dating is the consideration of *personality characteristics.* Although the listing in Table 15.1 supports the importance of physical attractiveness in choosing a date, the influence of personality characteristics is also evident. Men and women do not seem to differ significantly in their ranking of personality characteristic, although men tend to consider intelligence and companionship more important than women do, and women value thoughtfulness, consideration, and honesty more than men do.

Table 15.1

QUALITIES OF A DATE MOST VALUED BY COLLEGE MEN AND WOMEN

Rank	Women Desired in Men:	Men Desired in Women:
1	Looks	Looks
2	Personality	Personality
3	Thoughtfulness, consideration	Sex appeal
4	Sense of humor	Intelligence
5	Honesty	Fun, good companionship
6	Respect	Sense of humor
7	Good conversation	Good conversation
8	Intelligence	Honesty

SOURCE: From *The Individual Marriage and the Family*, Third Edition, by Lloyd Saxton.© 1977 Wadsworth Publishing Company, Inc. Belmont, California 94002. Reprinted by permission of the publisher.

Discovery Activity 15.1
DATING

To help you identify what you value in a date:

1. List five people you know personally and really like:

    a. _____

    b. _____

    c. _____

    d. _____

    e. _____

2. List five people you know personally and dislike:

    a. _____

    b. _____

    c. _____

    d. _____

    e. _____

3. List any traits (such as sense of humor) that at least three of the people you like have in common:

4. List any traits that at least three of the people you dislike have in common:

5. Of the people you dated this past year, which ones possessed the traits you identified in question 3 above, and which ones possessed the traits you identified in question 4 above:

    Traits liked   **Traits disliked**

6. Why do you think you dated those people who possess traits that are possessed by people you don't like?

Rank the following, assigning "1" to the most valued most, "2" to the next most valued and "3" to the least valued:

_____ physical appearance

_____ intelligence

_____ sense of humor

_____ going to a show

_____ going to a party

_____ having a private conversation

_____ shyness

_____ conceit

_____ clumsiness

_____ someone you can depend upon

_____ someone who is unique

_____ someone who is experienced

A close examination of your responses to these exercises may indicate why you date the people you do. Are there are some generalizations about dating *for you* that you can now make?

Check those questions you would answer yes to:

_____ 1. Sometimes I date because I'm lonely.

_____ 2. Sometimes I date because I'm bored.

_____ 3. Sometimes I date to be popular.

_____ 4. Sometimes I date because my parents want me to.

_____ 5. Sometimes I date because a friend wants me to.

_____ 6. Sometimes I have a date but don't want to keep it.

_____ 7. Sometimes I get nervous about an upcoming date.

_____ 8. Sometimes I am embarrassed by my behavior on a date.

_____ 9. Sometimes I'm disappointed in the person I've dated.

_____ 10. Sometimes I think about why and whom I date.

Most of us could answer yes to all but question 10. Perhaps if we could say yes to question 10, we wouldn't have to answer yes to so many of the others. ●

Love

Concept: Determining you're in love is more difficult than it at first appears.

For most of us, dating serves as preparation for a deeper form of intimacy, particularly for the feelings embodied in the word "love." Because love is the primary reason people marry in our society, it is important to try to understand what love is. Poets, philosophers, social scientists, and many others have tried to define love, but it is probably impossible to find a simple, all-inclusive definition, because when people talk about love, they may mean a variety of things. We all rec-ognize that different forms of love exist: parents' love for their children is obviously different from the passionate love between a man and woman, for example.

A useful way to get at the meaning of love is to consider it in relationship to the concept of liking. Psychologist Zick Rubin tried to do this by developing self-report scales of passionate love and of liking.[1] To develop his love scale, he studied a variety of descriptions of love and concluded that the major dimensions of romantic love are *attachment*—the bond between a couple based on mutual need—and *caring*—the desire to give to the other person, such that the other's needs are perceived as just as important as one's own. Rubin determined that the major dimensions to liking are *affection*—liking based on the way another person relates to you—and *respect*—liking based on another's admirable qualities in areas apart from personal relations.

When Rubin asked couples who were dating or engaged to complete the loving and liking scales, he found that the scores on the two separate scales were not related. This supports the premise that liking and loving are essentially different. Another finding was that high scores on the love scale were related to desire for marriage, but high liking scores were not. In addition, dating partners and best friends received high liking scores, but dating partners received much higher love scores. It would seem that liking is necessary for love to occur but that a love relationship involves more than simple affection and respect. Discovery Activity 15.2 includes a few items from Rubin's scale. If you want to know whether you are more "in like" or "in love" with someone you're seeing, complete this scale.

Concept: Love changes over time.

Romantic and conjugal love. In speaking of love, we should differentiate between conjugal love and romantic love. **Conjugal love** is a domestic, calm, solid, comforting love relationship developed over time. **Romantic love** refers to total absorption of partners with each other and is referred to by such statements as "Love at first sight," "True love comes only once," and "Love conquers all." Relationships which begin with romantic love will eventually develop into conjugal

Discovery Activity 15.2
LIKING AND LOVING

Complete the scale below by thinking of someone you wish to be the object of your love rating. Then answer the three questions in each column, summing up the totals to determine how much you love and how much you like this person. Score as follows, depending upon how strongly you feel: disagree—1, 2, 3; agree to some extent—4, 5, 6; agree completely—7, 8, 9.

Passionate Love Scale

1. I feel that I can confide in _____ about virtually everything.
2. I would do almost anything for _____.
3. If I could never be with _____, I would feel miserable.

Liking Companionate Love Scale

1. I think that _____ is unusually well-adjusted.
2. I have great confidence in _____'s good judgment.
3. _____ is one of the most likable people I know.

Answer Sheet

Loving scale	Liking scale
Your feelings	Your feelings
1. _____	1. _____
2. _____	2. _____
3. _____	3. _____

Now add them all up.

Total: _____　　　　Total: _____　●

SOURCE: Zick Rubin. "Measurement of Romantic Love," *Journal of Personality and Social Psychology* 16 (1970):265–273. Copyright 1970 by the American Psychological Association. Reprinted by permission of the publisher and author.

love if they are positive, healthy relationships. Conjugal love is created out of a sum of experiences between lovers and is therefore impossible for new lovers to experience.

Most of us recall a romantic love relationship as one that caused our hearts to beat whenever we were near, or even thinking of, our lover. As we grow older and our love relationships become more serious, we tend to shift from being romantic to valuing conjugal love, and our relationships become more realistic. Studies have shown that by college age, males and females alike have more conjugal than romantic attitudes toward love.

How love develops. Love is the result of several stages of growth in a relationship, leading to greater intimacy. As Thamm describes it, this process begins by knowing and loving oneself and subsequently behaving in a manner to satisfy one's needs. Next, close

How would you define love?

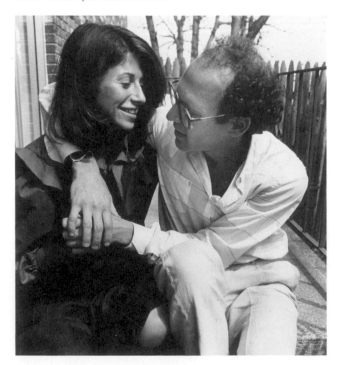

relationships with others develop, which help satisfy those needs (for example, understanding, touching, emotional closeness). The next stages of learning to love are accepting other people, developing empathy for others (understanding them), and being concerned with other people's needs and security. Lastly, we learn to gratify others' needs and feel rewarded for doing so.[2]

Love relationships, then, are the result of a growth process—a process described by one author as "an act of continuous creation."[3] Therefore, instead of "falling in love," we usually "grow in love."[4]

MARRIAGE

Concept: Marital relationships today are in the process of changing.

So much has been written about the difficulties of marriage and the high divorce rate that you may be surprised to learn that 96 percent of Americans will be married at some time in their lives. Despite the adjustments required in marriage, most people still believe that marriage provides the best opportunity to fulfill psychological, sexual, and material needs.

Married couples today face some unique concerns and challenges. Whether because of economic necessity or interest in pursuing a career, more and more married women are entering the work force. The two-earner family requires a sharing of household responsibilities (for example, cleaning, cooking, child care, and shopping). Consequently, many married couples today are working out flexible arrangements that fit their needs, rather than conforming to the stereotyped view of marriage. Decisions about having children and, if so, when to have them vary greatly between married couples. Two incomes also permit more options regarding the use of leisure time and have led to a greater emphasis upon companionship between marriage partners.

These changes have not occurred without problems. More flexibility has meant more negotiation of marital relationships, and some couples have not been up to that task. This, plus the emphasis upon meeting individual needs, has been a factor in the increasing number of divorces.

Factors Contributing to Marital Success

Concept: Successful marriages depend on several psychosocial variables.

Although there is no set formula for success in marriage, several elements that seem to be important have been identified. The most important factor is age at marriage. Statistically, couples who marry later (in their twenties or even thirties) have a much greater chance of success than those who marry young (in their teens). Probably one reason for this is that younger couples, especially those who haven't finished high school, experience more economic difficulties than couples in their twenties or thirties. Also, many teenage women marry because of pregnancy, which creates more stress for the couple.

Another important predictor of marital success is emotional maturity. Research has shown that couples who perceive themselves as emotionally mature, as measured by such words as "fair," "rational," and "competent," tend to be self-confident and have positive self-esteem. These qualities seem to make it easier to adjust to the demands of marriage.

Having similar ethnic, religious, social class, and educational backgrounds also seems to influence marital success. Couples whose socioeconomic backgrounds are similar apparently are better equipped to understand each other. In addition, they are less subject to external pressures, such as parental disapproval.

Finally, marriages are more likely to succeed when husband and wife share the same expectations about marriage. Marriages are based on a great many assumptions regarding the rights, duties, and role obligations of the partners. When couples think about and ultimately agree on these basic assumptions, they are more likely to avoid disillusionment or disappointment. Among the issues about which partners need to reach an understanding are personal and career goals, finan-

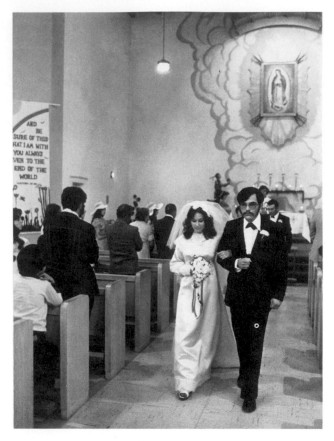

Coming from similar ethnic and religious backgrounds has been identified as contributing to the likelihood of marital success.

1. What are your expectations for job or career satisfactions? Will both of you work? If so, whose career will be more important?

2. How will you manage your income? What will be the rights of each partner in managing and spending money?

3. Where do you want to live? How will you make decisions about moving if one partner's career advancement calls for a change of residence?

4. How will you handle the management of the household? How will household tasks be divided?

5. What are your expectations for your sexual relationship? How frequently do you expect to have sexual intercourse? Will extramarital relationships be permitted?

6. Who will be responsible for birth control, if any?

7. Do you want to have children? How many? How will child care and parenting responsibilities be assigned?

8. How will you spend your leisure time and vacations?

9. What are your obligations to your respective families? Will you take an elderly or infirm parent into your home?

10. If you have been married before, how will you handle obligations to your former spouse and/or children from the previous marriage?

Communication in Marriage

Concept: Communication requires a good deal of work to be effective.

Earlier in the chapter we said that communication is an essential ingredient in achieving a satisfying intimate relationship. Research has shown that couples that are able to communicate well with each other are more satisfied with their marriages than couples that communicate poorly. In one study marriage and family counselors reported that nine out of ten couples who sought help for marital problems said they had trouble communicating with each other.

cial matters, household arrangements, sex, children, and relationships with kin and friends. The important point is not the particular goals and responsibilities a couple decides upon, but the fact that they are in agreement about these issues. Having similar expectations, they are less likely to experience conflict and more likely to feel secure about what to expect from each other.

The following questions may help you determine whether your expectations for marriage agree with those of a potential marriage partner. Both of you should answer the questions. Compare your answers. Do you have similar expectations for marriage?

According to a researcher who studied working class couples, many marital partners have trouble communicating because of the different socialization of men and women.[5] Men are traditionally socialized to be rational and unemotional, whereas women are encouraged to express their intuitive, emotional side. When they try to talk, the woman relies on her feelings, whereas the man becomes increasingly detached and reasonable. This can lead to fear, anger, or even despair. "He (or she) doesn't understand me" is a common complaint. The pattern does not apply only to working class couples; many middle-class couples experience the same difficulty.

How can couples be helped? For many, the answer may lie in becoming aware of the problem and being willing to change long-standing habits. There is some evidence that young people today want to communicate more openly and express more of their thoughts to an intimate partner. If this is true, it is probably because attitudes about gender roles are becoming less traditional.

Communicating effectively in a relationship cannot be learned overnight. It's a process that develops gradually over time. It depends on being aware of oneself, one's partner, and the relationship, and wanting to nurture the relationship and help it grow.

What exactly is effective communication? One researcher suggests that in order for a couple to communicate effectively, four components must be present: self-disclosure, confirmation, transaction management, and situational adaptability.[6]

Self-disclosure refers to revealing personal information about oneself, expressing what one is and what one feels. This does not have to mean telling the partner everything one feels; rather it means expressing one's feeling while at the same time being sensitive to how the disclosure will affect the other person. Whether partners are better off keeping some things to themselves or sharing all their feelings—positive and negative—probably depends on the degree of mutual trust and commitment.

Confirmation refers to the type of feedback partners give each other, the type of responses they make. Confirming responses are those that show acceptance of the partner, as well as of what he or she is saying.

Issues in Health
SHOULD TWO PEOPLE LIVE TOGETHER BEFORE THEY DECIDE TO MARRY?

Some say yes. They argue that you never know people until you live with them, but once you do, their likes and dislikes, moods, and expectations become apparent. The constant association brought about by living together serves as a trial period. It is easier to dissolve this relationship than a legal marriage, and there is little chance of having children, because not being married and living together might necessitate the use of contraception. If such a living arrangement works out, there is good reason to believe a marriage would be successful.

Others maintain that people are always changing, and there is no way of knowing if you can live with someone in the future—in spite of being able to live with that person right now. They argue that a successful living arrangement now doesn't imply a successful marriage later. They further oppose living together because sex before marriage is prohibited by religious teaching. Besides, they believe that this arrangement represents "playing at" marriage and is therefore immature.

What do you think? ●

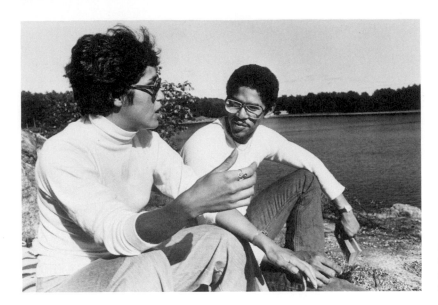

Effective communication is a gradual process of learning to be open and flexible, to set rules for interaction, and to accept the feelings of one's partner.

A spouse gives confirming feedback by being supportive and sympathetic rather than critical or judgmental.

Transaction management refers to the couple's ability to control their communication rather than be controlled by it by establishing realistic rules for interaction and keeping the communication moving toward desired goals. A couple has to decide, for example, whether it is permissible for them to shout when they are angry. If one partner is very upset by shouting, the couple would agree on another way of expressing anger and stick to the agreement. Managing communication also means not allowing it to get out of hand. In some cases this might consist simply of a husband telling his wife that he's afraid an argument is about to begin. Once the partners are aware of the situation, they can then decide to change their pattern of interaction if necessary.

Situational adaptability refers to flexibility in communicating, knowing that what is effective communication in one situation may not be appropriate in another. Adaptability requires being aware of when to bring up certain subjects and when not to. For example, if the wife is experiencing a personal crisis, the husband will delay discussing a problem he's having and instead offer sympathy and support.

Improving communication in a relationship isn't easy. It requires a great deal of awareness and commitment. But the effort can have very positive results. As partners learn to communicate better, their relationship has the chance to grow more intimate; as intimacy grows, communication improves.

Managing Marital Conflict

Concept: Marital conflict can be managed in a positive manner.

In all human relationships of any substance, conflict will arise from time to time. Marriage is no exception. Conflict is inevitable in marriage, but the partners can learn to manage conflict positively. The following suggestions apply to managing conflict of all types, including marital conflict.

1. *Express emotions but don't act out negative behavior.* It is all right to feel angry, for instance, but it is not all right to hit someone when you feel this way. Express your feelings and allow your partner to express his or hers.

2. *Use reflective listening.* When conflict arises, refrain from arguing your point of view until you understand your partner's and have let him or her know that you understand it. To do this it is helpful to paraphrase what your partner is saying so that he or she realizes that you understand his or her point of view. A clue here is to listen to the emotions behind the words, as well as the words themselves.

3. *Explain your position.* Once your partner realizes that you understand what you are being told and the feelings involved, he or she will then be ready to listen to your point of view. Describe your feelings and thoughts and the rationale behind them.

4. *Explore solutions.* Mention and analyze alternative solutions to the problem and their consequences. Choose a solution.

Consider the following description of how one couple handled a conflict.

John has worked hard all day and is very tired. His wife, Mary, had a difficult day with the children. John wants to spend a quiet, relaxing evening at home. Mary wants to get out of the house.

Mary: Let's go shopping tonight.

John: Are you kidding? I had a hard day at work. I wasn't home relaxing all day, like you were. I want to stay home, plop in front of the TV, and take it easy.

Mary: I was home all day relaxing? Are you serious? It's not easy to spend the day with toddlers making constant demands. I need to get out.

John: Forget it! No way! I'm staying home.

Mary: You're being inconsiderate. I don't think you even care about me.

John: Just leave me alone.

The result of this situation might be that John goes begrudgingly with Mary and complains the whole time. The shopping would not be enjoyable for either of them under these circumstances. Or Mary might go by herself but not have John's companionship. Another alternative would be for John and Mary to stay home, but Mary would complain and John would not be able to relax. Mary would also be unhappy.

Now consider how John and Mary could have responded to this conflict by employing the steps outlined above:

Mary: Let's go shopping tonight.

John: Sounds like you had a rough day and need to get out.

Mary: Rough? It was miserable. I get so keyed up having to watch the children constantly to make sure they don't get into everything or hurt themselves. I wish there was another adult I could talk to.

John: You feel pretty frustrated and keyed up. It must be hard not having some adult stimulation.

John has been paraphrasing to this point and trying to let Mary know that he understands her feelings as well as her words. They continue, and John now explains his position:

John: I had a rough day too. It seemed to be nonstop. I'm very tired and feel like a wound-up spring. I was looking forward to coming home and relaxing. Going shopping wouldn't be relaxing for me.

Mary: Gee, it sounds as though one of us will have to lose out on what we need.

John: Well, hold off a second. Let's see if there is some way we could both go out and yet make it relaxing.

Mary: Maybe we could go out for dinner or perhaps to a movie.

John: Yes, why don't we have dinner out. That way neither of us will have to cook and we can relax together. I'll call a babysitter.

The point here is that now they both get their way and both feel better about the situation. In the first situation described, although at first glance it appears that one person wins, both really lose. The shopping will be miserable for Mary because of John's complaining, or staying home will be unrelaxing for John because of Mary's complaining. In the second situation, although it first appears that no one wins, both really do. They neither go shopping nor stay home, but Mary gets her stimulation and John his relaxation.

This procedure for responding to conflict is appropriate for all kinds of relationships. The important thing to remember is to continue the reflective listening until the other person is ready to listen to you. The other person must believe that you have been listening and that you understand the feeling being expressed before being ready to listen to you.

In terms of marriage, mates should be concerned with each other's feelings. They should take the time to understand them and resolve conflict positively rather than with a "no win" posture. The procedure outlined here is designed to make conflict resolution a positive experience rather than a negative one, with the result being a better relationship.

Divorce

> **Concept:** Although divorce is painful for everyone involved, there are ways to heal the emotional wounds.

Divorce is a fact of our society. It is predicted that 38 percent of women now in their late twenties will have their first marriages end in divorce, and for those who remarry, 44 percent of their second marriages will also end in divorce.[7] Several factors are related to the high divorce rate:

1. More wives are working outside the home, making them less economically dependent on their husbands.

2. Divorce has lost the social stigma associated with it in the earlier part of this century.

3. The emergence of "no-fault" divorce, whereby one partner need not prove the other to be at fault for the dissolution of the marriage, has made divorce easier to obtain.

4. Some researchers believe Americans have idealistic and unrealistic expectations of what marriage should be like and are disappointed when these expectations are not met.[8]

5. A change in American values toward personal freedom and happiness and away from hard work and "stick-to-it-iveness" leads some to pursue these desires at the cost of their marriages.

When divorced people who had remarried were asked the reasons for the breakup of their first marriages, they responded in two ways: with the major reason and also with a list of other reasons (see Table 15.2).

The responses suggest that infidelity, no longer loving each other, emotional problems, financial problems, and sexual problems are the predominant factors contributing to divorce. Obviously, these reasons cannot be separated from each other; for example, infidelity and unhappiness in other areas of marriage are likely to be related. Similarly, financial problems can undermine affection.

Effects of divorce on children. In 1964 only 8.7 children per 1000 were from families that divorced that year. In 1979 that figure was 18.9. Obviously, divorce is affecting more and more children. In 1979 almost 1.2 million children were part of families in which the parents were divorced that year.[9]

The initial response that children have to divorce is one of great distress. Younger children are usually afraid the custodial parent will leave, as well as the absent parent. They may attempt to get their parents back together again and fantasize about the return of the absent parent. In addition, many children blame themselves for the divorce, not realizing that they may have been the reason the marriage remained intact as long as it did. Physical symptoms, such as stomach aches and sleeplessness, may also result, and many children experience difficulty in school.

In spite of the initial negative effects of divorce, in about one year most children adjust. There is still some sense of loss but little guilt or anger. To help them reach this point, children need the love and support of both parents, but in particular the parent with whom

Table 15.2
REASONS GIVEN AS MAJOR FOR FAILURE OF FIRST MARRIAGES
(490 RESPONDENTS)

Reason	Number of Times Listed First	Reason	Total Number of Times Listed
Infidelity	168	Infidelity	255
No longer loved each other	103	No longer loved each other	188
Emotional problems	53	Emotional problems	185
Financial problems	30	Financial problems	135
Physical abuse	29	Sexual problems	115
Alcohol	25	Problems with in-laws	81
Sexual problems	22	Neglect of children	74
Problems with in-laws	16	Physical abuse	72
Neglect of children	11	Alcohol	47
Communication problems	10	Job conflicts	20
Married too young	9	Other	19
Job conflicts	7	Communication problems	18
Other	7	Married too young	14

SOURCE: Stan L. Albrecht, "Correlates of Marital Happiness among the Remarried," *Journal of Marriage and the Family* 41 (Nov. 1979):857–867. Copyrighted 1979 by the National Council on Family Relations. Reprinted by permission.

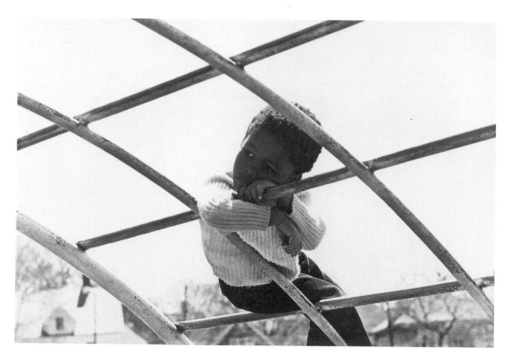

When divorce occurs, children need to be reassured that they are not to blame.

they live. Unfortunately, the parents are working through their own problems and feelings and sometimes have little emotional energy left for helping their children. In these cases, professional support—for example, from a psychologist—may be helpful. Older siblings, who tend to adjust to divorce sooner than younger children, can also help their younger brothers or sisters. And, most important, adjustment to divorce requires a relationship with *both* parents that encourages communication of feelings such as guilt, anger, frustration, or the sense of loss.

Getting over the pain of divorce. Divorce results in disequilibrium in the lives of all those involved: husband, wife, children, and close relatives and friends. If the husband and wife handle the divorce well, a new equilibrium will emerge for themselves, as well as for others affected. The following suggestions may help heal the emotional wounds of divorce:[10]

1. Do your mourning now. Don't pretend, deny, cover up, or run away from the pain. Everything else can wait. The sooner you allow yourself to be with your pain, the sooner it will pass.

2. Be gentle with yourself. Accept the fact that you have an emotional wound, that it is disabling, and that it will take a while before you are completely well.

3. If possible, don't take on new responsibilities. When appropriate, let employers and co-workers know you're healing.

4. Don't blame yourself for any mistakes (real or imagined) you may have made that brought you to this loss. You can acknowledge mistakes later, when the healing process is further along.

5. For a while, don't get involved in an all-consuming passionate romance or a new project that requires great time and energy.

6. Don't try against obvious odds to rekindle the old relationship. Futile attempts at reconciliation will only cause more pain, slow the process of healing and growth, and waste recuperative energy.

7. If you find photographs and mementos helpful to the mourning process, use them. If you find they bind you to a dead past, get rid of them. Put them in the attic, sell them, give them away, or throw them out.

8. Remember that it's okay to feel anger toward God, society, or the person who left you, but it is not okay or good for you to hate yourself or to act on your anger in a destructive way. Let the anger out safely: hit a pillow, kick the bed, sob, scream.

9. Watch your nutrition. Eat good foods and get plenty of rest.

10. Don't overindulge in alcohol, marijuana or other recreational chemicals, or cigarettes.

11. Pamper yourself a little. Get a manicure, take a trip, bask in the sun, sleep late, see a good movie, visit a museum, listen to music, take a long bath instead of a quick shower. As healing progresses, remember that it's okay not to feel depressed.

12. You might find it helpful to keep a journal or diary so that you can see your progress as you read past entries.

13. Heal at your own pace. The sadness comes and goes, but it comes less frequently and for shorter lengths of time as healing proceeds.

PARENTHOOD

Today, more than at any time in the past, it is no longer automatic that being married means having children. Most American couples now consciously decide how many children they want to have, and a small but growing number are choosing not to have any children.

Several factors have influenced couples to limit their family size. The most important is the development of effective methods of birth control, particularly the Pill. Social change has had an impact too. As a consequence of the women's movement, more women are seeking careers than ever before, and although a career and parenthood need not be mutually exclusive, women who work outside the home generally find that working and having children is not an easy combination to manage. A few career women, especially those who are highly educated, are deciding not to have children. Concern about overpopulation is another factor, as are economic conditions. Today the cost of rearing a child through the college years on a middle class income is over $85,000 dollars, a figure that does not include the earnings lost while a mother stays out of the work force. Economics, however, do not seem to deter couples from deciding to have at least one child. When researchers asked parents about the disadvantages of having children, parents mentioned emotional costs, such as worry and restrictions on their freedom, more often than the financial burden.

Making the Choice

The decision to have children is often made more on an emotional basis than a practical one. Many couples have rather romantic notions about parenthood and think that being a parent will be a lot of fun. Researchers suggest that these notions can lead to disappointment:

> Most American women view love, marriage, and children as the three great chapters in their lives. Of these three, children will probably be the most disappointing because most adults come to parenthood with over-romanticized fantasies and exaggerated expectations without realistic anticipation of the strain a child will bring to the marriage economically, psychologically, and sexually. There will be a decrease in the time one previously had for one's spouse. Letdown is inevitable.[11]

There is also evidence that having children can detract from, rather than contribute to, marital satisfaction:

> For both men and women, reports of happiness and satisfaction drop to average, not to raise again significantly until their children are grown and about to leave the nest.[12]

> The preservation of husband-wife intimacy tends to get more disciplined; some research has indicated that young parents talk to each other only one-half as much as newly married couples and when they do talk, they tend to talk about the children rather than themselves or their relationship.[13]

Despite the difficulties, however, most Americans still believe there are many satisfactions in raising children. Children fulfill important social, interpersonal, and psychological needs for their parents. Among the positive values of having children that were identified in a national survey of both parents and nonparents are the following, in rank order:

1. Children provide love and companionship and act as a buffer against loneliness.

2. Children bring stimulation, happiness, and joy to life.

3. Children help fulfill the need to find meaning and purpose in life and enable parents to attain a sense of immortality by having a part of the self live on after death.

4. Being a parent brings acceptance as a mature adult.

5. Having a child gives parents a feeling of creativity, and watching the child grow contributes to the parents' feelings of competence.

6. Children can offer an economic contribution to the family and security in old age.

7. Raising a child makes some parents feel they have become a better person.[14]

Of course, it is important to point out that the values people associate with having children aren't always the same as the motives individual couples have for becoming parents. Some couples have children because they assume it is expected of them. Some hope to save a troubled marriage, and others hope that children will fulfill the dreams they haven't been able to fulfill themselves. Clearly these are not the best reasons for having children. Like other health-related decisions, deciding whether or not to have children should be carefully thought out. Rather than trying to live up to others' expectations, decide for yourself what is best for you. Of course, it can be helpful to seek advice from others and discuss the issues involved. In the long run, however, it is you and your partner who will experience the benefits and disadvantages of parenthood. Are the economic burden, the restrictions on your time, and the responsibility involved worth the joys you will derive from parenthood? To help you think about whether you are good parent material, answer the questions in Discovery Activity 15.3, *Am I Good Parent Material?*

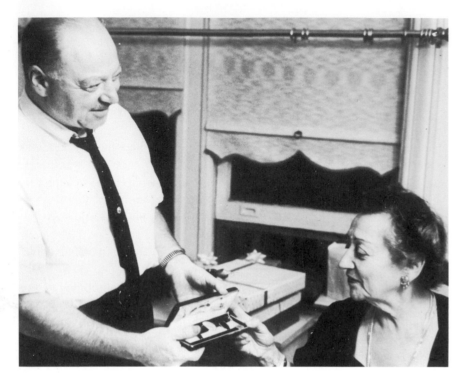

Parent-child relationships can continue to be a source of strength and support throughout life. This mother is giving her son a fiftieth birthday present.

Discovery Activity 15.3
AM I GOOD PARENT MATERIAL?

Does Having and Raising a Child Fit the Lifestyle I Want?

1. What do I want out of life for myself? What do I think is important?

2. Could I handle a child and a job at the same time? Would I have time and energy for both?

3. Would I be ready to give up the freedom to do what I want to do, when I want to do it?

4. Would I be willing to cut back my social life and spend more time at home? Would I miss my free time and privacy?

5. Can I afford to support a child? Do I know how much it takes to raise a child?

6. Do I want to raise a child in the neighborhood where I live now? Would I be willing and able to move?

7. How would a child interfere with my growth and development?

8. Would a child change my educational plans? Do I have the energy to go to school and raise a child at the same time?

9. Am I willing to give a great part of my life—AT LEAST 18 YEARS—to being responsible for a child? And spend a large portion of my life being concerned about my child's well-being?

Raising a Child? What's There to Know?

1. Do I like children? When I'm around children for a while, what do I think or feel about having one around all of the time?

2. Do I enjoy teaching others?

3. Is it easy for me to tell other people what I want, or need, or what I expect of them?

4. Do I want to give a child the love (s)he needs? Is loving easy for me?

5. Am I patient enough to deal with the noise and the confusion and the 24-hour-a-day responsibility? What kind of time and space do I need for myself?

6. What do I do when I get angry or upset? Would I take things out on a child if I lost my temper?

7. What does discipline mean to me? What does freedom, or setting limits, or giving space mean? What is being too strict, or not strict enough? Would I want a perfect child?

8. How do I get along with my parents? What will I do to avoid the mistakes my parents made?

9. How would I take care of my child's health and safety? How do I take care of my own?

10. What if I have a child and find out I made a wrong decision?

What's in It for Me?

1. Do I like doing things with children? Do I enjoy activities that children can do?

2. Would I want a child to be "like me"?

3. Would I try to pass on to my child my ideas and values? What if my child's ideas and values turn out to be different from mine?

4. Would I want my child to achieve things that I wish I had, but didn't?

5. Would I expect my child to keep me from being lonely in my old age? Do I do that for my parents? Do my parents do that for my grandparents?

6. Do I want a boy or a girl child? What if I don't get what I want?

7. Would having a child show others how mature I am?

8. Will I prove I am a man or a woman by having a child?

9. Do I expect my child to make my life happy?

Have My Partner and I Really Talked about Becoming Parents?

1. Does my partner want to have a child? Have we talked about our reasons?

2. Could we give a child a good home? Is our relationship a happy and strong one?

3. Are we both ready to give our time and energy to raising a child?

4. Could we share our love with a child without jealousy?

5. What would happen if we separated after having a child, or if one of us should die?

6. Do my partner and I understand each other's feelings about religion, work, family, child raising, future goals? Do we feel pretty much the same way? Will children fit into these feelings, hopes, and plans?

7. Suppose one of us wants a child and the other doesn't? Who decides?

8. Which of the questions listed here do we need to really discuss before making a decision? ●

SOURCE: National Alliance for Optional Parenthood, 2010 Massachusetts Ave., N.W., Washington, D.C. 20036. Used with permission.

SHOULD A SINGLE PERSON BE ALLOWED TO ADOPT CHILDREN?

Some people believe that a single person should not be permitted to adopt a child. They insist that a child needs both the warmth, love, and nurturance of a mother, and the strength, security, and independence in a father to model. With only one parent, only half these needs are met. Further, a single person will have to work and will not be able to give children the same amount of time that two parents can.

Others contend that love is the primary ingredient in parenting and that a single person can provide that love as well as any other family structure. They argue that just because people are married doesn't ensure that they will be good parents. Although the single person has to work and leave the child in the care of others for part of the day, it is the quality of the time spent with the child, rather than the quantity, that should be considered. Single persons can provide this quality as well as two parents.

What do you think? ●

Developing Parenting Skills

Concept: Parenting skills can be learned.

It has been suggested that parenting is too easy a job to get. Although all you need to become a parent is a reproductive system, it is becoming increasingly obvious that parenting requires skills and that, further, these skills can be learned. Consequently, parent-training courses are becoming popular. The largest of these programs is Parent Effectiveness Training (P.E.T.) which in 1978 was reported to have 8,000 instructors and 250,000 students of parenting. Other such programs are the Parent Involvement Program, Responsive Parent, and the Parenthood Education program, funded by the federal government and conducted in many public schools.

These programs have much in common. Though employing different philosophies, they consist of approximately 10 sessions in which techniques of communication and behavior modification are taught. Their goal is to improve the relationship between parent and child, while at the same time helping the child to develop and mature in a positive direction.

If you are contemplating parenthood, or have already decided that you want to be a parent, perhaps you should attend a parent education program. Many of us learn how to parent by observing the only role models we have—our own parents. Although we can learn many positive ways to parent from observing our parents, we can also learn inappropriate behavior.

Family Style

Concept: Family style tends to be repeated from one generation to the next.

The family in which you grew up has provided you with a model of family life. This model, often the only one with which you have a great deal of familiarity, will tend to be the one you adopt in your future family. So, for instance, parents who have been abused as children abuse their own children to a greater degree than those who were not themselves abused. Children who come from a family in which one parent was an alcoholic have a greater tendency to be alcoholics as adults. These are generalizations, of course, and need not be true for individuals. You can select the good aspects of your family life to model and reject the negative aspects. Simply stating that you will do so, however, may not result in this behavior. Serious thought must be given to your past and present family life in order to make sense of a future one. Try identifying the positive aspects of your family life that you want to repeat and the negative aspects you seek to avoid.

Child Abuse

One of the unfortunate realities of our society is that some parents act out their frustrations by abusing their children. The National Center for Child Abuse and Neglect estimates that 1 million children are physically abused by their parents or guardians in this country every year. This figure does not include those children who are psychologically abused by constant harangue, verbal assaults on their self-worth, and ridicule—not to mention outright neglect. Child abusers do not differ by race, socioeconomic status, or by profession. However, they do have some common characteristics. Parents who abuse their children are more likely to have been abused when they were children than parents who do not abuse their children. It seems that we learn our parenting style from our own parents, and if they were abusers, we are more likely to be abusers ourselves. Furthermore, abusing parents tend to be lonely and isolated; to lack trust in other people; to possess a poor self-image; and to use a strict, disciplinarian style of parenting.

In addition to the characteristics of the parents, the child and the family situation also contribute to child abuse. Some children are more disobedient, more stubborn, or slower than other children. Although there is no excuse for child abuse, these traits often contribute to the parent's frustration and anger. Research has also shown that a family crisis—for example, the father losing his job or the mother finding out her husband is leaving—often instigates the abuse.

Those in professions where they come in contact with children (for example, teachers) are both morally and legally required to report suspected instances of child abuse to the proper authorities. A national organization, Parents Anonymous, has been formed to help parents stop abusing their children.

Single-Parent Families

The single-parent family is becoming increasingly common. The U.S. Census Bureau reports that the number of families maintained by one parent increased by 80 percent between 1970 and 1980. By 1980, 19 percent of all families with children still at home were maintained by one parent. Data from the Census Bureau also confirm that the increase in one-parent families is the result of marital separation, divorce, and out-of-wedlock pregnancy, rather than the death of one parent. In the last decade the percentage of one-parent families maintained by divorced women rose from 29 to 38 percent, and the proportion headed by single women rose from 7 to 15 percent. However, the proportion of one-parent families maintained by widowed mothers decreased from 20 to 12 percent. Single parenthood is especially common in black families. In 1979 half the black families with children at home were maintained by one parent.

Single-parent families have particular financial, psychological, custodial, and other needs that are often more acute than the needs of two-parent families. The single parent must provide both financial and emotional support for their children single-handedly. Many single parents have the added responsibility of trying to provide role models for their opposite sex children.

Research suggests that coming from a single-parent family may create some problems for children during their formative years. A study by the Charles F. Kettering Foundation and the National Association of Elementary School Principals concluded that children from single-parent homes cause more discipline problems in schools and do worse academically than children from two-parent homes. The study showed that three one-parent children were disciplined by teachers for every two two-parent children disciplined. For every

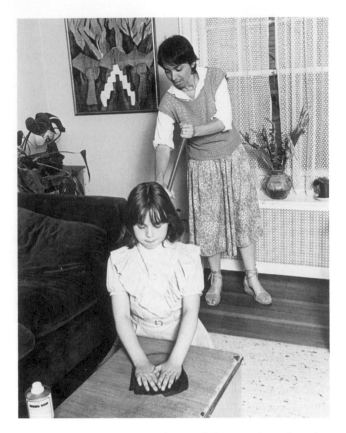

Single parenting requires resourcefulness and good coping skills on the part of both the parent and children.

five two-parent children dropping out of school, nine one-parent children dropped out. And for every two-parent child expelled from school, eight one-parent children were expelled.

Such research findings might seem discouraging, especially to those who are single parents themselves. We hasten to add that these findings refer to trends in groups. Children from one-parent families often adjust very well. Nevertheless, single parenthood does present special problems requiring care and consideration. Perhaps most important, the special needs of one-parent families should be understood both by family members themselves and by those with whom they interact (for example, teachers and employers). To meet this need for understanding, a group called Parents Without Partners serves as a sounding board and a source of counsel for single parents. In addition, many books and pamphlets are available to help people cope with marital separation and divorce. Some good sources are listed below:

Louise Montague Athearn. *What Every Former Married Woman Should Know*. New York: David McKay Co., 1973.

Barbara R. Hirsch. *Divorce: What a Woman Should Know*. Chicago: Henry Regnery Co., 1973.

Robert S. Weiss. *Marital Separation*. New York: Basic Books, 1975.

Richard A. Gardner. *The Boys' and Girls' Book about Divorce*. New York: Science Press, 1970.

Richard A. Gardner. *The Parent's Book About Divorce*. New York: Doubleday, 1977.

The Single Parent. Journal of Parents Without Partners, Inc.

ALTERNATIVES TO MARRIAGE

Concept: Cohabitation and singlehood are alternatives to marriage that have become increasingly popular.

Cohabitation

In the literal sense of the word, cohabitation means inhabiting, or living in, the same place as others. However, in the context of this book we define cohabitation as living together in a sexual relationship without being married. In the last two decades this living arrangement has become more common. According to the 1980 Census, in 1970, 1.1 million adults were cohabiting, but by 1979, the number had risen to 2.7 million. Cohabitation among college students is common. Macklin estimates that between 9 and 56 percent of college students live in cohabiting situations for some period of time.[15] Divorced or separated adults also make up a large percentage of cohabitants, and one out of ten cohabiting couples includes a partner 65 or over.

Until the early 1960s, cohabitation was practiced primarily by celebrities such as movie stars, and lower-class couples. During the 1960s, however, young, unmarried middle-class couples began to set up households. The availability of effective, easy-to-use contraceptives contributed to the trend by reducing the fear of pregnancy among couples who wished to live together but not start families. In addition, the social climate of the time, which rejected many traditional standards, was an important factor.

People choose to live together for a variety of personal reasons. According to Macklin, some college students cite sexual fulfillment as their reason for living with their partners.[16] The relationship often began with the couple's having sex together once or twice a week, then increasing the time they spent in a more regular pattern, and finally deciding that they might as well live together all the time. Other reasons for cohabiting cited by Macklin's subjects were that they found the dating process laborious, they found that a large university could be very lonely, they sought a more meaningful and fulfilling relationship, they felt a need for security, and they had begun to question the institution of marriage. Although many respondents wanted to test their suitability for each other, marriage was not their initial objective in taking on this lifestyle. Almost all Macklin's subjects reported that they were deeply involved with their mates emotionally, but none were ready or willing to make a total commitment to a permanent relationship, such as that required in marriage.

Couples who live together cite several advantages. First, they suggest that partners don't have to follow the traditional roles of husband and wife, although research suggests that roles in cohabitant relationships tend to be divided conventionally. Second, if the relationship breaks up, they do not have to go through the trauma of divorce. This does not mean that ending such a relationship is easy. Indeed, breaking up can be a very difficult experience, married or not. A third advantage of cohabitation is that it is more convenient

and less expensive to maintain than a conventional two-residence love affair.

Most of the negative aspects of cohabitation are related to society's disapproval of this lifestyle. Even though living together is more acceptable today than it was even 20 years ago, it still meets with some objections. Parents may object to the living arrangement. Clearly, a person faced with parental rejection experiences considerable stress. Employers may disapprove, especially in conservative corporations where the norm is marriage. Cohabitors also sometimes have problems in renting or buying a residence.

Singlehood

For some people who have never been married, singlehood is just a phase of their lives that they hope will culminate in marriage. For others who have been married but are no longer, singlehood may be an interlude that will end with their next marriage. However, there are also those for whom singlehood is the preferred lifestyle or who never marry because they never meet someone whom they want to marry. About 20 percent of those who are divorced never remarry.

Our society has traditionally disapproved of the single lifestyle. The agrarian society that characterized eighteenth and nineteenth century America valued families and, in particular, children, because of the pressing need for more workers. Singlehood, of course, worked counter to the need for large families. Today, however, singlehood is becoming a more acceptable choice.

Research suggests that several factors lead people toward singlehood and other factors lead them away. Peter Stein has described these as "pushes" to leave permanent relationships and "pulls" to remain single or return to being single (see Table 15.3).

In studies comparing single and married individuals, single men tend to score lower on intelligence tests than married men and achieve less occupationally. Single men tend to come from authoritarian, stressful homes where they have had poor relationships with their mothers. Single women, on the other hand, tend to be better educated and more career-oriented than

Table 15.3
PUSHES AND PULLS TOWARD SINGLEHOOD

Pushes (to leave permanent relationships)	Pulls (to remain single or return to singlehood)
Lack of friends, isolation, loneliness	Career opportunities and development
Restricted availability of new experiences	Availability of sexual experiences
Suffocating one-to-one relationship, feeling trapped	Exciting lifestyle, variety of experiences, freedom to change
Obstacles to self-development	Psychological and social autonomy, self-sufficiency
Boredom, unhappiness, and anger	Support structures: sustaining friendships, women's and men's groups, political groups, therapeutic groups, collegial groups
Role playing and conformity to expectations	
Poor communication with mate	
Sexual frustration	

SOURCE: Information from Peter Stein, "The Lifestyles and Life-Chances of the Never-Married," *Marriage and Family Review* 1 (July 1978): 4. © 1978 by The Haworth Press, Inc. All rights reserved.

married women. Those who have never married come from single-parent homes more frequently than those who do marry.

It is important to note in this discussion of singlehood that people who choose this lifestyle are not always unhappy or envious of their married friends. There are many happy, well-adjusted, productive people who simply prefer more independence than marriage allows.

CONCLUSION

We must all make decisions concerning dating, marriage, parenthood, and family life. We have presented information in this chapter to help you make these decisions. We have observed that the divorce rate is high, that many parents don't enter their roles with enough consideration of the tremendous responsibilities involved, and that some families' reactions to societal influences cause observers to speak in terms of "the family in crisis." Rather than an academic study of these topics, what is needed is for people to give some thought to their personal involvement in them. Analyze what you want *from* a family and what you are capable of giving *to* a family. What is right for *you?* Marriage or remaining unmarried? Parenthood or non-parenthood? There are choices to be made, and each of us must choose according to our own needs and values. The commonality of our decisions should not be in the end results, but rather in the rational process by which we come to them.

SUMMARY

1. Whether the initial purpose of dating is companionship, recreation, or courtship, it serves as a training ground for future intimate relationships, including marriage.

2. Dating decisions are related to three factors: prestige considerations, physical attractiveness, and personality considerations.

3. Men and women value similar personality characteristics in their dates, although men tend to value intelligence and companionship more than women do, and women tend to value thoughtfulness, consideration, and honesty more than men do.

4. Romantic love—total absorption of two partners with each other—usually characterizes beginning love relationships. Conjugal love—a domestic, calm, comforting relationship—develops over time in healthy love relationships.

5. Love is the result of several stages of growth: knowing and loving oneself, satisfying one's own needs, developing close relationships with others, accepting and developing empathy for others, being concerned with others' needs, and learning to gratify others' needs and feeling rewarded for doing so.

6. Successful marriages depend upon several factors, including age (couples who marry in their twenties and thirties have more successful marriages than those who marry in their teens), emotional maturity, self-confidence, and positive self-esteem.

7. Among the factors contributing to the high divorce rate are women's increased economic independence, the loss of social stigma previously associated with divorce, the emergence of "no-fault" divorce, and a change in American values toward personal freedom and happiness and away from hard work and "stick-to-it-iveness."

8. Divorce has some negative effects upon children, especially during the first year following the divorce, but with good communication between both parents and the children adjustment usually takes place.

9. There are many reasons why people decide to have children (for example, for love and companionship, to find meaning in life, or to feel creative), as well as many reasons why people decide not to have children (for example, children limit one's freedom, they don't want the responsibility for another person, or they don't want to take the time away from their careers).

10. Cohabitation and singlehood are two alternatives to marriage that have become increasingly popular. Many people choose to cohabit or remain single for some portion of their lives rather than permanently. Both options offer a chance to redefine oneself and one's relationships.

REFERENCES

1. Zick Rubin, "Measurement of Romantic Love," *Journal of Personality and Social Psychology* 16 (1970):265–273. Copyright 1970 by the American Psychological Association. Reprinted by permission of the publisher and author.

2. Robert Thamm, *Beyond Marriage and the Nuclear Family* (San Francisco: Canfield, 1975).

3. Emily Coleman and Betty Edwards, *Brief Encounters* (Garden City, N.Y.: Doubleday 1979), p. 50.

4. Gilbert D. Nass, Roger W. Libby, and Mary Pat Fisher, *Sexual Choices* (Belmont, Calif.: Wadsworth, 1981), p. 131.

5. Lillian B. Rubin, *Worlds of Pain: Life in the Working-Class Family* (New York: Basic, 1976).

6. Barbara M. Montgomery, "The Form and Function of Quality Communication in Marriage," *Family Relations* 30 (1981): 21–30.

7. Paul C. Glick and Arthur J. Norton, "Marrying, Divorcing, and Living Together in the U.S. Today," *Population Bulletin* 32 (5). Washington, D.C.: Population Reference Bureau, 1977.

8. Lillian E. Troll, Sheila J. Miller, and Robert C. Atchley, *Families In Later Life* (Belmont, Calif.: Wadsworth, 1979).

9. National Center for Health Statistics, "Advanced Report of Final Divorce Statistics, 1979," *Monthly Vital Statistics Report* 30 (May 29, 1981):4.

10. Melba Colgrove, Harold Bloomfield, and Peter McWilliams, *How to Survive the Loss of a Love: 58 Things to Do When There Is Nothing to Be Done* (New York: Bantam, 1979). Reprinted by permission of Leo Books, Allen Park, Michigan.

11. David J. Anspaugh and Vava Cook, "Nonparenthood," *Health Education* 8 (1977):21. Reprinted with permission of the American Alliance for Health, Physical Education, Recreation and Dancing.

12. Angus Campbell, "The American Way of Mating—Marriage Sí, Children Only Maybe," *Psychology Today* 9 (1975):37–43.

13. David Schulz and Stanley Rodgers, *Marriage, the Family and Personal Fulfillment* (Englewood Cliffs, N.J.: Prentice-Hall, 1975).

14. L. W. Hoffman and J. D. Manis, "The Value of Children in the United States: A New Approach to the Study of Fertility," *Journal of Marriage and the Family* 41 (August 1979):583–596.

15. Eleanor Macklin, "Review of Research on Nonmarital Cohabitation in the United States," in B. Murstein, ed., *Exploring Intimate Lifestyles* (New York: Springer, 1978).

16. Eleanor Macklin, "Unmarried Heterosexual Cohabitation on the University Campus," in J. Wiseman, ed., *The Social Psychology of Sex* (New York: Harper & Row, 1976).

Laboratory 1
RESPONSIBILITIES OF PARENTHOOD

Purpose To experience the restrictions that accompany parenthood.

Size of Group Total class.

Equipment A doll for each student in the class. If students can't provide enough dolls for those in the class, and college funds are not available for purchasing dolls, perhaps a nursery school or elementary school could help out.

Procedure

You are to be responsible for your baby (doll) from the last class meeting of the week until Monday of the next week. In this way a weekend will be included. The rules governing the care of your baby are:

1. You must feed your baby every six hours.
2. You must change your baby's diapers every three hours during the time that you are awake.
3. Your baby must never be left alone.
4. You must get a baby sitter one evening to watch your baby while you go out.

Results

The whole class should discuss the experiences and conclusions that pertain to caring for the baby (doll). Possible questions for discussion are:

1. What are some of the restrictions that go along with being a parent?
2. How would your experience have been different if you were married rather than a single parent?
3. You experienced the restrictions involved in parenting. What are some of the positive aspects of being a parent?
4. How would your experience have differed if you had other children to care for in addition to your baby? What if your baby was twins?
5. What are the economic considerations in parenting? Cost of food, diapers, etc.? How might these concerns be restrictive?
6. When is the right time to have children?

Laboratory 2
LOVE ANALYSIS

Purpose To learn of several different types of love and to identify whether you are well matched with the individual with whom you are in love.

Size of Group Done individually.

Equipment The Love Chart.

Procedure

1. The following handout is given to each student:

Some researchers have identified four basic types of love: erotic, ludic, storgic, and manic. *Erotic love* (eros) is a passionate, all-enveloping love. The erotic lover experiences a racing heart, a fluttering in the stomach, and shortness of breath. *Ludic love* (ludus) is a playful, flirtatious love. It involves no long-term commitment and is basically for amusement. Ludic love is usually played with several partners at once. *Storgic love* (storge) is a calm, companionate love. Storgic lovers are quietly affectionate and have goals of marriage and children for the relationship. *Manic love* (mania) is a combination of eros and ludus. A manic lover's needs for affection are insatiable, and he or she is often racked with highs of irrational joy, lows of anxiety and depression, and bouts of extreme jealousy. Manic attachments seldom develop into lasting love.

To find out what type of lover you are, answer each question as it applies to a current boyfriend or girlfriend, lover or spouse.*

A = almost always   U = usually   R = rarely   N = never (or almost never)

1. You have a clearly defined image of your desired partner.
2. You felt a strong emotional reaction to him or her on the first encounter.
3. You are preoccupied with thoughts about him or her.
4. You are eager to see him or her every day.
5. You discuss future plans and a wide range of interests and experiences.
6. Tactile, sensual contact is important to the relation.
7. Sexual intimacy was achieved early in the relation.
8. You feel that success in love is more important than success in other areas of your life.
9. You want to be in love or have love as security.
10. You try to force him or her to show more feeling and commitment.
11. You declared your love first.
12. You are willing to suffer neglect and abuse from him or her.
13. You deliberately restrain frequency of contact with him or her.
14. You restrict discussion and display of your feelings with him or her.
15. If a breakup is coming, you feel it is better to drop the other person before being dropped.
16. You play the field and have several persons who could love you.
17. You are more interested in pleasure than in emotional attachment.
18. You feel the need to love someone you have grown accustomed to.
19. You believe that the test of time is the only sure way to find real love.
20. You don't believe that true love happens suddenly or dramatically.

If you answered A or U to 1–8, you are probably an erotic lover. If you answered A or U to 3–4 and 8–12, your love style tends to be manic. If you answered A or U to 13–17 and R or N to the other questions, you are probably a ludic lover. If you answered A or U to 17–20, together with R or N for the other statements, your love style tends to be storgic.

2. If you are currently in love with someone, have that person also complete the love chart.

Results

Compare your type of love with that of the person you love. Do you both have the same expectations? Needs? What do you see as the future for this relationship?

*SOURCE: John Alan Lee, *The Colours of Love* (Toronto: New Press, 1973). Reprinted by permission of the author and New Press, Toronto, Canada.

diseases

Part Six

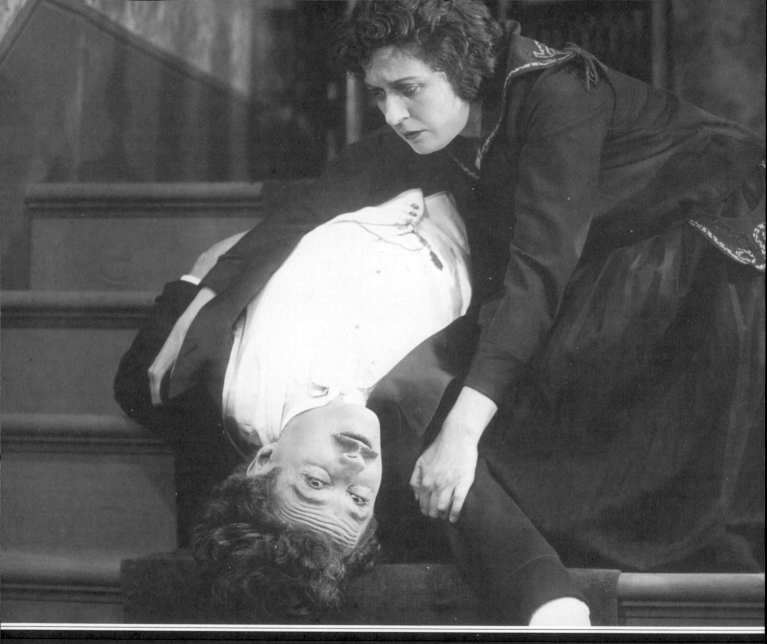

cardiovascular disease

- *heart disease*
- *theories explaining heart disease*
- *risk factors in heart disease*
- *prevention of heart disease*
- *stroke*

The dangers of cardiovascular disease and the fact that lifestyle is a significant factor in many forms of cardiovascular disease began to be the focus of considerable attention during the 1960s. Since that time, many Americans have altered their lifestyles: they no longer smoke, engage in regular exercise, control their blood pressure and blood fat levels, manage their diets more carefully, and maintain proper weight. It appears that these behaviors are having some effect. The number of deaths caused by cardiovascular disease has been declining, and recent advances in medical research suggest that the future may be even brighter. Nevertheless, cardiovascular disease is still the number one killer of American adults, both men and women.

The major diseases of the cardiovascular system include diseases of the heart valves, diseases of the electrical system (heart rhythm and heart block), high blood pressure, atherosclerosis, stroke, diseases of the heart muscle, rheumatic heart disease, congestive heart failure, congenital defects, and coronary artery disease. Coronary artery disease has reached almost epidemic proportions in some Western countries and is responsible for over one-half of all cardiovascular deaths, with strokes accounting for approximately one-fifth. Evidence is increasing to support the hypothesis that coronary artery disease can be delayed or prevented with early changes in lifestyle.

This chapter focuses on specific behavioral changes that can influence the pattern of heart disease. Major emphasis is placed upon providing information to increase your understanding of heart disease, to clarify the various theories concerning the causes of heart disease, and to aid you in making wise decisions to prevent heart disease.

HEART DISEASE

An explanation of the function of the heart is provided in Fig. 16.1. The heart muscle is rarely at fault in causing a heart attack; instead, inadequate supply of blood to the heart, usually as a result of clogged coronary arteries and their branches, causes tissue death in certain areas of the heart muscle. The heart receives nourishment from two main coronary arteries that branch off the aorta. The right coronary artery covers the back side of the heart by branching into smaller and smaller arteries that penetrate the wall of the heart, eventually branching into tiny **capillaries** to supply oxygen and nutriments to the heart muscle and its electrical conduction system. The left coronary artery is divided into two parts, which nourish the front and left side of the heart. Through these coronary arteries, the heart maintains its own nourishment. Unfortunately, these arteries are most susceptible to fatty deposit buildup and clogging.

Types of Heart Disease

Heart attack. A heart attack, or coronary, results from **coronary thrombosis,** a clot in a coronary artery. Artery closure may be caused by an accumulation of atheromas, fatty degeneration of the inner coat of the arteries (see Fig. 16.2). In most cases, only a branch of an artery supplying a portion of the heart muscle is affected (see Fig. 16.3). This may explain why many heart attacks are not fatal. Blockage in the larger sections of a coronary artery would diminish blood supply to a larger area and generally result in death. Figure 16.4 shows the progression of plaque buildup (fatty deposits) in a coronary artery over a 30-year period.

Angina pectoris. The condition known as **angina pectoris** is a symptom of oxygen deprivation to the heart muscle caused by diminished blood supply. When any muscle fails to receive an adequate blood supply (oxygen and nutriments), pain results. This condition is referred to as **ischemia.** When the heart muscle is involved, the victim experiences a tightness or pressure in the chest and pain that may radiate to the shoulders or arms. If angina is confirmed, a physician's care and changes in lifestyle are indicated.

Arteriosclerosis and atherosclerosis. The terms **arteriosclerosis** (hardening of the arteries) and **ather-**

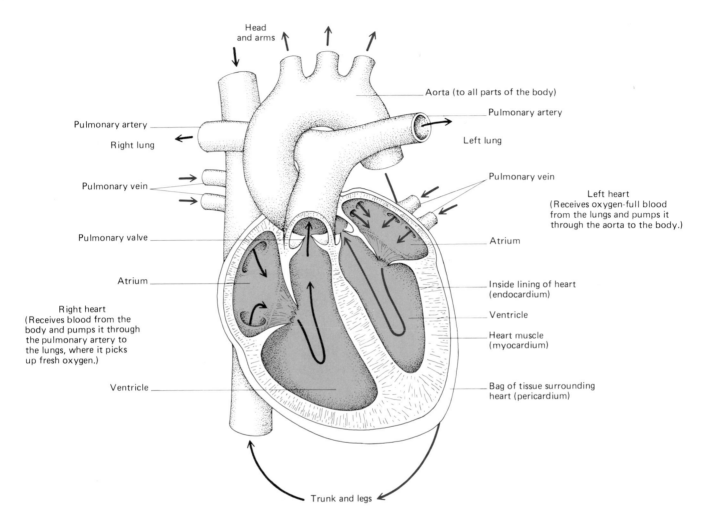

Head and arms

Aorta (to all parts of the body)

Pulmonary artery

Left lung

Pulmonary artery

Right lung

Pulmonary vein

Pulmonary vein

Left heart
(Receives oxygen-full blood
from the lungs and pumps it
through the aorta to the body.)

Pulmonary valve

Atrium

Atrium

Right heart
(Receives blood from the
body and pumps it through
the pulmonary artery to
the lungs, where it picks
up fresh oxygen.)

Inside lining of heart
(endocardium)

Ventricle

Heart muscle
(myocardium)

Ventricle

Bag of tissue surrounding
heart (pericardium)

Trunk and legs

Figure 16.1
Your heart and how it works. Your heart weighs well under a pound and is only a little larger than your fist, but it is a powerful, long working, hard working organ. Its job is to pump blood to the lungs and to all the body tissues.

The heart is a hollow organ. Its tough, muscular wall (myocardium) is surrounded by a fiber-like bag (pericardium) and is lined by a thin, strong membrane (endocardium). A wall (septum) divides the heart cavity down the middle into a "right heart" and a "left heart." Each side of the heart is divided again into an upper chamber (called an atrium or auricle) and a lower chamber (ventricle). Valves regulate the flow of blood through the heart and to the pulmonary artery and the aorta.

The heart is really a double pump. One pump (the right heart) receives blood that has just come from the body after delivering nutrients and oxygen to the body tissues. It pumps this dark, bluish red blood to the lungs where the blood gets rid of a waste gas (carbon dioxide) and picks up a fresh supply of oxygen that turns it a bright red again. The second pump (the left heart) receives this "reconditioned" blood from the lungs and pumps it out through the great trunk-artery (aorta) to be distributed by smaller arteries to all parts of the body.

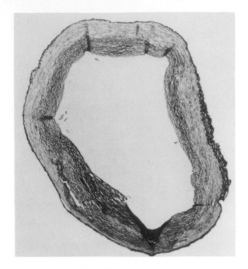

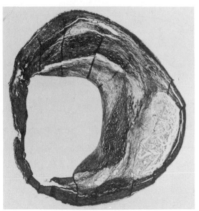

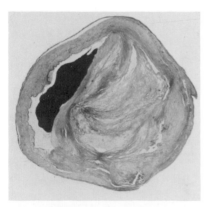

Figure 16.2
Development of atherosclerosis in an artery. The first frame shows a normal artery; the second frame shows an artery narrowing from atherosclerotic buildup; the third frame shows complete blockage.

SOURCE: © American Heart Association. Reprinted with permission.

osclerosis (plaque buildup inside arterial blood vessels) are used to identify a disease process occurring in the arteries of systemic circulation; rarely does the disease involve the veins or blood vessels to the lungs. If the arteries supplying the brain are involved, a stroke occurs; if the arteries supplying the legs are involved, leg pain (**claudication**) occurs; and if the coronary arteries are involved, chest pain (**angina pectoris**) and heart attack result. As shown in Figs. 16.2 and 16.4, atherosclerosis is a condition involving a progressive buildup of fatty material (**triglycerides** and **cholesterol**) inside arterial blood vessels, which narrows or blocks the vessels.

Congenital heart disease. Inborn heart defects, known as **congenital heart disease,** fall into four major groups: (1) narrowing or constriction of a blood vessel or a heart valve; (2) abnormal holes between the two blood vessels, in the muscle, or in the septum that

Figure 16.3
Clot or blockage in a branch of the coronary artery.
SOURCE: National Heart, Lung and Blood Institute, National Institutes of Health.

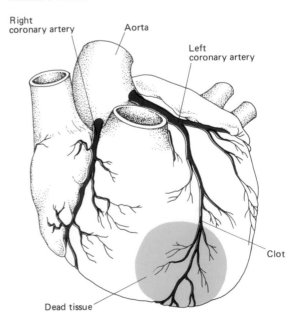

Right coronary artery

Aorta

Left coronary artery

Clot

Dead tissue

separates the two chambers of the heart; (3) a combination of (1) and (2); and (4) abnormal connections of the blood vessels leading to or from the heart. In most cases, these defects are correctable through surgery.

Heart rhythm disturbances. Irregular blood flow results in a **heart murmur,** which is a heart rhythm disturbance. The difficulty may be an impaired valve that fails to close completely or valve orifices that are narrowed and slow the flow of blood. In the case of valve defects, a greater load is placed on the heart,

heart walls may increase in size, and tension increases inside the walls. In effect, the heart is less efficient and, in a sense, has to regurgitate blood twice.

In what are termed **functional heart murmurs,** no structural defect is evident to account for the abnormal rhythm. In children, most heart murmurs are not indicative of disease or physiological impairment.

Rheumatic heart disease. Rheumatic fever is a leading cause of valvular or **rheumatic heart disease.** Generally regarded as a disease of children and young people, it accounts for approximately 95 percent of all heart disease in patients under 20 years of age. The condition may develop during the convalescent period following an upper respiratory streptococcal infection (commonly called strep throat). Inflammation occurs in several areas of the body, especially the joints, lungs, brain, and **endocardium** (lining of the heart). When the inflammation is in the heart, granular nodules develop on the cusps of the heart valves, with permanent connective tissue forming around the injured valve as a part of the healing. Damage may result in fatigue, shortness of breath, or serious valvular impairment.

Rheumatic heart disease is largely preventable. When severe sore throat persists for more than a few days, the individual should have a throat culture to determine whether there is a strep infection. If the infection exists, antibiotic therapy can prevent rheumatic fever and secondary valve damage.

Figure 16.4
Common progress of plaque buildup and a heart attack.

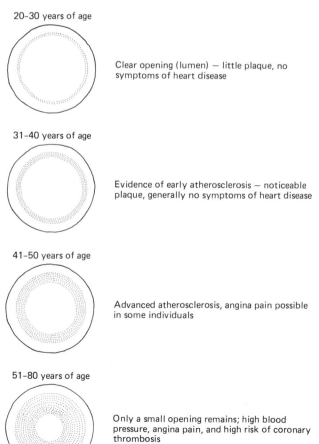

20–30 years of age

Clear opening (lumen) — little plaque, no symptoms of heart disease

31–40 years of age

Evidence of early atherosclerosis — noticeable plaque, generally no symptoms of heart disease

41–50 years of age

Advanced atherosclerosis, angina pain possible in some individuals

51–80 years of age

Only a small opening remains; high blood pressure, angina pain, and high risk of coronary thrombosis

Symptoms of Heart Attack

Concept: Chest pain may or may not be a symptom of a heart attack.

For the male over 30 years and the female over 40, any chest pain is often regarded as a sign of a heart attack. In actuality, however, apparent pain in the chest may be occurring in the chest wall (muscle, ligament, rib, or rib cartilage), the lungs or outside covering, the gullet, diaphragm, skin, or other organs in the upper part of the diaphragm. It is not easy to distinguish between chest pain associated with heart attack and other pains. Table 16.1 identifies the signals of a heart attack.

Table 16.1

What You Should Know About Heart Attack		The Signals of Heart Attack
An estimated 41,290,000 Americans have one or more forms of heart or blood vessel disease. As many as 1.5 million may have a heart attack this year; 550,000 will die— 350,000 of them before they reach the hospital. Many thousands of these might have been saved if the victims had heeded the signals. Delay spells danger. When you suffer a heart attack, minutes—especially the first few minutes—count.	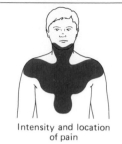 Intensity and location of pain	Uncomfortable pressure, fullness, squeezing, or pain in center of chest lasting two minutes or more. Pain may spread to shoulders, neck or arms. Severe pain, dizziness, fainting, sweating, nausea, or shortness of breath may also occur. Sharp, stabbing twinges of pain are usually not signals of a heart attack.

Adapted from *Heart Facts*, 1982. Reprinted with permission. Copyright © the American Heart Association.

Anyone who experiences heart attack symptoms should be transported immediately to the hospital, and his or her blood pressure, breathing, and heart rate should be monitored.

THEORIES EXPLAINING HEART DISEASE

Concept: Several theories attempt to explain the cause of heart disease.

Lipid Theory

The lipid theory is based on the premise that a high number of fatty particles in the blood stream called **hyperlipidemia,** causes atherosclerosis, the accumulation of these particles on the walls of the arteries. The more fatty particles in the blood, the greater the propensity for accumulation within the arterial walls. Eventually, circulation through an artery is blocked or partially blocked. Depending upon the body part supplied by this artery, heart attack, stroke, muscular weakness, senility, or a host of other ailments results. The process becomes more common with age, undoubtedly preceded by a long silent period of fatty deposit buildup beginning in the first decade of life.

The fatty particles that increase the tendency toward atherosclerosis are called **lipoproteins.** They consist of fat (triglyceride), a blood protein (to make the fat soluble in the water portion of the blood), and cholesterol. Blood measurements of triglycerides and cholesterol provide an index of the fatty particles in the blood stream. The lipoprotein fractions implicated in atherosclerosis are the β and pre-β types. The α lipoproteins are not implicated.

Blood serum cholesterol has also been analyzed for its percentage of HDL (high-density lipoproteins) and LDL (low-density lipoproteins). Coronary heart disease is inversely related to HDL and positively related to LDL. Individuals with high percentages of HDL are two or three times less likely to suffer from early heart disease than individuals with low percentages of HDL.

Total cholesterol is a combination of that formed by the liver and that ingested in food. Triglyceride levels increase after eating a meal high in animal fat, with elevation also related to excessive carbohydrates or protein in the diet. Of recent concern is the role of carbohydrates in the form of sugar.

Management of total serum cholesterol and the HDL concentration involves: (1) a reduction in body fat, (2) regular exercise, (3) cessation of smoking, (4) use of alcohol only in moderation (one to two drinks may elevate HDL), and (5) maintaining a ratio of polyunsaturated to saturated fats of at least two to one (see Chapter 6).

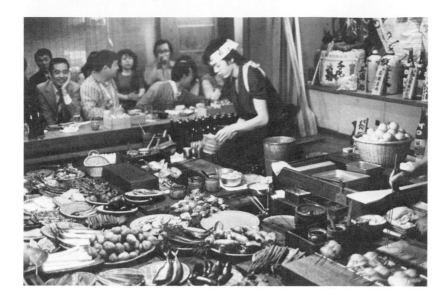

One significant piece of evidence supporting the lipid theory is that heart disease is uncommon in countries such as Japan where the traditional diet is low in fat and cholesterol.

There is considerable evidence to support the lipid theory: (1) heart disease is uncommon in countries where the people generally have low cholesterol and low triglyceride levels in the blood; (2) the disease is most common in countries where people's diets are rich in dairy and meat products (saturated fats); (3) individuals who have moved from the Orient and adopted the Western diet and lifestyle greatly increase their risk of heart disease; (4) genetic errors in fat metabolism causing elevated lipid levels may result in death from coronary heart disease in one's early twenties; (5) women develop coronary heart disease 10 to 15 years later in life than men, possibly because the female sex hormone tends to reduce lipid levels; (6) diet-induced elevated lipid levels in animals cause atherosclerosis; and (7) in males age 30 to 49 a blood cholesterol level of 260 mg per 100 ml of blood increases the incidence of heart disease to approximately three times that of men with levels below 180.[1] Nevertheless, not all individuals with high levels of blood lipids develop serious atherosclerosis, and additional evidence is needed to isolate the exact cause or causes of this disease.

Fibrin Deposit Theory

Somewhat similar to the blood lipid theory, the fibrin deposit theory states that the cause of atherosclerosis is fibrin deposits on the inside of the arteries that lead to a reduced flow of blood or a complete blockage. **Fibrin** is a tough, fibrous protein that combines with blood cells to form a clot in the healing of a wound.

Personality Behavior Theory

The idea that personality is an important factor in the development of heart disease was first advanced by Friedman and Rosenman in their research on Type A and Type B personalities. As was described in Chapter 4, the Type A individual is typically in a hurry, pressed for time, a clock watcher, competitive, aggressive, hating to lose, lacking patience, and having an underlying hostility. The Type B individual is typically unaggressive, not overly concerned with job advancement, not concerned with time pressures, more interested in family than career.

In the first edition of their book, Friedman and Rosenman stated: "In the absence of Type A Behavior Pattern, coronary heart disease almost never occurs before 70 years of age regardless of the fatty foods eaten, the cigarettes smoked, or the lack of exercise."[2] One might falsely conclude from this that Type B individuals can abuse their bodies by almost any known means because the cause of early heart disease is emotional stress.

Unfortunately there is little evidence to support the view that personality behavior type is the key to

379

heart attacks. Although some studies show a higher rate of heart disease among Type A persons, others do not.

In a revised edition of their book, Friedman and Rosenman expanded their description of Type A and Type B behavior patterns.[3] In addition to having the characteristics mentioned above, the Type A individual is described as one who eats a high-fat diet (including a high-cholesterol breakfast), has abnormally high blood cholesterol, has high blood pressure, does not exercise, and smokes over two packs of cigarettes a day. The Type B individual has normal weight and blood pressure, is a nonsmoker, consumes a diet low in both cholesterol and fat, and exercises regularly.

This revised description of the two behavior patterns suggests that Type A behavior in combination with other risk factors increases the chances of early heart disease. You can get an idea of your own personality behavior type by completing Discovery Activity 16.1.

Discovery Activity 16.1
PERSONALITY RATING TEST

INSTRUCTIONS: Opposing behavior patterns are presented in the left- and right-hand columns with a horizontal line between. Place a vertical mark across the line where you feel you belong between these two extremes. For example, most of us are neither the most competitive nor the least competitive person we know; we fall somewhere in between. Your task is to make a vertical line where you feel you belong between the two extremes. ●

1.	Never late	Casual about appointments
2.	Not competitive	Very competitive
3.	Anticipates what others are saying	A good listener, hears others out
4.	Always rushed	Never feels rushed, even under pressure
5.	Takes things one at a time	Tries to do many things at once, thinks about what to do next
6.	Emphatic speech (may pound desk)	Slow, deliberate talker
7.	Wants a good job recognized by others	Only cares about satisfying self no matter what others think
8.	Fast (eating, talking, etc.)	Slow doing things
9.	Sits on feelings	Expresses feelings
10.	Easy going	Hard driving
11.	Many interests	Few interests except work
12.	Satisfied with job	Ambitious
13.	Can wait patiently	Impatient when waiting
14.	Goes "all out"	Casual

SCORING: Using a ruler, one point is scored for each $\frac{1}{16}$-inch you fall from the Non–Type A behavior end of the $1\frac{1}{2}$ inch line to the point marked. Points are summed for all 14 questions. Items 2, 5, 10, 12, and 13 are measured from the left of the line to your mark; items 1, 3, 4, 6, 7, 8, 9, 11, and 14 are measured from the right of the line to your mark.

Type B average score: 178.21
Type A average score: 211.51

Reprinted with permission from *Journal of Chronic Disease 22*, R. W. Bortner, "A Short Rating Scale as a Potential Measure of Pattern A Behavior," Copyright © 1969, Pergamon Press, Ltd.

Risk Factor Theory

The risk factor theory suggests that heart disease is caused by several factors that appear to be additive. The presence of one factor in combination with others greatly increases the chances of heart disease. For example, individuals who have high blood pressure, smoke, and also have high cholesterol are eight times more likely to have a heart attack and have a death rate six times higher than individuals with none of these characteristics. To complicate the picture, the presence of Type A behavior in combination with other risk factors appears to compound the individual's chances of becoming a victim of early heart disease.

RISK FACTORS IN HEART DISEASE

Several factors have been linked with a high risk of heart disease. Among the factors that cannot be controlled are sex, race, age, and heredity. Controllable factors include hypertension, obesity, inactivity, hyperlipidemia, smoking, and diabetes. With normal blood pressure and lipid levels and in the absence of smoking and diabetes, the chances of a male having a heart attack prior to age 65 are fewer than one in 20. With one of these risk factors, the risk doubles; with two, the chances become one in two, or 50 percent.

Men have a higher incidence of cardiovascular disease than women, across all age groups. Although the rate of heart attacks in women increases after menopause—presumably because of hormonal changes—there is evidence that women are developing cardiovascular disease at an earlier age than in the past. Black Americans have a much higher risk of developing hypertension and are likely to suffer strokes at an earlier age than whites. Older people suffer more heart attacks than young people.

Hereditary Traits

The genetic tendency to develop atherosclerosis early in life greatly increases the risk of early heart disease.

Although a small percentage of individuals apparently develop little plaque buildup regardless of living habits, others develop large amounts very early in life. In the past decade several professional athletes between 23 and 39 years of age suffered serious heart attacks. Diagnosis by autopsy or by arteriography revealed advanced atherosclerosis. Apparently these young adults possessed the hereditary tendency to acquire plaque and hardening of the arteries. There is also some evidence that a tendency toward high blood pressure or hypertension is inherited. A history of early heart disease in your family is a signal for you to form healthy living habits and receive periodic physical examinations. This is especially important for individuals from families in which one or more parents or grandparents suffered a heart attack or stroke prior to age 60.

Hypertension

The condition known as **hypertension,** or high blood pressure, accelerates arteriosclerosis and atherosclerosis. It also forces the heart to work harder and can lead to kidney damage. Heart disease and high blood pressure are directly related. A nine-member group sponsored by the National High Blood Pressure Coordinating Committee has been working on a redefinition of normal and abnormal blood pressure based on recent research linking hypertension with cardiovascular disease (heart attack and stroke). Previously accepted normal ranges of 110 to 139 (systolic) and 60 to 90 (diastolic) are now considered too lenient. Individuals with a diastolic reading between 80 and 90 were found to have twice the risk of an individual with a reading below 80. It is expected that "intermediate" risk will be defined as a diastolic range of 80 to 90 and "definite" risk as a reading above 90. For those in the intermediate risk category, it is unlikely that medication will be prescribed; however, reduced salt intake, regular exercise, and weight control will be strongly recommended, because these three changes have been shown to lower blood pressure significantly.

Approximately one person in 10 has high blood pressure. As noted, hypertension is also more common among blacks than whites. Even among children, high blood pressure is not uncommon. In fact, some experts have suggested the use of mass screening programs in elementary schools to aid in the early identification and treatment of hypertensive youngsters.

Obesity or Overweight

These conditions are often accompanied by high fat levels in the blood, a higher incidence of arteriosclerotic disease, and high blood pressure. As a result, obesity is associated with a higher incidence of coronary artery disease.

Inactivity

This appears to contribute to early heart disease in a number of ways. Lack of exercise is often associated with obesity, high lipid levels, and plaque accumulation (see the next section: Prevention of Heart Disease).

Hyperlipidemia

This refers to high blood lipid levels. See our discussion of the blood lipid theory.

Discovery Activity 16.2
PULSE TAKING

Excess body weight causes the heart to work harder while the body does simple chores, such as walking, standing, and even sitting. To demonstrate this, record your resting pulse rate (the beats per minute) on a note pad. Now walk at a normal pace back and forth across the room exactly 10 times before immediately sitting down and taking your pulse rate again. Record this figure in beats per minute. Find an item weighing 15 to 20 pounds or several items of five pounds each. Carry the items with you as you again walk back and forth across the room 10 times. Sit down and take your pulse rate again. Compare the two pulse rates with and without the 15- to 20-pound weight. You can see how much additional stress an extra 15 to 20 pounds places on the heart. ●

Cigarette Smoking

Smoking, in combination with some of the other risk factors, is a strong contributor to heart disease. The smoker who also has high blood pressure runs a greater risk of heart attack than a nonsmoker. Statistically, the incidence of heart disease is 70 to 200 percent higher among smoking males. Recent data on female smokers also indicate a significantly higher incidence of heart disease. The risk of heart disease increases with the number of cigarettes smoked and the degree of inhalation habits. The risk is reduced when smoking is stopped. In a study supported by the U.S. Department of Health and Human Services, 2000 male smokers and 2000 male nonsmokers were examined on a regular basis for six to eight years. Signs of arteriosclerosis were absent when the study began. After six to eight years, three times as many smokers as nonsmokers had died from all causes, most from arteriosclerosis. Unfortunately, there is no accurate diagnostic technique

Smoking has been found to be a strong contributor to heart disease.

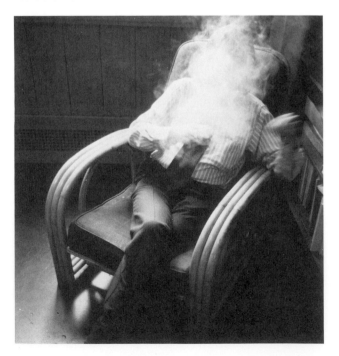

available, other than invasive methods that monitor the vessels after a dye is inserted, that could have been used in a study of this nature to determine the progress of arteriosclerosis over the eight-year period.

Cigarette smoking appears to produce several changes, each with implications for heart disease. The evidence so far indicates that smoking increases the amount of cholesterol deposited in the arteries; increases heart pain in heart patients; increases the clumping of **platelets** which may be associated with the tendency to form clots; elevates heart rate (15 to 25 beats per minute), systolic blood pressure (10 to 20 mm Hg), and diastolic pressure (10 to 20 mm Hg); and decreases tolerance of pain during exercise.

The Pill

The use of the contraceptive pill has been associated with a higher incidence of early heart disease. Women who have used the pill for 10 years or more could benefit from physician screening for symptoms of heart disease. Use of the pill in combination with moderate or heavy smoking significantly increases the risk.

Diabetes

Individuals who suffer from diabetes are more apt to suffer an early heart attack or stroke.

PREVENTION OF HEART DISEASE

Nutrition and Diet

Concept: Proper nutrition and diet can help prevent early heart disease.

Three risk factors identified by the American Heart Association (hyperlipidemia, diabetes, and obesity) can be changed or managed through diet modification. Well-documented studies have revealed that in countries where the diet is low in saturated fat and cholesterol there is a much lower incidence of coronary heart disease. Conversely, a diet high in saturated fat and/or

Issues in Health
DOES CONTROLLING CHOLESTEROL INTAKE HELP PREVENT HEART DISEASE?

High blood serum cholesterol has been strongly linked to heart disease. Children born with **familial hypercholesterolemia (FH)** (high levels of cholesterol) experience atherosclerosis, hardening of the arteries, and heart attacks as young adults. Individuals with high blood cholesterol at all ages are also more susceptible to heart disease than those with normal levels. The controversy concerns whether a diet that is low in saturated fat reduces blood serum cholesterol.

Cholesterol is supplied in the diet only from foods of animal origin; however, it can be synthesized in the body from carbohydrates and fats. In the absence of dietary cholesterol, the body produces its own to carry out critical functions. Cholesterol is an important part of certain organs, such as the coverings for nerve fibers; it facilitates the absorption of fatty acids from the intestines; and it is a precursor of sex hormones, adrenal hormones, and bile acids. Opponents of dietary regulations of cholesterol argue that cholesterol intake is necessary on a daily basis and that the body will produce a similar level regardless of animal food intake; therefore, it is senseless to be concerned about quantity.

Proponents of dietary regulation of cholesterol disagree, pointing to evidence that a high level of cholesterol intake is associated with high incidences of both stroke and heart attack. Therefore, they argue, any attempt to control cholesterol intake is desirable. We know that establishing correct eating habits early carries over into the adult years. Thus, individuals with appropriate eating habits are more likely to have normal cholesterol levels throughout life. Research has also shown that a reduction in saturated fat intake, accompanied by an increase in the consumption of polyunsaturated fats, significantly decreases blood cholesterol.

What do you think? ●

cholesterol, such as is prevalent in the United States, has been repeatedly linked to a high incidence of heart disease. The evidence is sufficient to warrant certain changes in the American diet at this time.

An effective diet for the prevention of atherosclerosis reduces serum lipids and is palatable, economically feasible and nutritionally adequate. The Prudent Diet discussed in Chapter 7 meets these criteria. Specifically, the American Heart Association recommends:

1. A caloric intake adjusted to achieve and maintain ideal weight. This means preventing obesity by establishing healthy eating patterns early in life.

2. A reduction of total calories in fat, achieved by substantially reducing intake of dietary saturated fatty acids. Total calories in fat should be reduced from 40 percent to 30 to 35 percent. In addition, total fat consumption should be managed by establishing a favorable ratio of polyunsaturated to saturated fats (see Chapter 7).

3. A substantial reduction in cholesterol intake—less than 300 mgs daily.

4. A modest increase in carbohydrates from vegetables, fruits, and cereals to make up for the reduction in dietary fat intake.

5. Reduced salt intake.

6. Control of alcohol intake.

There is substantial evidence that these diet suggestions and the Prudent Diet will aid in the control of serum lipid levels. Evidence also indicates that reducing blood lipids will also lower the risk of heart disease. These diets have been tested with no harmful effects uncovered. Vegetarians are unlikely to be afflicted with heart disease until approximately 10 years later than people on a typical American diet.

Early Diagnosis and Prevention

Concept: Prevention of heart disease is a pediatric issue and should begin in infancy.

Atherosclerosis is normally a silent process, until middle age, which affects 80 to 90 percent of the adult population. In some individuals, it appears as a heart attack or stroke in the late twenties or early thirties. Autopsy reports of young American and Korean soldiers suggest that the process can be quite advanced by age 20 to 25. There even is evidence of vascular fatty de-

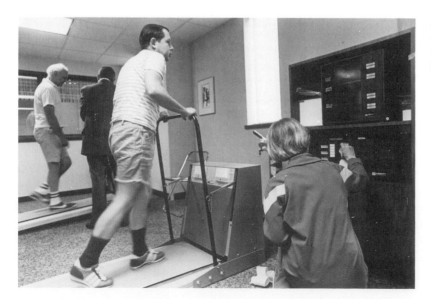

A treadmill stress test monitors the electrical activity of the heart during exercise. A diseased heart produces a different electrical pattern from that of a healthy heart.

posits in young children of school age. A preventive approach, which includes moderate fat intake and sufficient exercise, would have to begin almost at birth and continue throughout the adult years. Mass screening of elementary school children in the areas of blood pressure and blood lipid levels would greatly assist management of the problem throughout youth and the adult years.

Unfortunately, for more than half of all heart attack victims, the first sign of heart disease is sudden death. This situation need not be; physicians can assess an individual's risk potential by looking at the risk factors we described earlier. In addition to the use of a coronary risk profile, the American Heart Association suggests nine measures physicians should take to help prevent heart disease in their patients:[5]

1. Discontinue cigarette smoking.
2. Control hypertension.
3. Control blood lipids.
4. Encourage regular physical activity.
5. Identify ECG abnormalities.
6. Monitor use of oral contraceptives.
7. Identify Type A behavior.
8. Identify diabetes and gout.
9. Monitor intake of alcohol and coffee.

It is important to remember that multiple factors play interrelated roles in coronary heart disease. This principle also applies to preventive approaches. Application of only one or two of the above recommendations is likely to be ineffective; a total approach is needed. Although your physician can alert you to a potential problem, it is ultimately up to you to take responsibility for maintaining a healthy heart.

Exercise

Concept: The right kind of regular exercise plays an important part in preventing premature heart disease.

Exercise aids in the prevention of early heart disease by causing numerous physiological changes within the

Issues in Health
IS IT NECESSARY TO HAVE A PHYSICAL EXAMINATION BEFORE BEGINNING AN EXERCISE PROGRAM?

A rule of thumb in the past has been to recommend that the sedentary individual undergo a complete physical examination before starting an exercise program. Individuals who had been sedentary for a year or more and those over the age of 40 were told to see their doctors before exercising. This position has recently come under attack by the U.S. government, physicians, and exercise physiologists.

Advocates of the physician's examination point out that a good, thorough examination may detect illness or hidden signs of heart disease. Even if only one person in 1000 is diagnosed as unfit for exercise, the argument continues, the procedure is worth the effort. The examination also provides an opportunity for the physician and the patient to discuss exercise choices in light of the patient's history. The popular stress test (EKG), in conjunction with a heart disease risk profile (blood pressure, smoking, and exercise habits, drinking habits, diabetes, family history of heart disease, cholesterol analysis, personality type, body weight and fat), may identify hidden signs of heart disease and even predict difficulty in the future. In addition, older individuals who have been sedentary for years need careful guidance to guarantee their safe introduction to an exercise program and their safe progression to higher fitness levels.

Those who oppose a physician's examination argue that it is unlikely to reveal anything of value, with the exception of high blood pressure. A traditional physical (listening to the heart and lungs, eyeball examination of various body parts, and a few brief questions), with no blood work or heart monitoring during and after exercise, is a waste of a patient's time and money. Even when a stress test

(continued)

Issues in Health *(continued)*

is used, many young, highly conditioned individuals show false positive EKGs. Older individuals have also been given clearance to exercise following negative EKGs, only to have a heart attack several weeks later. Moreover, the physician's examination provides another excuse for some individuals to avoid exercise for another decade or so—one more hurdle that will never be crossed. In addition, the average physician is poorly informed on the principles of exercise and often incapable of preparing individualized programs in various activities.

Opponents of physical examinations agree that some people should see a physician before beginning an exercise program, including those who have had a heart attack; a heart murmur; frequently have pains or pressure in the left or midchest area, left neck, shoulder, or arm during or right after exercise; feel faint or have spells of severe dizziness; experience extreme breathlessness after mild exertion; or have been told their blood pressure is too high. Individuals over the age of 60 with a family history of heart disease or a medical condition, such as diabetes, should also consult a physician. Other people don't need a physical before beginning an exercise program.

What do you think? ●

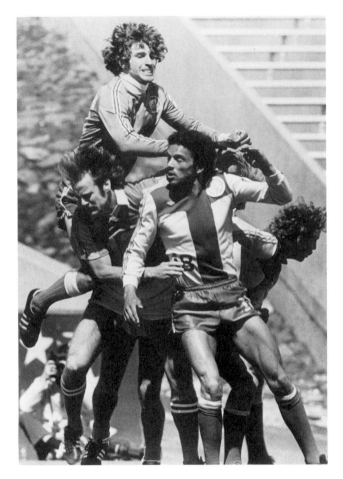

Regular exercise may reduce the risk factors in heart disease by lowering fibrin and lipid levels in the blood and aiding in the control of blood pressure.

body. It is important to remember, however, that *all* of the major risk areas cited previously must be regulated; that is, normal blood pressure, lowered blood lipid levels, and normal weight must be maintained, and smoking must be avoided. Regulation in only one or two areas does not afford great protection.

The active person is three or four times less likely ever to have a heart attack and three or four times more likely to survive, should one occur. The exercising cardiac patient who has suffered an attack is also less likely to have another. In addition, autopsy reports show less incidence of cardiovascular disease among those who were active prior to death. Numerous studies relate inactivity to early heart disease. Unfortunately, the so-called active person is classified by occupation in most studies. A carpenter, bricklayer, or construction worker, for example, is considered highly active when, in reality, such occupations do little to elevate heart rate or produce a training effect similar to that resulting from jogging, cycling, swimming, cross-country skiing, and other aerobic activities.

Exercise may aid in reducing the coronary risk factors associated with heart disease. Several of the risk factors are affected by regular exercise, as shown in Table 16.2. Reducing the risk in four or five areas identified as contributing to early heart disease can be extremely important. Evidence recently presented by Cooper suggests considerable regulation or control of the risk factors and lowered incidence of heart disease

among individuals of all ages (men and women) who can stay within the good-to-excellent category on the 1.5-mile test for their age group (see Chapter 6).

There is evidence that regular exercise relates in some way to each of the theories of heart disease discussed previously. First, exercise can help reduce lipid-deposit atherosclerosis. A reduction in triglyceride levels can be expected with regular aerobic exercise. Although we do not mean to suggest that an active person can continuously consume high-calorie, high-fat foods and expect that exercise will automatically regulate fatty particles in the blood, there is evidence that exercise is an important factor in maintaining lower blood lipid levels. Both pre-β and β lipoprotein fractions (both implicated in atherosclerosis) are lowered during exercise and lowered even further one week after exercise. In addition, recent studies have shown that individuals with large amounts of high-density lipoproteins (HDL) in the blood tend to be protected from early atherosclerosis and heart disease. Runners (joggers, distance runners, and competitive runners) possess 30 percent more HDL than the nonexercising population. Aerobic exercise greatly increases the amount of HDL in the bloodstream.

Exercise also helps reduce fibrin levels in the blood. Regular exercise has been shown to cause the breakdown of fibrin in the blood and to reduce fibrin blood levels, which in turn may decrease the chance of a blood clot and the development of fibrin atherosclerosis.

Exercise-induced **coronary collaterilization** (development of new arteries that bypass the clogged portion of an artery to continue nourishing that portion of the heart muscle) has been demonstrated in animals, but there is no creative evidence to show that exercise can cause collaterilization in humans. Collaterilization has been found in older men with chronic profuse organic heart disease, regardless of their exercise habits, and it is rarely found in younger men, even if they do exercise.

Finally, exercise may increase the diameter of the arteries. Some protection may result from posessing larger arteries, in that more fatty deposits can build up before causing occlusion.

Table 16.2
EXERCISE AND CORONARY RISK FACTORS

Risk Factor	Effect of Regular Physical Exercise
Obesity and overweight	Reduction of body fat, return to ideal weight
High lipid levels	Reduction of atherogenic fatty particles in the blood
Hypertension	Aid in the control of blood pressure
Tension and stress	Increased tolerance of stress, release of tension and nervous or emotional energy
Lack of physical activity	No longer a risk factor for the exercising person
Genetic history	No change
Smoking	Changes in smoking habits are likely to take place
Age	Slows aging process

Discovery Activity 16.3
PHYSICAL ACTIVITY
READINESS
QUESTIONNAIRE
(PAR-Q)*
A SELF-ADMINISTERED
QUESTIONNAIRE FOR
ADULTS

PAR–Q is designed to help you help yourself. Many health benefits are associated with regular exercise, and the completion of PAR–Q is a sensible first step to take if you are planning to increase the amount of physical activity in your life.

For most people physical activity should not pose any problem or hazard. PAR–Q has been designed to identify the small number of adults for whom physical activity might be inappropriate or those who should have medical advice concerning the type of activity most suitable for them.

Common sense is your best guide in answering these few questions. Please read them carefully and check the ☑ YES or NO opposite the question if it applies to you.

YES NO

☐ ☒ 1. Has your doctor ever said you have heart trouble?

☐ ☒ 2. Do you frequently have pains in your heart and chest?

☐ ☒ 3. Do you often feel faint or have spells of severe dizziness?

☐ ☒ 4. Has a doctor ever said your blood pressure was too high?

☑ ☒ 5. Has your doctor ever told you that you have a bone or joint problem such as arthritis that has been aggravated by exercise, or might be made worse with exercise?

☑ ☒ 6. Is there a good physical reason not mentioned here why you should not follow an activity program even if you wanted to?

☐ ☒ 7. Are you over age 65 and not accustomed to vigorous exercise?

If You Answered YES to One or More Questions

If you have not recently done so, consult with your personal physician by telephone or in person BEFORE increasing your physical activity and/or taking a fitness test. Tell him what questions you answered YES on PAR–Q, or show him your copy.

Programs

After medical evaluation, seek advice from your physician as to your suitability for:

• unrestricted physical activity, probably on a gradually increasing basis.

• restricted or supervised activity to meet your specific needs, at least on an initial basis. Check in your community for special programs or services.

NO to All Questions

If you answered PAR–Q accurately, you have reasonable assurance of your present suitability for:

• A GRADUATED EXERCISE PROGRAM—A gradual increase in proper exercise promotes good fitness development while minimizing or eliminating discomfort.

• AN EXERCISE TEST—Simple test of fitness (such as the Canadian Home Fitness Test) or more complex types may be undertaken if you so desire.

Postpone

If you have a temporary minor illness, such as a common cold.

*PAR–Q Validation Report, British Columbia Ministry of Health, May, 1978. Developed by the British Columbia Ministry of Health. Conceptualized and critiqued by the Multidisciplinary Advisory Board on Exercise (MABE).

STROKE

Concept: The causes of stroke are similar to those of heart attacks.

Like the heart, the brain must be continuously nourished. When blood supply to any portion of the brain is greatly reduced or cut off completely, nerve tissue in the brain is unable to function, and body tissue controlled by this nerve tissue also ceases to operate. This

Figure 16.5
Causes of a stroke.

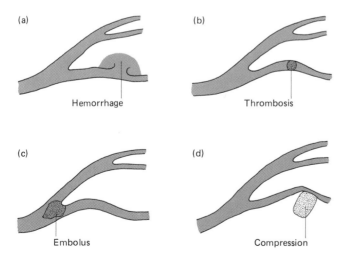

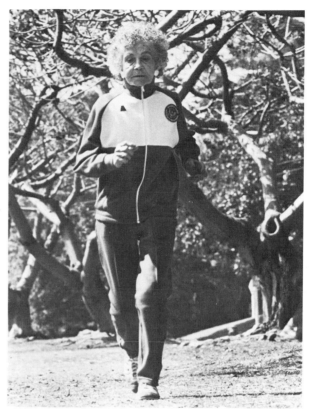

Eula Weaver used to jog two miles a day, but after recovering from a nearly paralyzing stroke she reduced her course to just a mile a day.

occurrence is known as a **cerebrovascular accident (CVA)** or **stroke.** Depending upon the portion of the brain affected, a victim may experience loss of speech, loss of memory, or partial paralysis. The four ways in which a stroke occurs are shown in Fig. 16.5. Fewer than 10 percent of strokes are caused by an **embolus,** or small clot from another body part (c). A much more frequent cause is atherosclerosis. The same fatty deposits that cause heart attacks also block the arteries supplying the brain.

A mild stroke occurs when the brain is deprived of adequate blood supply for a short period of time (**ischemia**). A **transitory ischemic attack (TIA)** often results in momentary periods of paralysis, vision problems, or inability to speak. Generally, the deeper brain cells are not permanently damaged, although repeated episodes can bring about personality changes. TIAs are warning signs of insufficient blood supply to the brain. Careful diagnosis and prompt action can prevent a stroke from occurring. Some 80 percent of victims survive the first stroke, with the likelihood of death increasing with age. Over 20 percent of those who recover have a second stroke within two years, and over half of the survivors eventually die from a heart attack. The warning signals of stroke are shown in Fig. 16.6.

Concept: A stroke affects different victims in different ways.

The most visible sign of a stroke is paralysis on one side of the body, or **hemiplegia.** Paralysis of the right side (right hemiplegia) indicates injury to the left side of the brain, whereas left side paralysis (left hemiplegia) indicates right brain injury. Left brain injury produces speech and language difficulties (**aphasia**) and results in slow, cautious, and disorganized behavior when the victim is confronted with an unfamiliar problem. Right brain damage causes difficulty with spatial-perceptual tasks (judging distance, size, position, rate of movement, form, and the relation of parts to wholes). Many stroke patients also experience "visual field cuts," producing vision similar to what you would see if you wore goggles with tape across half of each lens. Right hemiplegics tend to have right field cuts and left hemiplegics left field cuts. Patients learn to turn their heads to compensate, although not everyone makes this adjustment. Any patient who has suffered a stroke will show evidence of brain damage. Loss of memory, short attention span, difficulty with new learning, inability to generalize learning to new situations, and **emotional lability** (loss of emotional control) may occur.

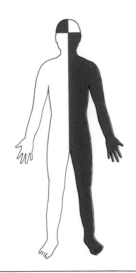

WHAT YOU SHOULD KNOW ABOUT STROKE

An estimated 1,840,000 persons are afflicted by stroke. Almost 200,000 suffered fatal strokes in 1975. Many fatal strokes can be prevented if high blood pressure, a leading cause of stroke, is diagnosed and controlled. Many major strokes are preceded by "little strokes" or warning signals experienced days, weeks, or months before the more severe event. Prompt medical or surgical attention to these symptoms may prevent a fatal or disabling stroke from occurring.

The warning signals of stroke

- Sudden, temporary weakness or numbness of the face, arm, and leg on one side of the body.
- Temporary loss of speech, or trouble in speaking or understanding speech.
- Temporary dimness or loss of vision, particularly in one eye.
- Unexplained dizziness, unsteadiness, or sudden falls.

Act immediately

Sometimes these symptoms subside, then return. When you experience one or more warning signs, call your doctor and describe these symptoms in detail. If he's not immediately available, get to a hospital emergency room at once. Be prepared to act. Instruct others to act if you cannot. Keep a list of numbers — doctor, hospital, ambulance, or other emergency services and police — next to your telephone, and in a prominent place in your pocket, wallet, or purse.

Figure 16.6

Practically all spontaneous recovery of intellectual abilities will occur in the first three to six months following the stroke. A stroke will not affect all areas of the brain equally, nor will all aspects of intellectual functioning be affected equally. Patients will behave differently depending upon the portion of the brain that has been injured, the severity of the injury, and the recency of the stroke.

Each stroke patient and the affected family have unique problems. Although a complete cure is unlikely, many stroke victims can adapt successfully.[7]

Reducing the Risk of Stroke

Concept: The risk of stroke can be reduced by preventive measures.

Reducing the risk of stroke involves prevention and control of atherosclerosis and high blood pressure. Specific measures include:

1. Elimination of tobacco smoking;

2. Elimination of alcohol consumption, coffee, and tea;

3. Elimination of obesity by controlling caloric intake, total fat, saturated fat, and cholesterol consumption;

4. Initiation of a sensible exercise program to control weight and maintain good circulation; and

5. Scheduling regular medical checkups for contributing factors, such as anemia, diabetes, high blood pressure, and compression on arteries in the neck.

CONCLUSION

Diseases of the cardiovascular system, particularly heart disease and stroke, represent major health problems in the United States. These chronic and degenerative diseases appear to begin in the first decade of life and slowly and silently progress until, much later, they take the form of heart attack and stroke. By the time first

symptoms appear, such as angina pains or high blood pressure, preventive techniques have lost much of their effectiveness, although lifestyle changes will still delay the onset of the disease.

Several factors contribute to cardiovascular disease: sex, race, obesity, high blood lipid levels, hypertension, stress, sedentary living, smoking, diabetes, genetic makeup, the Pill, and the aging process. Most of these factors are directly related to lifestyle and decisions you make about how you want to live. Only genetic makeup, sex, race, and the aging process are uncontrollable. Taking charge of your life can greatly reduce the risk of early coronary heart disease and stroke.

SUMMARY

1. The most common form of heart disease is coronary artery disease, resulting from plaque buildup in these two main arteries and their branches, which supply blood and oxygen to the heart muscle.

2. Clogging of the coronary arteries may result in a heart attack from artery closure or angina pectoris from a partial closure that limits oxygen supply to the heart and produces pain.

3. Heart problems in children generally involve congenital defects, heart rhythm disturbances, or damage to the heart muscle following rheumatic fever or prolonged upper respiratory streptococcal infections (strep throat).

4. The most common theories about the causes of heart attacks are the lipid theory, the fibrin deposit theory, the personality behavior theory, and the risk factor theory.

5. Use of the contraceptive pill, especially in combination with smoking, has been associated with a higher incidence of heart disease in women.

6. Early heart disease can be prevented through management of saturated and unsaturated fat intake, early diagnosis, and sound lifestyle choices (regular exercise, absence of smoking, maintenance of normal body weight and body fat, and a careful

diet). These lifestyle choices are most beneficial when begun early in life and continued throughout the adult years.

7. Exercise may contribute toward a reduction in the incidence of early heart disease by controlling body weight and fat, increasing the amount of HDL in the blood, reducing blood fibrin levels, increasing the diameter of the arteries, and improving the efficiency of the heart and circulatory system.

8. Both the causes and prevention of heart disease also apply to stroke (cerebrovascular accident).

9. A mild stroke occurs when the brain is deprived of adequate blood supply for a short period of time. Transitory ischemic attacks are warning signs of clogging in the vessels supplying the brain. Most victims of stroke make significant progress toward a complete recovery.

REFERENCES

1. Robert A. O'Rourke and John Ross, Jr., *Understanding the Heart and Its Diseases* (New York: McGraw-Hill, 1976).

2. E. H. Friedman, "Type A or B Behavior?" *Journal of the American Medical Association* 228 (1974):1369.

3. Glen M. Friedman and R. H. Rosenman, *Type A Behavior and Your Heart* (New York: Knopf, 1974).

4. American Heart Association, *Diet and Coronary Heart Disease*, 1978.

5. American Heart Association, *Risk Factors and Coronary Disease: A Statement for Physicians*, 1980.

6. Kenneth H. Cooper, *The New Aerobics* (New York: Bantam Books, 1970).

7. American Heart Association, Roy S. Fowler, and W. E. Fordyce, *Stroke: Why Do They Behave That Way?* 1974.

Laboratory 1
LOCATING YOUR CRITICAL THRESHOLD

Purpose To determine your "critical threshold," or minimum training necessary for cardiorespiratory development.

Size of Group Individually or in small groups of between three and five.

Equipment Watch with second hand.

Procedure

1. Select two of the following activities. Engage in each on separate days for the number of minutes suggested:

   Jogging (at your usual pace): 10 minutes

   Badminton (singles): 30 minutes

   Basketball: 15 minutes

   Bicycling: 15 minutes

   Golf: 9 holes

   Ice hockey: 15 minutes

   Rugby/Soccer: 15 minutes

   Swimming (lap, freestyle): 15 minutes

   Tennis (singles): 30 minutes

   Volleyball: 30 minutes

   Water polo: 15 minutes

   Weight training: 15 minutes

   Wrestling: 5 minutes

   Other:

2. At the end of the suggested time period, stop and take your radial pulse (wrist) for 30 seconds. Double this figure and record your beats per minute in the Results section.

3. Determine your maximum heart rate (220 − age = maximum heart rate) and record in the Results section.

Results

1. Complete the information below:

   a. Resting heart rate (60 seconds)

   b. Maximum heart rate for age

   c. Your critical threshold, or minimum heart rate needed to produce a training effect on the heart and lungs:

   CRITICAL THRESHOLD = 60 percent of distance between your "resting" and "maximum" heart rate.

For example, Lynne has a resting heart rate of 80 and a maximum heart rate for her 28 years of age of 200.

   Critical threshold = 200 − 80 or 120
   60% of 120 = 72
   80 + 72 = 152 beats per minute (critical threshold, or minimum heart rate elevation necessary to produce a training effect)

4. Heart rate following your activity sessions:
   Activity _____   Heart rate _____
   Activity _____   Heart rate _____

5. Did each activity elevate your heart rate to your critical threshold?

6. Was your activity continuous, forcing your heart rate to work at or above the critical threshold level for 6 to 10 minutes?

7. Was your activity one of intermittent exertion, causing only temporary rises to the critical threshold?

8. Evaluate the exercise programs listed in terms of ease of elevating heart rate to the critical threshold.

Laboratory 2
THE RISK OF EARLY HEART DISEASE

Purpose   To estimate your chances of suffering an early heart attack.

Size of Group   Between five and ten.

Procedure

Play the game of RISKO following the instructions in Fig. 16.7.

Results

1. Determine your exact score and rating. What changes do you feel are needed to reduce your chances of suffering an early heart attack?

2. Tabulate the number of students falling into each category. Place this information on the board for the entire class. Discuss the risk factors once again in terms of reducing the risk.

RISKO

The purpose of this game is to give you an estimate of your chances of suffering heart attack.

The game is played by making squares which —from left to right—represent an increase in your RISK FACTORS. These are medical conditions and habits associated with an increased danger of heart attack. *Not all risk factors are measurable enough to be included in this game.*

RULES:
Study each RISK FACTOR AND its row. Find the box applicable to you and circle the large number in it. For example, if you are 37, circle the number in the box labeled 31-40.
After checking out all the rows, add the circled numbers. This total—your score— is an estimate of your risk.

IF YOU SCORE:
6-11 — Risk well below average
12-17 — Risk below average
18-24 — Risk generally average
25-31 — Risk moderate
32-40 — Risk at a dangerous level
41-62 — Danger urgent. See your doctor now.

HEREDITY:
Count parents, grand-parents, brothers, and sisters who have had heart attack and/or stroke.

TOBACCO SMOKING:
If you inhale deeply and smoke a cigarette way down, add one to your classification. Do NOT subtract because you think you do not inhale or smoke only a half inch on a cigarette.

EXERCISE:
Lower your score one point if you exercise regularly and frequently.

CHOLESTEROL OR SATURATED FAT INTAKE LEVEL:
A cholesterol blood level is best. If you can't get one from your doctor, then estimate honestly the percentage of solid fats you eat. These are usually of animal origin—lard, cream, butter, and beef and lamb fat. If you eat much of this, your cholesterol level probably will be high. The U.S. average, 40%, is too high for good health.

BLOOD PRESSURE:
If you have no recent reading but have passed an insurance or industrial examination, chances are you are 140 or less.

SEX:
This line takes into account the fact that men have from 6 to 10 times more heart attacks than women of child-bearing age.

Figure 16.7
The game of RISKO.
Copyright © Michigan Heart Association.

RISK FACTOR						
AGE	**1** 10 to 20	**2** 21 to 30	**3** 31 to 40	**4** 41 to 50	**6** 51 to 60	**8** 61 to 70 and over
HEREDITY	**1** No known history of heart disease	**2** 1 relative with cardiovascular disease Over 60	**3** 2 relatives with cardiovascular disease Over 60	**4** 1 relative with cardiovascular disease Under 60	**6** 2 relatives with cardiovascular disease Under 60	**7** 3 relatives with cardiovascular disease Under 60
WEIGHT	**0** More than 5 lbs. below standard weight	**1** -5 to +5 lbs. standard weight	**2** 6-20 lbs. over weight	**3** 21-35 lbs. over weight	**5** 36-50 lbs. over weight	**7** 51-65 lbs. over weight
TOBACCO SMOKING	**0** Nonuser	**1** Cigar and/or pipe	**2** 10 cigarettes or less a day	**4** 20 cigarettes a day	**6** 30 cigarettes a day	**10** 40 cigarettes a day or more
EXERCISE	**1** Intensive occupational and recreational exertion	**2** Moderate occupational and recreational exertion	**3** Sedentary work and intense recreational exertion	**5** Sedentary occupational and moderate exertion	**6** Sedentary work and light recreational exertion	**8** Constant lack of all exercise
CHOLESTEROL OR FAT % IN DIET	**1** Cholesterol below 180 mg.% Diet contains no animal or solid fats	**2** Cholesterol 181-205 mg.% Diet contains 10% animal or solid fats	**3** Cholesterol 206-230 mg.% Diet contains 20% animal or solid fats	**4** Cholesterol 321-255 mg.% Diet contains 30% animal or solid fats	**5** Cholesterol 258-280 mg.% Diet contains 40% animal or solid fats	**6** Cholesterol 281-300 mg.% Diet contains 50% animal or solid fats
BLOOD PRESSURE	**1** 100 upper reading	**2** 120 upper reading	**3** 140 upper reading	**4** 160 upper reading	**6** 180 upper reading	**8** 200 or over upper reading
SEX	**1** Female under 40	**2** Female 40-50	**3** Female over 50	**5** Male	**6** Stocky male	**7** Bald stocky male

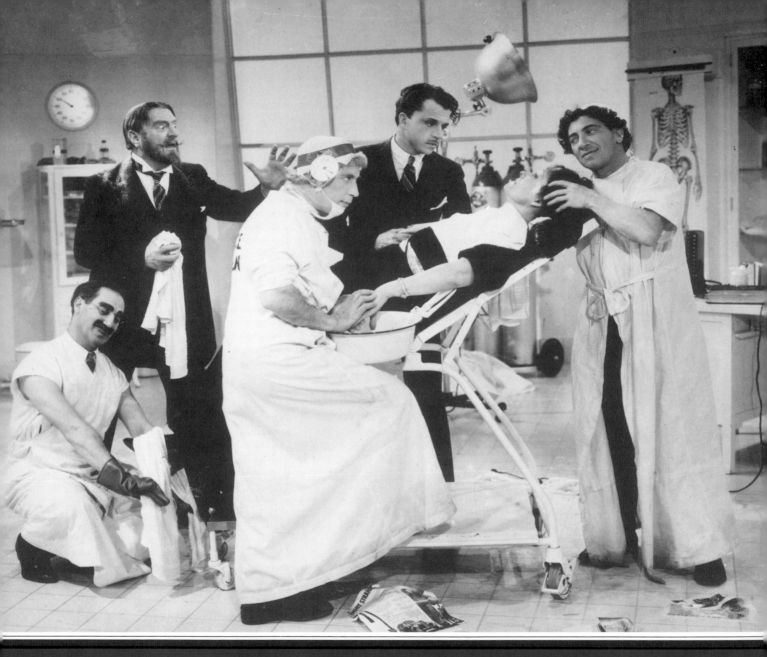

noncommunicable diseases

- *cancer*
- *diabetes mellitus*
- *disorders of the nervous system*
- *genetic diseases*
- *other noncommunicable diseases*

As we saw in Chapter 16, diseases of the cardiovascular system are the leading cause of death among adult Americans. When cancer is added to the list, we find that the cardiovascular diseases and cancer cause two of every three deaths in the United States (see Table 17.1). Although noncommunicable diseases occur more commonly among the older population, they are much more prevalent among children and young adults than most people realize. One way to reduce the incidence of some of these disorders later in life is to change one's living patterns, or lifestyle, at an early age.

A long life free from serious disease is not guaranteed to anyone. However, it is possible to minimize the risk of disease through proper diet, exercise, and avoidance of tobacco and alcohol. We will discuss these and other preventive measures in connection with particular diseases. This chapter attempts to provide you with a basic understanding of some of the major noncommunicable diseases, their prevention, and their treatment.

CANCER

> **Concept:** There are many forms of cancer, all of which can be labeled a disease of the body cells.

Cancer is not a single disease but rather a group of over 100 diseases involving abnormal cell growth. In normal body cells the rate of cell division is under precise control. Cancer cells, in contrast, grow wildly, divide rapidly, and assume irregular shapes; tumors develop and invade nearby normal tissue. These abnormal cells eventually spread to distant body areas via the blood and lymphatic system; this process of spreading is referred to as **metastasis.**

Cancer tumors may begin in epithelial cells, the cells that form the lining of the lungs, digestive organs, reproductive organs, and body cavities. These **carcinomas** tend to spread through the lymphatic system and can often be treated successfully if discovered early. A second major type of cancer arises from the cells that form the muscles, ligaments, and connective tissue. **Sarcomas,** as these are known, tend to spread through the blood stream and are more difficult to treat and control. Common sites for cancer and incidence by sex are shown in Fig. 17.1.

Discovery Activity 17.1
CANCER MISCONCEPTIONS

A complicated, baffling disease such as cancer is subject to considerable speculation and misinformation. To find out what you know about cancer, complete the following true–false test.

1. Cancer is contagious. T F
2. Cancer may be caused by a single injury to the body. T F
3. Use of aluminum cooking utensils causes cancer. T F
4. The chances of contracting cancer are increased by even light or moderate consumption of alcohol. T F
5. The use of synthetic or chemical fertilizers rather than organic types causes cancer. T F
6. Water fluoridation causes cancer. T F
7. Breast tumors are always malignant. T F
8. Vaccination for smallpox leaves one more susceptible to cancer. T F
9. Birth control pills cause cancer. T F
10. Cancer cannot be cured once it is discovered in the body. T F

Give yourself one point for each correct answer. If you marked all items false, you have a perfect score. Each of the statements is incorrect. ●

Table 17.1
MORTALITY FOR LEADING CAUSES OF DEATH: UNITED STATES, 1977

Rank	Cause of Death	Number of Deaths	Death Rate per 100,000 Population	Percent of Total Deaths
	All Causes	1,899,597	816.3	100.0
1	Diseases of heart	718,850	303.4	37.8
2	Cancer	386,686	168.4	20.4
3	Stroke	181,934	75.3	9.6
4	Accidents	103,202	45.4	5.4
5	Influenza and pneumonia	51,193	21.4	2.7
6	Diabetes mellitus	32,989	14.1	1.7
7	Cirrhosis of liver	30,848	14.0	1.6
8	Arteriosclerosis	28,754	12.0	1.5
9	Suicide	28,681	12.6	1.5
10	Diseases of infancy	23,401	13.0	1.2
11	Homicide	19,968	8.6	1.1
12	Emphysema	16,376	7.1	0.9
13	Congenital anomalies	12,983	6.8	0.7
14	Nephritis and nephrosis	8,519	3.7	0.5
15	Septicemia and pyemia	7,112	3.2	0.4
	Other and ill-defined	248,101	107.3	13.1

SOURCE: *Vital Statistics of the United States*, Washington, D.C., 1977

Figure 17.1
1981 estimates
SOURCE: American Cancer Society. Used by permission.

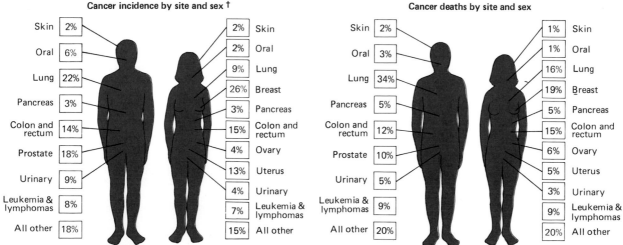

Cancer incidence by site and sex †

Skin 2%	2% Skin
Oral 6%	2% Oral
Lung 22%	9% Lung
	26% Breast
Pancreas 3%	3% Pancreas
Colon and rectum 14%	15% Colon and rectum
Prostate 18%	4% Ovary
	13% Uterus
Urinary 9%	4% Urinary
Leukemia & lymphomas 8%	7% Leukemia & lymphomas
All other 18%	15% All other

Cancer deaths by site and sex

Skin 2%	1% Skin
Oral 3%	1% Oral
Lung 34%	16% Lung
	19% Breast
Pancreas 5%	5% Pancreas
Colon and rectum 12%	15% Colon and rectum
Prostate 10%	6% Ovary
	5% Uterus
Urinary 5%	3% Urinary
Leukemia & lymphomas 9%	9% Leukemia & lymphomas
All other 20%	20% All other

†Excluding nonmelanoma skin cancer and carcinoma in situ.

399

Causes of Cancer

Concept: The immediate cause of the many different types of cancer is unknown.

Researchers theorize that cancer is produced from a basic change in the nucleic acid chain located in the nucleus of the cell. DNA (deoxyribonucleic acid) may control the rate of cell division. RNA (ribonucleic acid) appears to assist DNA with this control. It is believed that factors inside or outside the cell may act upon the DNA or RNA through a physical or chemical disturbance and result in abnormal, erratic cell division.

The World Health Organization estimates that up to 85 percent of all cancer cases are the result of exposure to environmental factors. Of the 1400 chemicals, drugs, and pollutants suspected of causing cancer, 22 have been declared carcinogenic to humans. Uncovering cancer-causing substances is no easy task and is complicated by three problems: The 20- to 35-year "latent" period between exposure and symptoms of the disease, the amount of exposure that produces cancer, and the controversy over whether animal test results can be applied to humans. Regardless of these obstacles, it is evident that the environment has become a major target of cancer researchers.

Concept: There are a number of agents that may attack the DNA and RNA within certain body cells and cause cancer.

Occupational agents. Certain physical and chemical environmental agents tend to contribute to cancer formation. In 1775 coal soot was identified as a contributor to cancer of the scrotum. One hundred years later, during the industrial revolution, a type of lubricating oil constantly sprinkled on men working beside cotton-spinning machines was linked to cancer of the scrotum. The air in mines contains a fine, radioactive dust, which can cause lung cancer in miners. During the 1920s bone cancer was observed in factory workers who painted numbers on the hands of watch faces with a radium compound to make the numbers

glow in the dark. By twirling the end of a fine brush in their mouths to acquire a "tip" before dipping the brush into the compound, the workers absorbed minute quantities of radium, which eventually worked into the bones.

Among the occupational agents suspected of contributing to cancer are asbestos, arsenic, tar, creosote oil, and crude paraffin oil. Asbestos chromate compounds, nickel carbonyl, tar fumes, and ionizing radiation (x rays and radium) increase the likelihood of cancer of the lungs. Nickel carbonyl, isopropyl oil, and radioactive dusts and gases are recognized as causes of cancer of the nasopharynx and sinuses. Aromatic amines (used in the manufacture of synthetic dyes) cause cancer of the bladder. Radioactive elements of radium and mesothorium produce sarcoma of the bone. Finally, benzene and ionizing radiations can cause the malignant disease of the blood-forming tissues (spleen, lymph nodes, bone marrow) called **leukemia.**

Environmental pollution. Many experts believe that some cancers are a product of our environment. Many blame high levels of hydrocarbons dumped into the air from automobiles and other vehicles for certain types of cancer. Absestos and radiation exposure, asphalt road and street surfaces, chemicals in some water supplies, some food additives or preservatives (such as nitrites), and insecticides are examples of contaminants that appear to have the potential to cause some types of cancer.

Pesticides are among many chemicals in the environment known to have carcinogenic properties.

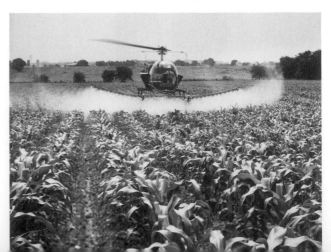

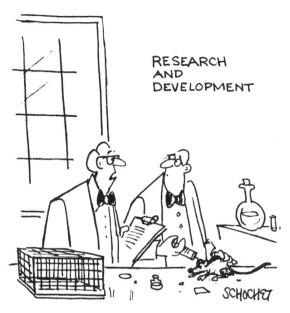

RESEARCH
AND
DEVELOPMENT

SCHOCHET

*"I think we should change our research
project to what doesn't cause cancer in rats."*

From *The Wall Street Journal.*
Permission-Cartoon Features Syndicate.

Scientists are concerned about an accumulative or multiplying effect from these environmental agents. Even if so-called safe levels are maintained, there may be an effect from daily exposure. There is evidence that some cancers develop after years of exposure to certain agents.

Chronic irritation or tissue damage.   Repeated low-grade tissue damage may lead to cancer. Gallstones on the lining of the gallbladder, some tissue injuries, a few chronic infections to certain organs, chronically infected scars (such as burn scars), repeated ulcerations, and bladder infections have been linked to cancer.

Viruses.   Some malignancies in animals may be caused by viral agents, and considerable research is underway to identify viruses related to cancer in human beings. Studies have linked acute leukemia, sarcoma,

and melanoma to viral agents. At one time it was believed that breast cancer might be caused by a virus; however, the majority of scientists today reject this view. As discussed in the next chapter, the virus known as herpes, type 2, has been linked to cancer of the cervix.

Radiation.   Rays of various types are known to cause leukemia and other forms of cancer, including thyroid and bone cancer. Repeated sunburn and overexposure to ultraviolet rays are the leading causes of skin cancer. Fair-complexioned individuals are much more vulnerable than those who have darker skin. In one experiment, nine out of 10 white rats exposed to the sun several hours daily for eight to 10 months developed skin cancer in areas where hair was sparse or absent.

X rays and radium rays can cause cancer. However, no evidence is available to link cosmic rays bombarding earth from outer space with cancer.

Skin cancer has been linked with prolonged exposure to the sun's ultraviolet rays.

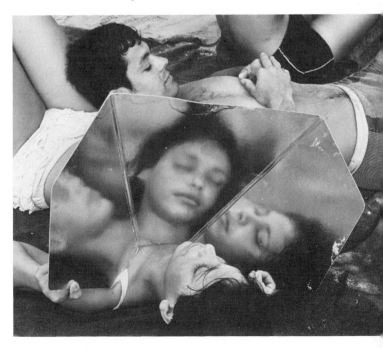

Issues in Health
ARE DIET AND NUTRITION RELATED TO CANCER?

In recent years researchers have advanced the theory that there is a connection between the foods we eat (in particular, cranberry juice, saccharin, and red food dye) and cancer. Many have noted that in cultures where the people have diets high in roughage there is an absence of cancer of the colon. Some have suggested that total absence of vitamin B (fresh fruits and vegetables) and protein from the diets of the South African Bantus and the inhabitants of Java is responsible for their high incidence of a type of liver cancer. Chemical substances added to food, candy, soft drinks, and other products for coloring, flavoring, sweetening, preserving, and moistening are suspected of causing cancer. Fatty diets have been linked to bowel and breast cancer; excessive alcohol to cancers of the mouth, throat, esophagus, larynx, and liver; and sodium nitrate and sodium nitrite (in bacon, ham, and smoked foods) to stomach cancer. The list goes on, and many believe that the link between diet and cancer is clear.

Despite these associations between cancer and a particular food or absence of food in the diet, there is no conclusive evidence that cancer of any type is actually caused by nutritional habits. No food dye or other additive certified for use in the United States has been shown to cause cancer in humans. Arsenic, found in traces in soil and in water, is related to some kinds of cancer. Eating a high number of calories (resulting in obesity) tends to be associated with cancer in mice.

Although a cause–effect relationship has yet to be shown, numerous studies have linked nutritional habits with certain types of cancer. Additional research is obviously needed.

What do you think? ●

Hereditary and congenital factors. Hereditary factors appear to be related to some cancers. For example, retinoblastoma, a malignant eye tumor occurring in infants and young children, has been found to be hereditary. More common, however, is a predisposition, or tendency, of members of a family to acquire a particular form of cancer. In some types of cancers, such as cancer of the breast, uterus, stomach, intestine, and colon, immediate family members face a greatly increased risk. However, it should be noted that a predisposition does not mean that a person will definitely develop the disease. It does mean that people in such families should be alert to signs of possible conditions, have regular checkups, and develop healthy eating and exercise patterns.

Congenital causes, or cancer occurring during the development of the embryo during the prenatal period, involve a few special groups of tumors affecting infants, children, and young adults. Congenital tumors (most are benign) account for only a small fraction of tumors and cancer.

Precancerous conditions. Some precancerous conditions—but not all—tend to develop into cancer, with the cause of cancer being the same as the cause for the precancerous condition. Benign tumors, a mass or overgrowth of cells in the mouth, lip, tongue, or cheek or a patch of cells on the skin (small scab, scaly patch, brown to black warts) fall into the category of precancerous conditions. Moles are not precancerous, and the average person has about 22 to 23 of them. A mole that is constantly irritated is much more likely to become malignant. Benign tumors should be removed as soon as possible, regardless of how low the probability of developing cancer is.

Tobacco use. There is a strong link between tobacco use and lung cancer; cancer of the lip and mouth; and cancer of the larynx, esophagus, pancreas, and bladder. The incidence of lung cancer is related to the number of cigarettes smoked, the degree of inhalation, and the number of years one has smoked. Giving up smoking at any time in one's life greatly reduces the risk of cancer. After 15 years as a nonsmoker, one's risk is identical to that of a person who has never smoked. The risk of developing lung cancer from pipe and cigar smoking is smaller than for cigarette smoking but much higher than for the nonsmoking population.

Individual susceptibility. The known and suspected causes of cancer discussed in this section account for only some of the cases of cancer that develop. Also, most people who are exposed even to recognized carcinogens do not develop cancer. It therefore appears that there exists within the living organism a quality of individual susceptibility. That susceptibility seems to be related to personality factors. A "cancer personality" has been identified, which is characterized as depressed, rigid, self-condemning, and unable to develop meaningful relationships with others. Scientists theorize that some people with this personality pattern are unable to release their pent-up feelings and turn them inward, thereby disrupting their hormonal levels or other aspects of metabolism. This theory is becoming an important focus of research.

Some Common Cancers and Their Detection

A list of seven warning signals for cancer has been developed by the American Cancer Society (see Table 17.2). These symptoms may be an indication of other, less serious ailments. Nonetheless, they should be brought to the attention of a physician immediately.

Early detection requires that you become alert to changes in your body and see a physician if you experience any of the seven warning signals. For people without symptoms of cancer, the American Cancer Society has developed guidelines for cancer-related checkups by age (see Table 17.3).

Concept: Suspected cancer at different sites requires different diagnostic procedures.

Pancreatic cancer now kills more than 20,000 Americans annually—double the rate of 20 years ago. Several chemical agents (cleaners, gasoline), as well as tobacco, coffee, alcohol, and tea, have been sus-

Table 17.2
SEVEN WARNING SIGNALS FOR CANCER

Warning Signals for Cancer
1. Unusual bleeding or discharge
2. A lump or thickening in the breast or elsewhere
3. A sore that does not heal
4. Persistent change in bowel or bladder habits
5. Persistent hoarseness or cough
6. Persistent indigestion or difficulty in swallowing
7. Change in a wart or mole

pected. Preliminary data of the type that first established the relationship between lung cancer and cigarette smoking have linked coffee to pancreatic cancer. A Harvard research team suggests that as much as one-half of all cases may be caused by coffee consumption of two cups or more per day. Pancreatic cancer is difficult to diagnose in its early stages and progresses rapidly, with few individuals surviving more than three years.

Cancer of the testis afflicts approximately 3500 men each year. It is most often found in men aged 20 to 35 and is the most common tumor in men aged 20 to 25. Testicular cancer is more likely to occur in men whose testes never descend to the scrotum or descend after the age of six. Testicular cancer is more common in white males, with the incidence in blacks and Orientals very low. The most common sign is a pea-sized lump, usually painless in the early stages. Other symptoms include enlargement of a testicle, a heavy feeling, accumulation of fluid, or blood in the scrotum. Testicular cancer is curable in most cases if treated early. Regular self-examination of the testicles (see Fig. 17.2 on page 405) is the most common and effective means of early detection.

Cancer of the prostate is prevalent in men over 55 years of age. Blood in the urine or in the ejaculate can be a sign, but more often such symptoms indicate a bacterial infection of the prostate or bladder.

Skin cancer, which generally affects the face, neck, and hands, is easy to diagnose and treat. Yet more than

Table 17.3
GUIDELINES FOR THE EARLY DETECTION OF CANCER IN PEOPLE WITHOUT SYMPTOMS.

Age 20–40	Age 40 and Over
Cancer-related checkup every 3 years	*Cancer-related checkup every year*
Should include the procedures listed below plus health counseling (such as tips on quitting cigarettes) and examinations for cancers of the thyroid, testes, prostate, mouth, ovaries, skin and lymph nodes. Some people are at higher risk for certain cancers and may need to have tests more frequently.	Should include the procedures listed below plus health counseling (such as tips on quitting cigarettes) and examinations for cancers of the thyroid, testes, prostate, mouth, ovaries, skin and lymph nodes. Some people are at higher risk for certain cancers and may need to have tests more frequently.
Breast <ul><li>Exam by doctor every 3 years</li><li>Self-exam every month</li><li>One baseline breast X-ray between ages 35–40. Higher Risk for Breast Cancer: Personal or family history of breast cancer, never had children, first child after 30</li></ul>	*Breast* <ul><li>Exam by doctor every year</li><li>Self-exam every month</li><li>Breast X-ray every year after 50 (between ages 40–50, ask your doctor) Higher Risk for Breast Cancer: Personal or family history of breast cancer, never had children, first child after 30)</li></ul>
Uterus <ul><li>Pelvic exam every 3 years</li></ul> *Cervix* <ul><li>Pap test—*after 2 initial negative tests 1 year apart*—at *least* every 3 years, includes women under 20 if sexually active. Higher Risk for Cervical Cancer: Early age at first intercourse, multiple sex partners</li></ul>	*Uterus* <ul><li>Pelvic exam every year</li></ul> *Cervix* <ul><li>Pap test—*after 2 initial negative tests 1 year apart*—at *least* every 3 years Higher Risk for Cervical Cancer: Early age at first intercourse, multiple sex partners</li></ul> *Endometrium* <ul><li>Endometrial tissue sample at menopause if at risk Higher Risk for Endometrial Cancer: Infertility, obesity, failure of ovulation, abnormal uterine bleeding, estrogen therapy</li></ul>
	Colon and rectum <ul><li>Digital rectal exam every year</li><li>Guaiac slide test every year after 50</li><li>Procto exam—*after 2 initial negative tests 1 year apart*—every 3 to 5 years after 50 Higher Risk for Colorectal Cancer: Personal or family history of colon or rectal cancer, personal or family history of polyps in the colon or rectum, ulcerative colitis</li></ul>

Remember, these guidelines are not rules and apply only to people without symptoms. If you have any of the 7 Warning Signals, see your doctor or go to your clinic without delay.

SOURCE: American Cancer Society, Inc., 1980. Used by permission.

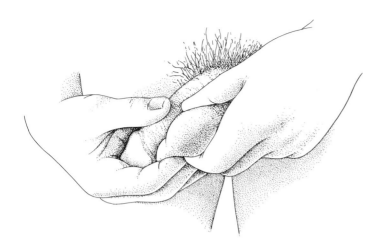

Figure 17.2
The best time to examine the testes is right after a hot bath or shower. Heat causes the testicles to descend and the scrotal skin to relax, making it easier to find unusual lumps. Each testicle is examined by placing the index and middle fingers of both hands on the underside of the testicle and the thumbs on the top. Gently roll your testicle between your thumb and fingers, feeling for small lumps. Changes or anything abnormal will appear at the front or side of your testicle.
SOURCE: American Cancer Society. Used by permission.

4000 people die unnecessarily from skin cancer each year, even though early diagnosis and treatment would almost certainly result in cure or control.

Lung cancer is difficult to diagnose in time for effective treatment, because the usual procedures call for X ray and examination of a portion of lung tissue. Persistent hoarseness, coughing, and spitting of blood are some of the more overt symptoms. In some cases, few symptoms appear until it is too late for treatment. Approximately 4 percent of males and 8 percent of females recover fully.

Stomach cancer has decreased by 40 percent in the past 25 years. Common symptoms include persistent indigestion and blood discharge with bowel movements.

Leukemia remains a leading cause of death in children aged 4 to 14. Affecting the blood-manufacturing organs, bone marrow, spleen, and lymph glands, this form of cancer is uncovered by blood analysis to detect large numbers of white blood cells or immature white cells.

Cancer of the lymph glands (Hodgkin's disease) generally strikes young adults aged 20 to 40. A common symptom is enlarged lymph glands over a period of several weeks.

Cancer of the colon or rectum may produce early symptoms, such as blood in stools (bright red or black) or changes in bowel habits (diarrhea or constipation,

abdominal discomfort or pain). Among the various diagnostic procedures available, a physician can feel for a tumor in the rectum, use a proctosigmoidoscope to see the lower 10 to 12 inches of the intestine, examine X rays of the large intestine following a barium enema, biopsy (examine microscopically) suspected tissue, examine the stools, or use a colonoscope to view the entire colon.

Bone cancer refers to malignant tumors developing in the skeletal system. The most noticeable symptom is pain, particularly pain that tends to worsen at night. The knee, thigh, upper arm, ribs, and pelvis are the most common sites of persistent pain. Swelling and fever may also be present.

Breast cancer is a leading cause of cancer deaths among women, in spite of the fact that early detection through breast self-examination is a rather simple procedure. Single women and married women who do not breast-feed their babies have the highest incidence of breast cancer. Symptoms include lumps or thickening in the breast, bleeding from the nipple, and swollen lymph nodes under the armpit. Most lumps in the breast are not cancerous; however, any lump should be carefully examined by a physician. Breast self-examination should take place monthly one week after the end of the menstrual period. It is important to complete the examination at the same time each month. Figure 17.3 shows how to perform a breast self-examination.

1. In the Shower. Examine your breasts during your bath or shower, since hands glide more easily over wet skin. Hold your fingers flat and move them gently over every part of each breast. Use the right hand to examine the left breast and the left hand for the right breast. Check for any lump, hard knot, or thickening.

2. Before a mirror. Inspect your breasts with arms at your sides. Next, raise your arms high overhead. Look for any changes in the contour of each breast: a swelling, dimpling of skin, or changes in the nipple.

Then rest your palms on your hips and press down firmly to flex your chest muscles. Left and right breast will not exactly match—few women's breasts do. Again, look for changes and irregularities. Regular inspection shows what is normal for

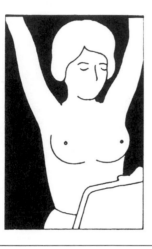
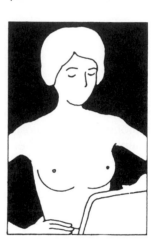

Figure 17.3
Breast self-examination.

Cervical cancer is now easily detected by the **Pap smear,** a microscopic examination of cells scraped from the cervix and body of the uterus. An estimated 54,000 new invasive cases of cervical cancer were reported in 1981, including 16,000 cases of cancer of the cervix and 38,000 cases of cancer of the endometrium (lining of the uterus). The death rate from cervical cancer has decreased more than 70 percent during the last 40 years, due mainly to the Pap test and regular checkups. Unusual bleeding or discharge may be early warning signals. Risk factors include first intercourse at an early age; multiple sex partners; history of infertility; failure to ovulate; estrogen therapy; late menopause; and a combination of diabetes, high blood pressure, and obesity. Figure 17.4 shows normal and cancer cells taken in Pap smears.

Treatment of Cancer

Concept: Cancer treatment involves surgery, radiation, or chemotherapy, or some combination of these procedures.

Cure rates for cancer have improved dramatically in the last generation. Whereas 30 years ago only 25 percent of cancer patients survived for five years (the cri-

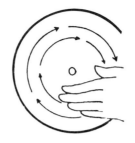

you and will give you confidence in your examination.

3. Lying down. To examine your right breast, put a pillow or folded towel under your right shoulder. Place your right hand behind your head; this distributes breast tissue more evenly on the chest. With the left hand, fingers flat, press gently in small circular motions around an imaginary clock face. Begin at outermost top of your right breast for 12 o'clock, then move to 1 o'clock, and so on around the circle back to 12. (A ridge of firm tissue in the lower curve of each breast is normal.)

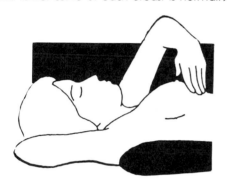

Then move 1 inch inward, toward the nipple and keep circling to examine every part of your breast, including the nipple. This requires at least three more circles. Now slowly repeat the procedure on your left breast with a pillow under your left shoulder and left hand behind your head. Notice how your breast structure feels.

Finally, squeeze the nipple of each breast gently between the thumb and index finger. Any discharge, clear or bloody, should be reported to your doctor immediately.

[1]From the American Cancer Society. Used by permission.

SOURCE: American Cancer Society. Used by permission.

terion used to define "cure") after treatment without recurrence of the disease, the overall cure rate today is 40 percent. Even more dramatic improvement in the survival rates for various cancers has occurred during the past decade, thanks to advances in chemotherapy (see Table 17.4 on page 408).

The three main forms of treatment for cancer are radiation, surgery, and chemotherapy. The choice of treatment (or treatments) depends upon the type of cancer and the extent to which it has spread. For example, surgery is most successful at treating cancers that have not spread beyond the original site, whereas chemotherapy and radiation are used to treat cancers that have spread into different areas of the body.

Radiation treatment involves using X rays, radium, and the betatron. Cancer cells are more vulnerable than healthy cells to X rays and radium. The ideal dosage would destroy cancer cells with minimal damage to normal cells. Often, however, the dose required to destroy cancer cells permanently damages surrounding normal cells. Some kinds of cancer can be entirely destroyed using radiation. High-voltage X rays have proved successful in treating cancer, as have streams of electrical charges from the atom-smashing betatron.

About six radioactive isotopes have been useful in treating cancer. Radioactive cobalt has been used with about as much success as supervoltage x rays. Isotopes ingested into the body by drinking the chemicals at-

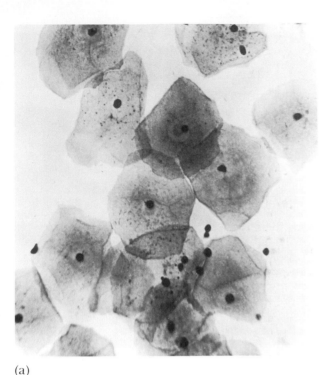

(a)

(b)

Figure 17.4
Normal (a) and cancer cells (b) taken in Pap smears of the cervix.
SOURCE: National Institutes of Health.

Table 17.4
THE ODDS ON SURVIVAL

Type of Cancer	1970	1980 (projected)
Hodgkin's disease	61%	80%
Lung	10	15
Breast		
Local	86	90
Disseminated	58	73
Stomach	12	20
Bladder	65	70
Colon	47	52
Prostate	60	65
Testicular	68	90
Uterine	69	73
Melanoma (skin)	70	75
Leukemia		
Chronic	35	40
Acute adult	3	15
Childhood	3	15

Note: Data apply to whites only and show five-year survival rates. Black patients average 5 to 10 percent lower survival rates for tumors, evidently because of delayed treatment.

tempt to single out malignant tissue and destroy it. Because only a few radioactive isotopes have been successful in doing this, isotopes play only a small part in cancer treatment at present.

Chemotherapy is a treatment that uses chemicals (drugs) to seek out and attack cancer cells. More than 25 drugs have been identified that will poison cancer cells and stop or slow their growth; all damage normal cells and cannot be used indefinitely. In addition, most of the drugs have serious side effects. The control of hormones in the body has been used with varying degrees of success in treating breast cancer and prostate cancer.

Recent Advances in Cancer Treatment

In recent years, dramatic advances have taken place in the area of chemotherapy. **Immunotherapy,** the stimulation of the body's own defense systems to attack cancer cells, appears to be a promising approach. Studies of **interferon,** a natural antiviral substance, are underway. Investigators believe that interferon fastens to cells and causes the release of enzymes that inhibit growth. Until recently, natural interferon could only be extracted in minute quantities from donated white blood cells. Today, however, enough interferon is now being produced in laboratories to permit an extensive study. **Monoclonal antibodies** represent perhaps the most promising immunological approach. These are antibodies made in the laboratory to seek out and react with malignant cells. It is hoped that they can be used to transport drugs or radioactive isotopes to tumors without harming healthy tissues.

Approved and experimental anticancer drugs fall into four main categories. *Alkylating agents* (Cytoxan, L-PAM, Myleran) interfere with the orderly pairing process to prevent successful cell division and inhibit cancer growth. *Antimetabolites* (methotrexate, 5-FU, and 6-mercaptopurine) are absorbed by the cell and disrupt its metabolic machinery. *Antibiotics* (bleomycin and Adriamycin) disrupt the synthesis of RNA, a substance

A young cancer patient undergoes chemotherapy.

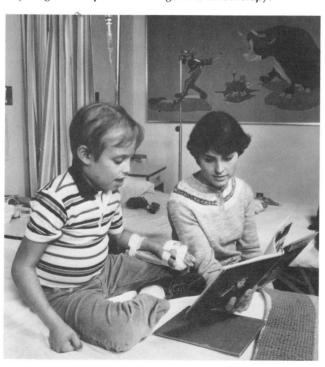

Issues in Health
SHOULD LAETRILE BE LEGAL?

Laetrile is a substance that falls on the borderline between a nutrient and a drug. Laetrile is purified from apricot pits and was originally packaged as a health food with the number 17 on the box. It later acquired the name B_{17}, as though it were a vitamin.

In laetrile clinics, such as the Contreras Clinic in Tijuana, Mexico, cancer patients receive several injections of laetrile daily and are told to stop all other medication for a complete cure. Laetrile, they are told, breaks down into several components when inside the human body. One of these components, a cyanide poison, chokes off the cancerous tumor. One investigator (reported in *Time Magazine*, April 12, 1971) has also claimed that cancer may be due to a nutritional deficiency and that the missing ingredient is laetrile. Prolaetrile groups argue that the cancer victim has the right to use any treatment that offers even the slightest hope of a cure. Of the more than 50,000 cancer patients who have received treatment in a clinic or through consumption of illegally purchased laetrile, some have given testimony of complete cures.

Opponents of laetrile argue that it is a toxicant because it contains the poison cyanide, and that it is not effective in cancer treatment. Autopsies have shown a progression of cancer in individuals treated with laetrile injections. Another argument against the legalization of laetrile is that it may sidetrack the cancer victim from getting proven, effective treatment. Hope of a miracle cure can delay needed early treatment, such as surgery, until the disease spreads to other body parts and is inoperable. Cancer can go into a state of remission, which may explain so-called cures following laetrile treatment. There are no documented five-year studies to support the effectiveness of laetrile as a cancer cure. Unless such studies are forthcoming, laetrile should not be legalized.

What do you think? ●

the cell needs to make essential proteins. *Steroids* (prednisone and estrogen) are thought to prevent the production of proteins or other key enzymes.

Most drugs must be given intravenously to avoid damage to the stomach or destruction by digestive enzymes. Additional research is also needed to determine the most effective way to use the arsenal of new drugs. The search continues for drugs that destroy cancer cells and leave normal cells unharmed, avoiding the side effects of chemotherapy, such as nausea, loss of appetite, hair loss, diarrhea, destruction of white blood cells, and damage to the heart muscle and nerve tissue. Unfortunately, drugs free of these side effects have not yet been found, although some drugs can be used to attenuate certain side effects. Marijuana derivates and other drugs can be used to control nausea, Adriamycin can help prevent hair loss, and transfusions of platelets and white cells help maintain the body's defense system.

Reducing the Risk of Getting Cancer

To date, there is no guaranteed way either to prevent or treat most cancer. This does not mean, however, that one should not try to reduce the risks. Enough evidence is now available in some areas to suggest certain precautions that should be taken throughout life:

1. Memorize the seven cancer danger signals and be alerted to these changes in your body.

2. Abstain from using tobacco.

3. Learn the breast self-examination technique (females), and use this method monthly.

4. Learn the testicular self-examination technique (males), and use this method monthly.

5. Examine your skin periodically for moles, lumps, and sores.

6. Avoid contact with known carcinogens whenever possible.

7. Maintain a healthy body at all times through proper eating, sleeping, hygiene, and exercise habits as outlined in Part III.

8. Avoid lowering your body resistance by "crash" dieting or placing unusually heavy demands on your body for prolonged periods of time.

9. Report any family history of cancer to your doctor.

Not all of the above suggestions can be substantiated by research, but all have implications for improved general health and early detection.

DIABETES MELLITUS

> **Concept:** Diabetes mellitus is a metabolic disorder that interferes with the body's ability to use glucose.

Diabetes is caused by insufficient production of the hormone **insulin** in the pancreas. All carbohydrates must be transformed into glucose before they can be used as energy. Lack of insulin interferes with the body's ability to use carbohydrates. When the body can no longer use glucose efficiently, the blood sugar level becomes extremely high, a condition called **hyperglycemia.** Without proper control, serious complications may develop. Some of the more common problems of untreated diabetes include vascular disease leading to heart attacks, heart pain, heart failure, strokes, senility, gangrene of the feet, blindness from damage to the arteries in the retina; liver and kidney damage, nerve damage, foot and leg ulcers, and susceptibility to infections.

With too much insulin in the blood, **insulin shock** may occur. The diabetic becomes very weak, skin is moist and pale, and tremors or convulsions may occur. Sugar (orange juice, soft drinks, granulated sugar on the tongue) can be given if the diabetic is conscious; sugar cubes can be rubbed on the tongue of the unconscious victim.

With insufficient insulin in the blood, generally caused by excessive ingestion of carbohydrates, **diabetic coma** may occur. The victim may have a fever, appear extremely ill, complain of intense thirst, and vomit. An acetone odor may be present on the breath. It is imperative that you call an ambulance or a doctor.

The victim should be kept lying down flat and covered with a blanket until a physician arrives. Fluids may be given to a conscious victim, providing they do not contain sugar or starches.

Diabetes may occur in childhood or adolescence (juvenile diabetes); the average age is 10 to 12 years. Juvenile diabetes is caused by a severe deficit in the synthesis of insulin by the pancreas. Adult diabetes is common in obese individuals over the age of 40. This form is caused by insufficient insulin rather than lack of insulin and is rarely as severe as juvenile diabetes.

Some of the more easily recognized symptoms of diabetes include excessive thirst and urination, unexplained weight loss, slow healing of cuts and bruises, excessive hunger, low energy level, intense itching, changes in vision, chronic skin infections, and pain in the extremities. If you possess any of these symptoms, see your physician immediately. Urine analysis will determine whether further tests are needed.

Factors in Developing Diabetes

Concept: Even with the hereditary tendency, diabetes may be prevented.

There is a genetic tendency to develop diabetes. One of every four people is a carrier of this tendency. The individual carrier does not have and will not develop diabetes. Being a carrier of the diabetic trait means that some close relative has or had diabetes. Possessing the diabetic trait means that at some time in one's life, some evidence of diabetes may develop. The genetic pattern can be predicted:

If both parents are diabetic, all their children will have the diabetic trait. If both parents are nondiabetic, none of their children will have the diabetic trait.

If one parent is diabetic and the other is a carrier, the probability that any one child will have the diabetic trait will be one in two.

If both parents are carriers, the probability that any one child will have the diabetic trait will be one in four.

If one parent is nondiabetic and the other is a carrier, it is unlikely that any of the children will have the trait.

If one parent is diabetic and the other is nondiabetic, the probability that any one child will have the trait will be one in four.

Possessing the diabetic trait is not the only determining factor. In studies of identical twins, researchers have noted that one may acquire diabetes much sooner in life than the other. Prevention centers around a number of factors. Because obesity is the single most common nongenetic factor, weight control is essential. In addition, infectious illnesses, accidental wounds, surgery, psychic stress, and emotional shock frequently seem to trigger diabetes in individuals who have the trait. Healthy eating habits and regular exercise aid in prevention by using calories and decreasing the need for insulin, preventing obesity, and lowering blood fat levels. Clearly, then, keeping in good physical condition is quite important. If insulin is needed, the level of exercise and diet should be consistent. Unaccustomed strenuous exercise will decrease the insulin needed and may cause insulin reaction. The diet described below for the diabetic should also be used as a preventive approach for those who may possess the diabetic trait.

Managing Diabetes

Concept: Proper management and control of juvenile diabetes requires some lifestyle changes.

Once a diagnosis of juvenile diabetes is confirmed, a few changes are needed immediately, but there is no reason why one's life must be drastically altered. Although there is no special diabetic diet, it is necessary to eat well-balanced meals with all the essential vitamins and minerals. Obesity must be eliminated, and this may erase many or all of the symptoms. The diet should be designed by a physician. Regular exercise is important in regulating body weight and blood fat levels and in decreasing the body's need for insulin.

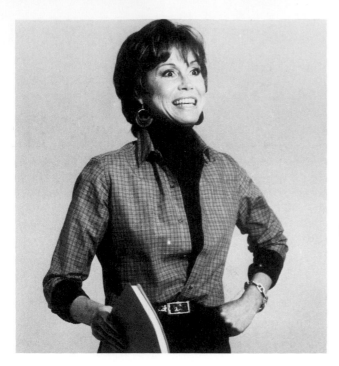

Careful control of her diabetes has enabled actress Mary Tyler Moore to pursue an active career.

Diabetics should stop smoking tobacco immediately. It has been found that they are already prone to heart disease and should avoid the added risk. In addition, smoking is a factor in stimulating blockage of circulation in the legs.

Diabetics should wear an identification bracelet that can be noticed easily. A bracelet with a warning phrase will guarantee proper diagnosis or treatment. In case of diabetic coma, the inscription can list the medicines one is taking, including the amount of insulin.

DISORDERS OF THE NERVOUS SYSTEM

There is much to be learned about the functioning of the brain and nervous system. Disorders of the nervous system are difficult to diagnose and treat. In addition, the causes of many disorders remain elusive. This section covers several of the better known disorders.

Epilepsy

There are many misconceptions about epilepsy. As a result, it is a disorder that many people fear unnecessarily. Before reading on, complete Activity 17.2, *What Do You Know about Epilepsy?*

Discovery Activity 17.2
WHAT DO YOU KNOW ABOUT EPILEPSY?

Epilepsy victims suffer considerable discrimination from a misinformed public. Circle each question True or False to rate your knowledge of this illness.

1. Epilepsy, if untreated, will lead to insanity. True False

2. A bystander should place an object between the teeth of a victim of convulsions in order to prevent the tongue from being swallowed. True False

3. It is important to prevent or restrain the jerking and rigidity of muscle groups that can occur during a seizure. True False

4. The best thing for a bystander to do for a person suffering a seizure is nothing. True False

5. Bystanders should attempt to make a person "walk it off" after suffering a grand mal seizure. True False

6. All seizures are indicative of epilepsy. True False

7. Epilepsy cannot occur after age 18. True False

8. Epilepsy is hereditary. True False

9. In most instances, epileptic seizures cannot be controlled. True False

Check your answers on page 414.

Recurrent seizures from any cause can be termed **epilepsy.** This condition affects approximately 0.5 percent of the population. The exact causes are unknown, although some factors have been identifed. Seizures of unknown cause generally appear from age 3 to 15. Seizures before age 2 are related to developmental defects, birth injuries, or metabolic diseases affecting the brain. Seizures appearing for the first time after age 25 generally are a result of cerebral trauma, tumors, or organic brain disease.

Five basic types of epileptiform attacks can be distinguished, each with unique traits and symptoms. The *grand mal* is of the *focal* or *jacksonian* seizure type, or the typical grand mal. Jacksonian seizures may begin in one part of the body and gradually move upward to other body parts. A so-called aura, referred to as a warning of an oncoming seizure, is actually part of the seizure. The aura directs attention to the portion of the brain where the attack originates. Loss of consciousness may or may not occur with this type. The *typical grand mal* may involve a cry; loss of consciousness; falling; and contractions of the muscles of the arms, legs, trunk, and head. The attack lasts between two and five minutes and may be followed by a deep sleep, soreness, and headache. Attacks can occur at any age and are often associated with organic brain disease.

Petit mal attacks usually involve some clouding of consciousness for 1 to 30 seconds, after which the patient recovers rather rapidly. Petit mal attacks are more common in children and often outgrown by midadolescence. Attacks may occur several times daily, generally when at rest. Seizures during exercise are rare.

Psychomotor attacks are usually minor seizures of one to two minutes in duration. The patient may stagger around and perform automatic movements, make unintelligible sounds, lose contact with the environment, and suffer mental confusion for a short period after the seizure ends. Psychomotor attacks are associated with brain damage and can occur at any age.

Treatment varies with the specific type of attack and may take the form of (1) eliminating the causative or precipitating factors (infections, endocrine abnormalities), (2) proper care during a convulsion, (3) maintaining emotional balance by leading a normal life, and (4) drug therapy. It is important that people understand this disorder. Epilepsy is in no way associated with mental illness, feeblemindedness, or intelligence.

Multiple Sclerosis

Concept: Multiple sclerosis is a progressive disease of the central nervous system that generally appears between the ages of 20 and 40.

Both the cause and the cure of **multiple sclerosis (MS)** are unknown, although recent findings suggest that a delayed action virus may be the cause. The disease affects the myelin sheath of the nerves. This sheath insulates nerve fibers and prevents the overflow and loss of nerve impulses. Many different (multiple) parts of the nervous system are attacked and left with scars (sclerosis).

Some minor symptoms may appear and disappear months or years before the disease is recognized. Minor visual disturbances, stiffness or fatigue in a limb, occasional dizziness, and mild emotional disturbances are some of the early warning signs. After diagnosis, the disease progresses differently from individual to individual; it is slow in some and more rapid in others; attacks are frequent in some, infrequent with many remissions in others. In the more advanced stages, the victim may experience partial or complete paralysis, numbness, double vision, slurring of speech, general weakness, loss of bowel control, and difficulty in swallowing. Life expectancy is shortened, although it is difficult to predict how the disease will progress in different individuals. Multiple sclerosis is uncommon in the subtropics, but moving to such a climate fails to slow the progress of the disease.

Cerebral Palsy

Concept: Cerebral palsy of children affects the motor area of the brain, leaving victims unable to control the voluntary muscles of the body.

There are more than half a million victims of **cerebral palsy** in the United States. The exact cause of this disease is unknown; however, some factors have been

Answers to Self-Test on Epilepsy

1. False. This myth developed many years before modern medicine determined what epilepsy is. Epilepsy will not lead to insanity.

2. False. It is difficult to open the jaws of a person having a grand mal seizure, and an object could damage the interior of the mouth. It is also impossible to swallow your tongue.

3. False. The more a person is restricted, the greater the chance of a repeat seizure of greater magnitude.

4. True. You need only protect the victim from being injured by objects in the room and from other well-meaning bystanders.

5. False. It is best to allow the victim to sleep as long as he or she desires and avoid talking about the seizure unless the victim initiates the discussion.

6. False. Factors such as illness and poison contribute to seizures.

7. False. Epilepsy can occur at any age; however, among adults it is often brought on by a head injury.

8. False. The likelihood that any epileptic will have a child who will become epileptic is very slim.

9. False. Medication greatly reduces the incidence of seizures. ●

isolated. Among those known to be related are rubella (German measles) when contracted during the first three months of pregnancy, birth trauma, anoxia (lack of oxygen), Rh factors, and possibly heredity.

Symptoms of the disease may be present from birth. In less severe cases, symptoms may not appear until the child fails to perform certain developmental tasks, such as sitting, crawling, walking, or talking. The *spastic* and *athetoid* types of cerebral palsy represent about 80 percent of the cases. Spastics experience muscle tenseness and excessive muscle contractions, which in turn make coordinated movements difficult. Symptoms of the athetoid type include slow, involuntary movements. A third type, *ataxia,* is characterized by difficulty with balance and frequent falls. Mixtures of the three basic types are common.

There is no sure means of preventing cerebral palsy. However, because factors related to pregnancy and birth are implicated in the disease, rubella screening in the mother is essential. In addition, steps should be taken to assure adequate oxygen to the baby during delivery.

GENETIC DISEASES

Diseases are passed on through the genes in one of four patterns: **dominant inheritance** (harmful gene is dominant and can be transmitted by only one parent), **recessive inheritance** (harmful gene is recessive and two genes, one from each parent, are necessary to transmit the gene), **sex-linked inheritance** (the female X chromosome carries the bad gene and the male child is affected), and **polygenic** or **(multifactorial) inheritance** (the interaction of several genes, with or without the influence of environmental factors, causes the defect). Some inherited diseases are evident at birth (PKU or cystic fibrosis); others show up during infancy (Tay-Sachs), during the teenage years (familial hypercholesterolemia), or in adulthood. There are over 300 inherited diseases. Most are considered inborn errors of metabolism or chemical mistakes. Some of the more common inherited disorders follow.

Sickle-Cell Anemia

Concept: Sickle-cell anemia is a hereditary disease affecting only the black population.

Approximately 2 out of every 25 black people carry the trait for **sickle-cell anemia,** although only 1 out of every 400 actually has the disease. When both parents are carriers, the probability is that of every four children, one will possess sickle-cell anemia, two will be

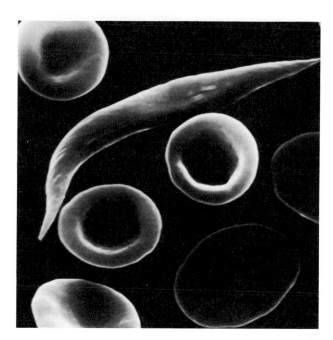

A red blood cell characteristic of sickle-cell anemia, surrounded by normal red cells. The elongated abnormal cell cannot transport oxygen efficiently.

carriers, and one will have neither the disease nor the trait. The Sickledex test lends itself to mass-screening methods. A positive reaction to the test means the person either carries the trait or possesses the disease. Further tests are then needed to confirm the disease.

In sickle-cell anemia, the abnormal structure of the hemoglobin causes red blood cells (oxygen carrying) to pucker and assume a sickle shape. These cells have difficulty passing through capillary walls and at times pile up to block the flow of blood to body tissues. In addition, because these cells possess a life span of 30 to 40 days, rather than the normal 120 days, they are easily destroyed. New cells are not produced as fast as old cells are destroyed, and anemia results. The so-called sickle-cell crisis results when blood flow to normal tissues is hampered from a blockage and excessive cell destruction occurs, causing severe pain, anemia, weakness, nausea, and jaundice.

Treatment methods have improved tremendously in past years. The disease is most severe in the young and much less so after adolescence. Most therapy focuses upon treating the symptoms. Patients should avoid high altitudes and unpressurized planes, because lower oxygen tension increases the sickling tendency.

Muscular Dystrophy

Concept: Muscular dystrophy is a hereditary disease characterized by weakness due to degeneration of muscle fibers.

Approximately 200,000 persons (half of them between the ages of 4 and 15) are afflicted with some form of **muscular dystrophy.** The causes have not been uncovered to date. The pattern of inheritance is sex linked and recessive. In one form, affecting only boys and involving pelvic-girdle weaknesses, symptoms of the disease tend to appear as the child starts to walk. Waddling, toe-walking, frequent falling, and difficulty in getting up occur at this stage, with symptoms progressing until adolescence, when the patient is usually confined to a wheelchair. In another form, affecting both sexes, the disease starts later in life, generally during adolescence. Progression of symptoms is slower and more variable from one patient to another. Some become disabled, whereas others are barely aware of symptoms throughout life. Because there is no known drug therapy, treatment focuses on physical therapy.

Down's Syndrome

Concept: Down's syndrome (formerly called mongolism) is a form of physical and mental retardation caused by abnormal chromosome formation.

One in 600 American babies born each year has **Down's syndrome.** This condition is caused by chromosome abnormality in which the individual possesses three instead of the normal two twenty-first chromosomes. Down's syndrome is much more common in children born to women over the age of 40 than it is in children born to younger women. For example, the risk of a

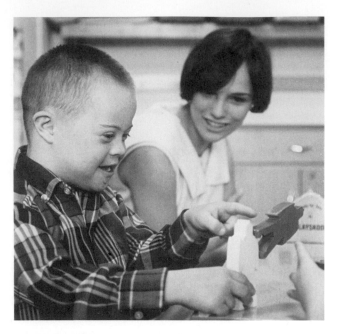

Down's syndrome is a genetic disorder that results in mental retardation and characteristic physical defects.

woman's giving birth to an infant with Down's syndrome is about 1 in 3000 prior to age 30, 1 in 300 at age 35, 1 in 60 at age 40, and about 1 in 40 over age 45.

Individuals with Down's syndrome exhibit such physical defects as slanted eyes, facial deformities, and short legs and torso. Mild to severe mental retardation occurs.

Down's syndrome can be detected by **amniocentesis,** in which amniotic fluid is extracted from the pregnant woman's uterus and analyzed. This procedure is recommended for all pregnant women over the age of 35.

Tay-Sachs Disease

Concept: Tay-Sachs disease is a hereditary disease caused by the absence of a key enzyme needed to break down fats.

The massive accumulation of fat lipids in the brain that occurs with **Tay-Sachs disease** leads to mental retar-

dation, blindness, and death at the age of 3 or 4. Approximately 85 percent of the victims are from Jewish families of eastern European origin. Prevention through genetic counseling has proven effective. Blood tests on both parents determine whether one is a carrier. If both parents are carriers, each pregnancy is monitored by amniocentesis.

Familial Hypercholesterolemia

Concept: FH is caused by an error of fat metabolism that first produces atherosclerosis, then heart attacks in young children and young adults.

Familial Hypercholesterolemia (FH) strikes about 1 in every 500 people in the United States, making it one of the most common genetic diseases. FH occurs in all segments of the population.

Most genetic diseases are recessive; a bad gene must be inherited from both parents before it is transmitted to the offspring. FH is a dominant genetic disease requiring only one FH gene to transmit the disease to an offspring. If both parents are carriers, the victim receives a double dose. FH victims are born with a cholesterol count 5 to 12 times the normal level. The molecules at fault are low-density lipoprotein (LDL) receptors. LDL receptors act as cellular gatekeepers and transmit needed cholesterol into the cell. If a cell is deficient in LDL receptors, it cannot remove the cholesterol it needs from the bloodstream and therefore makes its own. The liver cells, also suffering from the same genetic deficiency, receive no signal to stop production and therefore continue to produce and circulate cholesterol. The entire cycle burdens the blood with excess cholesterol it can't get rid of. FH homozygotes (both parents carried the gene) may show signs of the disease by age 5: yellowish lumpy areas loaded with cholesterol develop in the knees, elbows, heels, and between the fingers. The combination of diet and exercise has little effect on the cholesterol level of homozygotes, and symptoms of heart disease may appear before the age of 10 or in the teens. Few victims live beyond age 20. The prognosis for FH heterozgotes (one parent carried the gene) is much better because they have half the normal LDL receptors. Signs of early heart disease may appear by age 20 to 29, with the first heart attack normally occurring in the thirties or forties. Few victims live into their sixties.

Current research is focusing on genetic counseling and early screening. Drugs, careful diet, and altered lifestyles are then utilized in an attempt to lower the risk of heart attack to a normal level.

OTHER NONCOMMUNICABLE DISEASES

Arthritis

Arthritis in some form afflicts over 17 million people in the United States. Degenerative arthritis is common among the elderly. An estimated 4.5 million people suffer from **rheumatoid arthritis,** which causes chronic inflammation of the joints. Women are three to four times more likely than men to develop rheumatoid arthritis.

Treatment of arthritis is directed at controlling the symptoms, relieving discomfort, and preventing or correcting deformity. Drugs may be prescribed to relieve pain, and physical therapy and sometimes surgery can help to correct deformities.

Arthritis is often extremely painful, and as a result many sufferers are susceptible to the lures of quacks who promise miracle treatments. We'll discuss such quackery in Chapter 19.

Allergies*

Allergy affects approximately one out of every seven people in the United States today. Some 15 million people have asthma, and an additional 17 million suffer

*This section was prepared by G. E. Rodriguez, M.D., Associate Professor of Pediatrics and Director, Pediatric Chest-Allergy-Immunology, Medical College of Virginia, Virginia Commonwealth University, Richmond, Virginia.

Discovery Activity 17.3
DO YOU HAVE AN ALLERGY?

Check those items below that apply to you. Over the past 12-month period, have you had:

1. Three or more colds and sore throats?
2. Chronic, croupy cough?
3. Frequent runny nose?
4. Night cough?
5. Coughing bouts after exercising or laughing?
6. Repeated attacks of shortness of breath, wheezing, or itchy nose and palate?
7. Frequent sneezing attacks?
8. Itchy eyes?
9. Dark circles under your eyes?
10. Recurrent skin eruptions?

If you have had some of these symptoms, you may have an allergy. This can be confirmed by an examination of your nose, skin, and chest by a doctor, who will also order appropriate laboratory tests. ●

from hives, hay fever, eczema, or some other form of allergy. As a rule, allergies don't kill, but they certainly make life miserable. It is estimated that at least half of the people suffering from allergies are not aware of having the condition. They go through life at 60 percent efficiency. Yet in the great majority of cases, excellent allergic control can be achieved.

The term allergy was introduced by C. von Pirquet, a pediatrician, in 1966 to represent the concept of changed or "altered reactivity" as a result of contact with a foreign substance. Harmful allergic reactions are called **allergic hypersensitivity reactions.** Four different classes of hypersensitivity reactions are recognized. Some involve antibodies that "recognize" a particular foreign material and cause reactions between it and the cells of the body. Other reactions seem to involve only cells and foreign material. We will describe the most common form of allergy—**atopy.**

Concept: Atopy, or "reaginic antibody dependent reaction," is the most common form of allergy.

Common allergies. In atopy, target cells (in the nose for hay fever or in the lung for asthma) are coated with reaginic antibodies made elsewhere and interact with an allergenic foreign substance (allergen). The chemical response initiated results in the liberation of pharmacologically active substances (mediators) by the target cells. These chemical mediators are responsible for the symptoms of atopic allergy. For example, in the case of a skin test done in a ragweed-sensitive patient, ragweed introduced into the skin interacts with reaginic antibody fixed to tissue mast cells (target cells). As a result of this interaction, chemical mediators such as histamine and slow-reacting substances of anaphylaxis are released from the mast cells. The pharmacologic action of histamine and anaphylaxis on the blood vessels in the skin is responsible for the swelling and redness observed in the positive skin test. One can envision hives as occurring in the same way, but in multiple areas of the skin at the same time.

In **hay fever,** also known as allergic rhinitis, allergens such as house dust, plant pollen, or mold spores are blown through the air and collected on the mucous membranes of the nose and eyes, where they are absorbed. In a sensitized individual, reaginic antibodies on tissue mast cells combine with the allergens and cause the release of histamine and the other chemical mediators. The result is swelling and congestion of the mucous membranes, leading to such unpleasant symptoms as sneezing, itching, and runny nose, plus watering and swelling of the eyes.

Factors in allergic reactions. Heredity seems to be very important in the development of allergy. Other known factors include allergen concentration, time of exposure and of reexposure to allergens, quality and

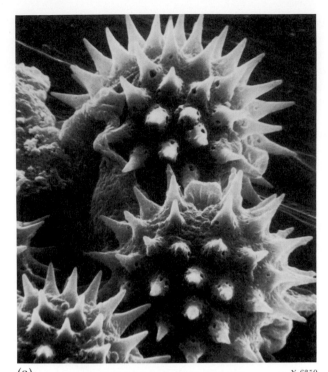

(a)   X 6350

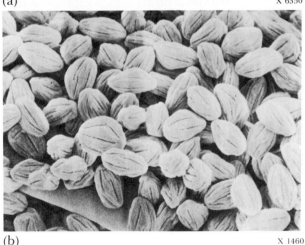

(b)   X 1460

(a) Plant pollen and (b) bread-mold spores may be absorbed into the mucous membranes of the nose and eyes. These foreign materials, or allergens, react with antibodies and cause target cells to release certain chemicals which can irritate sensitive body tissues.

quantity of reaginic antibody present, and the nonspecific simulation threshold required to induce symptoms. This last point, nonspecific stimulation threshold, means that a particular organ, such as the nose, can be stimulated by mediators to a certain point before symptoms are experienced. The degree of sensitivity in various organs of an allergic person determines what symptoms will occur.

Most children with asthma also have other allergies. Allergies, however, are only one way in which symptoms can be triggered. Other factors, such as weather changes, stress, air pollution, colds, and exercise, are nonallergic inducers of nasal symptoms or expiratory wheezing. Most adults have nonallergic asthma, although in some, allergic triggers are also important. Nonallergic hives, rhinitis, and eczema often occur in response to stress.

Treatment of allergies. Treatment of allergic conditions has two objectives: elimination or avoidance of the specific or contributory factors, and a change in the degree of sensitivity to them, usually accomplished by hyposensitization injections. Sometimes treatment with drug therapy is also required. Complete elimination of the offending allergen from the environment or diet is the ideal therapeutic method, because it makes further treatment unnecessary. However, complete avoidance is possible in only a few instances, such as removing a feather pillow or cat from the home. It is virtually impossible to avoid house dust, plant pollens, and atmospheric molds. Nonetheless, certain precautionary measures can significantly decrease the degree of exposure. All items that collect dust, such as rugs, drapes, old mattresses, upholstered chairs, and books, should be removed from the bedroom. Air filters, air conditioners, and zippered encasings for the mattress and pillow are also very helpful in decreasing the dust and mold concentration.

Any food that is known to cause symptoms should be avoided. Although most people usually do this, they may not realize that other food products can also contain the allergen. Therefore, it is important to read all labels before using new food products. **Hyposensitization,** or **immunotherapy,** is a specific form of treatment using an extract of the allergen to which the patient is reacting. The treatment consists of injecting gradually increasing amounts of the specific allergens until the maximum tolerated dose is reached, resulting in lessening of sensitivity. It takes several years of immunotherapy before all sensitivity is lost. The similarity of allergic reactions allows similar medicines or combinations or medicines to be employed in treating most patients. These are bronchodilators, corticosteroids, and antihistamines.

Dental Diseases

Concept: Dental diseases can be prevented.

Dental diseases are quite prevalent, as the following data suggest:

1. It is estimated that 95 percent of Americans will at some time have dental decay.
2. Nearly 23 million people in the United States have lost all of their teeth.
3. At least 34 percent of Americans between the ages of 12 and 17 have a gum disease.

Health scientists have identified the cause of dental diseases and have developed methods of preventing most of them from occurring.

Dental caries. Dental caries refers to tooth decay or cavities. Cavities usually occur in crevices, fissures, and surfaces that are in contact with other teeth, because these are the most difficult areas to keep clean.

Periodontal (gum) disease.[1] A condition frequently seen in both youths and adults, gingivitis is actually an early stage of most periodontal disease. At first there is mild inflammation and swelling of the gum tissue around one or more of the teeth. Later the redness and swelling become more pronounced, and the gums tend to bleed easily. Bleeding while toothbrushing is one of the earliest signs of gum disease. During these changes, the gums may or may not feel tender. Thus there may be no warning that disease is present. If the inflammation is not controlled, it usually progresses to the more severe condition called periodontitis, which includes bone destruction.

Periodontitis (pyorrhea) is the most common form of destructive periodontal disease. The gums gradually become detached from the teeth, and pockets develop, sometimes progressing to a depth of one-half inch or more. As the gums recede, some of the roots of the teeth are exposed. Eventually, the connective-tissue fibers that fasten the teeth to bone are destroyed, and much of the bone socket gradually disintegrates. The tooth loosens and is eventually lost.

Periodontosis is a more rare and puzzling condition, which afflicts adolescents and young adults. Little inflammation or discomfort is associated with it. The first sign of trouble is loose teeth. X rays will reveal that some of the bone around the roots of the molar teeth and upper incisors has been destroyed. Yet the mouth appears healthy, and the teeth are undamaged. Current treatment for this condition is surgery with antibiotic supplementation.

Acute necrotizing gingivitis is an acute infection in which the tissue is ulcerated and dying. This disease is associated with the presence of two specific types of bacteria. The condition is usually painful, and the inflamed, tender gums make eating a problem. It is likely to develop in times of severe stress and often occurs in students and soldiers. Dentists find that removal of the bacteria and dead tissue, good nutrition, rest, hygiene, and sometimes a short course of an antibiotic usually control this type of periodontal disease.

Causes and prevention. The cause of dental caries and most periodontal disease is **plaque.** Plaque is "a sticky, colorless layer of harmful bacteria that is constantly forming on your teeth."[2] These bacteria change the sugar in the foods we eat into acid, and the sticky bacterial plaque holds the acid to the tooth surface. The greatest damage to the tooth enamel occurs within the first 20 minutes of ingesting foods that contain sugar. After many acid attacks, a portion of the tooth enamel becomes demineralized, and a cavity is formed. Because the acid attack is strongest during the first 20 minutes, how *frequently* throughout the day you eat sugary foods is more important than the quantity of sugar in the foods eaten.

If plaque is not removed from the teeth, within 24 hours it will become a hard, mineralized deposit known as **calculus** or tartar. Calculus makes the removal of plaque from the teeth more difficult, and thus increases the risk of periodontal disease.

Dentists suggest that the daily removal of plaque by brushing and flossing will prevent most dental disease. Limiting the number of times you snack each day and eating sugary foods only with meals will also help. And lastly, fluoridation has a profound effect on dental decay. Fluoride in your water supply (one part per million) can significantly reduce dental decay. In its absence, topical fluoride applied to your teeth by a dentist can help.

CONCLUSION

Cancer is the second leading cause of death in the United States. In addition, other noncommunicable diseases afflict millions of people. The majority of nongenetic diseases and disorders can be prevented, delayed, or managed through regular exercise, proper nutrition, regulation of body weight and fat, cessation of tobacco use, moderate use of alcohol, and avoidance of known carcinogens. The best protection against passing on potentially harmful genetic traits is screening. Although there is no guarantee of a lifetime free from noncommunicable diseases, you can greatly reduce the risk.

SUMMARY

1. Cancer is responsible for more than 386,000 deaths each year. It is estimated that approximately 85 percent of these cases are the result of exposure to environmental factors.

2. Cancer has been associated with carcinogens, environmental pollution, chronic irritation, viruses,

radiation, hereditary factors, tobacco use, precancerous conditions, and diet.

3. Cancer can be detected in its early stages through an awareness of the seven warning signals and a regular schedule of physician examination and self-examination. With early detection, the cure rate for cancers of all types continues to rise.

4. There are three main forms of treatment for cancer: surgery, radiation, and chemotherapy. Modern advances in cancer treatment include the use of immunotherapy, stimulation of the body's own disease defenses to attack cancer cells, and approved and experimental anticancer drugs.

5. The risk of getting cancer can be reduced through certain lifestyle changes.

6. Diabetes mellitus can be prevented and managed through healthy eating habits, regular exercise, and control of body weight and fat.

7. Diseases of the nervous system are difficult to diagnose and treat, and their causes are often unclear.

8. Genetic diseases are passed on through dominant inheritance, recessive inheritance, sex-linked inheritance, or polygenic (multifactorial) inheritance. Of the more than 300 hereditary diseases, most are considered inborn errors of metabolism or chemical mistakes.

9. Rheumatoid arthritis affects approximately 4.5 million people. Women are three to four times more likely to get arthritis than men.

10. One of every seven people in the United States suffers from some type of allergy. Treatment consists of eliminating the contributing factors and changing the degree of sensitivity to them through hyposensitization injections.

11. Dental diseases can be prevented through proper care of the teeth and gums and proper nutrition.

REFERENCES

1. National Institute of Dental Research, *Periodontal (Gum) Diseases*. Department of Health, Education and Welfare, Pub. No. 76-1142.

2. American Dental Association, *Cleaning Your Teeth and Gums* (Chicago: American Dental Association, 1972), p. 2.

Laboratory 1
CANCER AND OUR ENVIRONMENT

Purpose   To determine exposure to known carcinogenic agents.

Size of Group   Four to five per group.

Equipment   None.

Procedure

1. Each student is assigned the task of determining the exposure of the typical college student to potential carcinogenic agents in one of the following areas:

   a. Nutritional patterns
   b. Outside air
   c. Inside air (including smoke-filled rooms)
   d. Recreational habits

2. Suggest changes in the lifestyles of college students that can reduce exposure.

Results

One member from each group is selected to report the findings to the entire class.

Laboratory 2
FAMILY TREE OF LIFE AND DEATH

Purpose   To determine the cause of death resulting from chronic or degenerative diseases within families.
To determine the average life span in specific families.
To determine the tendency toward hereditary diseases within families.

Size of Group   Students work alone, consulting parents and grandparents when necessary.

Equipment   None.

Procedure

1. Complete the family tree in Fig. 17.5, indicating date of birth (born), date of death (died), cause of death, and age. Consult parents and grandparents if possible for exact information.

2. When "Cause of death" or "Date of death" is not known, write "unknown" and skip that relative.

3. If death was caused by an "accident," indicate "accidental death" on the chart.

Results

1. What was the average age at death among relatives who died from natural causes?

   a. Number of relatives dying from natural (nonaccidental) causes   _____

   b. Total years lived of these relatives (add all years)   _____

   c. Average age of relatives dying from natural causes (divide the answer in *a* into the answer in *b*)   _____

2. List the chronic and degenerative diseases causing death in your family.

Disease:

Number of Relatives Afflicted:

3. What diseases appear more than once in your hereditary line?

4. Are any of the above diseases hereditary?

5. What preventive action can you take to reduce the possibility of acquiring this disease later in life?

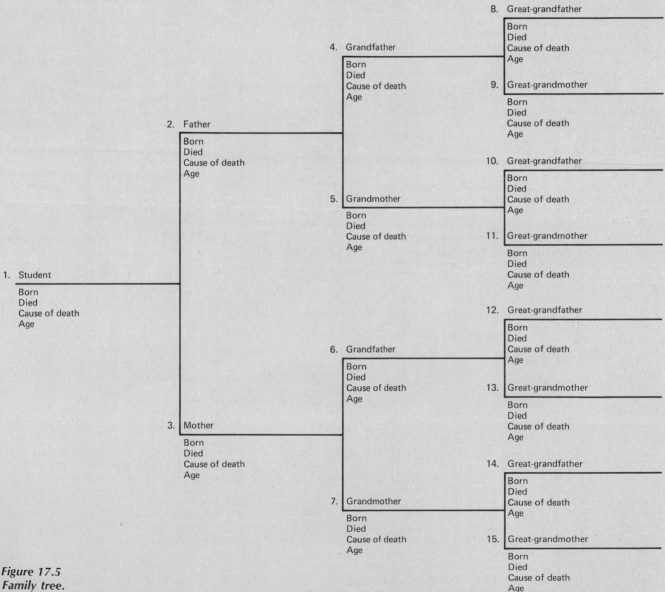

Figure 17.5
Family tree.

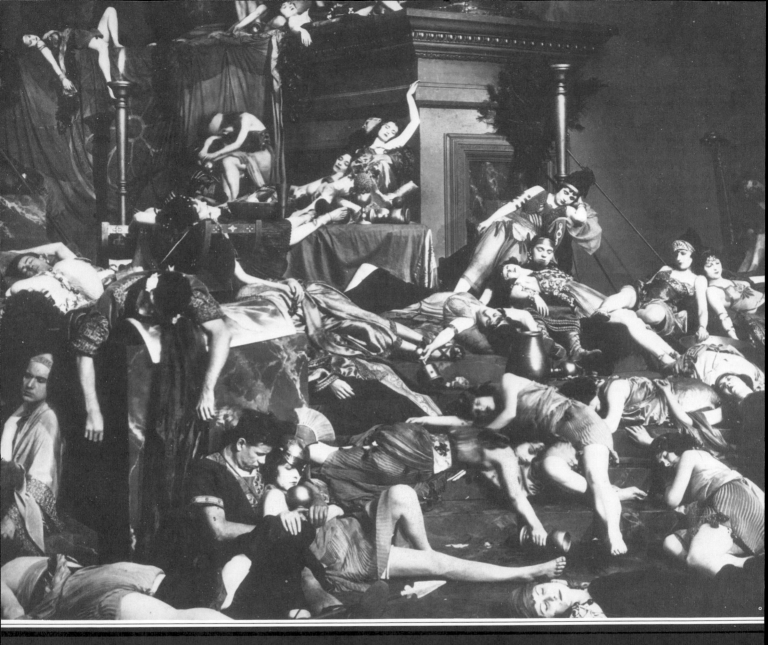

chapter

18

communicable diseases

- *mechanisms of defense*
- *epidemiology: studying disease patterns*
- *disease control*
- *common communicable diseases*
- *sexually transmitted diseases*

This chapter was written by Dr. Albert J. Banes,
Surgery Department and Dental Research Center,
University of North Carolina, Chapel Hill.

All living creatures have been plagued with disease since the beginning of recorded history. Both humans and other animals have carried their characteristic communicable diseases for thousands of years. Rabies, a lethal viral disease, was reported by the Egyptians as early as 5000 B.C.; hieroglyphics of a rabid dog predate Louis Pasteur's vaccination treatment for rabies by 5000 years. Modern analysis of mummified humans from 4000 B.C. indicates that tuberculosis and other infectious diseases were early health problems among North and South American Indians, as well as among the Egyptians.

The early Egyptians attempted to understand the disease process by studying human corpses. Over three-quarters of a billion bodies were examined by embalmers during the centuries of Egyptian rule. Most of the information amassed by the Egyptians was subsequently lost for thousands of years, until the Greeks began to dissect human corpses and collect medical information from autopsies. Much descriptive anatomy of the normal and diseased body was committed to illustration at this time. However, the significant advances toward an understanding of the function of the human body and the role that communicable diseases play in threatening life were initially made between 1840 and 1900. During the latter period, Louis Pasteur, Robert Koch, and others proved the germ theory of disease; Joseph Lister began the practice of antiseptic treatment before and during surgical procedures; bacteria were grown in pure culture; immunization against specific diseases (rabies, anthrax, and diphtheria) was begun; and viruses were discovered.

During the first half of the twentieth century, Ehrlich, Fleming, Domagk, and others greatly advanced the field of chemotherapy, particularly in the development of antibiotics.

After the production of the first electron microscope in the 1930s, a new miniworld was opened to the scrutiny of scientists. Now bacteria and viruses could be observed on the ultrastructural level.

In 1949 mammalian cells were grown successfully outside the body in cell cultures, inaugurating a new

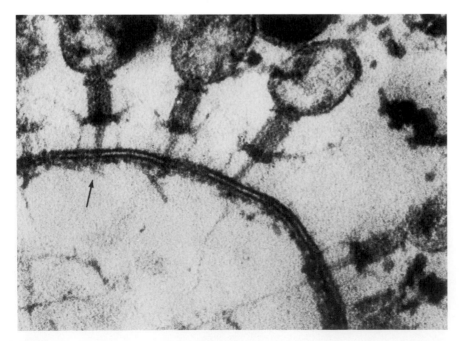

Electron micrograph of the edge of a cell with virus particles attached. Viruses cannot reproduce on their own; they must use the host cell's enzymes and nourishment. The virus attaches itself to the host by its tail and injects a single molecule of DNA. Inside the host, the DNA disrupts normal cell activity and commands the cell to produce new virus particles. Eventually, the host cell is destroyed and the new viruses burst out ready for another round of infection.

era in molecular biology and vaccine research. In 1954 the structure of DNA (deoxyribonucleic acid) was elucidated, and in the next ten years tremendous advances were made in comprehending the functions of living cells: how cells divide, synthesize proteins and nucleic acids, and metabolize compounds, and how bacteria and viruses effect their damage on the molecular level.

We are rapidly approaching the time when scientists will discover the precise biochemical mechanisms by which most infectious diseases occur. Some mechanisms are already known in detail. The next step in the campaign against the spread of infectious disease is to prevent disease selectively by disrupting a single step in the life process of the infectious organism without affecting the host metabolism. During the next 50 years medical science will pursue research of this type.

In this chapter we'll examine some of the mechanisms the body uses to defend against infection by communicable diseases, how these diseases spread, and how they can be controlled or prevented. We'll give special attention to sexually transmitted diseases, because their incidence has risen alarmingly and their consequences can be extremely serious.

MECHANISMS OF DEFENSE

Concept: A microorganism must penetrate the individual's external defenses before infection can occur.

A communicable disease is one that can be transmitted from person to person. Six factors are necessary to produce infectious disease in humans. These are outlined in Table 18.1 on page 428.

Infection occurs when a microorganism successfully penetrates the host's defense barriers and multiplies. Disease is caused when microorganisms destroy tissue and/or utilize large quantities of host nutrients to sustain infection. As normal, healthy humans, we all carry infections continually; for instance, over 90 percent of throat cultures taken at random contain *Streptococcus viridans,* a bacterial organism. Such infections, however, are usually not sufficiently debilitating

to cause discomfort. When they do cause noticeable discomfort, fever, and malaise, we use the term **disease** to characterize the symptoms.

Microorganisms can enter your body through the skin, respiratory tract (mucous membranes of the nose, throat, and lungs), gastrointestinal tract (oral cavity, esophagus, stomach, and alimentary tract), urogenital tract (bladder, ureters, penis, vagina), the eyes, and ear canals. When one of these physical barriers is broken, the infectious organism is said to have penetrated the body's first line of defense.

Lines of Defense

Concept: Once it has entered the body, the organism must confront internal defenses.

After the organism penetrates the body's external defenses, it encounters the second line of defense. Various enzymes and other compounds in blood can kill an infectious organism by causing it to break open, destroying its cell wall, or preventing it from multiplying. Special white blood cells, called **phagocytes,** engulf and digest bacteria. Larger phagocytic cells, called **macrophages,** are contained in the body's tissues, and these too fight off bacteria, so that the offending organism may never be able to establish a foothold. If the invader does become established, the body then resorts to a third line of defense in which tissue fluids, along with antibacterial and antitoxin proteins, accumulate. The body's fight to repel the disease microbe becomes evident through inflammation of the infected area and accompanying discomfort. Fever is another sign that the body is fighting the infection.

If the third line of defense is penetrated, the infection may spread through the body tissues and perhaps into the blood stream. If this happens, the infection becomes very serious. If instead the infection remains localized, an **abscess** may form as more and more tissue in the infected area is destroyed. An abscess is a cavity filled with fluid, white cells battling the disease microbe, and pus (dead white cells). The body returns to normal only when enough of the infection organisms are killed or rendered inactive.

Table 18.1
SIX FACTORS NECESSARY TO PRODUCE INFECTIOUS DISEASE IN HUMANS

Factor	Interpretation	Examples	Comments
A causative agent	A living organism must exist (pathogen) that is capable of invading the body and causing disease.	Viruses, bacteria.	Viruses and bacteria that cause disease are in the environment at all times.
A reservoir	The pathogen must have a place to live and multiply until it is passed on to a host, such as a human being.	Humans: infected human or someone who is a carrier and is not affected; or an animal, insect, or bird.	Animal diseases that are transmitted to humans are generally not transmitted from human to human.
A means of escape	The pathogen must have a means of escape from the reservoir.	Through the respiratory tract (nose, throat, lungs, bronchial tree via coughing, sneezing, or breathing); the digestive tract (feces, saliva, vomitus, contaminated items); open sores, wounds, and lesions.	Each disease has a period when the pathogen is most likely to escape (infectious period) and infect another human. Quarantine during this period reduces the risk of spreading the disease.
A means of transmission	The pathogen must have a means of contacting a host.	Body to body (kissing, touching, sexual contact), animals and insects; inanimate objects (clothing, eating utensils, tissues, toilet articles).	Pathogens that can survive outside a host pose the greatest threat to humans.
A means of entry	The pathogen must have a way to enter the host.	Respiratory tract (breathed in), digestive tract (swallowed), breaks in the skin (cuts, abrasions), or mucous membranes (lining of the mouth, nose, eyes, vagina, anus).	Hand-to-mucous membrane contact is a common way the pathogen enters the human body.
A host that is susceptible to the pathogen	The host must receive the pathogen.	Strong body defenses or immunity can fight off the pathogen before the disease occurs.	The period between entry of the pathogen and the disease's first symptoms is called the incubation period. It is easier to eradicate the disease during this period than during subsequent stages of the disease.

Thus far we have been referring primarily to defenses against bacteria. When the invading organism is a virus, the body produces the protein interferon in the infected cells. Interferon does not protect the infected cell itself, but rather protects the healthy cells surrounding it by blocking viral invasion.

The Immune Mechanism

Another way in which the body fights infection is by producing specific proteins called **antibodies.** Antibodies are produced by **lymphocytes,** types of white blood cells formed in the bone marrow. B lymphocytes play the primary role in manufacturing antibodies. Antibodies are found principally in the blood, but are also present in mucous membranes in the respiratory, urogenital, and gastrointestinal tracts. They are very important both in preventing initial infection and in preventing the subsequent spread of infectious agents.

Antibodies are produced in response to foreign substances, or **antigens.** The antibodies react specifically with the antigen that elicited their production. A

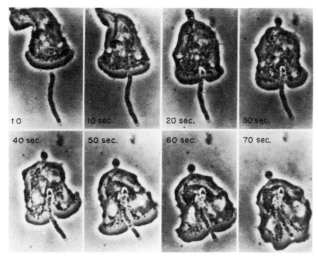

(a)

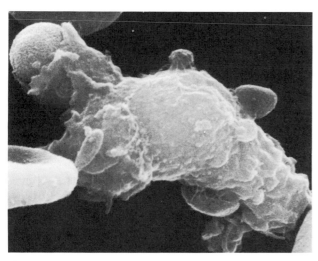

(b)

(a) A human white blood cell destroying a bacterium. White blood cells can move amoebalike and pass through blood-vessel walls into tissue spaces. Some specialize in producing antibodies; others hunt out and engulf foreign material, such as bacteria, as shown in these photos. (b) A scanning electron micrograph gives a three-dimensional view of the white blood cell at work. In this photo, it is engulfing a particle of yeast (the small sphere in the upper left corner).

practical example of an antigenic stimulus is toxin, produced during a bacterial infection. Your immune system recognizes the toxin (antigen) as foreign, and antibodies produced in response to the toxin (by plasma cells), either in the past or during the present infection, combine chemically with the toxin. The resulting aggregation of toxin and antibodies is engulfed by immune cells, metabolized, and excreted. Thus the primary role of antibodies is to combine with a specific antigen and aid in the clearance of antigens from your body. Once you have been exposed to an antigen, you retain the ability to respond to it for a period of months or years.

Primary and Secondary Immune Responses

Concept: The body has primary and secondary immune responses.

The first time you are infected with a virus—influenza, for example—you react immunologically to antigens produced by the virus. A virus is usually inhaled in mucus droplets from an infected person (for example, after a sneeze); it is absorbed in the mucous layer of the respiratory tract; penetrates susceptible cells in the nose, bronchi, or lungs; and multiplies. While infection is continuing, macrophages in the infected area are engulfing virus particles. Macrophages then present some form of the virus protein to a B lymphocyte that is predetermined to produce an antibody to that antigen. The B lymphocyte then produces an antibody (IgM) to influenza virus.

Up to this point, the virus has had one to two days to incubate in the respiratory tract. During this time you may have chills, aching muscles, and fever. Fever may continue for several days. As soon as enough virus is present to be detected by your immune cells, you begin your defense against the infection. Within 24 hours after immune cell recognition of the viral antigen, you may produce some specific IgM. Within seven days after antigen recognition, you have a high level of IgM in your blood, and some IgG, another antibody, is being produced. Within two weeks after antigen recognition, you have a high level of IgG in your blood; it is this IgG that can protect you from subsequent influenza virus infections. This is your primary immune response.

When infected a year later with similar influenza, you have an antibody present in your blood that can react with the virus (and macrophages) to aid in clearance of the virus from your body. At this time, some of your plasma cells, which were previously committed to making the specific antibody to influenza A virus, recognize the antigen of this year's virus (A group). These committed cells are now ready to commence production of IgG directly, and do so immediately. The second dose of natural influenza virus antigen acts like a vaccination that stimulates your immune cells to produce an influenza-specific antibody.

EPIDEMIOLOGY: STUDYING DISEASE PATTERNS

Concept: The goal of epidemiologists is ultimately to prevent disease by gathering and analyzing data.

Epidemiology is the study of the causes and means of controlling disease. Epidemiologists study particular populations affected by infectious disease and gather information on the frequency of the disease, its distribution, and causes.

When a particular disease has been localized in a geographic area for years, the disease is said to be **endemic** to that area. In an endemic disease zone, one can expect that a certain percentage of people will contract the disease in any given year; the segment of the population that contracts the disease comprises the **susceptible hosts.** The number of susceptibles that contract the disease is recorded as the percent **morbidity,** or percent diseased, people in the area per year. The number of individuals that die from the disease each year is referred to as the percent **mortality,** or percent deaths, that occurred. A large segment of the popula-

tion will not contract the disease because either they are immune (not susceptible) or they were not infected.

Keeping records of the percent morbidity and mortality in a population for a given disease in a given geographical area helps health professionals establish zones of endemicity. When the percent morbidity and mortality for an area increases over the expected level for a given year, the disease is said to occur in **epidemic** proportions (epidemic: *epi*—above; *demos*—the world). Thus an epidemic occurs when high levels of an infectious agent circulate in the population of susceptible people, causing an increased percentage of illness and death. When illness and death caused by a disease occur all over the world, the disease is said to be **pandemic** (*pan*—across; *demos*—the world).

Factors Influencing Endemicity

Concept: Characteristics of the infectious agent, vector, host, and environment influence the endemicity of a disease to a geographic area.

The infectious agent must have a suitable **vector** population (mosquitoes, for example), as well as a host reservoir, to survive in an area. In addition, the agent must be able to survive in a host during unfavorable periods, that is, when the possibility for transmission is low. For example, some viruses live during winter in snakes, mosquito eggs, or migratory birds. When conditions are favorable for replication and transmission, the infectious agent reproduces and is transmitted to humans and/or other animals.

The quality of the climate in a particular area determines the extent to which an agent can survive and be transmitted. In temperate or tropical climates, during warm weather, people are more likely to contact polluted water used for swimming and drinking, thus contracting and transmitting agents that cause gastrointestinal disorders. In addition, in warm climates many insect vectors take blood meals on hosts, thus increasing the chance for infectious disease to spread.

In cold weather climates, large groups of people collect in confined areas, increasing the incidence of

Discovery Activity 18.1
YOUR COMMUNICABLE DISEASE PATTERN

List below those communicable diseases you remember having contracted over the past year. Indicate the time of year you contracted the disease, as well as the type of climate you live in. Can you find a pattern?

Disease	Season	Climate
1. _____		
2. _____		
3. _____		
4. _____		
5. _____		●

airborne transmission of disease. In addition, during cold weather the lack of humidity indoors causes mucous membranes in the respiratory tract to dry out. Dry mucous membranes do not offer the protection (physical trapping in moist, mucous membranes) against airborne microorganisms that mucus-coated membranes do. Thus colds and influenza are common in such climates.

Yellow Fever: A Case in Point

Concept: Yellow fever is an endemic viral disease that has been controlled but not eradicated.

Yellow fever is a classic viral disease whose epidemiology has been fully investigated (see Fig. 18.1). The virus of yellow fever is transmitted to humans by the bite of an infected mosquito. The virus infection does not kill the mosquito. The **incubation period** (time from infection to onset of symptoms) for yellow fever is between three and six days, after which time the individ-

ual exhibits fever, chills, muscle aches, and headache. At this time, the virus is reproducing in the liver, and degenerative changes also occur in the kidney, spleen, lymph nodes, brain, and heart. The patient experiences severe nausea and vomiting. By the fourth day after onset of symptoms (between seven and ten days after infection), the patient has black vomit, caused by the presence of hemoglobin from lysed (destroyed) red blood cells. After this stage, the patient usually dies. If the disease doesn't reach this stage, the patient may recover from infection without experiencing malaise.

Yellow fever occurs in two forms: (1) urban, epidemic yellow fever; and (2) jungle yellow fever. It is

Figure 18.1
Life cycles of yellow fever virus.

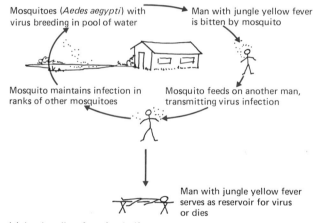

Mosquitoes (*Aedes aegypti*) with virus breeding in pool of water

Man with jungle yellow fever is bitten by mosquito

Mosquito maintains infection in ranks of other mosquitoes

Mosquito feeds on another man, transmitting virus infection

Man with jungle yellow fever serves as reservoir for virus or dies

(a) Jungle yellow fever (cycle 1)

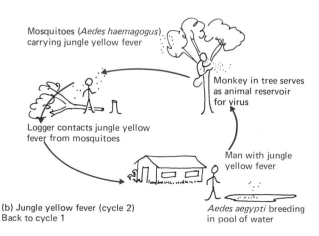

Mosquitoes (*Aedes haemagogus*) carrying jungle yellow fever

Monkey in tree serves as animal reservoir for virus

Logger contacts jungle yellow fever from mosquitoes

Man with jungle yellow fever

(b) Jungle yellow fever (cycle 2)
Back to cycle 1

Aedes aegypti breeding in pool of water

prevalent in warm climates (Africa, South America, southern parts of Asia) where there is a great deal of rainfall. The mosquitoes multiply in swampy areas around human settlements. Mosquitoes are infected after feeding on humans that have yellow fever virus circulating in their blood. The infected mosquitoes then transmit the virus to susceptible individuals.

Jungle yellow fever is primarily a disease of monkeys and is transmitted from monkey to monkey by mosquitoes that inhabit exclusively the tops of trees. Humans that come in contact with the infected monkeys can contract jungle yellow fever, which follows the same course as urban yellow fever. It is very difficult to control a disease that has a large virus reservoir among wild animals. One can attempt to eradicate the vector for urban yellow fever, but yellow fever virus can always reinfect humans via the second cycle (jungle yellow fever).

How is yellow fever controlled? Attempts have been made to eradicate the vector, by draining swamps and spraying pesticide (DDT) to remove the mosquitoes' breeding grounds, and to protect susceptible hosts through mass vaccination programs. Surveillance of the population for new outbreaks of the disease and regular vaccination of susceptible people with a live vaccine strain of yellow fever have greatly reduced morbidity and mortality rates.

DISEASE CONTROL

Concept: Vaccination programs have been successful in controlling infectious disease.

Vaccination

The term vaccination is derived from the word *vaccinia*, or cowpox. Edward Jenner performed the first vaccination against smallpox in 1798. He noted that milkmaids rarely contracted smallpox and wondered why this was so. He found that milkmaids did contract a disease from cows (cowpox) but that the illness was not serious and left no disfiguring marks. He prepared

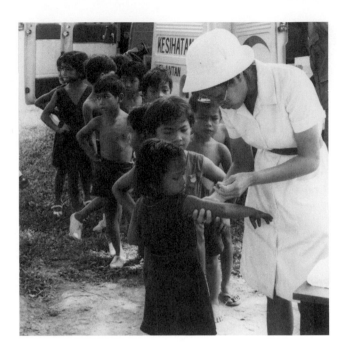

School children in Thailand receive a smallpox vaccination from members of a mobile health team.

an inoculum from the pustule of a milkmaid with cowpox, inoculated susceptible humans, and found that these vaccinated individuals did not contract smallpox, even when challenged by virulent smallpox virus.

Since Jenner's time, medical professionals have prepared vaccines against many different infectious agents. A **vaccine** is a preparation of an antigen or antigens from an infectious agent that, when injected into a normal, susceptible human, initiates an immune response against a subsequent infection by the organism. A vaccine consists of live organisms that retain their antigenic properties and can replicate in the body but will not cause severe illness, killed organisms that retain antigenic properties but will not replicate in the body and will not cause severe illness, or pure antigens.

Many successful vaccine preparations have been developed over the years, particularly to combat virus infections. Some of these are polio, rubella (German measles), measles, mumps, adenovirus, smallpox, and influenza. Table 18.2 indicates the principal vaccines used in preventing human viral diseases.

Table 18.2
PRINCIPAL VACCINES USED IN PREVENTION OF HUMAN VIRUS DISEASES

Disease	Source of Vaccine	Condition of Virus	Route of Administration
Recommended immunization for general public (in USA and other developed countries)			
Poliomyelitis	Tissue culture (human diploid cell line, monkey kidney)	Live	Oral
Measles[a]	Tissue culture (chick embryo)	Live	Subcutaneous[b]
Mumps[a]	Tissue culture (chick embryo)	Live	Subcutaneous
Rubella[a,c]	Tissue culture (duck embryo, rabbit, or dog kidney)	Live	Subcutaneous
Immunization recommended only under certain conditions (epidemics, exposure, travel, military)			
Smallpox	Lymph from calf or sheep (glycerolated, lyophilized	Active	Intradermal: multiple pressure, multiple puncture, or (with specially prepared vaccine) by jet injection
	Chorioallantois, tissue cultures (lyophilized)	Active	
Yellow fever	Tissue cultures and eggs (17D strain)	Live	Subcutaneous or intradermal
Influenza	Chick embryo allantoic fluid (formalinized or UV-irradiated, concentrated by various processes)	Inactive	Subcutaneous
	Highly purified or subunit forms recommended where available	Inactive	Subcutaneous
Rabies	Duck embryo treated with phenol or ultraviolet light	Inactive	Subcutaneous
Adenovirus[d]	Monkey kidney tissue cultures (formalinized)	Inactive	Intramuscular
	Human diploid cell cultures	Live	Oral, by entericcoated capsule
Japanese B encephalitis[d]	Mouse brain (formalinized), tissue culture	Inactive	Subcutaneous
Venezuelan equine encephalomyelitis[e]	Guinea pig heart cell culture	Live	Subcutaneous
Eastern equine encephalomyelitis[d]	Chick embryo cell culture	Inactive	Subcutaneous
Western equine encephalomyelitis[d]	Chick embryo cell culture	Inactive	Subcutaneous
Russian spring-summer encephalitis[d]	Mouse brain (formalinized)	Inactive	Subcutaneous

[a]Available also as combined vaccines.

[b]With less attenuated strains, gamma globulin is given in another limb at the time of vaccination.

[c]Neither monovalent rubella vaccine nor combination vaccines incorporating rubella should be administered to a postpubertal susceptible female unless she is not pregnant and understands that it is imperative not to become pregnant for at least three months after vaccination. (The time immediately postpartum has been suggested as a safe period for vaccination.)

[d]Not available in the USA except for the Armed Forces or for investigative purposes.

[e]Available for use in domestic animals (from the U.S. Department of Agriculture) and for investigative purposes.

SOURCE: E. Jarvetz, J. L. Melnick, and E. A. Adelberg, *Review of Medical Microbiology*. Los Altos, Calif.: Lange Medical Publication, p. 323. Used by permission.

Discovery Activity 18.2
YOUR VACCINATION RECORD

Which diseases have you been vaccinated against? Consult with your family physician or your university health service to obtain access to your medical file.

Vaccinations	Dates Vaccinated
1. _____	_____
2. _____	_____
3. _____	_____
4. _____	_____
5. _____	_____
6. _____	_____
7. _____	_____
8. _____	_____
9. _____	_____
10. _____	_____ ●

The vaccines most commonly used to protect against bacterial infections are diphtheria, pertussis, and tetanus toxoid (the latter to protect against infection by *clostridium tetani,* the causative agent of lockjaw). Although there are thousands of strains of bacteria, only a few bacterial vaccines have been developed, because most bacterial infections are readily controlled through the use of antibiotics. In contrast, most viral infections cannot be controlled by drugs; therefore, immunization by vaccination is of more benefit.

Antibiotics

Concept: Antibiotics have been vitally important in controlling bacterial infections.

Chemicals had been used to combat infectious diseases for hundreds of years before Paul Ehrlich made chemo-therapy a science. In 1903 he developed Salvarson, a drug containing arsenic, which is effective against the causative agent of syphilis. In 1929 Sir Alexander Fleming discovered that a compound (later shown to be penicillin) produced by a fungus could inhibit the growth of certain bacteria. In 1940 Chain and Florey reported that penicillin could be used to treat humans with bacterial infections. Domagk, in 1935, discovered sulfonamides and their inhibitory action on bacterial multiplication. Once these compounds had been discovered, advances in antimicrobial chemotherapy were rapid. **Antibiotic** (*anti*—against; *bios*—life) was originally a term used to mean natural products of microorganisms, but now it includes synthetic compounds (for example, synthetic penicillin, ampicillin) as well.

Antibiotics can successfully control several major bacterial diseases, such as strep and staph infections, bacterial pneumonia, and many of the sexually transmitted diseases. However, these drugs cannot treat viruses. Although antibiotics have made a vital contribution, some problems are associated with their use, including allergic reactions and the development of strains resistant to the drugs (see the Issue on page 438).

COMMON COMMUNICABLE DISEASES

Measles

Concept: Measles is a serious disease, but it can be prevented.

Measles is a highly contagious disease caused by measles virus. Airborne virus enters the upper respiratory tract, where it replicates and is spread via blood, mucus, or secretions throughout the respiratory tract. A red rash appears in the mouth and on the skin. The rash is caused by serum seepage from the blood and dead or dying cells forming discrete spots on the skin.

The incubation period is 10 days from the time of initial infection until the individual becomes feverish. Two weeks after fever, the rash appears, but fever and malaise continue for an additional 48 hours. The rash progresses, spreading over the body in two to four days, declining in severity in five to ten days.

Measles is a serious disease and, under certain circumstances, can lead to inflammation of the brain, or **encephalitis.** It is a common disease: over 80 percent of individuals over age 20 have an antibody to the virus. A measles vaccine is available for children and adults; infants are usually protected by the maternal antibody until six months of age and should be vaccinated at 15 months.

Mumps

> **Concept:** Mumps virus infection causes swelling of the parotid glands.

Mumps virus exists in only one form. After inhalation of virus, infection may proceed in the outer layer of cells of the respiratory tract or through the oral cavity into the parotid glands, located in the tissue in the floor of your mouth to either side of the tongue. Once virus replicates and enters the blood, it can localize in salivary glands, reproductive organs (testes and ovaries), pancreas, thyroid, and brain.

The incubation period is 12 to 35 days, and the disease is characterized by swelling of the parotid glands, fever, and general malaise. In adults the reproductive glands can be affected: 20 percent of males around the age of puberty develop a swelling of the testes, but this does *not* generally lead to sterility. You may have heard that if only one side of your face swells during mumps infection, you could contract mumps again. This is not true. Once you have had mumps virus infection in one or both parotid glands, with or without swelling of the reproductive glands, you are protected against a future mumps infection.

A good vaccine is available to protect against mumps infection. For children, a combined vaccine against measles, mumps, and rubella is usually administered at 15 months.

Rubella

> **Concept:** Rubella infection during early pregnancy may cause birth defects.

Rubella is generally a disease of childhood. The rubella virus infects the outer layer of cells of the upper respiratory tract but may replicate in the cervical lymph nodes. Virus appears in the blood about a week after infection and persists for an additional two weeks. A characteristic skin rash develops when the antibody appears in the blood. Once you have contracted the rubella virus, you are generally immune. However, reinfection may occur in some cases, due to inadequate levels of the antibody.

Rubella infection may have serious effects if contracted during early pregnancy. Infection during the first 10 weeks of pregnancy can lead to birth defects in the fetus.

Children are generally given the combined measles, mumps, and rubella vaccine at 15 months. Adults may be immunized at any time, although the great majority of adults are already immune, even if they

Childhood immunization programs have been crucial in reducing the incidence of many communicable diseases.

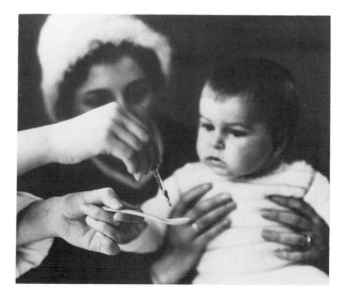

Table 18.3
**RECOMMENDED SCHEDULE FOR ACTIVE
IMMUNIZATION OF NORMAL INFANTS
AND CHILDREN**

Recommended Age	Vaccine(s)
2 mo	DTP,[1]OPV[2]
4 mo	DTP, OPV
6 mo	DTP (OPV)
12 mo	Tuberculin Test[3]
15 mo	Measles, mumps, rubella (MMR)[4]
18 mo	DTP, OPV
4–6 yr[5]	DTP, OPV
14–16 yr	Td[6]

[1]DTP—Diphtheria and tetanus toxoids with pertussis vaccine.
[2]OPV—Oral, attenuated poliovirus vaccine contains poliovirus types 1, 2, and 3.
[3]Tuberculin test—Mantoux (intradermal PPD) preferred. Frequency of tests depends on local epidemiology.
[4]MMR—Live measles, mumps, and rubella viruses in a combined vaccine.
[5]Up to the seventh birthday.
[6]Td—Adult tetanus toxoid (full dose) and diphtheria toxoid (reduced dose) in combination.
SOURCE: *Report of the Committee on Infectious Diseases,* 19th edition, 1982. Copyright © American Academy of Pediatrics, 1982.

have no history of the disease. If a woman is pregnant and there are unimmunized children in the household, those children should be vaccinated, as they are the most likely rubella carriers. Table 18.3 indicates the recommended schedule for immunization of infants and children against a number of viral diseases.

Herpes Simplex, Type 1

Concept: Herpes, type 1, virus causes cold sores and fever blisters.

Herpes is a virus that occurs in two types: **herpes, type 1,** causes cold sores and fever blisters; herpes, type 2, is a sexually transmitted disease and will be discussed in that section.

Although cold sores may disappear rapidly, the herpes 1 virus remains in a dormant state until triggered to appear again at a lesion site. You may have had a cold sore on your lip and recall that it hurt and looked unsightly, and you were quite relieved when it was gone. The bad news is that it isn't really gone. The virus is still with you in a latent or dormant form, just waiting for the proper stimulus (sunburn, nervous tension, hormone imbalance) to reappear as a lesion. Infection recurs in spite of high levels of antibody and good, cell mediated immunity, because the virus leads a relatively sheltered existence in a part of your nervous system where antibody and immune cells can't reach it. Your immune system can only act on the virus after your skin has been traumatized.

The Common Cold

Concept: The common cold is caused by one of more than 100 different viruses.

Contrary to popular belief, you cannot "catch" a cold from a draft, wet feet, a chill, or going outside in inclement weather without a hat. The infection can, however, be transmitted by direct contact, such as handshakes or kissing, through mucus droplets coughed or sneezed into the air, and through contact with soiled tissues used by an infected person. There is currently no known means of preventing, curing, or shortening a cold, but the symptoms can be treated with aspirin (for headache, fever, and body aches); a humidifier; saltwater gargle or lozenges (for sore throat); limited use of nasal decongestants; and fluids, such as juice, tea, or soup. Antibiotics are ineffective in treating a cold virus, and the value of taking massive doses of vitamin C to prevent or cure a cold is still debated.

Colds are more prevalent during the winter months, when people spend more time indoors. Preventive measures include avoiding carriers (particularly during the first 24 hours of symptoms, when the virus is most contagious), avoiding handshakes, avoiding hand contact with the mucous membranes, and practicing proper hygiene (washing hands and face frequently).

Influenza

> **Concept:** The flu is more serious and more contagious than the common cold.

Influenza (flu) is caused by three types of viruses (A, B, and C), and each has several strains that tend to change slightly from year to year. Type A occurs in epidemic cycles every 10 to 12 years and is the most serious. Type B produces a milder virus but can also reach epidemic proportions. Epidemics of Type C virus do not occur. Because so many different strains of flu exist, a vaccine must be repeated annually and may not offer protection unless the specific type of flu virus is identified. The elderly and the chronically ill may benefit from vaccination against Type A virus.

Treatment involves bed rest until body temperature is back to normal along with symptomatic treatment similar to that described for the common cold. If complications develop, such as earache, sinus pain, persistent cough, sore throat, a physician should be consulted.

Mononucleosis

> **Concept:** Mononucleosis tends to be a disease of young people.

Infectious mononucleosis can be transmitted in the saliva during kissing or in a manner similar to the common cold. The highest rate of occurrence is in the 15 to 19 age range, followed by the 20 to 24 age range. Symptoms appear from two weeks to two months after exposure: fever, sore throat, enlargement of the spleen and other lymph glands, headache, and fatigue. Serious complications occur in only a small percentage of cases, but the disease is debilitating and requires several weeks to months for full recovery.

Treatment is similar to that for a common cold; the course of the disease is not altered. Bed rest may be required in the early stages. There is currently no known prevention, although a vaccine is under development at this time.

Hepatitis

> **Concept:** Hepatitis, a viral inflammation of the liver, can be prevented.

Infectious hepatitis (Type A) is caused by fecal contamination of food or the environment and is easily preventable by proper hygiene. **Serum hepatitis (Type B)** accounts for only 10 percent of the cases and is often transmitted when the blood of an infected person enters another individual's blood stream. It is commonly caused by unclean needles, sharing of needles for injecting narcotics or amphetamines, tattooing, or ear piercing. Hepatitis B can also be transmitted by bodily secretions, such as saliva and semen. It is commonly transmitted by sexual contact. Symptoms of hepatitis appear 10 to 50 days after exposure and include fever, weakness, loss of appetite, nausea, abdominal discomfort in the upper right quadrant, and sometimes jaundice (yellowing of the skin and eyes). The most contagious period is from the last half of incubation to a few days after jaundice appears. Recovery is very slow, even with proper treatment, and may require several months. The disease is fatal to approximately 1 percent of those afflicted. It is possible to receive temporary protection or immunity through injections of gamma globulin.

Bacterial Infections

> **Concept:** Spherical bacteria can cause pus-forming infections that can be treated with antibiotics.

Staphylococci are bacteria that can be present on the skin without causing serious infection. But once infection begins, the bacteria multiply and produce the various toxins and enzymes that allow it to spread to the blood stream causing *bacteremia,* or bacteria in the blood. In the central portion of the lesion the tissue dies and is used to nourish the bacteria. Thus, an abscess is formed, leading to breakage at the point of least resistance (skin), or to internal drainage of abscess con-

ARE ANTIBIOTICS OVERPRESCRIBED?

Many physicians prescribe antibiotics to treat the common cold. This practice is currently under attack by experts in various health fields, because antibiotic therapy is of no value in treating viruses.

Those who favor antibiotic therapy indicate that such an approach controls secondary bacterial infections that may occur with colds, flu, and other viruses. In addition, it is felt that many patients who visit a physician are suffering from a combination of cough, stuffy nose, swollen glands in the neck, and earache—symptoms of secondary bacterial complications. For these patients, antibiotic therapy is certainly indicated. Antibiotic therapy catches the disease early and prevents secondary bacterial infections in many people. It may be better to prescribe antibiotics immediately than to wait for the results of a throat culture. The time required for the culture allows the disease to gain momentum, produce additional symptoms, and become more difficult to treat.

Opponents of indiscriminate use of antibiotics argue that a throat culture should always be taken before prescribing an antibiotic to make certain that the invading organism can be destroyed by the drug. The costs of a throat culture and an antibiotic are about the same; no additional financial burden is placed on the patient. Studies have also indicated that only a small number of patients with symptoms of the common cold actually have or develop a secondary bacterial infection. Thus there is no need to prescribe antibiotic therapy for every patient.

Overuse of antibiotic therapy can lead to the growth of resistant strains that require higher doses to control. This has already occurred in the treatment of some strains of gonorrhea. Overuse also makes one less likely to respond to the drug in the future. Also, drug reactions can be very serious; the indiscriminate use of antibiotic therapy increases the number of reactions and results in unnecessary deaths.

What do you think? ●

tents in deep tissue infections. You may have seen a dog suffering from an abscess acquired in a fight with a cat. Or you may have had a group of staph-infected hair follicles (pimples) appear on your cheeks and chin just in time to embarrass you for a Saturday night date. The pus pockets forming in response to infection should be drained, flushed with an antibiotic, and allowed to continue draining to promote healing.

Staph organisms are everywhere and can be transmitted by contact with contaminated material (for instance, blankets) or in the air (sneeze droplets). Newborn babies are particularly at risk and can develop an infection if skin breaks due to diaper chafing.

Streptococci cause sore throats, ear infections, nasopharyngitis, tonsilitis, impetigo, bacterial endocarditis, and can lead to rheumatic fever and even tooth decay. Infection in wounds (skin abrasions or surgical wounds) is caused by Group A streptococci, as are many sore throats and ear infections. Impetigo is a Group A skin infection, usually prevalent among children, and is extremely infectious. Gymnasts and wrestlers can contract the disease after exercising on contaminated mats. Like staph infections, strep infections respond well to antibiotic treatment.

SEXUALLY TRANSMITTED DISEASES

Before you read this section, complete Discovery Activity 18.3.

Sexually transmitted diseases (STDs) are bacterial or, in the case of herpes, viral infections that attack the genital areas and may cause serious complications elsewhere in the body. The organisms thrive on warm, moist body surfaces, such as the mucous membranes that line the reproductive organs, mouth, and rectum. STDs are transmitted via sexual contact. There is no evidence that they can be contracted from toilet seats, drinking cups, wet towels, and the like.

Until the 1970s these infections were called venereal disease (named for Venus, the goddess of love).

Discovery Activity 18.3
TEST YOUR KNOWLEDGE ABOUT STDs

Complete the true–false test below to discover how much you know about sexually transmitted diseases. Circle either T or F and score your test from the answers on page 440.

1. Syphilis can be acquired by coming in contact with a contaminated toilet seat.   True   False

2. Pubic lice can be transmitted only through sexual contact.   True   False

3. Gonorrhea is easily eradicated through the use of penicillin.   True   False

4. STDs cannot be transmitted from one partner to another unless one or both reach orgasm.   True   False

5. Some people have developed an immunity to STDs and need not take precautions.   True   False

6. Gonorrhea is easily detected in the female.   True   False

7. Syphilis can be transmitted by kissing an infected person.   True   False

8. STDs are uncommon and there is generally no need for precautionary measures.   True   False

9. If one partner is infected with gonorrhea or syphilis, the other partner has only a slight chance of acquiring the disease during sexual contact.   True   False

10. Genital herpes is easily cured with antibiotic therapy.   True   False

Recently, however, the term sexually transmitted diseases has come into use because it is thought to be more descriptive. Medical knowledge about STDs has increased dramatically in recent years. In the past, venereal disease referred to five types of infections, the most important being syphilis and gonorrhea. Today, however, it is known that over 20 different organisms are linked to STDs. Among the STDs that are the focus of recent research are nongonococcal urethritis (NGU), resistant strains of gonorrhea, and Herpes simplex, type 2.

Why should you be concerned about STDs? A major reason is that the incidence of these diseases has been skyrocketing in recent years. The U.S. Department of Public Health considers the problem not just an epidemic but a pandemic. An estimated 2.5 million

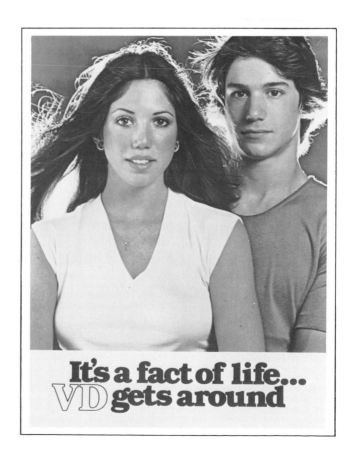

It's a fact of life... VD gets around

Answers to self-test on STDs:

1. False. Highly unlikely and nearly impossible.

2. False. Pubic lice are commonly spread through use of contaminated towels, clothing, or linen.

3. False. Some strains of gonorrhea are extremely resistant to penicilin and very difficult to eradicate with other antibiotics.

4. False. Reaching orgasm has nothing to do with the spread of STDs.

5. False. One cannot develop a natural immunity to STDs.

6. False. Gonorrhea in the female is difficult to detect and may exist for months prior to any noticeable symptoms.

7. True. A person with a chancre sore on the mouth could transmit syphilis to a partner through kissing.

8. False. STDs are quite common among all socio-economic groups and all age groups.

9. False. The probability of acquiring an STD from an infected sexual partner is quite high.

10. False. At present, there is no known cure for genital herpes. ●

Answers: 9–10 correct—Excellent; 7–8 correct—Good; 5–6 correct—Poor; fewer than 5 correct—Very poor

new cases of gonorrhea occurred in 1979, and the actual number is probably much higher because so many cases go unreported. Although anyone can contract a venereal disease, more than half of the victims of gonorrhea are between the ages of 15 and 24, and many of these cases are repeats. Many bacterial types of STD can be treated with antibiotics, but untreated cases can lead to a variety of serious health problems. There is increasing attention among medical specialists toward the role of STDs in causing birth defects, infertility, and long-term disability. Particularly alarming is the discovery of new forms of STD that have caused deaths among homosexual males. Let's examine how the STD pandemic occurred and then consider the major types of STDs, prevention, and treatment.

Historical Background

Sexually transmitted diseases were mentioned in the Old Testament as early as 1500 B.C. The first epidemic of venereal disease was blamed on Christopher Columbus's crew, who were said to have brought the diseases back from the New World. In the modern era, the first worldwide epidemic of gonorrhea took place during and after World War I. With the introduction of sulfa drugs in the 1930s and penicillin in the 1940s, both gonorrhea and syphilis seemed to have been checked and appeared headed for eradication. This apparent victory resulted in reduced research dollars, less emphasis on prevention, and lack of follow-up on the sexual partners of treated patients. As a result, hundreds of thousands of people infected with STDs unknowingly transmitted the diseases to others.

Several social factors contributed to the growing incidence of STDs, which by the 1960s had begun to reach epidemic proportions. The introduction of birth control pills and IUDs decreased the use of condoms, which had provided good protection against some STDs. Changing sexual standards meant that people were engaging in sex at younger ages and with more partners than in the past. Many people felt complacent about contracting an STD because they assumed that the disease could be easily treated. Others were reluctant to seek treatment, fearing the social stigma associated with STDs. In addition, strains of gonorrhea appeared that were resistant to treatment with penicillin. Even in strains that responded to penicillin, larger dosages of the drug were required. Since the 1950s, an injection four times more powerful in men and ten times more powerful in women has been required to elicit a cure. And even though new antibiotic treatments are being explored, experts are concerned that strains might develop that are resistant to these treatments.

Gonorrhea

Gonorrhea, popularly known as "clap," is caused by the **gonococcus** bacterium and is transmitted by intercourse, and by oral-genital and anal-genital contact. It affects the urogenital tract in both sexes—the urethra in males and the urethra, vagina, and cervix in females.

The symptoms are somewhat different in men and women because of their different anatomies. The early symptom in men is a milky, bad-smelling discharge from the penis. Beginning three to eight days after exposure, urination may become compelling and be accompanied by a burning sensation. If the infection goes untreated, it can cause swelling of the testicles and damage to the prostate gland, resulting ultimately in sterility. Further complications may include bladder or kidney conditions.

Whereas infected men are usually aware that something is wrong with them, women may not notice the early signs of gonorrhea. The symptoms are similar to those in common vaginal infections—a slight burning sensation in the genital area and a mild discharge from the vagina. It is estimated that 80 percent of women who have gonorrhea are unaware of it until the disease has become more severe. If left untreated, gonorrhea invades the uterus, Fallopian tubes, and ovaries. Pelvic infection may result, causing sterility or requiring surgical removal of the pelvic organs.

Gonorrhea can be passed from an infected mother to her infant as it passes through the vaginal canal during delivery, often resulting in blindness. To prevent this from occurring, the eyes of newborns are routinely treated with silver nitrate or penicillin.

Diagnosis of gonorrhea is not as simple as it is for syphilis. It requires laboratory examination of a sample taken from the infected area with a cotton swab or growing the bacteria under laboratory conditions. The disease usually responds to penicillin treatment or, if the victim is allergic to penicillin, to tetracycline drugs. As mentioned earlier, researchers have recently uncovered a new strain of penicillin-resistant gonorrhea. This development has prompted interest in using tetracycline drugs rather than penicillin in the initial treatment of gonorrhea.

Syphilis

Syphilis is caused by an organism called a **spirochete** and is transmitted from open sores during intercourse, during oral-genital or genital-anal contact, or by kissing a person who has a syphilic chancre in the mouth region. The disease progresses through four stages. In

Issues in Health *(continued)*

that may be detrimental to the child's health and emotional well-being.

The problem of a minor contracting an STD can provide an opportunity to open the lines of communication and pave the way toward improved parent-child relationships in the future. Family problems may worsen if parents discover the problem months after treatment. Until a child reaches the age of majority, it is argued, parents have the obligation and responsibility to be informed and aware of all the child's problems. Most parents want to be involved and are deeply hurt when they are not consulted.

What do you think? ●

Stage One (primary stage) a painless sore, called a chancre ("shanker"), appears three to four weeks after the spirochete enters the body. The chancre looks like a pimple or wart and appears where the spirochete entered the body, often on the penis, the lips, or the vaginal wall. The chancre may go unnoticed in women or may be ignored in men, because it is painless and disappears in a few weeks without treatment.

Stage Two (secondary stage) occurs about six weeks after contact. Symptoms may include a rash over the entire body, welts around the genitals, low-grade fever, headache, hair falling out, and sore throat. These symp-

Microscopic examination reveals the corkscrewlike appearance of the syphilis spirochete.

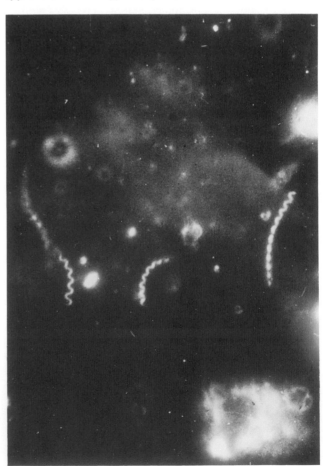

toms also disappear without treatment. However, if the symptoms are noticeable to them, most victims see a doctor. Thus, it is uncommon for cases of syphilis in the United States to progress to the third stage.

Stage Three (latency stage) begins about two years after contact (and up to five years in some people). After one year, the victim cannot transmit the disease to anyone else. The only exception is that a pregnant woman can transmit the disease to her fetus through the placental wall. Latency may last for 40 or more years. During this time the organism infects the heart, brain, and other organs. By Stage Four (tertiary stage) the disease may lead to heart failure, blindness, other organ damage, and finally death.

Syphilis can be detected by means of a simple blood test. Because it is such a potentially dangerous disease and can be transmitted to unborn babies, most states require a blood test for syphilis prior to marriage and, in pregnant women, during the prenatal period. Syphilis generally responds well to penicillin or, in some cases, to other antibiotics. Because no immunity develops to the disease, prompt diagnosis and treatment after any possible exposure are essential.

Herpes Simplex, Type 2

Genital herpes is a viral infection caused by the virus **herpes simplex, type 2.** As noted earlier, the virus is related to herpes simplex, type 1, which causes cold sores or fever blisters. Whereas type 1 herpes affects the mouth region, type 2 herpes affects the genital region and is transmitted through sexual contact. Herpes type 2 now rivals gonorrhea as one of the most common sexually transmitted diseases in this country. The Center for Disease Control estimates that over 20 million Americans have been exposed to herpes type 2.

The major symptom, which appears two to six days after contact with an infected person, is an outbreak of very painful sores on the genitalia. Other symptoms may include fatigue, swelling of the legs, watery eyes, and painful urination.

Herpes has potentially more harmful effects for women than for men. It has been found that women who have herpes, type 2, are eight times more likely to develop cervical cancer than noninfected women. If a pregnant woman has an outbreak of herpes at the time her child is delivered, she runs a risk of one in four that the newborn will contract the disease and suffer damage or even die. Thus the wisest course of action for pregnant women with herpes is to be delivered by cesarean section.

Unlike gonorrhea, herpes cannot be cured. Once the virus is in the body it remains in the body, and outbreaks can occur periodically, spreading the disease. Symptoms can be alleviated by soaking the genital area in hot water, then keeping it clean and dry, or with a new drug called acyclorir. In case of severe outbreaks, a doctor should be consulted.

Nongonococcal Urethritis

Urethritis refers to an infection of the urinary tract. **Nongonococcal urethritis (NGU)** is urethritis that is caused not by the gonococcus bacterium but by some other organism. It has been found that about half of the cases of NGU are caused by the organism **chlamydia trachomatis.** In males NGU causes a discharge, as in gonorrhea, but in females there may be no symptoms. As a result many cases go undiagnosed.

Most patients who are treated for NGU are young, white, single, sexually active, and affluent. NGU is probably the most common form of urethritis seen in student health centers and by private physicians. Whereas gonorrhea usually responds to treatment with penicillin, NGU responds to other antibiotics (usually tetracycline). Often NGU is recognized in cases when gonorrhea is not identified as the problem or when penicillin treatment for gonorrhea proves ineffective.

Although our discussion of STDs has covered the most common forms, there are others as well. See Table 18.4 for information about other STDs.

Homosexuals and STDs

The greatest increase in STDs in recent years has occurred among homosexuals. Male homosexuals account for the majority of this increase. Only a small percentage (less than 4 percent) of male homosexuals

Table 18.4
PREVALENT SEXUALLY TRANSMISSIBLE DISEASES

Disease	Estimated Number of Persons Affected Yearly	Signs a Woman May Notice	Signs a Man May Notice	Consequences of Prolonged Infection	Special Considerations
Gonorrhea	3,000,000	Puslike vaginal discharge, vaginal soreness, lower abdominal pain, painful urination.	Puslike urethral discharge.	Pelvic inflammatory disease (PID)—tubal damage, pelvic adhesions and tubo-ovarian abscesses, tubal pregnancy, which can lead to pathological sterility.	Even if the original gonoccocal infection is cured, PID may predispose the body to repeated episodes of pelvic inflammation caused by a variety of organisms.
Syphilis	More than 400,000	Rashes appearing almost anywhere on the body, including palms of hands and soles of feet. Chancre (lesion) on or in vagina, anus or mouth.	Rashes or hair loss in the same pattern as in women. Chancre on or around penis.	Brain or heart damage.	An infected pregnant woman may pass syphilis to a developing fetus, which could lead to a variety of birth defects.
Sexually Transmitted Nongonococcal Urethritis/Cervicitis	3,000,000	Symptoms similar to those caused by gonorrhea.	Occasionally, heavy puslike discharge. More frequently, a mild watery discharge.	Pelvic Inflammatory Disease. (See Gonorrhea)	Like gonococcal PID, nongonococcal PID could lead to repeated episodes. Organisms which cause this disease can infect a newborn infant during the birth process and may result in pneumonia or eye infection.
Genital Herpes	Between 5,000,000 and 20,000,000	Painful, blisterlike, fluid-filled lesion (or cluster of lesions) on, in or around vagina. Often accompanied by swollen glands in groin area.	Same as in women, only on or around penis.	Under study at this time. Genital herpes has been implicated with a form of meningitis and associated with cervical cancer.	Genital herpes may be passed from an infected pregnant woman to her newborn during birth, causing infant death or neurological damage.

Trichomoniasis	3,000,000	Heavy, frothy, often yellow, foul-smelling vaginal discharge. Vaginal itching, often severe and continuous.	Most often, none. Occasionally, mild urethral discharge.	The consequences of repeated infection are under study. There are indications that repeated trichomoniasis may damage cervical tissue.	The venereal nature of trichomoniasis often is misunderstood or denied, even by doctors. Male partners often are ignored in the treatment process, leading to reinfection of the female.
Pubic lice	Unavailable	Intense itching in pubic hair or other hairy areas.	Intense itching in pubic hair or other hairy areas.	Skin rash, infection.	Pubic lice are transmitted through sexual contact, clothing, or linen. Cream, lotion, or shampoo preparations of gamma benzene will eliminate the adult lice and their eggs.
Scabies	Unavailable	Blisterlike vesicles appear on the skin surface, developing into papules, pustules, and an itchy rash.	Same as in women.	Infection.	Parasites invade the genital area, as well as the hands and feet. Can be transmitted through sexual contact or contact with clothing or linen.
Genital warts	Unavailable	Wart on lower part of the vaginal opening.	Wart on glans, foreskin, opening, or shaft of the penis.	Additional warts may appear, infection may occur.	Caused by a virus similar to those causing skin warts; usually transmitted by sexual contact. Chemical treatment or surgery successfully removes the warts.
Nonspecific vaginitis	Unavailable	Blisterlike vesicles appear on skin surface, developing into papules, pustules, and an itchy rash.	Infection.		Parasites invade the genital area, as well as the hands, wrists, and feet.

SOURCE: American Social Health Association, 1981. Reprinted by permission.

who contract gonorrhea name another man as the infectious contact, whereas 12 to 18 percent of males with syphilis indicate the disease was spread by another male.

One of the hypotheses about the prevalence of sexually transmitted diseases in the homosexual population relates to the number of sexual contacts. Because some homosexuals have sexual contact with many partners, their chances of contracting STDs are greater.

There has also been recent speculation and some evidence that the immunological system of homosexuals may play a role in their vulnerability to STDs. According to the Center for Disease Control, during the summer of 1981 a surprisingly large number of young homosexuals contracted a rare form of pneumonia and a rare form of skin cancer, called Kaposi's sarcoma. These conditions are known to be a result of damaged immunological systems, and it is suspected by some that homosexuals may have less effective immunological systems than heterosexuals. If this is so, perhaps the prevalence of STDs in the homosexual population is partly a function of the inability of the immunological system to respond to the organisms causing the STDs.

Prevention of STDs

Concept: Most cases of sexually transmitted diseases could be prevented.

In view of the prevalence and potential seriousness of STDs, it might seem that the only wise course of action would be to abstain from sexual activity altogether. Of course, this solution would never be acceptable to most people, so it is necessary to consider more practical approaches.

Obviously, the number one preventive measure is to avoid sexual relations with someone who might have an STD. Thus, being selective in your sexual activity by "knowing your partner" is extremely important.

The use of condoms is another good preventive approach. Used properly, condoms prevent many venereal disease germs from traveling from one partner to another. After intercourse, the penis should be withdrawn slowly while holding the ring of the condom to prevent it from slipping off. Condoms should never be used more than once or lubricated with vaseline or other ointments, which damage and weaken the rubber.

Hygiene can also be helpful in STD prevention. Men should wash the genitals with soap and water after sex. Women should cleanse the genitals before and after sexual contact.

If you have sexual relations with several partners, you should have periodic screening for STDs. This is especially important if you experience any persistent symptoms. If you do have an STD, it is essential that your sexual partners be notified and that they receive screening and, if necessary, treatment.

Finally, because STDs can be transmitted to an unborn fetus or to a newborn, prenatal screening for women is important.

CONCLUSION

Many communicable diseases can be prevented through vaccination and the body's immune mechanism or through drug therapy, such as antibiotics. There is no known prevention for the common cold, mononucleosis, or some types of flu, although precautionary measures can reduce the risk.

Wise health decisions can completely eliminate the risk of acquiring an STD. You also have the power to decrease the risk of acquiring most other communicable diseases by practicing proper health habits. Once again, your personal health practices can make a difference in leading a more healthy life.

SUMMARY

1. Certain factors must exist for a communicable disease to occur in humans: a live virus or bacteria (pathogen) must be present; the pathogen must be able to live, multiply, escape from the reservoir,

contact and enter a host (human); and the host must receive the pathogen.

2. The body's immune system can prevent several communicable diseases from recurring.

3. The body's mechanism of defense generally fights off microorganisms before severe infections occur.

4. Antibiotic therapy has no effect on viral infections; it does control many secondary bacterial infections that penetrate the body's mechanisms of defense.

5. Vaccination can prevent several childhood communicable diseases, including polio, measles, mumps, rubella, and diphtheria.

6. The common cold cannot be prevented or cured.

7. Millions of people in the United States contract STDs. STDs can be prevented by proper hygiene and screening.

8. New strains of gonorrhea are appearing that are extremely resistant to penicillin; other antibiotics are now being tried on these strains.

9. There is no known cure for genital herpes.

10. Left untreated, STDs cause permanent damage to the human body and, in some cases, death.

Laboratory 1
YOUR COMMUNICABLE DISEASE RECORD

Purpose To identify and date the communicable diseases contracted in your lifetime.
To analyze potential communicable disease hazards for your future.

Size of Group Subjects work alone in their seats.

Equipment None.

Procedure

1. Complete the chart below, identifying the communicable diseases you have contracted. Record the date (year and month) the illness occurred.

2. Record vaccination or inoculation dates for diseases or illnesses where applicable (e.g., tetanus injection).

Illness (disease)	Date	Comment (include vaccination date, inoculation, number of bouts per year)
1. Bronchitis		
2. Chicken pox		
3. Cholera		
4. Cold (most recent)		
5. Diphtheria		
6. Hepatitis		
7. Influenza		
8. Malaria		
9. Measles (2 weeks)		
10. Measles (German, 3 weeks)		
11. Mononucleosis		
12. Mumps		
13. Polio		
14. Rabies		
15. Rheumatic fever		
16. Scarlet fever		
17. Smallpox		
18. Strep throat		
19. Tetanus		
20. Tuberculosis		
21. Typhoid fever		
22. Whooping cough		
23. Yellow fever		
24. Other:		

Results

1. List the communicable diseases you have contracted to date.

2. List those from which you are now protected through vaccination or natural immunity from having previously contracted the disease.

3. List those for which there is no protection (immunity).

4. List those diseases for which vaccinations are available that you have not received.

5. What common childhood diseases did you avoid that you could eventually contract? What special difficulties would you anticipate if you contracted these diseases as an adult?

6. Analyze your future in terms of contracting communicable diseases.

Laboratory 2
COMMUNICABLE DISEASES—CONTROL IN VARIOUS SETTINGS

Purpose To identify common problems in the home and the university that contribute to the spread of communicable disease.

Size of Group Between three and five students per group.

Equipment None.

Procedure

1. Each group meets in a separate section of the room.

2. Five primary sites commonly used in daily routines by the students in the group are identified (e.g., cafeteria, dormitory or bedroom, kitchen, classroom, automobile).

3. Each student is assigned one primary site for intensive study.

4. For the next 15 to 20 minutes, the entire group "brainstorms" each area to provide assistance to each individual. Groups are looking for behavior or environmental conditions in their setting that contribute to the spread of disease, such as:

   a. shaking hands
   b. touching the eyes, inside the nose
   c. sneezing
   d. poor ventilation
   e. drinking out of the same cup
   f. sharing towels
   g. hygiene practices

5. For the next three days, each student studies his or her assigned area carefully, building a list of suggested changes in that setting to help prevent the spread of disease.

Results

One member from each group is chosen to summarize the suggestions for each setting.

health
and
society

Part Seven

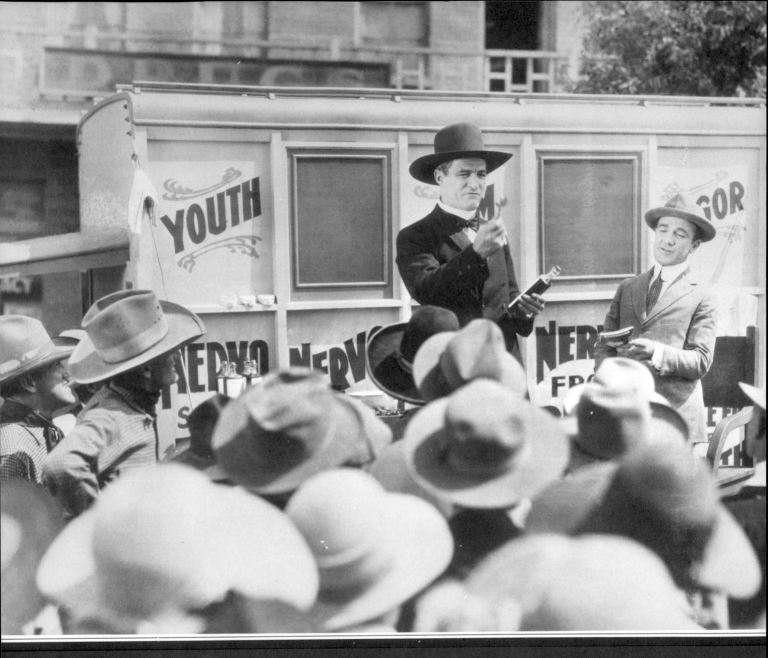

chapter *19*

health and
the consumer

Each individual in our society is the guardian of his or her own health. This basic responsibility requires a careful examination and analysis of health-related products before coming to a conclusion about their safe, beneficial use. The current consumer movement encourages individuals to become "healthy skeptics" as they evaluate the many scientific claims and counter-claims about the health-related products they use.

The voice of the individual consumer can make a difference. In fact, the majority of investigations of health-related products are initiated by consumer complaints. It is impossible for the various government and private agencies to monitor the influx of new products; each individual must therefore assume this responsibility by asking hard questions about safety, advertising claims, and cost.

This chapter provides information on several health-related products and suggests ways the consumer can evaluate advertising claims and take action through federal, state, or private agencies.

QUACKERY

Misrepresentation of health products and services is a profitable con game that drains the American public of billions of dollars each year. **Quacks** are people who use false advertising and a variety of other lures to entice consumers to spend their money on drugs, mechanical devices, foods, and other products that do no good and can be harmful.

The quack has existed for millennia and continues to thrive for several reasons. People fear pain, illness, aging, and death. Those who have a serious disease that modern medicine cannot cure may be especially vulnerable to health quacks. And, unfortunately, every new legitimate achievement of modern medical research makes it easier for quacks to convince people that they too have developed a cure. Also, many people suffer from conditions that will eventually improve without any treatment. Ailments of this sort disappear by themselves during the course of a quack's expensive treatment, and the quack gets the credit and the publicity. Finally, a quack can label any condition "cancer," prescribe some special cure, and win over a host of new patients—who may actually have cancer.

Mail-Order Quacks

Mail-order quacks promote drugs; food fads; and devices to energize, revitalize, develop, or cure just about anything imaginable. Drug advertisements focus on cures for cancer, diabetes, arthritis, constipation, and many other health problems. Food fads are currently one of our major quackery problems; the number of new books by so-called nutrition experts continues to increase, each promoting a special diet or special approach to weight loss. Mail-order quackery is typified by advertisements promoting the copper bracelet as a cure for arthritis. Such quack advertisements make their way into the home through all types of media, both print and visual. The days of the traveling medicine show may be gone; however, the huckster is still very much with us in quack advertisements.

One of the most extensive investigations of mail-order health advertising was conducted by the Pennsylvania Medical Society in 1977. Five hundred nationally circulated magazines were surveyed, one-fourth of which were found to carry mail-order ads for health products. Typical products included bust developers, weight reducers, hair loss remedies, blemish removers, longevity formulas, aphrodisiacs, sexual pleasure devices, penis enlargers, and impotency cures. Practically all the ads shared one characteristic, according to the Pennsylvania Medical Society: they were misleading.[1]

The problem of mail-order quackery is widespread and can be policed only by the consumer. It is a mistake to assume that advice published in magazines or books is legitimate or that ads appearing in reputable magazines are accurate. Ad space is sold in most publications with little concern for the accuracy of the claims.

Very few ads are unacceptable to publishers, as long as they receive payment for the advertising space.

Recognizing Quackery

How can you tell if you're dealing with a quack? Some tip-offs include:

1. Promise or guarantee of a quick cure;
2. Use of a "secret remedy" or unorthodox treatment;
3. Use of advertisement to gain patients, especially ads in sensational magazines, such as those related to faith healing;
4. Use of testimonials of patients who have been cured;
5. Claims that a product will cure a wide variety of ailments;
6. Request for payments in advance;
7. Use of scare tactics, such as warnings of harmful consequences if a product being promoted isn't used; and
8. Claims from the sponsor of the product that the medical profession is against them.

Quackery endangers both your pocketbook and your health. Fake treatments may delay early and accurate diagnosis and treatment until the problem is very serious. Your best protection is to analyze carefully all products or treatment methods you are considering. In most cases using good sense is enough. Sometimes it may be necessary to contact your doctor or a reputable agency or nonprofit organization. One good resource for information on drugs is a publication called *The Medicine Show,* an unbiased report on numerous products by the editors of *Consumer Report.*[2] Other sources of health-related consumer information are the National Health Council; the World Health Organization; the Food and Drug Administration; the U.S. Department of Health and Welfare; and various nonprofit associations, such as the American Heart Association, the American Lung Association, the American Cancer Society, and the American Medical Association.

Issues in Health
SHOULD ADVERTISEMENTS FOR HEALTH-RELATED PRODUCTS BE MORE STRICTLY CONTROLLED?

Thousands of worthless and potentially dangerous products are sold each year through misleading advertising. Many of these products appeal to basic human needs. Some purport to cure serious diseases; others claim their use will result in renewed energy, a slowing of the aging process, rejuvenation of aging skin, weight loss, and numerous other benefits. For the most part, the products are merely expensive and ineffective. Sometimes, however, they are harmful. The fact remains that the consumer is bombarded with such advertisements through magazine, newspaper, radio, and TV ads. Some people feel that stricter control of advertising is needed to protect the consumer's health and pocketbook.

Ideally, consumers should be able to analyze the worth and safety of a health-related product. In reality, however, many individuals do not possess the necessary judgment to make wise decisions in this area. These individuals, it is argued, need protection through stricter legislation governing ads for health-related products.

Vagueness and indirect suggestion of unfounded claims represent false advertising. Individuals afflicted with a serious disease or disorder cannot be expected to resist the hope of a miracle cure, regardless of the cost. These individuals, many of them from the elderly population, may stop effective treatment in favor of a "miracle" approach that endangers their health or life. For these individuals, stricter control is necessary. Advocates of stricter control argue that fines are needed to discourage the use of deceptive advertisement. To date, fines are imposed only as a result of criminal prosecution,

(continued)

Issues in Health (continued)

and only a few cases reach the courts. Civil penalites, it is argued, would be less cumbersome, less expensive, and more expedient in dealing with advertising fraud.

Opponents of stricter control of advertising point out that the media have the First Amendment right of freedom of speech and, short of libel, cannot be told what to print and what not to print. Publishers also contend that screening ads is time-consuming, expensive, extremely difficult, and often outside the competency of their staff. The selling of advertising space or time is an essential part of media work, providing valuable revenue to supplement subscription sales and keep the publication financially solvent. With stricter control of advertising, considerable revenue might be lost and more publications would fold. Opponents of stricter control feel that consumers should decide for themselves whether a product is valuable, safe, and effective. Consumers can consult their family physician or consumer agency for advice before making purchases.

What do you think? ●

Miracle Cures That Aren't

Concept: There is no known cure for rheumatoid arthritis.

Arthritis "remedies." Approximately 12 to 15 million Americans suffer from some form of arthritis or inflammation, pain, stiffening, swelling, and aching in the joints. Rheumatoid arthritis, one of the world's most crippling diseases, frequently occurs in young people. Arthritis victims are the easiest prey for quacks proposing all kinds of expensive remedies, including special gadgets, painkillers, dietary cures, clinics, and spas. Among the most common quack "cures" is a copper bracelet, which is claimed to treat arthritis magnetically. Another device is a vibrator, which supposedly relieves muscle pain. There is no evidence that these methods work. Americans spend $400 to $500 million annually on such worthless and often harmful cures. Most arthritis victims find that pain and stiffness disappear from time to time. When this happens, many sufferers credit the copper bracelet or vibrator. The truth is that the symptoms would have disappeared anyway, only to return again later.

Numerous types of arthritis exist, and medical diagnosis is needed in order to determine the appropriate treatment. In general, rheumatoid arthritis can best be managed by rest and aspirin to control pain and reduce inflammation.

Concept: There is no evidence that laetrile can cure cancer.

Cancer "cures." At this writing, the causes of various types of cancer are uncertain and there is no single cure for this disease. Even so, many desperate people spend huge sums of money for special ointments, pills, injections, diets, and mechanical treatments, thereby bypassing more promising medical treatments. The quack plays on the cancer patient's fear and promotes an unorthodox or "natural" remedy.

Unfortunately, many victims stop beneficial treatment in favor of the unproved method. The disease of cancer is ideal for quackery, because a remission will occur in many cases, with or without treatment. When remission occurs, the patient is encouraged to give credit to the quack remedy.

Table 19.1 summarizes some unproven remedies identified by the American Cancer Society that are purported to help cancer patients. Of these approaches, **laetrile** has received considerable attention in recent years. An estimated 75,000 cancer patients have used laetrile (a derivative of apricot pits) as part of their treatment; some have abandoned standard cancer treatments to do so. Public interest in laetrile peaked with

the case of Chad Greene, age 3, whose parents violated a court order to continue standard cancer treatment and instead took him to a laetrile center in Tijuana, Mexico. Chad died in Tijuana in October 1979.

The findings of the first scientific study (a $500,000 National Cancer Institute project) on the effectiveness of laetrile in treating cancer patients are now available. The study, sponsored by the National Cancer Institute and the FDA, involved 178 cancer patients, ranging in age from 18 to 84, with cancer of the lungs, stomach, colon, breasts, and other organs. Laetrile injections and pills were combined with "metabolic therapy," the use of high doses of vitamins, pancreatic enzymes, and a special diet. Over 150 patients have died, and the mean

Table 19.1
SOME UNPROVEN METHODS OF CANCER TREATMENT

Type Remedy	Basic Ingredients	Therapy Regimen	Evaluation
Bonifacio Anticancer Goat Serum	Intestinal villi of goats	0.5 ml every 48 hrs for 2 injections, increased to 1 ml after 48 hrs.	Invalid therapeutic evidence
Cancer Lipid Concentrate	Equine antibodies	Unable to determine	Research support
Malignancy Index Diagnostic Test	Unable to determine	Unable to determine	Ineffective treatment
Chaparral Tea	Leaves and stems of Larrea divaricata	Orally	Without therapeutic evidence
Chase Dietary Method	Food buffers—raw fruits and raw salads	Orally and via enema	Without therapeutic evidence
Fresh Cell Therapy	Fresh embryonic animal cells of organ or tissue with dysfunction	Injection	Without therapeutic evidence
Livingston Vaccine	Vaccine and antisera of pleomorphic microorganism	Injection twice a week for an indefinite time	Without therapeutic evidence
Orgone Energy Devices	Absorption of "blue bions" or "cosmic orgone energy" from the atmosphere	Accumulators for patients; materials approximately 2–4 inches from surface of body	Without therapeutic evidence of treatment or diagnosis
Revici Cancer Control	Adjustment of the acid–alkaline level through lipids	Biologically guided chemotherapy	Without therapeutic evidence
Zen Macrobiotic Diet	Yin and yang	Balance ratio 5 to 1: Yin to yang	Not beneficial as treatment, hazardous to health

Adapted from *Unproven Methods of Cancer Treatment*, American Cancer Society, 1975. Reprinted by permission.

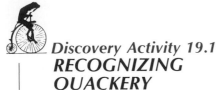

Discovery Activity 19.1
RECOGNIZING QUACKERY

Identify a product advertised in a magazine or newspaper that you suspect is not as effective or safe as claimed. List the clues that arouse your suspicion. Some health products commonly advertised are rubber suits and weighted belts to lose weight, pulley devices to get fit, vitamins and minerals to improve your health and vitality, pills or candy to depress appetite, creams to improve your complexion, and special gadgets to increase the size of various body parts.

Product   **Questionable Claims and Phrases**

Is the product safe? What potential dangers exist for users? Do you think the product works? How can the consumer recognize such unfounded claims? ●

survival time has been less than five months. Cancer worsened in all patients in spite of the laetrile treatment. It was concluded that laetrile is useless against cancer; it neither prevents the disease from spreading nor relieves pain or discomfort. In addition, laetrile was found to be toxic, producing cyanide levels high enough to kill animals and nearly high enough to kill humans. Investigators believe the findings are conclusive enough to close the books on laetrile and file it with other useless quack approaches.

Mail-order epilepsy treatments. The mail-order treatment of epilepsy is thriving. Those who respond to magazine ads are sent questionnaires seeking information about their condition along with a booklet praising the firm's product. If they write for the product, they receive a monthly supply of medicine for $10.00

or more. The active ingredient in the drug is generally **phenobarbital,** which has been used to control epilepsy for years. The problem is that phenobarbital is not adequate drug therapy for all patients. It is also a habit-forming depressant. Again, there is no magic cure for epilepsy: Effective management of the condition calls for individualized drug therapy under medical supervision. Another technique that has been successful is surgical removal of abnormal brain tissue in which the seizure originates.

COMMON NONPRESCRIPTION MEDICATIONS: HOW EFFECTIVE?

Aspirin: Brands Don't Matter

Concept: The only significant differences among brands of aspirin—plain, buffered, or in combination with other drugs—is price.

Any brand of **aspirin** is effective in providing some relief from fever, aches, grippe, flu, and tension headaches. To save money, ask your druggist for the least expensive generic aspirin. Using any of the highly advertised products will only relieve your pocketbook of a little more money.

Aspirin is the most commonly used medicine in the American household. Follow these suggestions for proper use:

1. Avoid aspirin if you react with hives, swelling of the mucous membranes, or asthma.

2. If you suffer stomach upset from taking aspirin, take it immediately after eating, and always drink a full glass of water with each dose.

3. Discard aspirin that has been in your medicine cabinet longer than two or three months. High humidity and moisture cause a chemical decom-

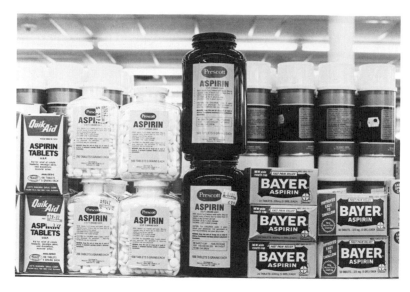

The only real difference among the scores of brands of aspirin is price.

position of the tablets. If aspirin have a vinegary odor or crumble when held between the fingers, discard them immediately. In this condition they are less effective and much more likely to irritate the stomach.

4. Avoid purchasing special-flavored children's aspirin. Any medicine that tastes like candy increases the risk of aspirin poisoning.

5. Avoid using aspirin for extended periods of time without medical supervision. See a physician if symptoms continue for more than 10 days (5 days in children under 12) or if new symptoms develop.

6. Read the label carefully and follow directions.

7. Avoid aspirin if you are allergic to it or if you have ulcers or a bleeding problem.

8. Seek medical assistance immediately if you experience any bleeding or vomiting of blood after taking aspirin.

9. Avoid administering aspirin-containing products to a child who has cold or flu symptoms or chicken pox. Give the child acetamenophen instead. Some children who are given aspirin appear to be more likely to develop **Reyes syndrome.** This is an acute illness in children up to 12 years of age that often follows the flu or other viral infection and affects the upper respiratory tract. Vomiting, progressive damage to the central nervous system, and fatty liver symptoms may occur, with 30 percent of the victims dying from cerebral damage.

Antacids

Concept: Highly advertised antacids for the treatment of indigestion, other than simple antacids, are expensive and unnecessary.

There are hundreds of **antacids** on the market to treat indigestion. Nothing is more effective than precipitated chalk (precipitated calcium carbonate U.S.P.), which can be purchased cheaply at any drugstore. If constipation occurs, use magnesium carbonate U.S.P. instead, or combine precipitated chalk with magnesium oxide U.S.P. Sodium bicarbonate (baking soda), a common home remedy, is safe and effective for indigestion if used sparingly. The closer a product is to a simple antacid, the more effective it is. If you purchase antacid tablets, make sure you suck or chew them thoroughly so that they are dissolved in the stomach before moving into the small intestine.

Sleep Aids

Concept: Occasional mild insomnia is normal and need not be treated with special drugstore remedies.

People of all ages have difficulty sleeping at times. Sleeplessness is often caused by tension or stress; only rarely is it caused by some physical disorder. There is no evidence that lack of sleep by itself is detrimental to health. Even people who have been deprived of sleep for long periods suffer no long-term ill effects once they are permitted to sleep again. Nevertheless, many people believe that if they lose sleep, their functioning will be impaired. Thus, they respond to occasional sleeplessness by using over-the-counter sleep remedies.

These nonprescription sleep aids contain small amounts of antihistamine and a painkiller (aspirin). Used infrequently, they offer little danger, providing the user follows directions and does not take stronger doses than are recommended. Overuse of sleep preparations containing antihistamines can produce side effects, such as dizziness, lack of coordination, blurred vision, skin rashes, and possibly blood changes. If loss of sleep is only occasional, medication is not recommended. If it becomes chronic, a physician should be consulted, because the condition may indicate other problems, such as stress or depression.

Cough Medicine

Concept: Cough medicine, over-the-counter or prescription, is of little or no value in relieving a cough caused by the common cold.

Coughing is a reflex action controlled by a cough center in the brain. It is nature's response to irritation in the respiratory tract or pleural lining of the lungs. Coughing is often caused by the common cold and can also be associated with a bacterial infection, pneumonia, and tuberculosis.

More than a hundred over-the-counter remedies are available to the consumer. All have one thing in common: they do not work. Most contain sugar, alcohol, antihistamines, salts, chloroform, and flavoring. Only **codeine** and **dextromethorphan,** contained in some prescription cough medicines, mildly depress the cough center with only a slight effect upon the cough. The only apparent benefit of over-the-counter cough medicine, as indicated in carefully controlled studies, is that one thinks the cough is easing up and adapts somewhat. Candy drops, hot drinks, vaporizers, or steam inhalation offer the most effective, safe relief. If a cough continues for more than a few days, a physician should be consulted.

Nasal Decongestants

Concept: Overuse of nasal sprays can actually worsen the condition and lead to addiction.

Many people use nasal decongestants for stuffiness related to colds and allergy. Nasal **decongestants** shrink small swollen blood vessels inside the nose. As the decongestant effect wears off, these capillaries begin to swell once again. A rebound nasal congestion may occur that is actually worse than the original stuffiness, and a vicious cycle is in effect, with the decongestant bringing on the very symptoms it was supposed to eliminate.

Labels on all decongestants warn against use for more than three days, yet the typical container has 0.5 fluid ounces, enough for three or four weeks. Unfortunately, many people ignore this warning. Many severe sufferers greatly exceed the recommended maximum use of twice per day. Breaking the habit requires withdrawal over a period of several weeks. If this procedure doesn't work, an ear, nose, and throat specialist can provide special medication and advice.

Discovery Activity 19.2
THE HOME MEDICINE CABINET

Other than first aid equipment, only a small number of safe supplies are needed in the home medicine cabinet to treat common ailments not requiring a physician:

1. Aspirin—Buy the cheapest brand available that meets U.S.P. standards in the 25- or 100-tablet bottle.

2. Sodium bicarbonate or calcium carbonate—Use to treat heartburn and simple indigestion.

3. Calamine lotion—Use to relieve itching of mild skin eruptions from mosquito and other insect bites and poison ivy.

4. Phenylephrine hydrochloride solution $\frac{1}{4}$ percent U.S.P.—Nose drops to reduce stuffy nose from a common cold.

5. Milk of magnesia U.S.P.—Use as a mild laxative.

6. Rubbing alcohol (70 percent isopropyl alcohol)—Use as an antiseptic for minor wounds.

Prepare a list of the items in your home medicine cabinet, and complete the information below:

Item	Cost	Purpose	Effectiveness

Circle the unnecessary, unsafe, or ineffective items. Are you spending your health dollars wisely or being influenced by advertising? ●

Issues in Health
CHILDREN'S HEALTH— WHO DECIDES?

In spite of a court order from the Commonwealth of Massachusetts to continue with chemotherapy, the parents of Chad Greene discontinued that treatment in favor of laetrile. Chad, age 3, subsequently died. Doctors who had treated Chad with chemotherapy felt that he would have had a good chance of cure had he not been removed from traditional therapy. There are other cases on record of parents refusing treatment or utilizing untested methods or spiritual healing for their child. The question arises whether parents have the right to refuse accepted medical treatment for their child in favor of unproven procedures, in cases where medical practitioners believe that the child's health will be threatened by the nonstandard treatment.

Parents who refuse treatment or resort to unconventional therapy usually do so because of religious beliefs or a lack of faith in accepted medical practices. Parents who refuse medical treatment for their children on religious grounds contend that interference by the state with their religious beliefs is unconstitutional. Therefore, parents have the right to refuse medication, transfusions, and the like for their children when these practices interfere with their religious beliefs.

In the case of Chad Greene, the second factor mentioned above was prominent. The Greenes did not belong to a religious group that promoted spiritual healing. Rather, they argued that they had no faith in the standard cancer treatments, that these treatments offered no guarantee that their child would be cured, and that chemotherapy in particular was painful and they wanted to spare their child from unnecessary pain. They believed that laetrile offered a cure for their child and that they had the right to select a treatment they believed in.

(continued)

Issues in Health (continued)

Opponents of the right of parents to refuse accepted treatments in cases such as Chad's contend that the overriding factor in such cases is the well-being of the child. They contend that parents cannot necessarily make sound decisions in areas requiring medical expertise and should not be permitted to jeopardize their child's life or health. Children are not the property of their parents. They have an inalienable right to life, and parents must not be permitted by the judgments they make to gamble with their child's life or health.

What do you think? ●

Laxatives

Concept: A laxative is not needed for mild constipation.

TV advertisements try to convince us that we all need a laxative from time to time. This is certainly not true. In fact, bowel habits vary greatly from one person to another. A movement once or twice a day may be common for one individual, whereas once every three days may be perfectly normal for another. Constipation is generally not accompanied by stomach pain. If you skip a day, this is not necessarily an indication that constipation is developing. For occasional, temporary constipation, a laxative is not needed. If an uncomfortable feeling persists, a very mild laxative, such as milk of magnesia, may be used. For chronic constipation, add roughage to your diet (fruits, vegetables, whole grain cereals), drink plenty of fluids, and see your physician.

DRUGS AND THE CONSUMER

The High Cost of Drugs

Many drugs have both a trademarked, **brand name** and a **generic name.** The generic name refers to the chemical ingredient in the drug. Generic drugs cost much less than brand name drugs. Any physician can prescribe drugs by the generic name; however, drug companies try hard to have the more expensive brand name used. A drug containing the same active ingredient often is put out in many forms, combinations, and brand names. Keeping up with this endless drug market is nearly impossible for the physician, who therefore tends to rely on medical advertisements supplied by the drug industry. Expensive advertisements—not research, as claimed by the drug industry—have pushed up the cost of all drugs. In addition, there is a tremendous cost difference from store to store, from locality to locality, and from one drug company to another. In U.S. Senate hearings, the following price inconsistencies were uncovered:

- One company sold 100 tablets of Darvon (a painkiller) to a U.S. druggist for $7.03. The same drug was sold for $1.66 in Ireland and $1.92 in England.

- A druggist paid $39.50 for 1000 tablets of Serpasis (used to lower blood pressure). The same drug, when purchased by the generic name (Reserpine) by the U.S. Department of Defense cost 60 cents per 1000.

- A major U.S. drug company buys the raw material for two brand name manufacturers and for use in the tablets it sells. The company was found to be purchasing the drug in bulk at 87 cents a pound and selling to domestic manufacturers at $23.80 a pound, representing a markup of 2600 percent.

Price fixing is difficult to control. Osco Drug, Inc., a retail chain of 178 pharmacies in 17 states, began to post its prices for prescription drugs in drugstore windows. This honest approach was attacked vigorously by rival pharmacies. The board of pharmacy of one state attempted to suspend the licenses of Osco pharmacies on grounds of gross immorality, and the pharmacy associations of several states threatened to demand revocation of licenses.[3] According to the American Pharmaceutical Association, posting of prices is inconsistent with its code and prohibited for the benefit of economic gain. As a result, selecting a drugstore is a difficult task and requires some shopping around to compare prices.

Industry-Related Problems

In general, the American public has a great deal of faith in the drug industry. Unfortunately, there are several problems with the industry, including inadequate testing of new drugs, withholding of clinical testing data, biased studies, and publications with an interest in the sale of a product. To complicate the picture, new drugs enter the market at a fantastic rate; many of them con-

tain the same basic ingredient plus a new brand name. At the center of all these problems is the physician, who is the target of practically all market strategy in drug advertising.

Dr. Walter Modell, one of the country's leading pharmacologists, believes that we should screen out all drug duplication (same basic ingredients with different brand names), all useless drugs, and all ineffective drugs and then add only those new drugs that are proven to be beneficial.

Protect Yourself: Read Labels

Concept: Your best protection against false claims and improper use of a drug is a careful study of the label.

Federal law requires that labeling of over-the-counter drugs provide all necessary directions for use by the consumer, including conditions under which the drug should not be taken (special instructions for infants, children, the elderly, pregnant women, or under certain medical conditions). These labeling standards are very thorough and cover several points that will help ensure better protection for the user, such as directions for use, warnings, drug interaction precautions, and active ingredients (see Fig. 19.1 on page 464).

COSMETIC PRODUCTS: MYTHS AND FACTS

Skin Products

Concept: Rapid, easy cures for acne do not exist.

Acne preparations. **Acne** refers to skin blemishes that form when canals, through which oil sebum flows to the surface of the skin, become blocked and infected. The pimples are caused by the action of the white blood

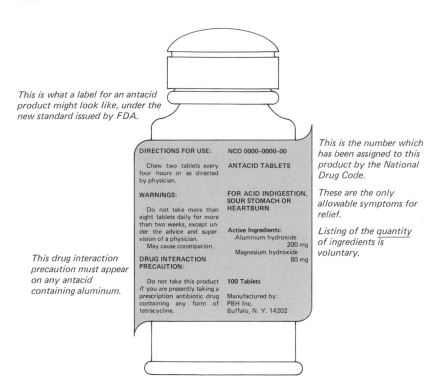

This is what a label for an antacid product might look like, under the new standard issued by FDA.

DIRECTIONS FOR USE:	NCD 0000-0000-00
Chew two tablets every four hours or as directed by physician.	ANTACID TABLETS
WARNINGS:	FOR ACID INDIGESTION, SOUR STOMACH OR HEARTBURN
Do not take more than eight tablets daily for more than two weeks, except under the advice and supervision of a physician.	
May cause constipation.	Active Ingredients:
	Aluminum hydroxide 200 mg
DRUG INTERACTION PRECAUTION:	Magnesium hydroxide 80 mg
Do not take this product if you are presently taking a prescription antibiotic drug containing any form of tetracycline.	100 Tablets
	Manufactured by: PBH Inc. Buffalo, N. Y. 14202

This is the number which has been assigned to this product by the National Drug Code.

These are the only allowable symptoms for relief.

Listing of the <u>quantity</u> of ingredients is voluntary.

This drug interaction precaution must appear on any antacid containing aluminum.

Figure 19.1
Sample label under the new FDA standard.
SOURCE: FDA *Consumer*, July–August 1974.

cells on the sebum and bacteria. A blackhead also occurs from a clogged pore of a **sebaceous gland** that is capped with a blackened mass of debris. Acne is a common adolescent disease, and although some adults have acne problems, the condition usually clears up by the age of 23 (with or without treatment). The exact cause of acne is unknown, but several factors may be related: heredity, emotional stress, and certain cosmetics and drugs. Foods (sweets and greasy, fried foods) and unwashed skin do not cause acne in most people.

To control mild acne:

1. Avoid using the many ointments, powders, and vitamin supplements advertised as fast cures.

2. Keep the skin as clean as possible. Wash your face before applying any medication that your physician prescribes.

3. Use soap and water instead of face creams for cleansing; creams close the pores.

4. Remove blackheads with a blackhead extractor after applying hot, wet compresses for 10 minutes; avoid squeezing blackheads.

Severe acne should be treated by a dermatologist.

Concept: There is no cosmetic product in existence that can improve the beauty of the skin or restore aging skin.

Skin rejuvenation.   Americans spend millions of dollars each year on skin products that claim to restore a youthful appearance to aging skin. Unfortunately, these products don't work. Studies of products containing hormones, turtle oil, shark oil, buttermilk, and so forth, reveal the same thing—no change in skin properties. Because hormones can be absorbed through the skin, they are unsafe and particularly dangerous to individuals with a family history of breast disorders or

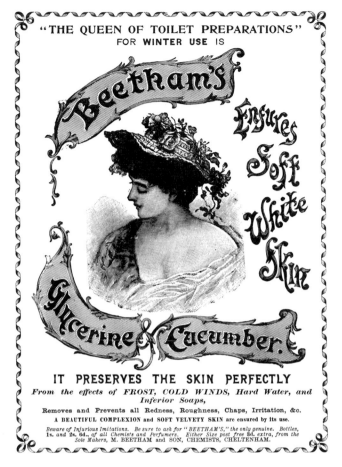

"THE QUEEN OF TOILET PREPARATIONS"
FOR **WINTER USE** IS

Beetham's

Ensures Soft White Skin

Glycerine & Cucumber.

IT PRESERVES THE SKIN PERFECTLY
*From the effects of FROST, COLD WINDS, Hard Water, and
Inferior Soaps,*
Removes and Prevents all Redness, Roughness, Chaps, Irritation, &c.
A BEAUTIFUL COMPLEXION and SOFT VELVETY SKIN are ensured by its use.

*Beware of Injurious Imitations. Be sure to ask for "BEETHAM'S," the only genuine. Bottles,
1s. and 2s. 6d., of all Chemists and Perfumers. Either Size post free 3d. extra, from the
Sole Makers, M. BEETHAM and SON, CHEMISTS, CHELTENHAM.*

*Advertisers have always had a ready market for products
that promise to preserve a youthful complexion.*

cancer of the genital organs. All such products are less
effective than old-fashioned emollient cream.

Concept: Suntan products vary greatly in cost,
protection against sunburn, and tanning effect.

Suntan products. There is some evidence that the
sun speeds up skin aging by causing degenerative
changes, resulting in wrinkles and coarsening of the
skin texture. Overexposure to the sun is also a common
cause of skin cancer. The skin's main protections against
solar radiation are hair and **melanin.** Tanning occurs
as increased amounts of melanin are formed to protect
against solar radiation. It takes greatly increased amounts
of ultraviolet light to burn a tanned skin.

The most effective lotion to prevent sunburn is a
sunscreen containing para-aminobenzoic acid (PABA)
in alcohol, which helps block the harmful ultraviolet
rays of the sun. Lotions with PABA also have a reservoir
effect, forming a semipermanent shield against the sun
by chemically bonding with the skin.

Concept: Both deodorants and antiperspirants
assist in controlling body odor.

Deodorants and antiperspirants. Body odor occurs through the action of bacteria on secretions from
the skin's glands. The best natural protection against
odor is bathing with an ordinary toilet soap. Following
the bath, a **deodorant** (to mask body odors) or **antiperspirant** (to reduce perspiration) may be applied. No
product prevents profuse sweating during vigorous exercise or in hot, humid weather. Sweating is a natural
process that is important to body functions and should
not be totally prevented. If you have an odor problem,
bathe regularly and use a deodorant or antiperspirant.

Hair Products

Concept: Unwanted body hair can be permanently removed only by electrolysis.

Hair removers. In our country it is considered
unattractive for women to have body or facial hair.
There are basically two approaches to the removal of
such hair: temporary treatments that must be repeated
and a permanent, "one treatment" method.

The following methods are temporary. Because
they remove hair above the root level, the hair will
grow back.

1. Chemicals soften and dissolve the hair shaft without disturbing the root. Skin reactions to these chemicals are common.
2. A wax stick composed of resin and turpentine, warmed and applied to hairy areas, tears the hair away from the roots when the wax hardens.
3. Tweezers pluck out hair; however, this method is painful and runs the risk of infection from unclean skin and tweezers.
4. A fine pumice stone, if used daily and rubbed against soap-lathered hair, prevents hair from appearing above the skin.

Some women prefer to remove facial and body hair permanently. **Electrolysis** is the only method that can permanently remove unwanted hair. The hair follicle is completely destroyed by injecting a fine electric needle down the root of the follicle and providing low electric current. A dermatologist can recommend a trained electrolysist. The procedure requires patience, good eyesight, coordination, and time. To reduce chances of infection, only a few hairs on the upper lip are removed at one visit.

If unusual hair growth exists, consult your physician. He or she will make a proper examination and identify the cause. Otherwise, live with it and resort to a safe method, such as shaving for legs and underarms and waxing for facial hair. Shaving will *not* coarsen hair or increase its growth.

Concept: Hair dyes, rinses, and bleaches may produce skin reactions.

Hair color products. Products that change the color of the hair either penetrate the hair shaft and remain until the hair grows out or remain only until the hair is washed. The majority of these products can produce skin irritations and require some caution. Before you use one, try this test: put a small amount of the product behind one ear or on the inside of an elbow. Allow to dry and do not wash this area for 24 hours. If itching, burning, swelling, or any other irritation occurs, avoid this product. If you should happen to use a product on the hair and get an irritation, shampoo again with soap and water, follow with hydrogen peroxide, and follow once again with a soap shampoo. All hair color products should be kept away from the eyes.

Products for Teeth and Eyes

Concept: Mouthwashes and gargles are of little value in alleviating a sore throat or bad breath.

Mouthwashes and gargles. Sore throats are a result of bacteria or virus infection. It is impossible to destroy the many types of viruses found in the throat. Millions of bacteria exist in the mouths of healthy individuals. Killing off some can offer no protection or cure for a sore throat. Even if you could gargle deep into the stomach, germs deeper in the tissues would be untouched. Throat infections can lead to acute nephritis or rheumatic fever. If a sore throat is accompanied by a fever, see your doctor immediately. In such cases, seeking temporary relief through a home remedy can delay proper diagnosis and treatment.

Unpleasant mouth odor, produced from eating garlic or onions or from smoking, does not originate in the mouth. The aroma is carried from the intestines to the lungs and expired into the air. Very little odor exists in particles that remain in the mouth and teeth. Therefore, gargling has little effect other than to mask the unpleasant odor with a pleasant smell, such as mint. It is not possible to absorb the odor, in spite of what the ads for some products claim. To limit the bad morning taste, brush thoroughly before going to bed, upon arising, and after meals. To mask breath odor after eating a strong smelling food, chewing on a mint is the least expensive choice.

Although mouthwashes may taste good, there is no evidence that they are any more effective in treating a sore throat or eliminating bad breath than pure water. In fact continuous use of mouthwash can actually cause excessive drying of the mucous membranes of the oral cavity.

Concept: Any low-abrasive, fluoride toothpaste will help prevent cavities.

Toothpastes. Tooth decay is most common among children and young adults. After age 30 to 35, tooth loss is generally a result of gum disease. If you live in an area with fluoridated water, brushing your teeth with water or baking soda will give the same results as toothpaste, providing you brush properly and use dental floss. Otherwise, choose a fluoride toothpaste or ask your dentist for a fluoride treatment. Do not spend money on toothpaste products that guarantee "whiteness." These have abrasives that can cause excessive wear on the teeth.

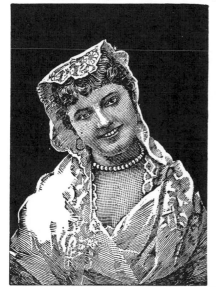

PEARLS IN THE MOUTH

BEAUTY AND FRAGRANCE
Are Communicated to the Mouth by
SOZODONT,
Which renders the teeth WHITE, the gums ROSY, and the breath SWEET. It thoroughly removes tartar from the teeth and prevents decay.
Sold by DRUGGISTS and FANCY GOODS DEALERS.

Discovery Activity 19.3
ARE YOU A BIG HEALTH PRODUCTS CONSUMER?

To determine whether you are a big consumer of health products, write down what you would do in the following situations:

You have indigestion or _____
stomach upset.
You have had trouble _____
sleeping for several nights.
You have a cold with _____
stuffiness.
You have dandruff. _____
You have a headache. _____
You have recently noticed _____
that your breath seems
bad.
You have a mild cough. _____
You have an outbreak of _____
blemishes.
You want a quick suntan. _____
Your eyes are bloodshot _____
from lack of sleep.

Did most of your answers involve using a health product? If so, are you satisfied that you're making wise choices? Given what you've learned, will you change your purchasing habits when it comes to health-related products? ●

Concept: Normal eyes do not need cleansing with any special chemicals.

Eye washes. The most effective way to remove irritating material from the eye is through natural tears. Frequent use of eye drops may delay early diagnosis of a serious disorder, such as **glaucoma,** which causes 15 percent of all blindness.

Eye discomfort can result from visual problems, eye fatigue, bacteria and viruses, or allergic sensitivity to dust or pollens. If these symptoms persist for more than two or three days, consult a physician. For relief of simple eye irritation, apply iced, wet compresses for 15 minutes or place several drops of cold water in the lower lid with an eye dropper. If eye irritation continues, consult your physician or ophthalmologist.

For Women Only

Concept: The risk of toxic shock syndrome (TSS) can be reduced by taking precautions in the selection and use of tampons.

Tampons and toxic shock syndrome. **Toxic shock syndrome (TSS)** was first recognized as a disease in 1978, although it wasn't until June 1980 that an association was made between TSS and young women using tampons continuously throughout their menstrual periods. TSS victims experience flulike symptoms in the early stages: fever (102°F or higher), vomiting, diarrhea, sore throat, and in some cases headache and muscle ache. These symptoms later disappear and are replaced by a sunburnlike rash and shock, involving a rapid decrease in blood pressure, kidney failure, and heart irregularities.

The exact cause of TSS and the specific role tampons may play in increasing susceptibility to the disease are unknown. It is hypothesized that the tampon acts as a growth medium for a bacteria (*Staphylococcus aureus*) releasing a toxin that is absorbed through the vaginal walls and into the bloodstream. The bacteria may enter through small abrasions caused by the tampon. A second theory places the blame on the new superabsorbent tampon fibers, because the appearance of TSS coincided with the introduction of these new products, especially Proctor and Gamble's Rely. In addition, information on the original patent of Rely clearly indicates that the fibers used in this tampon have a potential for toxicity.

A woman has about 15 chances in 100,000 of contracting TSS (less than 0.5 percent). This low incidence has prompted the Center for Disease Control in Atlanta to state that it seems "unwarranted to recommend that use of tampons be discontinued." Many women, however, feel that any risk is too high. To reduce the chances of contracting TSS, the following suggestions are offered:

1. Select your tampon very carefully. Avoid the superabsorbent tampons, and use the traditional cottonlike materials until further evidence is available. Sea sponges, which some women use, may be contaminated with ocean pollutants and are suspected in several cases of TSS.

2. Avoid changing the tampon too often. Repeated insertion and removal may irritate the vagina and provide additional entry points for TSS bacteria.

3. Switch to maxipads at bedtime and minipads as the flow tapers; avoid continuous use of tampons throughout menstruation.

4. If you use maxipads, avoid those with superabsorbent fibers.

5. Avoid using tampons to catch nonmenstrual secretions or to hide vaginal odor.

NUTRITION AND THE CONSUMER

Minimizing the Risks of Food Poisoning

Concept: Wise food handling and purchasing can prevent food poisoning.

Practically any food, perishable or nonperishable, carries the potential for food poisoning. For food to transmit disease, it must contain a disease-producing agent (bacteria, toxin-forming mold, virus) or be contaminated through handling, and it must be consumed in sufficient quantity to cause symptoms. The food must also provide an environment in which the agent may survive or reproduce. Should these factors exist, illness may or may not occur. Highly susceptible people, such as infants, the elderly, the incapacitated, or those already ill, could become mildly or fatally ill. The problem of food poisoning in the United States is not uncommon.

To reduce the risk of food poisoning, purchase, handle, and store foods carefully. Consider these suggestions:

Shopping:

1. Examine each item to detect signs of spoilage, such as a torn package, imperfect seal, or bulging can.

2. Avoid buying food stored above the "frostline," or load line, in supermarkets.

3. Avoid purchasing perishable products, such as milk, meat, or desserts, that are not adequately refrigerated.

4. Purchase perishable foods in small quantities.

5. Read labels at home for special storing instructions.

6. Transport food immediately from the store to your home; never leave groceries in a hot car, where disease-producing bacteria can multiply. Make the grocery store your last stop before returning home.

Cooking and storing:

1. Avoid tasting any food that appears spoiled; use the odor or appearance as your guide, discarding anything that is suspect.

2. Avoid storing food in a cabinet with a drainpipe, such as under the kitchen sink.

3. Avoid leaving leftover food on the table after a meal while you socialize; store in the refrigerator immediately.

4. Wash your hands after diapering a baby or visiting the bathroom.

5. Avoid using the same knife to cut uncooked meats and other foods; contamination can be transmitted from one food to another.

6. Discard any perishable food that was not refrigerated.

7. Devise a system to identify the time of storage; use older items first.

8. Examine foods carefully before cooking.

9. Follow the rules of personal hygiene in the kitchen at all times.

10. Cook pork, stuffed turkey, and other meats until the inner part reaches a temperature of 165°F to kill infectious microorganisms; use a thermometer to determine when this temperature is reached.

11. Serve cooked foods as soon as possible.

Product Labeling

Concept: Nutrition labeling is a valuable aid to the consumer.

The information on food products is your guide to wise food purchasing. It helps you choose foods low in sodium, saturated fat, and sugar; high in fiber; and with the proper vitamins, minerals, and number of calories. In addition, the U.S. Recommended Daily Allowances (RDAs) allow you to compare the nutritive value and relative costs of different foods.

Any food label providing nutrition information must include:

1. Net contents—number and size of servings per container (weight, fluid measure, and/or numerical count).

2. Ingredients—listed by common name in order of the largest percentage; for example, if sugar is listed first, the primary ingredient is sugar; number of calories, amount of protein, carbohydrates, fat, and sodium (in grams) per serving; amounts of eight nutrients (protein, vitamin A, thiamin, riboflavin, niacin, vitamin C, calcium and iron) in one serving expressed as a percentage of U.S. RDAs.

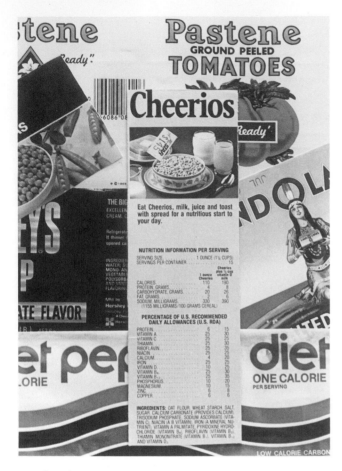

Nutrition information panel from a Cheerios box:

NUTRITION INFORMATION PER SERVING

SERVING SIZE .... 1 OUNCE (1¼ CUPS)
SERVINGS PER CONTAINER 15

	1 ounce Cheerios	Cheerios plus ½ cup vitamin D milk
CALORIES	110	190
PROTEIN, GRAMS	4	8
CARBOHYDRATE, GRAMS	20	26
FAT, GRAMS	2	6
SODIUM, MILLIGRAMS	330	390

(1155 MILLIGRAMS/100 GRAMS CEREAL)

PERCENTAGE OF U.S. RECOMMENDED
DAILY ALLOWANCES (U.S. RDA)

PROTEIN	6	15
VITAMIN A	25	30
VITAMIN C	25	25
THIAMIN	25	30
RIBOFLAVIN	25	35
NIACIN	25	25
CALCIUM	4	20
IRON	25	25
VITAMIN D	10	25
VITAMIN B₆	25	30
VITAMIN B₁₂	25	35
PHOSPHORUS	10	20
MAGNESIUM	6	15
ZINC	6	8
COPPER	6	6

INGREDIENTS: OAT FLOUR, WHEAT STARCH, SALT, SUGAR, CALCIUM CARBONATE (PROVIDES CALCIUM), TRISODIUM PHOSPHATE, SODIUM ASCORBATE (VITAMIN C), NIACIN (A B VITAMIN), IRON (A MINERAL NUTRIENT), VITAMIN A PALMITATE, PYRIDOXINE HYDROCHLORIDE (VITAMIN B₆), RIBOFLAVIN (VITAMIN B₂), THIAMIN MONONITRATE (VITAMIN B₁), VITAMIN B₁₂ AND VITAMIN D₂.

Reading food labels can be an eye-opening experience. Many processed foods contain unnecessarily high levels of sugar and sodium.

PROTECTING THE CONSUMER: YOUR ADVOCATES

Federal Agencies

The Food and Drug Administration. Approximately 4500 employees of the **Food and Drug Administration (FDA)** are faced with the nearly impossible task of surveying thousands of food, drug, and cosmetic companies in the United States. This organization operates in four main areas.

1. The Bureau of Drugs verifies the safety and effectiveness of all drugs. Companies must submit information on new drugs for investigation before they can be used in human tests.

2. The Bureau of Foods and Pesticides attempts to assure safe, pure, and wholesome foods. Food plants are inspected, ingredients of food products examined, and packaging and labeling checked. Safe levels for chemical food additives, such as preservatives, flavoring, and coloring, are established.

3. The Bureau of Veterinary Medicine enforces similar requirements for veterinary drugs and devices for optimum animal health and safety.

4. The Office of Product Safety enforces the Federal Hazardous Substances Act to protect the public from accidents involving chemicals.

The Federal Trade Commission. The agency known as the **Federal Trade Commission (FTC)** is required by law to keep competition free and fair. Key areas of concern for the consumer are the Fair Packaging and Labeling Act, the Trademark Act, the Truth in Lending Act, and the Fair Credit Report Act. The majority of violations are *misrepresenting* and *mislabeling* of products. The FTC will initiate action against a violator if the product is not what the label proclaims or implies, or if it is incorrectly labeled. You can file a confidential complaint with the FTC by explaining the facts in a letter and enclosing as much supporting evidence as possible. The FTC will initiate an investigation and take action, forcing the practice to discontinue through an informal settlement or a formal complaint in court. Fines, imprisonment, or seizure of the product may ensue.

The Consumer Product Safety Commission. The Consumer Product Safety Act of 1972 led to the formation of the **Consumer Product Safety Commission.** This act was designed to protect the public against unreasonable risks of injury associated with consumer products, to help consumers evaluate the safety of products, to develop uniform safety standards for consumer products, and to promote research on the causes and prevention of product-related deaths. The main goal of the commission is to reduce the more than 20 million annual injuries associated with consumer products by issuing and enforcing safety standards for over 10,000 products. The Flammable Fabrics Act, the Federal Hazardous Substances Act, the Poison Prevention Packaging Act, and the Refrigerator Door Safety Act are also the responsibility of the commission.

U.S. Postal Service. The U.S. Postal Service is responsible for protecting the health and well-being of the nation by investigating mail fraud and attempts to sell harmful or worthless merchandise or medicines through the mail, and by protecting the consumer from harassment, pornography, and some types of junk mail. Responsibility for initiating a complaint rests with the consumer. The Postal Service can only take a case to court with the evidence and witnesses you supply.

Private Agencies

Better Business Bureau. The **Better Business Bureau** in your community is a private, nonprofit corporation supported by private business. It assists you by mediating misunderstandings between consumers and businesses, investigating advertising misinformation and questionable activity, and supplying factual information on thousands of businesses in the United States. You can call your local office for the leaflet entitled, "What Is a Better Business Bureau?" which describes the services provided.

Chamber of Commerce. Your local **Chamber of Commerce** also acts as a liaison between the business community and the consumer and is supported by businesses within your community. The Chamber of Commerce functions similarly to the Better Business Bureau and performs most of its work at the local level.

Medical, dental, and other agencies. Other independent agencies that serve as watchdogs for the consumer include the State Medical Association and the State Dental Association (dental and medical ethics), the Legal Aid Society and the Legal Services Organization (advice on consumer problems and legal representation for those with limited income), the State Bar Association (advice and literature on common legal problems), the State Nursing Home Association (standards of care and services), the State Pharmaceutical Association (druggists, drugs, and prescriptions), the State Department of Mental Health (care and services), and the State Retail Council (liaison between retailers and consumers).

LEARNING TO JUDGE ADVERTISING

Concept: All health-related advertisements should be carefully analyzed.

Advertisers spend a lot of time and money analyzing the American people. They know what motivates different people to try different products. They know what words and pictures will sell a product. You are at the mercy of the advertiser unless you learn to judge commercials. Here are some questions to keep in mind:

1. Is the product objectively presented without appealing to basic human needs, such as fear, love, and security? If not, you should be skeptical.

2. If research findings are cited, were they performed by health scientists (not independent testing laboratories, which may need to show favorable results to stay in business) and published in a recognized medical journal?

3. Does the commercial make unsupported claims?

4. Does the advertiser use endorsements from individuals who are not scientists? Such endorsements indicate only that the company has enough money to hire a celebrity to read a script.

5. Are the findings consistent? Have other investigators in other areas found the same thing?

6. Is unclear information used, such as "Hospital tests showed . . .", "Doctors recommend . . .", or "A major study revealed . . .", without the hospital, doctors, or study being identified?

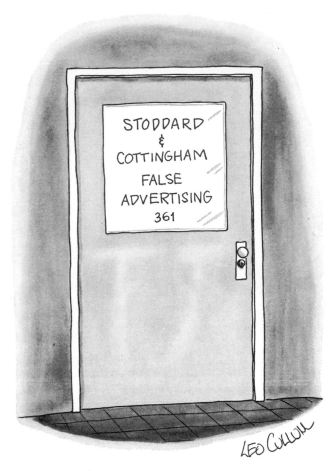

Drawing by Leo Cullum; © 1977 The New Yorker Magazine, Inc.

Probably your best protection is not to buy health-related products you see advertised in magazines or on TV unless you first check with your doctor or pharmacist. They can tell you whether the product has any benefit.

CONCLUSION

Quackery is ever-present in the United States in the treatment of illnesses and the sale of consumer products. A rather gullible public willing to spend billions of dollars on quick, easy approaches to practically anything guarantees its existence. False advertising in all forms of media remains a strong obstacle to the elimination of quackery. Fortunately, the public is slowly becoming wiser. Consumers are beginning to ask for hard evidence and to question the value of products and claims by advertisers. The FDA and other government agencies are also increasing their scrutiny of consumer products and advertising claims. The fact remains, however, that many over-the-counter medicines, cosmetics, special foods, and gadgets are a worthless waste of hard-earned money. Some are even hazardous to health. When in doubt about any product capable of affecting your health, it is wise to consult a physician before initiating any home treatment.

SUMMARY

1. There are two basic approaches to the control of quackery: the legal and the educational. Both approaches are the responsibility of the consumer.

2. Each individual in our society is the guardian of his or her own health and must become healthy skeptics in their evaluation of health-related products.

3. The quack has existed for millennia and will continue to prey on the unwise consumer. Mail-order quackery relies on unfounded claims; indirect suggestion of cures, remedies, and rejuvenation; and the consumer's attraction to fast, easy solutions to complicated health problems.

4. Consumers must become aware of the numerous cues that indicate that they are dealing with a quack or worthless product. There are no miracle cures for such serious disorders and diseases as cancer, arthritis, and epilepsy; nor are there quick, safe approaches to weight loss, insomnia, acne, skin rejuvenation, baldness, bad breath, enlarging body parts, or revitalizing your sex life.

5. Laetrile treatment for various types of cancer has been found to be completely useless, dangerous, and expensive.

6. Nonprescription medicines are not meant to—and do not—cure disease. They should be used only for temporary relief of minor symptoms. Improper use of over-the-counter drugs may irritate symptoms or mask a condition needing physician attention.

7. Over-the-counter drugs that claim to relieve more than one symptom, such as alleviating acid indigestion and headache, should be avoided if you have only one of the symptoms. Choose a drug that focuses on your specific symptom.

8. Overuse of nasal decongestants is a common problem among cold and allergy sufferers. Follow directions on the label carefully, using the nasal decongestant no more than twice per day and for no longer than three days. If the condition persists, see a physician.

9. To save money, ask your physician and druggist to provide you with the least expensive generic name (refers to the chemical ingredient in the drug) rather than the highly advertised product.

10. Your best protection against false claims and improper use of all over-the-counter drugs is a careful study of labels.

11. Women should be extremely careful in their selection and use of tampons to reduce the risk of Toxic Shock Syndrome.

12. The risk of food poisoning can be greatly reduced by wise purchasing, storing, and cooking practices. Your best guide to wise purchasing (cost and nutritive value) is the food label. Choose foods low in sodium, fat, and sugar; high in fiber; and with the proper vitamins, minerals, and calories.

13. More than 20 million injuries each year are associated with consumer products. Federal agencies rely on the consumer to provide valuable testimony on the dangers of such products and to work with them to prosecute or remove the product from the market. Other agencies, such as the Better Business Bureau, Chamber of Commerce, and State Medical and Dental Associations, advise consumers on health-related goods and services.

14. Wise consumerism also carries the responsibility of learning to evaluate and judge advertising claims before making the decision to purchase a health-related product.

REFERENCES

1. Warren E. Schaller and Charles R. Carroll, *Health Quackery and the Consumer* (Philadelphia: W. B. Saunders Co., 1976).

2. *The Medicine Show* (Mount Vernon, N.Y.: Consumers Union, 1974).

3. *Drug Industry Antitrust Act,* Hearings, Subcommittee on Antitrust and Monopoly: Committee on the Judiciary, 87th Congress, 1st Session; Part I, American Medical Association and Medical Authorities, p. 320.

LABORATORY 1
FACIAL CREAM AND SKIN CARE

Purpose   To determine the effects of any brand-name facial cream on the condition of the skin.*

Size of Group   Two groups of any size.

Equipment   Any brand of skin cream found in the house.

Procedure

1. Each female student is assigned to one of two groups:
   Group I: Agrees to wash one side of the face with soap and water and the other side with facial cream (any brand available in the home) for the next two weeks.
   Group II: Agrees to wash one side of the face with both soap and water and facial cream and the other side with only soap and water for the next two weeks.

2. No student in either group is permitted to reveal to anyone which side of the face is being cleansed with facial cream or soap and water or both.

3. After two weeks each student is evaluated (by group members only) for skin softness, smoothness, and cleanness, using the form shown below.

Results

1. Complete the form below. If one side of the face looks smoother or cleaner than the other, place a (1) in the appropriate column. In the example below for Scott, five students checked the left side,

*Long-term two-week experimental use of facial cream by females. Both males and females perform the in-class evaluation and complete the results section of the experiment.

three the right, and four no difference. DO NOT REVEAL HOW YOUR FACE WAS CLEANSED UNTIL EACH STUDENT HAS HAD AN OPPORTUNITY TO RECORD AND COMPARE HIS OR HER OBSERVATIONS.

	Side of Face Softer, Smoother, or Cleaner			
Name	*Left*	*Right*	*No difference*	*Treatment*
1. Scott	11111	111	1111	
2. Jones				
3. Smith				
4. Bell				
5. Hall				

2. Evaluate the data above by filling in the final (Treatment) column, stating the manner in which the different sides of the face were cleansed.

3. What cleansing method was most effective?

_____ Soap and water only—More evaluators checked the side of the face cleansed with soap and water as being cleaner, softer, or smoother. Discuss.

_____ Facial cream—More evaluators checked the side cleansed with facial cream. Discuss.

_____ Soap and water plus facial cream—More evaluators checked the side cleansed with both soap and water and facial cream. Discuss.

Laboratory 2
TRUTH IN ADVERTISING

Purpose To determine the accuracy of advertising claims.

Size of Group Five to seven students per group.

Procedure

1. Each group chooses one of the topics listed below:

   Nutrition

   Weight control

   Disease

   Tobacco and alcohol

   Human sexuality

2. Over a two-week period, 6 to 10 ads are clipped that promote a product or service in the area chosen.

3. Each student is responsible for writing the company for more information about the product or service.

Results

1. Compare the implied claims in each ad to the actual effect of the product or service. Use the information received from the company, information in your textbook, and interviews with physicians, health educators, and fitness experts to determine the accuracy of the advertisement.

2. Each group reports its findings to the class.

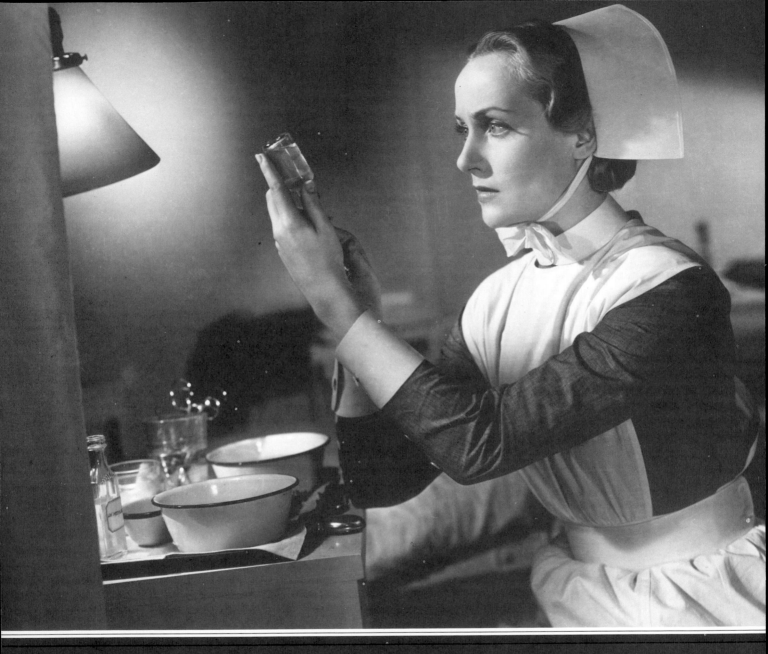

chapter 20

choosing medical services and health insurance

- *preventive health care*
- *making medical care work for you*
- *alternative approaches to health care*
- *health insurance*

Although the United States is among the most modern, technically advanced countries in the world in medical science, the health services available to some Americans are inadequate. In addition, medical care for a substantial portion of the population is a tremendous burden on the family budget. We are also facing a health care crisis in terms of personnel and cost. At present, approximately 98 percent of physicians specialize and only 2 percent have a general practice, with first patient contact and diagnosis. Medical care costs continue to rise at a much faster rate than the cost of living and at a greater rate than the average take-home pay increases of blue- and white-collar workers.

In view of this situation, securing and paying for high-quality medical care requires careful planning. Each individual or family needs to know what kind of health plan to have, how to select a physician, and how to monitor his or her health or the health of family members. This chapter offers some guidelines for choosing appropriate medical services for you.

PREVENTIVE HEALTH CARE

The Self-Care Movement

The self-care movement places the responsibility on the individual for maintaining good health and detecting and treating minor ailments. Self-care requires individuals to learn about their bodies, to monitor their bodily functions, and to determine when and how to use medical resources (doctors, hospitals, clinics, and the like). In addition, self-care carries with it the responsibility of taking care of one's own body by establishing a healthy lifestyle. This involves regular exercise; proper nutrition; maintenance of normal body weight; minimal stress; avoidance of tobacco smoking; and moderate use of alcohol, over-the-counter drugs, and prescription drugs. In recent years self-care has gained widespread acceptance. Many people believe

that requiring each individual to take more responsibility for his or her own health is the most effective form of preventive medicine.

An important part of self-care includes learning about the symptoms of common complaints and knowing when to treat yourself and when to seek help from medical practitioners. Several self-care books are available that provide health information in terms that any consumer can understand. For example, *Take Care of Yourself* and *Taking Care of Your Child* describe a large number of common ailments and tell you when you can safely treat yourself (or your child) and when you should call a doctor. Two other useful books are *The People's Pharmacy* and *How to Be Your Own Doctor Sometimes.*

Self-medication, which is a part of self-care, involves using over-the-counter drugs to relieve symptoms, such as headache and cold symptoms. However, self-medication can be abused, particularly if people rely on it too much, do not inform themselves about the effects of drugs, misdiagnose their ailment, or are unaware of their own reactions to particular medications. A study conducted by the U.S. Senate Committee on Aging revealed some interesting findings on self-diagnosis and self-treatment of ailments.[1] Despite the encouraging trend toward adequate self-care, dangerous abuses were noted: (1) 10 to 20 percent (16 million) of those who were self-medicating for asthma, allergy, and hemorrhoids indicated that a physician had never diagnosed the condition; (2) 4 percent (9 million) of those reporting heart trouble, high blood pressure, and diabetes had never seen a physician; and (3) approximately 16 million people indicated that they would medicate for longer than two weeks for such ailments as sore throat, cough, sinus trouble, head cold, hay fever, skin problems, sleeplessness, and acid or upset stomach. Prolonged self-medication for any of these ailments is dangerous. Moreover, five of them (heart disease, diabetes, high blood pressure, asthma, and allergies) have no cure; they can only be managed, and a physician must be involved for optimum protection of health. According to the findings of the survey, many people expect cures from self-medication.

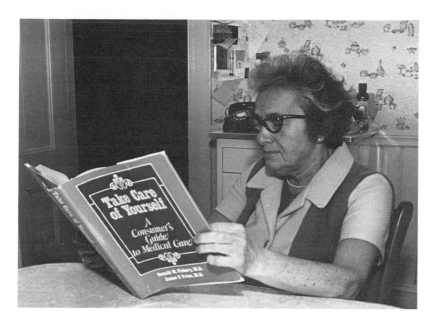

A basic principle of self care is that the individual has the primary responsibility for his or her own health. This responsibility includes learning when to safely diagnose and treat oneself and when to consult a doctor.

When to Seek Help

To take care of your health, you need to know when to seek help. In general, a visit to your doctor is indicated when any of the following occurs:

1. oral temperature above 101°F,
2. severe pain that is persistent or recurrent,
3. abdominal pain persisting for more than three hours or accompanied by nausea,
4. repeated digestive upset,
5. fatigue over a long period with no apparent cause,
6. unanticipated weight loss or gain,
7. dizziness or fainting,
8. bleeding without trauma,
9. personality changes without any apparent explanation,
10. any of the seven warning signals of cancer,
11. headache persisting for more than one day,
12. joint pain persisting for more than a few days,
13. shortness of breath,
14. unusual discharge from some body part.

Self-Care Skills

Concept: Preventive medicine requires careful monitoring of one's own body.

With minimum practice and time you can learn to identify changes in your health and determine when you should report these findings to your physician and when you can safely treat yourself. Careful observation of your body will help you decide whether to see a physician for diagnosis.

1. Temperature. Purchase a thermometer and master the proper technique of taking accurate temperature readings. Report the exact temperature to the physician rather than relying on "feel." Several types of forehead thermometers are available for use with young children that provide "ball park" readings. It is recommended, however, that a rectal or oral thermometer also be used and exact readings reported to the physician.

2. Pulse. Learn to count your rate accurately using the carotid or radial pulse. It is important to remain quiet in a sitting or lying position for five minutes prior to counting your pulse. The **radial pulse** is taken by placing the index and middle fingers of the left hand in the hollow of the wrist at the base of the thumb. Move the fingers around until you find a strong pulse. The **carotid pulse** is taken by placing these same two fingers in the hollow of the neck on the left side (under the jaw bone). Only gentle pressure should be applied. The number of beats should be counted for 30 seconds, then multiplied by 2. Learn to recognize a regular and irregular beat, such as skipping or palpitating, and describe the problem accurately to your physician. Record your normal resting pulse to provide some basis for comparison.

3. Breast.   Learn the breast self-exam (for women), and do it monthly. Men should learn to perform the testicular self-exam (see Chapter 17).

4. Body weight and fat.   Weigh yourself periodically at the same time of day and under the same conditions. In addition, it is helpful to pinch yourself in the abdominal area, thighs, and back of arms as a crude measure of body fat (see Chapter 8 for skinfold measures). Be able to provide accurate data on weight loss or gain over a specific period of time.

5. Blood pressure.   **Blood pressure** refers to the pressure of the blood against arterial walls during the beating or **systolic** stage and during the resting or **diastolic** stage. A nine-member group sponsored by the National High Blood Pressure Coordinating Committee, a government-backed board, is currently working on a redefinition of high blood pressure. Recent findings on the association of hypertension and cardiovascular disease suggest that blood pressure readings previously considered normal (110 to 139 systolic and 60 to 90 diastolic are too lenient. New standards are expected to place the cutoff for "minimal" risk at a diastolic of 80. (The diastolic, or lower, reading is generally used as an indicator of high blood pressure.) A doubling of risk occurs in the range between 80 and 90, which was previously considered normal but will probably now be associated with "intermediate" risk. A reading above 90 will be considered a "definite" risk.

Coin-operated blood pressure machines can be used for a rough indication of blood pressure but not as the basis for self-medication, altering therapy, or ignoring the instructions of a doctor. It is important to realize that machines may be inaccurate and that your blood pressure can vary from day-to-day as the result of emotions, bladder distention, climate changes, exertion, pain, and medication. Therefore, a single blood pressure reading may not accurately characterize your blood pressure. If you do not have a **stethoscope** and **sphygmomanometer** or do not know someone who can use this equipment properly, use the coin-operated machine to estimate your pressure, and consult a physician if you are outside the suggested ranges. The reading will be more accurate if you first rest in a sitting position for 5 to 10 minutes. Also, it is very difficult to take your own blood pressure unless you are extremely adept at the procedure.

6. Throat.   Learn what a healthy throat looks like so that you can recognize the symptoms of a problem. Inflammation, swelling, and white or yellow patches at the back of the throat are all indicators of infection. Examining the throat yourself is useful, but it may not reveal whether the infection is bacterial (strep throat) or viral. If someone in your family has a persistent sore throat, you should call your doctor to determine whether an office examination is indicated. The doctor can take a throat culture to determine if bacterial infection is present. You can also have a throat culture taken at a medical laboratory, if this is more convenient. If the culture is positive, your physician will start antibiotic therapy. If the culture is negative, you can treat the problem at home with throat lozenges, aspirin, and salt water gargle. Using a humidifier or vaporizer is also helpful, because the humid air will keep the throat from drying out.

7. Eyes.   Eye pain may be caused by injury, infection, or disease, such as glaucoma. Tiredness in the eyes after a long period of close work is normal. Severe pain behind the eye may be a symptom of a migraine headache. Pain below the eye may be caused by sinus problems. Pain in both eyes upon exposure to bright light is a common symptom of some viral infections and will disappear as the infection improves. A physician should be consulted if pain is severe and persists for more than 48 hours. If pain is associated with tiredness or flu, home treatment can be used (resting the eyes, taking aspirin, and avoiding bright light).

For vision problems, such as temporary blindness (partial or complete), blurred vision, blocked vision, or changes in vision, an ophthalmologist should be consulted.

Eye burning, itching, and discharge are generally symptoms of **conjunctivitis** (pink eye). Wearing dark glasses or goggles at work to avoid a particular allergic exposure may help. If the condition remains, the discharge gets thicker, eye pain develops, or vision is impaired, see an opthalmologist.

MAKING MEDICAL CARE WORK FOR YOU

Selecting a Doctor

Concept: Choosing the right doctor can affect the level of treatment and the recovery.

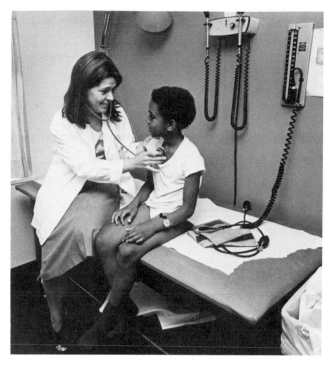

Many families select a family physician to care for most of their health problems. More serious ailments are usually referred to a specialist.

Practically everyone needs a **primary care physician,** or family medicine physican, as the new specialty is called. Your family physician will refer you to the appropriate specialist, should the need arise. If you belong to a health maintenance organization, you must choose a doctor in that program. One method of locating a physician is to ask your friends about the care they receive in terms of expertise and commitment to the patient. Another method is to identify the medical school and its hospital affiliation in your area. Call the school and ask for a list of doctors who see patients. You may also secure valuable suggestions by calling the resident on call at the local emergency room. First-year residents have had an opportunity to evaluate doctors in various situations and will generally be happy to suggest names. Keep in mind that teaching hospitals (those associated with a medical school) generally have the most advanced care and facilities; patients of doctors at these hospitals receive considerable attention from the medical personnel.

A wise choice for family health care is often a well-established group practice, in which three or more physicians work together in their various specialties. Records on patients are available to each physician, on-the-spot consultation is provided, and a physician who knows your health history is always available or on call nights and weekends. In addition, physicians pool their economic resources to purchase expensive equipment, hire auxiliary health staff, and reduce fees.

The county medical society will also provide you with a list of physicians and information on medical schools, residency programs, and whether boards were taken. You may also want to consult friends or neighbors who have lived in the area for several years and are familiar with medical care. Similar procedures can be used in locating a dentist.

After making your choice, call the doctor's office to be certain new patients are being accepted and to check on office hours, fees, and other information. It is also helpful to inquire about the physician's approach to preventive medicine (regular examinations, consultations, and vaccinations). Avoid making your final de-

Table 20.1
SPECIALISTS AND AREAS OF TREATMENT

Area of Specialty Treatment	Medical Specialist
Body reactions and hypersensitivity to drugs, pollens, food, and animals	Allergist
Heart disease	Cardiologist
Skin disease	Dermatologist
Internal secretions of the ductless glands	Endocrinologist
Preventive medicine for the family	Family physician
Diseases of the digestive system	Gastroenterologist
Diseases and changes in old age	Gerontologist
Illnesses of a nonsurgical nature in adults	Internist
Diseases of the nervous system	Neurologist
Care during pregnancy and in childbirth	Obstetrician
Refractive errors of the eye	Ophthalmologist
Diseases of joints, bones, and spine	Orthopedist
Diseases of the ear and larynx	Otolaryngologist
Diseases of the ear	Otologist
Diseases in children	Pediatrician
Correction of deformed or damaged body parts	Plastic surgeon
Diseases of the colon, rectum, and anus	Proctologist
Mental and personality disorders	Psychiatrist
Disorders of the nose	Rhinologist
Diseases of the genitourinary tract	Urologist
Diseases of the nerve of a tooth	Endodontist
Correction and prevention of teeth irregularities and malocclusion of the jaw	Orthodontist
Dental ills in children	Pedodontist
Gums and supporting tissue of the teeth	Periodontist
Construction of dentures, bridges, and crowns	Prosthodontist
	Nonmedical Specialist
Grinding and setting lenses to the prescription of an oculist	Optician
Measures visual acuity, prescribes glasses	Optometrist
Correction of defects through eye exercises	Orthoptist
Diseases, defects, injuries of the foot	Podiatrist
Applies scientific methods to the study of human behavior	Psychologist

cision until after your first or second visit. If you sense a communication problem or notice questionable practices, continue your search.

Types of Doctors

The five clinical specialties are internal medicine, surgery, pediatrics, obstetrics and gynecology, and psychiatry. There are other specialties; however, the patient rarely goes directly to such physicians without a recommendation from the family doctor. Table 20.1 lists common specialists and their treatment areas.

You need to decide whether the family physician should handle the health of the entire family. A pediatrician may be desirable for children of both sexes, a gynecologist for girls over the age of 12 or 13. Most people need a primary care (family) physician who handles the majority of the family health problems, including referral to an appropriate specialist when necessary.

Checkups and Screening

Concept: The annual checkup may be less important than periodic screening for major diseases.

The annual physical examination was once a major feature of preventive medicine in the United States. In recent years, however, the annual physical has been criticized as an unnecessary expense. Particularly when a person is in good health, the annual physical is not the best means of preventive care. A more useful approach is periodic screening for major diseases. Table 20.2 provides information on the most important screening tests. As for physicals, the American Medical Association recommends scheduling complete medical examinations according to age:

Prenatal	Monthly or biweekly examination of mother
1–6 months	Bimonthly
1–2 years	Every three months

Table 20.2
SCREENING TESTS FOR MAJOR DISEASES

Disease	Test	Screening Schedule
Hypertension (high blood pressure)	Measured by simple instrument; readings can be done at free screening stations	If screening indicates high blood pressure, consult physician to work out management program
Cervical cancer	Internal exam and Pap smear, performed in a doctor's office	Every two or three years for women over 25; annually for women with herpes, type 2
Breast cancer	Breast self-exam (steps outlined in Chapter 17)	Monthly, a week after menstrual period
Testicular cancer	Testicular self-exam (steps outlined in Chapter 17)	Monthly, right after a hot bath or shower
Glaucoma (an eye disease)	Examination by a physician	Regular screening after age 40
Tuberculosis	Skin test done in doctor's office	Every three or four years; annually for people who may have been exposed

2–6 years	Twice each year
6–15 years	Every two or three years
15–35 years	Every two years
35–60 years	Annually
60 and over	Twice each year

Regular dental checkups are important at all ages, and are critical during adolescence and the late teens, when a high rate of dental decay and periodontal disease is common. A minimum of one visit every six months is recommended for college-age students, as well as for all adults. Preventive dentistry is a very effective means of protecting against tooth and gum diseases later in life.

Discovery Activity 20.1
YOUR LAST PHYSICAL EXAM

Think about your last physical examination. How long ago was it? The areas listed below represent the major aspects recommended for a complete examination. What key areas were neglected? Do you have any symptoms that suggest a need for consultation in any area? How thorough was your physician? Did your consultation include suggestions for changes in lifestyle (exercise, smoking, eating, sleeping habits)?

_____ 1. Complete medical history, including chief complaints and present illnesses

_____ 2. Review of health habits (eating, sleeping, exercise, smoking, anxieties)

_____ 3. Exercise EKG or stress test

_____ 4. Exercise evaluation—body fat (skinfold measures), abdominal strength, aerobic capacity (from known 1.5-mile run, 2-mile time, Cooper's 12-minute test, or Master's Step Test administered in the office)

_____ 5. Heart disease risk profile

_____ 6. Pulse, respiration, and blood pressure

_____ 7. Blood work—including cholesterol and triglycerides

_____ 8. Rectal examination

_____ 9. Skin inspection

_____ 10. Ear, nose, and throat

_____ 11. Lymph nodes

_____ 12. Chest X ray or skin test for tuberculosis

_____ 13. For women, pap smear, breast and reproductive system examination

_____ 14. For men, examination of external genitalia

_____ 15. Test for glaucoma (after age 40)

_____ 16. Urinalysis, urine cultures, and tests for blood in the stool after age 30.●

How to Talk to Your Doctor

Concept: It is the patient's responsibility to provide the doctor with key information and to insist on direct, accurate answers.

Your doctor will first want to know the main reason you scheduled your visit—your primary complaint, specific symptoms (temperature, blood pressure, heart rate, swelling, redness, type of pain, etc.), medications taken, and the kinds of physical activity you are still participating in. Your doctor will also need information about previous illnesses, surgery, and treatment, as well as allergies and reactions to medication. During the physical examination, you should help the doctor by pointing out pains, lumps, growths, or previous injuries that occasionally produce pain, discomfort, or concern. On the initial examination, your doctor is trying to learn as much about your body as possible to aid diagnosis and treatment in the future.

It is up to you, the patient, to be direct and assertive, asking any question that occurs to you, no matter how trivial it may seem. Will this drug have side effects? What are they? When should I check back? How soon can I expect these symptoms to disappear? Should I go to work or school? Unless you ask, it is unlikely that the doctor will volunteer this information. To avoid forgetting important concerns, write them down prior to your visit and bring the list with you. Anything that concerns you is a fair question. Don't be hurried or permit the doctor to brush you off with a few sentences before rushing to the next patient. Do not leave the office until you are satisfied that the doctor has answered your questions. If you are hurried, treated like a child, or cannot secure direct answers about your condition, change doctors.

Selecting a Hospital

Concept: Choosing the right hospital affects the level of health care.

Those who are fortunate enough to live in an area with more than one hospital have an opportunity to select the one best suited for their needs. Hospitals vary tremendously in terms of available equipment, competency of physicians and other personnel, ability to administer sophisticated tests, treatment, and surgery. General medical and surgical hospitals diagnose and treat a wide variety of health conditions, generally for short periods of time. Specialty hospitals admit patients with specific conditions or diseases, generally for long periods of time.

Hospitals are also classified according to financing: voluntary, government, and private (see Fig. 20.1). Voluntary hospitals are public, nonprofit hospitals managed by philanthropic institutions or individuals. Financial assistance is often provided by local groups and the federal government. Government hospitals are supported by federal, state, county, or city government and are generally equipped to handle long-term illnesses. Care is provided for military and Public Health Service personnel and families and for American Indians, veterans, and merchant seamen. Private hospitals are owned by individuals or corporations with the

Figure 20.1
Types of hospitals.

SOURCE: Medical Care Expenditures, Prices, and Costs: Background Book (Department of Health, Education, and Welfare, Social Security Administration, Office of Research and Statistics, September 1973).

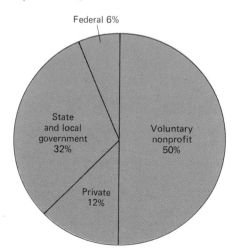

Federal 6%

State and local government 32%

Voluntary nonprofit 50%

Private 12%

Total hospitals: 7061

Discovery Activity 20.2
ARE YOU GETTING THE MOST FROM YOUR DOCTOR VISITS?

Consider the last time you went to the doctor for help with a health problem. Then answer the following questions:

1. Did you think about the reasons for your visit so that you could convey them to the doctor clearly?

2. Did you tell the doctor all your symptoms, or did you try to underplay some of them?

3. Assuming that the doctor was able to diagnose your ailment, did he or she give you an understandable and satisfactory explanation of it?

4. Did the doctor answer all your questions fully and clearly? If unable to answer a question, did he or she say so?

5. Did the doctor treat you like a responsible adult, or did you feel intimidated?

6. Did you report to the doctor any medications you take or allergies and other reactions you may have to medications?

7. If the doctor prescribed a medication, did you ask about how to take it and possible side effects?

8. If you left with a prescription, did you have it filled and take it as directed for the full time period directed?

9. If the doctor told you to check back within a certain time period, did you do so?

If your response to any of these questions was negative, you may not be getting the most out of your doctor visits. What steps could you take to improve your doctor/patient relationship? ●

intention of producing a profit. Consequently, private hospitals are often smaller, less well equipped, understaffed, lacking in facilities, and weak in handling emergencies. Emphasis is placed on patients with short-term illnesses who are unlikely to develop complications and are capable of making payment. The larger private hospitals maintain generally high standards and avoid most of the difficulties of the smaller hospitals.

Before choosing a hospital, consider the following six factors:

1. *Accreditation status.* Hospitals accredited by the Joint Commission on Accreditation have met certain standards in all phases of hospital care: selection and training of staff, equipment, facilities, food service, pharmacy, record keeping, and medical staff. Accreditation does not guarantee a perfect hospital, nor can one be assured that broad certification of staff is required. In general, however, a voluntary hospital is superior to a private or government-funded hospital and adheres more strictly to accreditation standards.

2. *Affiliation with a medical school.* Teaching hospitals are generally equipped to provide excellent medical care for practically any illness or ailment. Only hospitals with extremely high standards are associated with medical schools. You can be relatively sure these hospitals will have a well-trained staff of experienced physicians and most modern equipment.

3. *Size.* Small hospitals (200 beds or fewer) offer a narrow range of services, have few specialists, and may not be equipped to handle serious illnesses. In general, larger hospitals offer the best and most comprehensive health care.

4. *Location.* Depending upon the illness, it is desirable to choose a hospital within a reasonable distance from your home. Emergency room treatment varies considerably from one hospital to another, suggesting the need to investigate this area of health care.

5. *Cost.* Cost of private and semiprivate rooms and medical services varies from hospital to hospital.

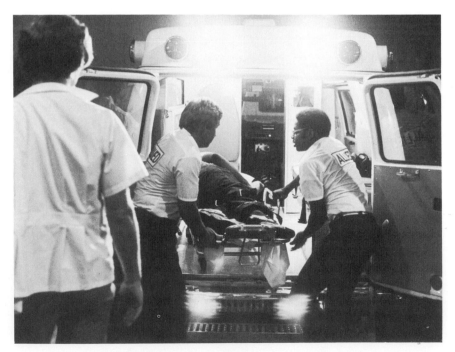

Hospitals vary greatly in the competence of their personnel, their ability to provide emergency care, and the range of services they provide.

It is helpful to consult your health insurance plan and discuss cost with the hospital of your choice.

6. *Ownership.* According to Consumers Union medical consultants, the voluntary hospital is your best choice.

A hospital should be used only when absolutely necessary. Many services can be provided outside the hospital for much less cost. The hospital should not be used for rest or for convenience. It is a noisy, unfamiliar environment with continuous interruptions. It is often not the best place to conduct screening tests. In addition, treatment for some ailments is more effective in a home environment that cannot be duplicated in the hospital.

Patient's Bill of Rights

Concept: The Patient's Bill of Rights sets forth guidelines for good, personal hospital care.

The American Hospital Association has devised a document listing the rights of hospital patients. You should receive your copy of this **Patient's Bill of Rights** when you are admitted to a hospital that belongs to the association. Although the Patient's Bill of Rights is not a legal document, it does set forth standards that member hospitals are expected to follow.

The Patient's Bill of Rights contains the following provisions.[1]

Discovery Activity 20.3
EVALUATING HOSPITALS

Using the text discussion and the chart, evaluate two local hospitals. If you don't know the answers to some items, ask your doctor for the information. List the major strengths and weaknesses of each hospital. ●

Criteria	Hospital 1	Hospital 2
Accreditation (Joint Commission on Accreditation)		
Emergency-room treatment capabilities		
Personnel (size of staff)		
Size (small or large)		
Ownership (voluntary, government, or private)		
Location (from home)		
0–5 miles (excellent)		
6–10 (very good)		
11–15 (fair)		
16–20 (poor)		
21–over (very poor)		
Capabilities for treating		
minor ailments		
major ailments		
Affiliation with medical school		

Rating: 5—Excellent   4—Very good   3—Fair   2—Poor   1—Very poor

1. Considerate and respectful care.
2. The right to obtain complete information concerning your diagnosis, treatment, and prognosis, in terms you can understand.
3. The right to all the applicable information you need to give informed consent (risks, benefits, alternative treatments), prior to treatment.
4. The right to refuse treatment, once you are aware of the facts, to the extent permitted by law.
5. Privacy and confidentiality (refusal to be examined in front of people who are not involved in your case, confidentiality of records).
6. A reasonable response when you ask for help, including evaluation, service, and referral as indicated by the urgency of the case.
7. Information about any possible conflicts of interest (hospital ownership of labs evaluating your tests, professional relationships among doctors who are treating you).
8. The right to be told if the hospital plans to make your treatment part of a research project or experiment.
9. The right to an explanation of your hospital bill.
10. The right to know what hospital rules apply to your conduct as a patient.
11. The right to expect good follow-up care.

Awareness of your rights as a patient is a first step toward getting the quality of care you need. It is your personal responsibility to look out for yourself, insisting on good care and expressing your needs and concerns freely.

Community Health Care

Concept: Free or inexpensive, confidential medical care is available in most cities and counties.

Community health resources are available to all. State health departments and county or city health units exist to assist residents with specific health problems. Al-

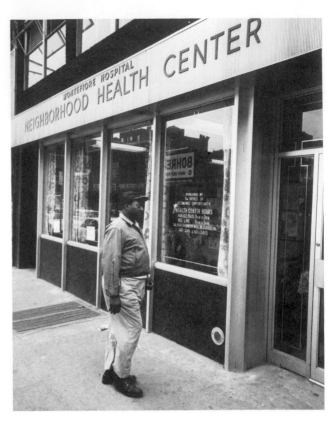

Free clinics provide essential services and information to the poor.

though the most important function of city and county health departments is the education of the public, direct medical services are provided to members of the community. Immunization centers for disease control, special clinics for sexually transmitted diseases, and maternal and child health services are generally available.

In most cities, "free clinics" have evolved to treat or counsel people for undesired pregnancies, sexually transmitted diseases, and drug use. Many of these clinics treat all ailments for those who cannot afford regular medical care. Minimum funding and a shortage of personnel restrict medical services to a small number of patients and reduce services considerably; however, sympathetic care and sincere interest are provided. With more community support, free clinics could provide a real contribution to the modern medical care system.

ALTERNATIVE APPROACHES TO HEALTH CARE

Acupuncture

Acupuncture is a method of eliminating pain using needles inserted at specific points on the body. This technique has been practiced in China for thousands of years and attracted the attention of medical practitioners in the West beginning in the 1970s. Using acupuncture, Chinese surgeons have been able to perform operations of the head, chest, and abdomen without anesthesia. The advantages of acupuncture anesthesia are numerous: the patient is able to remain conscious during surgery, there is no risk of side effects or possible death from general anesthetics, the danger of blood clotting after surgery is reduced, and the patient does not have to spend time in a recovery room while anesthesia wears off.

Considerable scientific investigation is under way to determine the therapeutic value of acupuncture as a treatment for nerve deafness, narcotics withdrawal, and pain. Acupuncture has been used successfully as a surgical anesthetic for root canal therapy, skin grafts, tumor biopsies, and minor surgical procedures, and it appears to be useful in abortions and childbirth as well. To date, the reasons acupuncture seems to work are unclear. The major danger with the treatment is its use by quacks who have no training. If you plan to look into the technique, seek out a licensed physician performing acupuncture under the auspices of a hospital or medical school.

Chiropractic

Because **chiropractic** is a controversial treatment method, we discuss it in the Issue on pages 490 and 491.

HEALTH INSURANCE

Concept: People of all ages need the financial protection provided by health insurance.

Health insurance is an absolute necessity in the United States today. Given the extremely high costs of medical care, the alternative—direct out-of-pocket payment by the patient—can pose a tremendous financial burden. Several kinds of group and individual health insurance plans are available. The major components of the ideal policy are : (1) hospital insurance to cover hospital bills, (2) surgical insurance to cover doctors' operating fees, (3) regular medical insurance to pay for nonsurgical doctors' fees in and out of the hospital, (4) major medical insurance to cover a percentage of expenses incurred above a certain cost in case of major illness or injury, and (5) disability or lost-income insurance to pay for living expenses if the family breadwinner is incapacited. Few things that you buy require such serious consideration and review on your part.

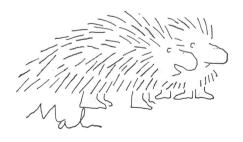
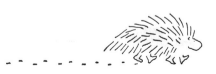

"My son, the acupuncturist."

Insurance Providers

Independent insurance plans. More than 500 independent insurance plans are available in the United States. Some are joint ventures between union and management; others provide benefits through prepaid group practice plans. Several of these plans are nonprofit service corporations allowing a free choice of medical personnel and providing service benefits.

Commercial insurance plans. Profit-making companies write both group and individual health insurance policies. Life insurance, disability insurance, and major medical insurance can also be acquired as part of a complete package. Major medical policies are designed to handle expensive medical costs not ordinarily covered by typical insurance. Maximum benefits range from $2000 to $40,000 or more, with a "deductible" and a "coinsurance" clause. The patient pays the deductible amount before any costs are paid by the company. The higher the deductible, the lower the premium. A coinsurance clause states that a specified percentage of the cost must be borne by the patient after the deductible amount is subtracted. A policy, for example, may pay a maximum benefit of $10,000, with a deductible clause of $500 and a coinsurance clause of 20 percent. If a portion of a total bill of $10,000 ($1200, for example) is paid by a basic plan, the patient presents a bill of $8800 less $500 (deductible), or $8300. This $8300 is subject to coinsurance (20 percent), with the patient responsible for paying $1660. Actual reimbursement from the major medical plan amounts to $6640 ($8300 minus $1660). In the case of prolonged hospital care and serious illness, a coinsurance clause can mean substantial cost to the patient.

Disability insurance. During hospitalization and convalescence, loss of income due to unemployment and expiration of accumulated sick leave threatens family security. Such a dangerous risk makes disability insurance a must for most families. Premiums are paid to insurance companies that, in cases of disability, pay 75 percent or more of the patient's regular monthly income. Policies are also designed to provide lump-sum benefits for loss of a limb or part of a limb, or to survivors in case of accidental death.

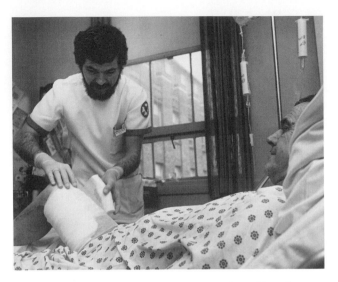

Major medical insurance, such as that offered by Blue Cross, is intended primarily to cover major medical needs, particularly hospitalization.

Blue Cross and Blue Shield. Blue Cross was founded by hospital officials during the Depression to keep hospitals from going bankrupt. A small premium (about $1.00 per month) was paid in return for a specified number of days of hospital care. Every member paid the same premium, regardless of age, sex, or health status. Blue Cross gave no cash to policyholders; instead, hospitals were paid for services rendered and generally kept their charges within the ranges provided by the Blue Cross plan. As hospital workers began to demand higher wages, expensive diagnostic and treatment equipment was invented, and hospital and physician costs soared, Blue Cross premiums increased tremendously. The plan was no longer an inexpensive, simplified answer to health insurance. Industry soon discovered that it was possible to purchase policies from private companies at lower rates, particularly when their work force consisted predominantly of young male (no pregnancy risk) workers. Faced with the threat of losing its healthiest members, Blue Cross began setting premium rates by classes and selling policies based upon actual risks.

Today, about 75 Blue Cross plans offer service benefits and provide compensation for a specified number of days in a hospital, generally covering the majority of costs (from the first dollar) of an average stay. Blue Cross/Blue Shield is a plan that primarily serves major medical needs, such as hospitalization and major surgery. Smaller medical expenses, such as physicians office visits and prescription medications, are covered in part and only after payment of a deductible (usually paid quarterly). No emphasis is placed on preventive care; routine physical examinations and periodic screening (Pap smears and the like) are not covered. All Blue Cross plans must meet the approval of the American Hospital Association's Blue Cross Commission and exist as a nonprofit organization—profits must be used to improve the plan. Surgical and medical benefits are obtained through Blue Shield, which covers bills in full only for patients up to certain income levels. Many hospitals accept Blue Shield allotments for different surgical and medical procedures and do not make added charges. Rates are increased to reflect increases in hospital, surgical, and medical costs.

Health maintenance organizations. The health care system in the United States has traditionally focused on treatment of the sick. When a patient notices some symptoms, the physician springs into action, and a health plan reimburses the patient for all or part of the costs for most illnesses. Little emphasis has been placed on preventive measures, because the typical health plan does not cover regular checkups, screening, and the like. **Health maintenance organizations (HMOs)** are different in that they provide comprehensive medical coverage, from a routine checkup to major surgery, from a physician visit to hospitalization, in exchange for advance payment of a fixed monthly fee. HMOs are designed to encourage subscribers to cut their costs by preventing illness. Both the physician and the patient share the financial risk of ill health. Unlike conventional health plans, HMOs guarantee that services will be made available to the consumer.

HMOs are group practices that also give doctors some incentive to keep people well; to treat illnesses early, before hospitalization is necessary; and to prac-

Issues in Health
THE CHIROPRACTIC PROFESSION—SCIENCE OR QUACKERY?

Chiropractic was originated in 1895 by David Palmer, labeled a "magnetic healer." Palmer performed manual adjustments of the vertebrae in order to cure deafness and heart trouble. From his experiences evolved the theory that partly dislocated (subluxated) vertebrae emit heat from pressure on the nerves, and these pressures cause practically all diseases. The R. J. Chiropractic Clinic was developed by Palmer's son as a model for future offices. Proponents of chiropractic support the modern-day theoretical basis of the profession and the following four principles:

1. Anatomical disrelation can create functional disturbances in the body.
2. Disturbances of the nervous system are primary factors in the development of many diseases.
3. Spinal subluxations are a specific cause of nerve irritation or interference.
4. The viscero-spinal principle: nerve irritation at the spine may lead to a disturbance in the function of one or more internal organs of the body.[2]

Opponents cite three main areas of controversy and criticism: lack of support for the theoretical basis of chiropractic clinics, inadequate education and training of the chiropractic, and unsupported claims of cures for practically any disease or ailment. In spite of numerous patient testimonials, there is no valid evidence that subluxation is a key factor in the disease process. Manipulation may be helpful in relieving pain due to loss of mobility in joints, muscle spasms, or minor backache, but research support is lacking.

Colleges of chiropractic offer a four-year training program. That there are weaknesses in the basic sciences is evident from the high rate of failure in the science-licensing examination; 84.5 percent of

(continued)

Issues in Health (continued)

chiropractic students fail on the first attempt, compared to only 18.6 percent of medical students.[3] In addition, considerable training is devoted to manipulation, massage, and business management. An HEW study of chiropractic education in 1968 revealed a lack of qualified faculty, low admission requirements, high student–faculty ratios, poor facilities and libraries, minimum hospital/patient exposure, and lack of basic scientific research on the part of the faculty.[4]

Chiropractors treat a wide range of ailments, including asthma, bronchitis, allergies, and others. Some chiropractors even advocate the elimination of certain inoculations—to be replaced by spinal manipulation.[5] There is no evidence that these ailments are successfully treated or that immunity is provided through manipulation.

Statements characterizing the chiropractic profession as unscientific, nonmedical, and lacking the body of basic knowledge related to disease and health care widely accepted by the scientific community have been made by HEW,[7] the College of Physicians and Surgeons of the Province of Quebec,[8] and the American Medical Association. Based on the findings of HEW in 1968, it was recommended that chiropractic services not be covered in the Medicare program.

According to the chiropractic profession, the American Medical Association and most physicians have unjustly condemned their mode of treatment. It is true that the quality of chiropractic training programs has greatly improved in recent years. The fact that more and more insurance companies now include coverage of chiropractic services in their health plans demonstrates a new faith in the profession. In addition, the profession is flourishing because many people believe the approach has helped them.

What do you think? ●

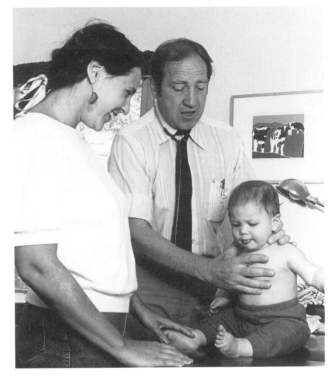

Health maintenance organizations focus heavily on preventive care by covering the cost of routine screenings, physical exams, well baby checkups, and the like.

tice preventive medicine. Although physicians associated with HMOs are salaried, their annual bonus is based on a percentage of the profits. The cost of office staff, equipment, buildings, and malpractice and other insurance is borne by the health maintenance organization. An administrative staff also handles much of the paper work which can consume 15 to 25 percent of a private physician's time. This frees the doctor to spend more time with individual patients. Doctors can order lab tests or admit patients to a hospital without concern over whether an insurance plan will cover the expense. HMO physicians also enjoy all the advantages of a typical group practice.

For the patient, HMOs offer a less expensive approach to medical care. A patient is also encouraged to seek early treatment, because the prepaid monthly fee covers all services. In addition, physicians, labs, and pharmacies are sometimes organized under one roof, saving the patient valuable time. A physician is usually on call 24 hours a day.

Over 6 million people in the United States are HMO subscribers in over 300 separate health maintenance organizations. There is evidence that this new approach is reducing medical costs for the consumer and providing adequate medical care. It also appears to be contributing to the health of its members by emphasizing preventive care. HMOs attract a younger, healthier individual than the general population. Some companies offer employees a choice between a conventional health plan and an HMO. Some states even permit Medicaid recipients to join. Table 20.3 makes some comparisons between traditional health insurers, such as Blue Cross, and HMOs.

Medicare and Medicaid. Congress amended the Social Security Act in 1965 to include Title 18 (**Med-**

icare) and provide a program of health insurance to individuals 65 years of age and older. Two programs were established: (1) compulsory hospital insurance financed by Social Security taxes to cover hospital care, extended-care facilities (nursing homes), and outpatient diagnostic services; and (2) voluntary medical insurance financed by individual premiums and matching funds from the government to pay doctor bills and other services not covered by hospital insurance.

The Social Security Act was also amended to include Title 19 (**Medicaid**), providing federal grants to the states to operate a medical assistance program for those already receiving public assistance from the federal government (including the elderly, blind, disabled, and families with dependent children); to assist those who have enough income to live on but not enough to cover medical expenses; and to provide help for all children under age 21 whose parents cannot afford medical expenses.

Medicare, with its unique feature of combining compulsory and voluntary methods of payment, has

Table 20.3.
TRADITIONAL HEALTH INSURERS AND HMOs: SOME COMPARISONS

Fee-for-Service Plans. (Blue-Cross/Blue Shield)	Prepaid Plans (HMOs)
Provide health care services for a *major part* of medical expenses on a fee-for-service basis.	Provide *comprehensive* health care services in return for a prepaid monthly fee.
Typically require a quarterly deductible for small medical expenses, such as doctor's visits or prescription drugs. Some plans also require clients to pay approximately 20 percent of expenses above the deductible.	No deductible for smaller medical expenses.
Provide 100 percent coverage for major medical expenses (hospital and surgical).	Provide 100 percent coverage for major medical expenses (hospital and surgical).
Do not encourage preventive care, because routine and preventive services are not covered.	Encourage preventive care, because routine and preventive services are covered (e.g., physical exams, Pap smears, well baby care).
Client may select *any* participating physician or medical facility.	Client must select a *specific* HMO primary care physician and use hospitals associated with the HMO.
Client must submit claim forms to be reimbursed for some smaller services, such as physician's office visits.	Virtually no claim forms or bills are incurred by the client.
Client must secure the medical services and submit the costs for reimbursement.	Client is guaranteed that services will be made available.

resulted in improved and extended health care to millions of Americans who previously could not afford to pay for medical services. The plan removes the elderly, or high-risk group, from the health insurance market. It is estimated that the government now has taken over approximately 90 percent of medical costs for persons over the age of 65. Unfortunately, the program is not without problems, as reports of abuses by physicians and patients increase and costs continue to rise, placing a heavier burden on tax dollars.

Evaluating Before You Buy

Concept: Before making a purchase, evaluate the policy with extreme care.

Examine your policy carefully to secure accurate answers to the following key questions:

1. Is there "first dollar" coverage?

2. How does a deductible of $100, $500, or more affect premiums? What amount is suited to your income?

3. Is disability or lost-income protection provided? What portion of your monthly salary is involved? For how long? Is there provision for permanent disability?

4. Is there a lump-sum payment to dependents in case of death?

5. Is full coverage provided for hospital, medical, and surgical costs? What dollar restrictions are placed on length of stay, costs for various surgical and medical procedures, cost of drugs, and special treatments? Are physicians' costs covered both in and out of the hospital?

6. Is major medical insurance available for serious illnesses or accidents?

7. Are expenses for care during pregnancy and delivery covered?

8. Are reduced rates available for policyholders not in need of coverage for pregnancy? Are reduced rates available to nonsmokers? Nondrinkers? Individuals in good health?

9. Is this a "commerical policy" (one that can be canceled if the holder becomes a bad risk after the claim for the current illness is paid); a "guaranteed-renewable" policy (the holder has the right to continue until age 65, as long as premiums are paid on time; and premiums cannot be raised unless they are increased for everyone in the insured's classification); or a "noncancellable guaranteed-renewable" (the insured can keep the policy until age 65 or, in some cases, for life, without any change in provision, including rates). Premiums rise with both the noncancellable guaranteed-renewable and the guaranteed-renewable policies.

10. Is a group policy available? Group rates are generally lower, and health risks are accepted into the plan that ordinarily are not handled on an individual basis.

11. Is coverage provided for mental and emotional disorders?

12. Does your policy use the terms "accidental bodily injury" if it covers expense sustained as a result of accident (this wording tends to guarantee coverage for injuries by a willful attempt to cause you bodily harm).

13. Is coverage provided for dental care?

14. What provisions are available for coverage of dependents?

15. What is the grace period for late premiums before cancellation occurs?

16. Do any restrictive clauses eliminate payment for previously existing illnesses or require a waiting period before such illnesses are covered?

Your state insurance department can also be of assistance. It will provide an analysis of any policy, explain its terms, provide information on the ease or difficulty of securing payment on claims, and clarify any feature of the policy you don't understand.

CONCLUSION

A health care crisis in the United States cannot be too far in the future. Rising medical costs are already so high that some families avoid or delay treatment. The introduction of Medicaid and Medicare has been of some help; however, Social Security costs have soared as a result. Moreover, sickness and disease may increase if the widespread physical abuse and sedentary life-styles of the American public continue. Any significant change in longevity and quality of life will come from two areas: the improved physical fitness of the nation and the improved health care of individuals through early detection of disease. The first area is completely free of cost; the second has the potential to drain family finances. A comprehensive health insurance plan is imperative for individuals of all ages to avoid bankruptcy due to illness. Such a plan, coupled with an awareness of body changes and certain lifestyle changes (sound nutrition, abstention from smoking, regular exercise) can result in a life relatively free from disease.

SUMMARY

1. Each individual is responsible for maintaining good health and for detecting and treating minor illnesses and injuries. To provide proper self-care, individuals need to learn more about their bodies, monitor bodily functions on a regular basis, and be capable of deciding when and how to use medical resources.

2. Self-medication is an important part of self-care. Over-the-counter drugs must be carefully selected and used to treat minor illnesses and injuries, not to cure disease. If the symptoms of an illness persist, a physician should be consulted.

3. Each individual should carefully select a primary care (family) physician to handle family needs and

Issues in Health
SECURING ADEQUATE MEDICAL CARE—A PRIVILEGE OR A RIGHT?

Soaring medical costs may eventually make health care a privilege only the upper-middle and upper classes can afford. The less economically fortunate would then be forced to use the services of public health agencies and special free clinics. Expenditures for medical care in the United States have mounted rapidly (see Fig. 20.2). In 1976 the figure was $139 billion, in 1978 it was more than $180 billion, and in 1980 it exceeded $200 billion. Increases in private physician, hospital, and insurance

Figure 20.2
The annual cost of medical care rose dramatically between 1950 and 1980—and it is still rising.
SOURCE: U.S. Department of Health and Human Services.

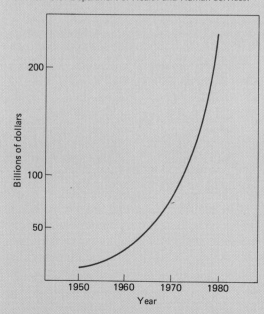

(continued)

Issues in Health (continued)

fees for the individual are staggering. If the trend continues, only a small percentage of the American people will be capable of financing health care for their families.

The view that every citizen has a right to adequate medical care is gaining support. More than a dozen national health insurance bills have been proposed by congressional representatives and interested groups. The Kennedy–Corman plan proposes shifting the financing of health care to the government and doing away with private health insurance firms. The plan is based on the idea that significant changes must be made not only in the financing of health care, but in the way medicine is practiced, hospitals are run, and costs are controlled. A 1 percent income tax, an employer's tax, and money from the general revenues would be used to finance the plan.

The most radical plan is a bill proposed by Representative Ronald Dellums (D-Calif.) to create a national health service similar to the one in England. By nationalizing the health care industry, this plan would eliminate fees for services; pay the salaries of doctors, who would work for the government; and provide government control of all hospitals.

Many medical personnel are skeptical about such plans. They point out that in other countries with government health services efficiency has declined, costs have risen, and taxpayers have had to support an evergrowing bureaucracy.

In spite of these concerns, the demand for change is spreading to the grassroots. Most advocates of reform agree that health insurance should be mandatory and should protect every citizen and cover the costs of all forms of illness. A broad health care program will be expensive and out of the reach of most citizens unless some form of government plan is initiated.

What do you think? ●

make referrals to specialists whenever needed. A physician should only be chosen after you have consulted your friends or neighbors, the local medical school, or the county medical society.

4. Each individual is responsible for periodic screening for hypertension, cervical cancer, breast cancer (for women), testicular cancer (for men), glaucoma, and tuberculosis.

5. It is the patient's responsibility to be direct and assertive in communicating with the doctor. It is also the patient's right to receive direct, honest answers about his or her condition.

6. Patients should select a hospital carefully, considering such factors as accreditation status and affiliation with a medical school.

7. Acupuncture, an alternative approach to medical care, eliminates pain by inserting needles at specific points on the body. The practice remains controversial. If you want to explore this treatment method seek out a licensed physician performing under the auspices of a hospital or medical school.

8. Chiropractic, another controversial alternative approach to medical care, uses manual adjustments of the vertebrae to cure various conditions and ailments. More and more insurance companies are including coverage of chiropractic services.

9. Fee-for-service health plans, such as Blue Cross, provide health care services for a major part of medical expenses by reimbursing all or part of the expenses associated with hospitalization and major surgery. Coverage is not provided for routine physical exams and screening. Health maintenance organizations offer comprehensive health care in return for a fixed monthly fee. There is no deductible for small medical expenses. HMOs encourage preventive care.

10. It is important to evaluate the services of a health plan carefully before choosing one—to determine if your anticipated needs and those of your family will be met with limited additional cost to you.

REFERENCES

1. Maxine Phillips, *Getting Health Care* (New York: New Readers Press, 1980).

2. John A. Conley, "Another Look at the Chiropractor," *Health Education* 7 (Jan./Feb. 1976):22.

3. R. L. Smith, "Chiropractic: Science or Swindle," *Today's Health* 43 (1965):60.

4. "HEW Rejects Chiropractic," *Today's Health* 47 (1969): 54.

5. Ralph L. Smith, *At Your Own Risk: The Case Against Chiropractice* (New York: Trident Press, 1969), p. 151.

6. "Chiropractic and Naturopathy," *American Journal of Public Health* 60 (1970):13.

7. W. T. Jarvis, "Chiropractic: A Challenge for Health Education," *Journal of School Health* 44 (1974):210.

LABORATORY 1
FREE HEALTH CARE IN YOUR COMMUNITY

Purpose To identify the free health care services available in your community.

Size of Group Five to seven students per group.

Procedure

1. Each group chooses one of the following:
   Health maintenance organizations,
   Mental health clinics,
   Medical clinics (including abortion, treatment of
   STDs),
   Other free clinics.

2. Each group prepares a list of all the free clinics within the area chosen and assigns one or two clinics to each group member.

3. Students visit the clinics and health maintenance organizations and complete the information on the chart that follows.

Results

1. Each group prepares copies of its findings (chart) for distribution to the entire class.

2. One student from each group is selected to summarize findings to the class.

COUNTY AND CITY HEALTH CLINICS/AGENCIES PROVIDING FREE SERVICES

Name of Clinic	Location	Telephone	Primary Services Rendered	Cost	Who Is Eligible

LABORATORY 2
YOUR COLLEGE HEALTH SERVICES

Purpose   To become familiar with the college health services available to you.

Size of Group   Complete the information requested on your own, asking for assistance should you be unfamiliar with the health care system. Visit the health care area.

Equipment   None.

Procedure

Fill in the following information about your college health services:

1. Location: _____

2. Medical personnel available:
   _____ Physician (part time)
   _____ Physician (full time)
   _____ Nurse (part time)
   _____ Nurse (full time)
   Hours:

3. List the special equipment located in the health care area:

4. Check the types of services offered:
   _____ Treatment for minor illnesses and injuries (outpatient)
   _____ Treatment for minor illnesses and injuries (infirmary)
   _____ Referral to private physicians, surgeons, clinics, hospitals
   _____ Health guidance and counseling
   _____ Psychological examinations and mental health guidance
   _____ Cooperation with college health council, food services, housing, athletics, student organizations, buildings and grounds, to provide a safe environment
   _____ Treatment of athletic injuries (including physical education, recreation)
   _____ Other (list):

5. List the step-by-step procedures for using the college health services should you be injured. (Who is called first? What first aid policies are in effect? etc.)

6. Describe your college health insurance plan, including cost and services.

Results

In paragraph form, evaluate all the services provided by your college or university in caring for your health needs.

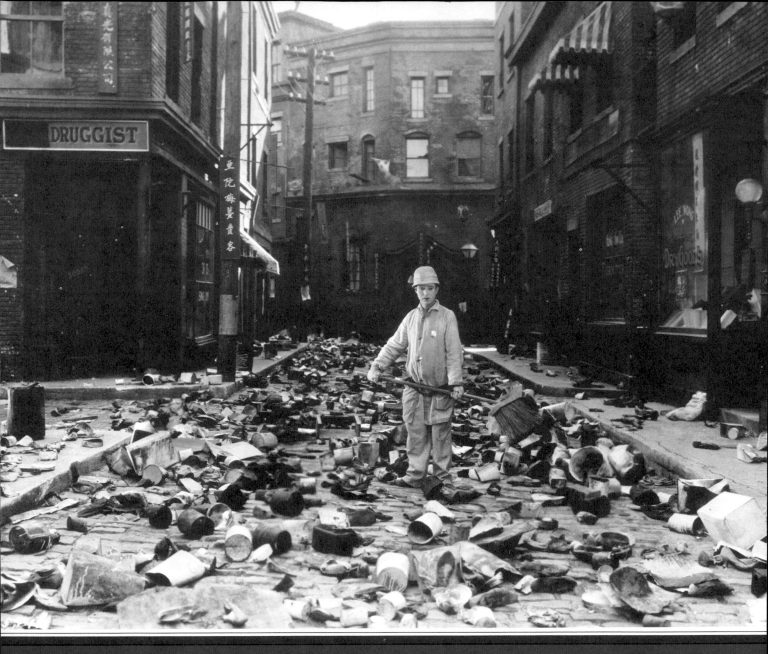

your environment

Over the past two decades it has become more and more evident that environmental pollutants pose a serious threat to the human body, plant and animal life, and even the human mind. Pollution of air, land, and water is a serious threat to the earth's very survival. Although some changes have been initiated, little improvement has been accomplished. A much more concentrated effort on the part of government, industry, and the private citizen is needed to reverse unfavorable trends and safeguard what is not yet contaminated. In addition to discussing some specific sources of environmental pollution, our primary emphasis here will be on the changes needed to halt the onslaught on our nation's air, land, and water—changes that can be brought about through the collective efforts of government, industry, and individuals. As you read this chapter, consider what you can do to help ensure a healthier environment in which to live.

AIR POLLUTION

Polluted air affects the health of human beings and is responsible for a significant number of deaths and illnesses (see Fig. 21.1). According to Dr. Herbert Schimmel, a biophysicist at the Albert Einstein College of Medicine, air pollution caused approximately 28 deaths daily from 1963 to 1972 in New York City alone. About 800 million tons of pollutants enter the atmosphere each year, consisting of approximately 38 percent carbon monoxide, 22 percent sulfur oxide, 17 percent particulate matter, 14 percent hydrocarbons, and 9 percent nitrogen oxides. Automobiles, factories, and power-generating plants, in that order, are the major sources of air pollution. These sources also produce chemical reactions from pollutant contact with sunlight, heat, and air. In addition, trash and garbage disposal, energy sources (coal and oil), and industrial chemical by-products complicate the problem.

Polluted air makes the eyes water, burns the throat, and irritates the respiratory system, causing coughing, chest discomfort, and impaired breathing. Carbon

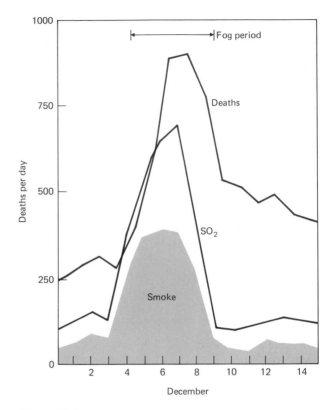

Figure 21.1
Deaths per day occurring during a "killer smog" that covered London in December 1952.

SOURCE: Committee on Air Pollution, *Interim Report* (London: Her Majesty's Stationery Office, December 1953). Used by permission.

monoxide interferes with the ability of the blood cells to carry oxygen and impairs the function of the central nervous system. Air pollution also causes serious problems for those with preexisting conditions, such as asthma, heart disease, chronic bronchitis, and emphysema. Asbestos fibers in the air have been associated with bronchogenic cancer, mesothelioma, and other forms of malignancy. Airborne mercury, used in batteries, mildew proofing, and the production of paint, pulp, and paper, affects the central nervous system.

Approaches to the Problem

Concept: Air pollution can be reduced through the cooperative efforts of government, industry, and the individual.

Because automobiles and industrial plants have been major sources of air pollution in the United States, environmentalists pressed Congress to pass a series of Clean Air Acts in 1963, 1965, and 1970. These laws required car manufacturers to cut auto emissions drastically and encouraged states and cities to set up programs to reduce pollution from stationary sources. Emission control devices on automobiles have had a beneficial effect. According to the Environmental Protection Agency (EPA), from 1972 to 1977, even though more people were driving, smog levels remained stable. Unfortunately, the same cannot be said for pollution from industrial sources. In general, industrial plants have resisted antipollution standards, because these measures tend to raise costs and lower profits.

Several solutions to the problem of air pollution have been proposed. One idea is to impose economic sanctions on industries responsible for pollution. Although fines have been imposed on industrial polluters, for many big industries they have amounted to little more than paying for the privilege of polluting the air.

Another suggestion is to ban the production of big cars, manufacture engines that cause less pollution, and switch to alternative fuels that do not cause such heavy emissions. As it happens, the public demand for more fuel-efficient cars has already caused auto makers to make drastic cuts in the number of large cars they produce. In addition, better engines and alternative fuels are being investigated, but immediate breakthroughs that are economically feasible are unlikely.

Political controls, such as the clean air laws, have been fairly effective in protecting the environment from even higher levels of air pollution. However, it is up to environmental groups and concerned individuals to continue pressing the government to enforce antipollution laws.

One way of continuing to stress the problem of air pollution is to do more research on the effects of pollution on health. Although it is widely acknowledged that air pollution is harmful to older individuals and those with preexisting respiratory and circulatory ailments, evidence linking pollution and disease among

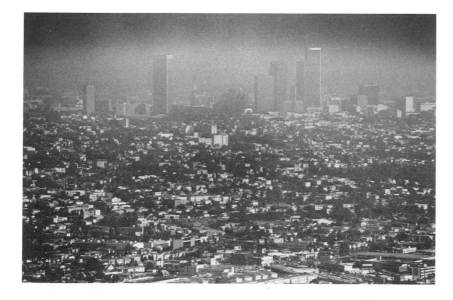

Automobile emissions have been a major source of air pollution from smog.

the healthy population is lacking. As a result, many people do not believe air pollution is really harmful. More medical research data might do much to increase public awareness of the problem.

It is likely that mandated action will be required if we are ever to have really clean air. Nevertheless, individuals do have an important role to play. Discovery Activity 21.1 asks you to consider what you could do.

Discovery Activity 21.1
HOW CAN YOU HELP CLEAN UP THE AIR?

Before reading the suggestions that follow, write down as many ways as you can think of to contribute to cleaner air. You might consider your driving and car care habits, whether or not you smoke, and what role you could play in keeping the pressure on politicians.

_____

_____

_____

_____

_____

_____

_____ ●

Clean Air: Your Responsibility

Although it might seem that the problem of air pollution is insurmountable, you can make a difference. Consider the following possibilities, which are under your control:

1. *Bicycling, walking, and using other nonpolluting transportation.* Evidence linking exercise and health is additional encouragement to walk, jog, run, or bicycle to work, if you live only a few miles away.

2. *Using public transportation (buses, subways).* This approach would reduce the number of autos on the highway.

3. *Purchasing a smaller car or one with a four-cylinder engine.* Small autos burn less fuel and produce less pollution than large cars.

4. *Tuning your automobile engine frequently.* A well-tuned engine using lead-free gasoline emits fewer harmful by-products.

5. *Owning one car instead of two.*

6. *Joining a carpool.*

7. *Avoiding open trash and incinerator burning.*

8. *Abstaining from smoking tobacco; lobbying for no-smoking sites in public places.*

9. *Reducing the use of volatile chemicals and cleaners in the home.* Household dust should be emptied into a receptacle to avoid dispersion in the air.

10. *Using the fireplace sparingly; burning dry wood instead of cannel coal.*

SOLID WASTE POLLUTION

Solid wastes produced by the household and industry amount to approximately four or five pounds per person each day. In our nation's cities, the majority of this material is burned in large incinerators, while waterfront and harbor debris is carried out to sea and burned by private contractors. In some cities as much as 40 percent of the municipal solid wastes are transported to dumps and landfill sites without passing through any incinerators. Another approach is to dump demolition materials into marshlands. As a result, it is estimated that cities use up land for solid wastes at a rate of one to two square miles per year. Most methods of handling solid waste today pollute the air, land, and water.

The general classification of solid waste materials, shown in Table 21.1, demonstrates the magnitude of the problem. These many sources of solid waste pollution have led to the serious pollution problems in the United States that are summarized in Table 21.2.

Table 21.1
GENERAL CLASSIFICATION OF SOLID WASTE MATERIALS

Category	Description		Source
Garbage	Wastes from the preparation, cooking, and serving of food Market refuse, waste from the handling, storage, and sale of produce and meats		Households, institutions, and commercial concerns (hotels, stores, restaurants, markets, etc.)
Rubbish	Combustible (primarily organic)	Paper, cardboard, cartons Wood, boxes, excelsior Plastics Rags, cloth, bedding Leather, rubber Grass, leaves, yard trimmings	
	Noncombustible (primarily inorganic)	Metals, tin cans, metal foils Dirt Stones, bricks, ceramics, crockery Glass, bottles Other mineral refuse	
Ashes	Residue from fires used for cooking and for heating buildings, cinders		
Bulky wastes	Large auto parts, tires Stoves, refrigerators, other large appliances Furniture, large crates Trees, branches, palm fronds, stumps, flotage		
Street refuse	Street sweepings, dirt Leaves Catch basin dirt Contents of litter receptacles		Streets, sidewalks, alleys, vacant lots, etc.
Dead animals	Small animals: cats, dogs, poultry Large animals: horses, cows		
Abandoned vehicles	Automobiles, trucks		
Construction and demolition wastes	Lumber, roofing, and sheathing scraps Rubble, broken concrete, plaster Conduit, pipe, wire, insulation		
Industrial refuse	Solid wastes resulting from industrial processes and manufacturing operations (food-processing wastes; boiler house cinders; wood, plastic, and metal scraps and shavings; etc.)		Factories, power plants, etc.
Special wastes	Hazardous wastes: pathological wastes, explosives, radioactive materials Security wastes: confidential documents, negotiable papers		Households, hospitals, institutions, stores, industry, etc.
Animal and agricultural wastes	Manures, crop residues		Farms, feed lots
Sewage treatment residues	Coarse screenings, grit, septic tank sludge, dewatered sludge		Sewage treatment plants, septic tanks

SOURCE: U.S. Environmental Protection Agency, Publication No. 2084, *Guidelines for Local Government on Solid-Waste Management* (Washington, D.C.: Government Printing Office, 1971), p. 42.

Table 21.2
LAND-RELATED PROBLEMS IN THE UNITED STATES

1. 4 billion tons of sediment are washed into streams annually as a result of land use or misuse.

2. 32 million tons of fertilizer, 235,000 tons of insecticides, and 90,000 tons of herbicides are applied annually to the land.

3. 130,000 acres of rural land are paved over annually for airports and highways.

4. 300,000 acres of rural land are consumed annually for reservoirs and flood control projects.

5. 1,687,288 acres of wildlife habitat have been destroyed by surface mining.

6. 281,116 surface acres of water have been adversely affected by mining.

7. 3,187,825 acres of land have been disturbed by surface mining.

8. 17,197,531 acres of wetlands have been destroyed in seven states alone (45.7 percent of the wetland area of Arkansas, California, Florida, Illinois, Indiana, Iowa, and Missouri).

9. 730,000 acres of agriculture land are consumed annually by urban sprawl.

10. 25 million tons of logging debris are left in forests every year.

11. 4.1 million acres of forested wetlands were cleared and drained for soybean production in the lower Mississippi valley and southern Florida from 1950–1969.

12. 4 million acres of right-of-way are traversed by over 300,000 miles of overhead transmission lines.

13. 1 billion (approximately) acres of forests are clearcut annually.

14. 4 billion tons of raw material are consumed annually in U.S. production, most of which are eventually disposed of as waste on the land.

15. Millions of tons of dredge spoil, industrial sludge, fly ash, and sewage sludge are land-deposited every year.

SOURCE: Environmental Protection Agency, Office of Public Affairs, *Land Use and Environmental Protection* (Washington, D.C.: Government Printing Office, 1974), pp. 4–5.

Mercury

Concept: Large accumulations of mercury in the human body are harmful to health.

Although the human body can adapt to the trace concentrations of inorganic mercury found in the natural environment, it is unable to cope with the large amounts of organic mercury introduced into the environment by human technology. Mercury is a metal that has thousands of uses in agriculture and industry, such as protection of seeds against fungus growth, control of microorganisms that cause machinery damage, and control of mildew and bacteria growth. It is also used in paints, floor waxes, furniture polish, plastics, fluorescent lamps, tooth fillings, and many other products. According to the National Institute of Occupational Safety and Health, approximately 150,000 people in the United States are routinely exposed to mercury on the job.

Numerous cases of mercury poisoning have been documented. Perhaps the most tragic incident occurred in Japan during the 1950s. Residents of a small fishing village contracted a serious, often fatal disease, which was characterized by neurological damage, numbness, loss of coordination, blindness, mental retardation, and emotional disturbance. It was discovered that the illness, which was later named **Minimata disease,** was caused by mercury wastes dumped from a chemical plant into Minimata Bay. A similar incident occurred in Canada in the early 1970s. Fortunately, no major outbreak of mercury poisoning has occurred in the United States. However, high levels of mercury in many American waterways have led to environmental regulation and concern over possible mercury poisoning resulting from consumption of contaminated seafood.

Inorganic mercury causes damage to the liver, kidneys, and small intestine and creates difficulties in reabsorption and secretion. Organic mercury affects the parts of the brain controlling vision, hearing, and balance. Symptoms of mercury poisoning are muscle weakness, loss of coordination, paralysis, blindness, deafness, and mental retardation. Children and developing embryos are most affected because of rapid cell growth.

There is some disagreement over the level at which mercury in the body is potentially harmful to health. Additional research is needed to determine the life span of mercury in the environment, to find ways of dissipating environmental mercury once it is discovered, and to determine mercury levels in the human body and in the environment.

Lead

Concept: Lead in the environment is among the most serious pollution problems facing us today.

It is estimated that over a million tons of lead are used in the manufacture of metal products, batteries, pesticides, solder for sealing food cans, and gasoline. **Lead poisoning (plumbism)** occurs as lead accumulates in the human body from the air, food, and water. The chief victims are children who live in older dwellings where the walls have been coated with lead paint. Small children have been poisoned from eating the lead-based paint flakes.

Symptoms of lead poisoning include weakness, loss of appetite, and anemia. Unfortunately, these early symptoms are also indicative of some other forms of illness and may not be diagnosed as lead poisoning until more severe, irreversible symptoms appear, such as brain damage, mental retardation, or miscarriage.

The high lead content in the environment is a problem that was created by and can also be solved by humans. Mandatory use of lead-free gasoline in newer model autos, removal of lead paint in old buildings, and stricter control of industrial wastes are already helping to alleviate the problem. Individuals can also reduce the risk of lead poisoning by washing all fruits and vegetables carefully to remove traces of airborne lead dust, not purchasing food in cans sealed with lead soldering, not storing food in the original can (air deteriorates the soldered seam), preventing children from playing near heavily traveled roads where lead-loaded dust may be present, and covering walls that may contain lead-based paint with wallpaper.

Chemical Wastes

Concept: It is an enormous task to undo the damage already done by indiscriminate disposal of hazardous chemical wastes.

More than 1000 new chemicals are produced each year, bringing the current total to more than 50,000 chemicals. Many of these products have been a boon to humanity, contributing to longevity, decreased suffering, and the prevention and treatment of disease. Unfortunately, some 35,000 chemicals are classified by the Environmental Protection Agency as either definitely or potentially hazardous to human health. Of particular concern is the disposal of toxic wastes from mining and industry. It is estimated that only 10 percent of hazardous chemical wastes are being disposed of in a safe manner. The remaining 90 percent are being dumped indiscriminately and are certain to pose serious health problems in the future.

Investigators have uncovered some shrewd, but extremely hazardous methods of disposing of dangerous chemicals:

- Metal barrels were buried in unmarked areas, only to decay and leak into the environment years later.
- Nearly 66 companies dumped approximately 10 million gallons of contaminated waste water daily into 11 municipal sewerage systems on Long Island; few of these sytems were capable of treating toxic wastes.
- In a wooded area of New Jersey (the Pine Barrens) 100 wells were poisoned by chemicals leaking from a 135-acre Jackson Township dump.
- Wastes polluted ground water at 300 sites in Michigan.
- In Charles City, Iowa, wells located downstream from a chemical dump showed traces of contamination; 6 million pounds of arsenic were found at the waste heap.
- A field in Illinois that was empty one week contained 20,000 barrels of dumped wastes a week later.

- Hundreds of toxic drums discarded by truck drivers have been found in various sites throughout the United States.

- Dangerous chemicals have been tossed into leaky burial pits.

- Farmers have been paid to allow handlers of toxic wastes to hide 55-gallon drums on unused land.

- Companies have paid haulers to get rid of their toxic wastes with no questions asked; some haulers have merely released the chemicals into ditches on rural roads.

- Poisonous chemicals have turned up near home plate at New York City's Shea Stadium, in the marshes around New Jersey's Meadowlands sports complex, and in abandoned shafts and tunnels in the hills above the Susquehanna River in Pennsylvania.

There is no way to determine just how many illegal toxic waste dumps exist. It is estimated that there are approximately 50,000 dump sites in the United States, about 2000 of them posing serious health problems. Many are revealed only after flash floods, soil erosion that exposes rusting drums, or excavation.

The Love Canal story gave the public its first look at the serious health hazards posed by uncontrolled dumping. In 1976 at the outskirts of Niagara Falls, New York, residents of houses built on a landfill began to notice oozing slime and a terrible stench. They learned that the landfill contained drums loaded with chemical wastes that had been buried there years before. Residents of Love Canal experienced a high incidence of cancer, birth defects, and respiratory and neurological problems and had to be relocated. More recently, other incidents have occurred. In April 1980 residents of Elizabeth, New Jersey, and Staten Island, New York, were exposed to toxic fumes caused by explosions from a dump storing over 50,000 barrels of chemicals. Similar incidents on July 4 and July 7, 1980, resulted in explosions, fires, and release of toxic fumes in Carlstadt and Perth Amboy, New Jersey.

The problem of toxic waste disposal is enormously difficult and will require concerted action by the federal and state governments. Severe penalties must be placed on industrial offenders who fail to comply with safe disposal techniques. At present, fines are not high enough to discourage risk taking and use of inexpensive, hazardous methods of disposal. In addition, more government personnel are needed to enforce EPA regulations, visit industrial sites, and educate the business community on the least expensive and safest alternatives. New, inexpensive methods for safely disposing of chemical wastes must be found in the near future if the problem is to be remedied. Industry should be provided with the financial incentive to conduct independent research in this area.

Solid Wastes: What You Can Do

Concept: Resolving the problem of solid wastes requires a cooperative effort on the part of government, industry, and the private citizen.

A variety of approaches are needed to protect the nation's land from further contamination. The first step is to salvage and recycle solid wastes (industrial and household) rather than dumping them.

Many communities have programs to recycle newspaper, and a few states have passed laws requiring that bottles and aluminum cans be returnable. These states have reduced their litter problem considerably, without putting many people out of work, as lobbyists for the bottling industry claimed would happen. If your state does not have a "bottle bill," you should join with others to bring pressure for such legislation.

Better designed incinerators can reduce air pollution from solid wastes. The remaining 10 to 20 percent by volume that cannot be incinerated must be buried on land or dumped at sea. One sound approach to landfill is careful selection of future recreational sites that are first used for several years for sanitary landfill. With proper planning, landfill actually improves these areas as future golf courses, parks, and green belts.

Manufacturers should also be encouraged to produce items (such as cans) capable of being reused, recycled, or disintegrated when attacked by invading bacteria. A "biodegradable" beer can should be de-

Discovery Activity 21.2
ARE YOU A POLLUTING CONSUMER?

Make a list of products you ordinarily use that you know contribute to pollution or waste disposal problems. Some examples might be nonbiodegradable detergents, soft drinks in plastic bottles, lawn products that contain nonorganic chemicals, and plastic containers. What could you substitute for these products?

_____

_____

_____

_____

_____

_____ ●

veloped that can provide adequate shelf life yet still disintegrate when discarded. Aluminum cans do not have this property, and the only solution to aluminum can disposal would seem to be recycling.

Government incentives might be provided to encourage the recycling of junked automobiles. The cost of collecting, transporting, and processing is now about twice the price of No. 2 steel—a strong disincentive for recycling.

The individual can influence the production of various types of packaging and containers for food products through wise purchasing. Consumers can avoid products that are not biodegradable or reusable, or that cannot be recycled. Consumers could also avoid products in fancy packages, giving first choice to products packaged in recycled material and products that do not need packaging. Such an effort, if undertaken by enough people, would eventually bring about a change in the kinds of containers produced by manufacturers. Individuals can also continue their efforts to eliminate litter. Beer cans and other garbage thrown onto the roadside,

into wooded areas, and onto beaches not only destroy the appearance of the land, but also are harmful to wildlife. Vigorous enforcement of litter laws would be helpful in this regard.

WATER POLLUTION

Public water supplies are provided from rivers, lakes, underground waters, and various upland sources. Water quality from the remote upland sources tends to be excellent since it often travels hundreds of miles through unpopulated areas. Unfortunately, this is not true of our rivers and lakes, into which modern industrial society has introduced the discharge of domestic sewage, industrial wastes (toxic chemicals), and agricultural wastes (animal excrement, fertilizers, insecticides, and liquid wastes from slaughter houses and canning and packing plants). In addition, the runoff of precipitation from the land (referred to as silt) provides a naturally occurring discharge into the stream bed. Silt can keep

Discharge of industrial chemicals into water systems poses a serious threat to all forms of life.

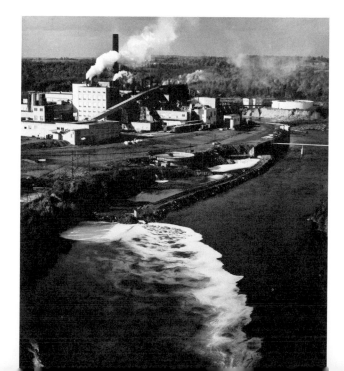

out needed sunlight or smother the bottom-dwelling organisms. Oil spillage from the more than 1 billion tons shipped by sea each year is also a major source of water pollution (approximately 1 percent, or 1 million tons, is lost at sea). Spillage causes damage to marine and bird life, and certain approaches to cleanup cause even greater damage to plants and animals.

Although pesticides control insects and thus contribute to improved food production, they also pose a serious threat to health. Pesticide residues are present in most surface waters and in many seafoods. With a high enough exposure level, damage occurs to the nervous, respiratory, and digestive systems; the eyes; the skin; the visceral organs; and even the brain.

More than 50,000 chemicals enter our nation's streams and rivers, and eventually enter the oceans of the world. According to oceanographer Jacques Cousteau, we will see the death of the world's oceans in fewer than 50 years unless a cooperative effort is launched by all industrialized countries. Cousteau pointed out to a Senate Subcommittee on Oceans and Atmosphere that ocean floors, free of chemicals only 20 years ago, are now almost devoid of living organisms.

Several poisonous and carcinogenic chemicals have been identified in drinking water. Sewage discharges place harmful bacteria and viruses in water, sodium levels are rising, and oil concentrates fat-soluble poisons and permits pollutants to be ingested by organisms that are part of our food chain.

Between 1961 and 1973, more than 200 known outbreaks of disease (muscle weakness, vomiting, diahrrea, kidney damage, higher incidence of cancer, skin rashes, viruses, etc.) or poisoning were caused by contaminated water, resulting in 22 deaths and 55,000 illnesses. It is estimated that 10 times as many incidents go unreported. The health consequences of contaminated water are frightening, yet a survey completed a little over a decade ago revealed that of 969 public water supply systems, 56 percent had facility deficiencies, 77 percent of the plant operators were poorly trained in microbiology, and 46 percent were poorly trained in chemistry. In addition, 79 percent of the systems had not been inspected by state or county au-

thorities during the preceding year. In the years to come water use, and conflicts over different uses, will be one of the nation's most critical problems.

Approaches to the Problem

Concept: Water pollution can be controlled only if existing legislation is enforced.

Drinking water standards (taste, odor, color, turbidity; chemical, radiological, and bacteriological) have been established by the U.S. Public Health Service. Water treatment plants provide clean water relatively free from health hazards.

Protection from waterborne infection is achieved either through purification of water supplies or treatment of waste before it enters water bodies. Purification has received the most emphasis to date, and improvement of waste treatment facilities is anticipated in the next decade. Strict enforcement of existing legislation and heavy fines could reduce contamination from industrial waste, agricultural waste, and oil spillage. There should also be increased emphasis on reuse of water, use of upstream land, restoration of land, land treatment, forest replenishment, topsoil conservation, and conversion of sea water to drinking water.

In the meantime, individuals can help by not throwing trash into lakes, streams, or oceans. Boaters should purchase self-contained toilets (now required on newer model boats) rather than dumping waste into the water. Another good practice is to use biodegradable detergents.

NOISE POLLUTION

Concept: Continuous exposure to noises exceeding 120 decibels can cause physical harm.

The American public is exposed to several sources of potentially harmful loud sounds. Urban dwellers live with the unpleasant sounds of jackhammers, garbage trucks, and sirens, and many suburbanites have to endure the sound of freeway traffic, airplanes taking off and landing, and power mowers.

Some people don't seem to be bothered by loud noise, whereas others experience both physical and psychological stress. At what point is noise so loud as to be dangerous? The pressure of sound on the ear is measured in decibels, an arbitrary unit based on the faintest sound that a person can hear. The scale is logarithmic, so that an increase of 10 dB means a tenfold increase in sound intensity, a 20 dB rise a hundredfold increase, and a 30 dB rise a thousandfold increase. Prolonged exposure to sounds above 90 decibels can result in hearing damage.

Figure 21.2 lists decibel ratings for some common sounds. Rock music (110 to 120 decibels at a distance of four to six feet), which is capable of causing permanent hearing impairment, may be the single most hazardous noise for today's youth, both listeners and performers.

Evidence suggests a loss of hearing sensitivity among youth. Such a loss in the early years may result in more serious problems later in life. Hearing damage among employees in industry is also common, costing millions of dollars each year in industrial compensation.

Rock music played at a high volume can seriously impair hearing.

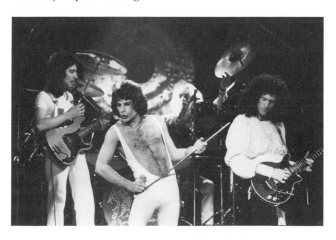

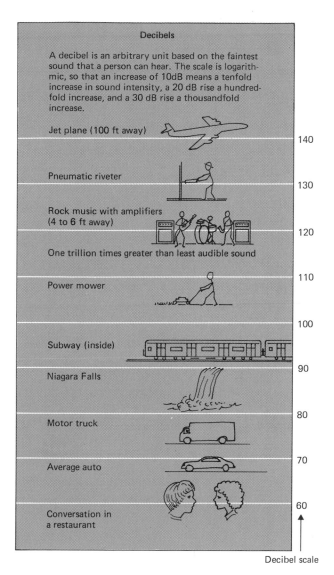

Figure 21.2
Common sounds and their decibel rating.

Individuals can reduce noise levels and protect their hearing by taking a few precautions:

1. Use cotton or ear muffs if your job requires constant exposure to loud noises.

2. If you're at a rock concert, sit as far away as possible from the band.

3. Learn to enjoy listening to music at home at moderate volume.

4. Put drapes over windows to reduce street noises.

5. Choose acoustical tile for ceilings and walls when building a house or adding a room.

6. Use floor carpeting or select an apartment with carpeting in all rooms adjacent to other units.

7. Locate noise-making appliances away from bedrooms, den, and living room.

8. Select home sites or apartments away from truck routes, airports, industry, and business areas.

RADIATION

Concept: Everyone is exposed to low-level radiation each day.

Humans have always been exposed to small amounts of radiation in nature. About 58 percent of our exposure comes from natural sources (radioactive gases released by soil and rock formations, cosmic rays, and radioactive agents in the atmosphere from sun flares), and about 41 percent comes from human-made sources (X rays, luminous wristwatches, color TV, radar, nuclear weapons testing, uranium mines, mills and fabrication plants, and various electronic devices). Nuclear power plants account for less than 0.15 percent of human-made radiation, and about 1 percent comes from nuclear fallout. The greatest single source of human-made radiation is medical X rays. Radiation is beneficial in medical diagnosis, treatment, and research. Unfortunately, its use carries some health risk to the patient, technician, and researcher.

Three types of radiation are harmful to health: (1) alpha particles are potentially dangerous, but they cannot penetrate the skin or body except through inhalation or a cut; (2) beta particles can penetrate the skin but not deeply enough to damage internal organs; (3) gamma rays (similar to X rays) pose the main threat to

human health because they can easily penetrate the body and its major organs.

Little is known about the long-term effects of repeated exposure to low-level radiation. It is generally accepted, however, that even small amounts of radiation can cause damage to genetic cells. Low-level radiation is also suspected of causing skeletal abnormalities, bone marrow damage, eye damage (cataracts), leukemia, and other types of cancer. Exposure to large doses of radiation damages human tissue, affects white blood cells (reducing natural defenses against invading microorganisms), and results in radiation sickness (nausea, fatigue, sore throat, anemia, diarrhea, loss of hair) and even death. There is also concern over potential damage to reproductive cells, alteration of genes, chromosome damage, and the possibility of mutations. It is impossible to determine whether such effects will occur in current or future generations. The extent of harm from radiation exposure depends upon the type of exposure (alpha, beta, or gamma rays), the potency of exposure, the part of the body exposed, the duration of exposure, and the rate at which the radioactivity was received by the body.

It is possible to protect yourself from certain types of radiation. Pregnant women, for example, should avoid X rays during the first trimester of pregnancy and, ideally, throughout pregnancy. One should avoid having dental X rays more frequently than once a year. Annual chest X rays are also questionable, due to radiation exposure. Finally, some individuals have moved away from nuclear power plant communities because of low-level radiation leaks.

A PLAN TO
REDUCE POLLUTION

Concept: Progress is being made, but your help is needed.

Important legislation has been passed in the areas of forestry, energy planning and conservation, coastal protection, smog, and auto emissions. The Environmental Protection Agency, created in 1970, has done much to protect health and the environment. Some states have also taken a leading role. Oregon, for example, received the first Citation for Excellence in Environmental Protection and Improvement for achieving federal water quality standards, passing an antilitter beverage container law, removing billboards, and funding bicycle paths. At present, more vigorous enforcement of the law is needed and local efforts must gain momentum. A few suggestions follow.

What You Can Do

1. Study the problem.   Joining an environmental group, such as the Sierra Club or Friends of the Earth, is a good way to keep informed about important environmental issues.

2. Call the problem to the attention of those who can help.   The editor of the newspaper, conservation groups, and city hall are sources you may want to contact. Be certain to point out that you are keeping a diary of all your efforts, including witnesses and photographs in such cases as improper solid waste disposal. Keep in mind that authorities depend upon responsible citizens to combat pollution. Letter-writing campaigns to senators and representatives can be effective. If a senator or representative receives enough letters, they can affect how he or she votes on particular bills or prompt an investigation into a situation the public is concerned about. Letter writing provides a permanent record and is preferable to a telephone call. A brief personal letter should be sent when the issue is hot; it should refer to the bill by name and number, point out how the bill affects the state or community, and state reasons for supporting or opposing the bill.

3. Consider taking legal action.   Under the Federal Refuse Act of 1899, attorneys have the responsibility of prosecuting those who pollute. To make a citizen's arrest, you need merely identify the site of pollution and include supporting documents, such as photos or letters from a local conservation officer. Action can be taken when either an individual or industry is violating the Refuse Act.

Issues in Health
NUCLEAR POWER PLANTS: ARE THEY REALLY WORTH THE RISK?

The amount of nuclear power generated in the United States is increasing tenfold every 6.5 years. In the near future a large amount of our energy, particularly electrical power, will come from nuclear power. To produce electrical power, nuclear fission generates heat; heat turns water into steam; and steam spins an electrical turbine, which in turn spins a generator to produce electricity. To date, there is no cheaper way to turn water into steam.

Debate continues over the need for nuclear power in the United States. Proponents argue that nuclear power must be used for beneficial purposes (generating electricity; propelling ships, submarines, and rockets) at a time when our energy sources are being depleted and our needs are increasing. Without nuclear power, it is argued, energy costs would soar, and millions of people would be without electricity for heat, light, and other uses.

According to the Nuclear Regulatory Commission, considerable safety is built into the construction of all nuclear power plants, and the probability of an accident is very low. The commission feels that the public greatly overestimates the risk of a catastrophe and fails to see the benefits of adequate power at reasonable costs.

Opponents of nuclear power reactors express concern on several grounds: the health risks from radiation leakage, the problem of disposal of hazardous nuclear wastes, and the danger of a catastrophic accident.

The incident at Three Mile Island in 1979 and other nuclear-related mishaps have raised questions about the safety of nuclear power plants. Opponents argue that the price of a major disaster, in terms of loss of life, property, and money, makes even the slightest risk of an accident unacceptable. If the probability of an accident is so low, it is argued,

(continued)

Issues in Health (continued)

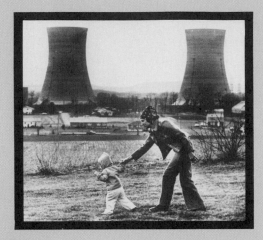

why does the largest insurance company in the western hemisphere refuse to underwrite more than 1 percent of the potential liability for a major nuclear power plant accident? Unfortunately, the cost of such an accident would be paid for by the American public from the U.S. Treasury's sum of $478 million dollars. No further compensation would be made to the victims.

In addition to questioning the safety of nuclear power plants, opponents point out that there is still no safe, permanent means of disposing of radioactive wastes. The extent of the problem becomes evident when one realizes that plutonium (one of the isotopes released during nuclear fission) has a half-life (time needed to reduce its radioactivity to one-half the original amount) of 24,000 years and that such products must be stored for periods of time up to 10 to 20 times their half-lives for optimum safety. Wastes are currently buried in concrete vaults, or geological strata, or even submersed in the sea in concrete containers. Each of these techniques requires continuous monitoring for leakage, which has occurred. In sum, opponents of nuclear power plants believe that the potential risks are not worth the possible benefits and that other solutions to the problem of energy supplies should be pursued.

What do you think? ●

Discovery Activity 21.3
TAKING ACTION

Think about the topics we've discussed in this chapter—the various dangers from environmental pollutants, radiation, and the like. Then select an issue that is of particular concern to you and compose a letter to the editor of the city newspaper. Outline your concerns and suggest what you think ought to be done. Be sure to do some research on the issue so you can back up your statements. Then send it off. You may be surprised to find that your letter is published! ●

4. Exercise your voting rights.   Groups that voice their intention to vote for leaders who will work to save the environment will get some action. Legislators are apt to make some promises and compromises if there is a danger of losing votes.

5. Exercise your consumer power.   When American consumers band together, things happen. If consumers purchased only environmentally safe products (reusable bottles, biodegradable cans and containers, recyclable packages, etc.), industry would produce only these items. Refusal to purchase from the known polluters in industry, as well as refusal to purchase energy-inefficient products and short-lived items, would bring about mass changes in manufacturing.

POPULATION AND HEALTH

Concept: Population growth has a significant impact on human health and the environment.

Many environmental problems are closely related to the world's population growth. It wasn't until the year 1830 that world population totaled 1 billion, yet 100 years later the population had doubled, and only 40 years

Table 21.3
RATE OF POPULATION INCREASE AND YEARS
REQUIRED TO DOUBLE PRESENT POPULATION

	Increase (percent)	at Present Rate
Canada	1.1	67
United States	0.9	83
The World	2.1	32
Africa	2.7	26
East Asia	2.3	31
Europe	0.7	95
Latin America	2.9	24
Near East	2.6	27
South Asia	2.8	25

SOURCE: World Population Data, Agency for International Development, Washington, D.C.

after that, in 1970, it had grown to an estimated 3.5 billion. The population passed the 4 billion mark on April 1, 1975, well ahead of population projections. At the present rate, it is projected that there will be 7 billion people on earth by the year 2000, with an additional billion added each subsequent five years (see Table 21.3).

In the United States population growth has been slowing as birth rates per family have dropped; however, the number has not declined. The U.S. population grows by approximately 3 million people, or the number of inhabitants of the city of Chicago, each year. Population growth in the United States is likely to continue because many deadly communicable diseases are now under control, the infant mortality rate is decreasing, and individuals are living longer as a result of improved medical procedures and lifestyle changes.

In most countries birth rates continue to exceed death rates by more than 50 percent (see Table 21.4). Population growth in the developing countries of Latin America, Africa, and Asia has been nothing short of spectacular. In poorer countries population has increased as fast as or faster than food production, resulting in malnutrition and starvation.

Unchecked population growth affects health in several ways. The most serious, as already noted, is

Issues in Health
IS STRICT ENVIRONMENTAL PROTECTION WORTH THE ECONOMIC BURDEN?

The technology needed to provide clean air and water and undefiled land is already available. Unfortunately, the elimination of pollution would involve substantial costs (in the form of higher taxes and higher prices for goods and services) at a time when economic considerations have a higher priority than the quality of health and environmental protection. Those who emphasize the health of the individual argue that a complete change in philosophy is needed. An economy based on consumption and waste that is detrimental to health is unsound. The public needs to become more aware of the causes of pollution and then to take action. Large corporations need to be forced into greater environmental responsibility. The creation of a clean, healthy environment must take precedence over the profit motive.

Opponents of strict environmental control argue that the impact of such policies on profits and taxes makes them impossible to implement. They argue that environmental standards cause too much economic displacement. Although the implementation of environmental control does increase the need for goods and services and create jobs, the economy suffers. The minimum improvement in the quality of life and health is not worth the economic setback that is certain to take place.

What do you think? ●

Table 21.4
BIRTH RATES AND DEATH RATES

	Birth Rate (per 1000 Population)	Death Rate (per 1000)
Canada	18	7
United States	18	9
The World	36	15
Africa	48	21
East Asia	41	18
Europe	17	10
Latin America	39	10
Near East	42	16
South Asia	44	16

SOURCE: World Population Data, Agency for International Development, Washington, D.C.

Unchecked population growth, particularly in the developing countries of the world, has produced malnutrition and starvation. This young mother is only 13 years old.

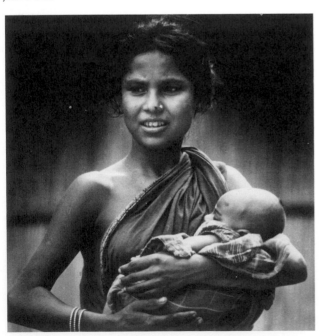

that food shortages produce hunger and starvation. The American trend toward urbanization has brought its own problems. Today more than 70 percent of the U.S. population lives on only 1 percent of the land. Urbanization is a prime contributor to environmental pollution of all types—air pollution from smog, water pollution, solid and chemical wastes—and to energy shortages. In addition, there is evidence that crowding, in combination with other factors, such as poverty, contributes to stress, disease, mental illness, and crime.

It is well known that although Americans comprise only 6 percent of the earth's population, they consume 40 percent of its resources and create over 50 percent of the world's waste. Unless waste and overconsumption are checked, the result will be more despoiling of our resources and more health-related problems.

Approaches to the Problem

Concept: A vital component in reducing health and environmental problems related to population growth is fertility control.

An obvious approach to solving the problems related to population growth is to produce fewer offspring. Many countries are moving in this direction through education, legislation, or incentive programs. The distribution of condoms and birth control pills in many countires has had some impact. In China the approach has been to institute strict government policy. The Chinese government issued a series of laws designed to reduce the birth rate by the year 2000. One law raised the minimum ages for marriage; another provides that the monthly allowance for one child be cut off if the family has a second child; a third law gives preference to first children in admissions to nurseries, hospitals, and schools. Governments in some countries, such as South Korea, Taiwan, India, Pakistan, and Egypt, have initiated birth control programs that encourage the use of IUDs and vasectomies. The results have been mixed. In India, for example, there has been strong resistance to birth control by certain groups that regard large families as a measure of wealth and prestige.

Research is needed to determine how to motivate people from different cultural backgrounds to want fewer children. Some countries see population growth as essential to economic development, because it adds workers to the labor force. Some Third World countries strongly oppose population policies, viewing them as a threat to their very survival. Nevertheless, a lowering of fertility rates is essential. The problem is how to break through centuries of tradition to convince individuals and countries to take action.

CONCLUSION

A clean environment is the responsibility of every human being. It starts with each person doing his or her part to avoid polluting the air, water, and land. It also involves insisting on a clean environment from industry, agriculture, and government; not contributing to the problem of over population; and keeping the pressure on the current political administration. It is up to the consumer to maintain the proper balance between environmental and economic issues. Hopefully, with enough individual concern and pressure, salvaging and recycling will replace dumping as the primary means of disposing of waste.

SUMMARY

1. Environmental pollution poses a serious threat to the human body, plant and animal life, and even the human mind.

2. Individuals can make a difference in reducing air, water, solid waste, and noise pollution. A clean environment is the responsibility of the individual; if individuals follow sound environmental practices and police industry, agriculture, and others, improvement will take place.

3. Research is needed to uncover more effective means of handling solid wastes that do not contaminate the land, air, and water, or slowly use up our precious land.

4. The identification and removal of illegal dump sites (for chemical wastes) will take many years. The task of this generation is not just to locate and remove these sites but also to see that no new sites are created through indiscriminate, illegal dumping.

5. The consumer can have a significant impact on the production of solid waste by purchasing foods only in biodegradable or recyclable containers.

6. Protection from waterborne infection is achieved through prevention, purification of the water supply, or treatment of waste before it enters water bodies. In the future much more emphasis must be placed on prevention. This will also require stricter enforcement of individual, agricultural, and industrial dumping.

7. Consumers have the responsibility to insist on the enforcement of existing legislation to keep the air, water, and land clean and uncontaminated.

8. Noises exceeding 90 decibels, such as rock music, can result in permanent hearing loss. It is the individual's responsibility to avoid continuous exposure to loud noises.

9. The individual can greatly reduce radiation exposure by avoiding frequent dental and medical X rays and using adequate protection when working near X ray equipment.

10. Individuals need to become involved in all areas of environmental pollution and exercise their right to a clean environment. Consumers should exercise their voting and consumer power, and even take legal action, if necessary, to eliminate contamination of the environment.

11. Population growth is directly related to environmental pollution; each additional human being contributes to the problem of pollution.

REFERENCES

Environmental News, Office of Public Affairs (A-107), U.S. Environmental Protection Agency, Washington, D.C. (December 1974):11.

LABORATORY 1
AUTO USE TRENDS AMONG COLLEGE STUDENTS

Purpose   To identify efforts by college students to reduce air pollution and conserve energy.

Equipment   None.

Size of Group   Between eight and ten students.

Procedure

1. Using the chart below, fill in the appropriate information for each student who drives an automobile.

2. Bring one member from each group together and combine all information onto one data sheet. Place this information on the board.

Results

1. What trends are evident in auto purchasing or use by these students?

2. Were autos purchased with energy conservation in mind? Air pollution control?

3. How energy and pollution conscious is this group based upon auto purchasing? Based on auto use?

Student	Automobile (make/model)	Size*	Cylinders 4 6 8	City mileage	Reasons for Use or Purchase

*S—Small, C—Compact, M—Midsize, F—Full size.

LABORATORY 2
HOW POLLUTED IS YOUR COMMUNITY?

Purpose   To analyze the air, water, and noise pollution in your community.

Size of Group   Three groups of 8 to 12 students each.

Procedure

1. Each group chooses one of the following areas of pollution: water, noise, air.

2. Groups send for a test kit for air, water, and noise. (Write for the free catalog of the Edmund Scientific Co., 100 Edscarp Blvd., Barrington, New Jersey 08007; or write to Urban Systems Inc., 1033 Mass. Ave, Cambridge, Mass. 02138.)

3. Test kits are used to evaluate the air, water, and noise pollution on the college campus and in the adjacent communities:

Water—Samples are taken at different times of the day from different buildings (including the cafeteria).

Air—Samples are taken at different times of the day and night.

Noise—Decibel levels are measured at functions, such as dances, athletic contests, and concerts.

Results

1. Each group compares its findings to EPA acceptable standards and reports to the class.

2. What suggestions do you have for improving the water, air, and noise pollution problems on your campus?

appendix A:
the body systems*

In order to make decisions related to your health, it is very useful to understand how your body functions. This appendix provides you with some basic information about the body systems. We don't expect you to become an expert about how your body works, but we do think some basic knowledge can help you understand some sections of the text. In addition, a greater familiarity with your body can help you know what to look for when you have a particular health problem.

THE SKELETAL SYSTEM

Your skeleton (see Fig. A.1) is composed of 206 bones. These bones have four basic functions: to support and protect the other body systems, to store minerals, and to produce cells for the circulatory system.

Support and protection. In order for your skeleton to provide support for the other systems of the body, it must be strong enough physically to hold the other systems in position, and it must be light enough to permit movement with as much efficiency as possible. Therefore, most bones are composed of two types of bony tissue—a firm, compact external layer and a

*SOURCE: Contributed by Dr. Fred Browning.

porous internal portion. Covering the bone is a layer of tissue called the periosteum. It aids bone growth (thickness or circumference) and provides tissue for the attachment of ligaments, tendons, muscles, and cartilage.

Protection of the other body systems is assured by the strong structure of the skeleton and the various cavities within or framed by the bones. The skull and vertebral column, for example, protect the brain and spinal cord; the pelvic girdle and rib cage help protect the intestines, heart, lungs, and other vital organs.

Storage of minerals. The bones of the skeletal system contain 95 to 98 percent of the body's calcium supply and approximately 80 percent of its phosphorus. These minerals are essential to life.

Production of cells. The skeleton produces the components of blood: red corpuscles, leukocytes, and platelets. Red corpuscles transport oxygen and carbon dioxide, leukocytes (white blood cells) fight infection, and platelets aid in blood clotting. The cavities within the bones are filled with either yellow marrow or red marrow. Yellow marrow is found in the shafts of the long bones, red marrow is found in the ends of the long bones, in short and flat bones, and in the vertebral bodies. Of particular importance is the red marrow, where the red corpuscles, leukocytes, and platelets are produced. Bone is living tissue.

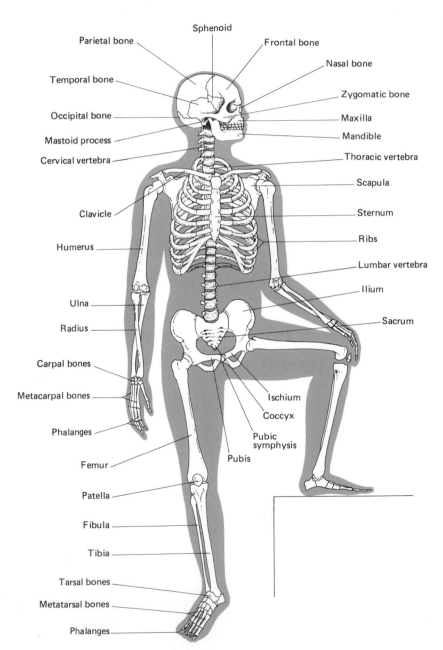

Figure A.1
The skeletal system.

THE MUSCULAR SYSTEM

The muscles of your body (see Fig. A.2) are classified as striated or nonstriated. The striated group includes both skeletal and cardiac muscle. The nonstriated group, also called smooth muscle, includes the walls of the blood vessels and the tissues of the internal organs, particularly the gastrointestinal tract. All muscle tissue has the same function: to create force so that you can move.

Although most muscles attach to the skeletal system via tendinous tissue, several connect directly to

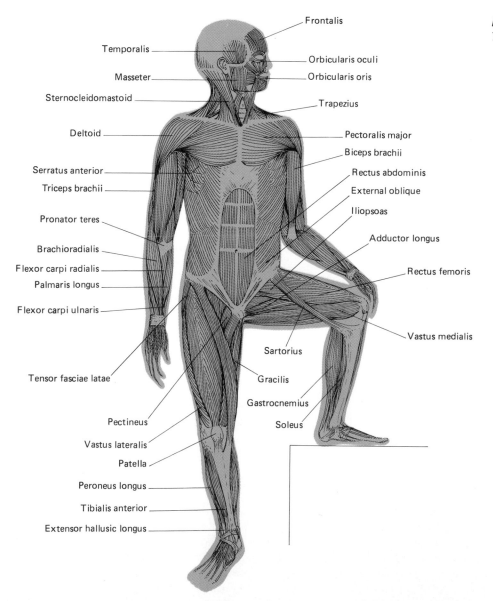

Figure A.2
The muscular system.

Frontalis
Temporalis
Orbicularis oculi
Masseter
Orbicularis oris
Sternocleidomastoid
Trapezius
Deltoid
Pectoralis major
Biceps brachii
Serratus anterior
Rectus abdominis
Triceps brachii
External oblique
Iliopsoas
Pronator teres
Adductor longus
Brachioradialis
Flexor carpi radialis
Rectus femoris
Palmaris longus
Flexor carpi ulnaris
Vastus medialis
Sartorius
Tensor fasciae latae
Gracilis
Gastrocnemius
Pectineus
Soleus
Vastus lateralis
Patella
Peroneus longus
Tibialis anterior
Extensor hallusic longus

the bone. These attachments allow two possibilities through muscle shortening: movement or the stabilizing of a joint or body segment. Thus it is possible to create force or perform work through movement of the body or body segments.

THE NERVOUS SYSTEM

The nervous system is as important to the body as the telephone system is to the life of a city. It receives and sends messages throughout the body, informing the brain of the welfare of the total organism. Interoceptors, located within the tissue of the body, respond to internal stimuli; exteroceptors, located on or near the surface of the body, respond to external stimuli.

Exteroceptors consist of organs, such as the eyes, ears, taste buds, nose, and sensors of touch and temperature within the skin. Most of these organs receive stimuli from far and near. We hear loud sounds from a distance or nearby; we view objects from afar or near; we smell distinct odors of various kinds; and we sense changes in temperature. Interoceptors receive stimuli from within the tissues (and skin) of the body and keep us informed of such things as pain, pressure, body position, movement of the body, and spatial orientation.

Anatomically, the nervous system consists of the cerebrum (two hemispheres housed within the skull), the midbrain stem (including the pons and the medulla), the cerebellum, the spinal cord, 12 pairs of cranial nerves, and 30 pairs of spinal nerves (see Fig. A.3). The brain and spinal cord are usually considered the central nervous system, and the pairs of cranial and spinal nerves are the peripheral nervous system. The central nervous system operates as a storage system (computer) to interpret the environment. Nerve cables extending from the brain and spinal cord convey electrical nerve impulses to and from every part of the body. The peripheral nervous system senses and responds to these impulses and works with the central nervous system as one unit to keep the organism alive and well.

The entire nervous system regulates other body systems. It makes the individual aware of changes occurring within the body. It also provides an awareness of changes in the external environment, through the special senses of vision, hearing, and taste and through such general sensations as pain, touch, temperature, and pressure. It provides spatial orientation and controls the activities of units, parts, or entire organs.

The entire nervous system is composed of neurons. These neurons are similar to other cells and have the special property of conduction, which allows an impulse to be passed from one point to another, establishing a method of communication for the entire body. For example, if you step on a nail, the pain receptors in your foot send an impulse to the brain for further consideration, and the brain simultaneously sends an impulse to the lower limbs, causing the injured foot to withdraw and the opposite lower limb to extend.

The following is a summary of some of the things that are known about the nervous system and the transmission of nerve impulses:

1. Neurons are either resting or sending impulses to other neurons; that is, they obey the all-or-none law.

2. Neurons generate impulses that may activate or inhibit other neurons.

3. Neurons conduct impulses in only one direction.

4. Larger neurons conduct impulses faster than small neurons. Myelinated neurons (those sheathed by a special white, fatty material) conduct impulses faster than nonmyelinated neurons.

5. The brain can store information, generate thoughts, create and control mood, and determine how we react to situations.

6. The spinal cord and brain stem convey impulses to and from the brain, as well as control most of the involuntary functions of the body through the autonomic nervous system. The autonomic nervous system controls the functions of the heart, gastrointestinal tract, and other organs.

7. The cerebellum functions as a modifier of motor functions, helping the body to coordinate movements. The cerebrum (consisting of left and right hemispheres) controls speaking, walking, and performance of other conscious acts, as well as perception of sensation and memory.

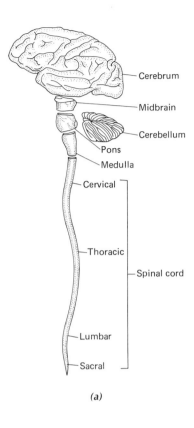

Cerebrum

Midbrain

Cerebellum

Pons

Medulla

Cervical

Thoracic

Spinal cord

Lumbar

Sacral

(a)

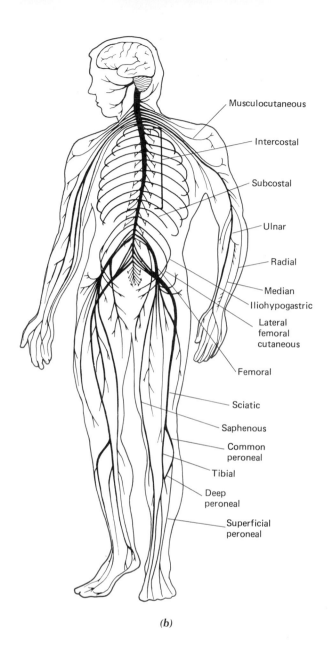

Musculocutaneous

Intercostal

Subcostal

Ulnar

Radial

Median

Iliohypogastric

Lateral
femoral
cutaneous

Femoral

Sciatic

Saphenous

Common
peroneal

Tibial

Deep
peroneal

Superficial
peroneal

(b)

Figure A.3
*Central (a) and peripheral (b) portions of the nervous
system.*

8. The brain allows for selective consideration and
   response. The spinal cord is capable of responding
   only as predetermined by reflexes or as com-
   manded by the autonomic and/or voluntary centers in the brain and brain stem.

9. Blood circulation to the brain must be constant
   whether a person is resting or working. Too little
   blood flow will cause dizziness, fainting, or permanent damage. Excessive blood flow may cause
   headaches or cerebral hemorrhage.

   In summary, the nervous system keeps us in touch
   with our external environment and our internal needs
   and provides the opportunities for action and reaction,
   which are necessary to survival.

525

THE CIRCULATORY SYSTEM

The circulatory system consists of the heart, blood vessels, lymph vessels, blood, and lymph (see Fig. A.4). It has the capacity to increase its work (total blood flow) to approximately six times the resting level.

The heart is a muscular organ lying just beneath the breast bone in a diagonal plane. It is controlled largely by hormones and the autonomic nervous system and, to a lesser extent, by metabolism and bodily movements. The heart pumps the blood throughout the body, and the blood and lymph vessels keep it circulating.

Figure A.4
The circulatory system.

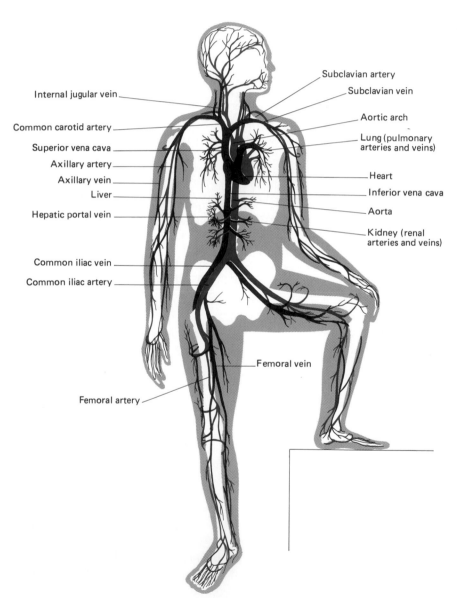

Internal jugular vein

Common carotid artery

Superior vena cava

Axillary artery

Axillary vein

Liver

Hepatic portal vein

Common iliac vein

Common iliac artery

Femoral artery

Subclavian artery

Subclavian vein

Aortic arch

Lung (pulmonary arteries and veins)

Heart

Inferior vena cava

Aorta

Kidney (renal arteries and veins)

Femoral vein

The heart is divided into right and left sides, and the two sides function as two separate circulatory systems (see Fig. A.5). In pulmonary circulation the right ventricle contracts, sending blood out via the pulmonary artery into the lungs. After passing from the lungs, the blood is returned to the left atrium of the heart via the pulmonary arteries.

Simultaneously, as the right ventricle contracts, the left ventricle also contracts, sending blood into the aorta and throughout the rest of the body. Blood leaving the left ventricle goes to the head, body, and limbs via arteries, arterioles, and capillaries; venules and veins

Figure A.5
Pulmonary and systemic circulation.

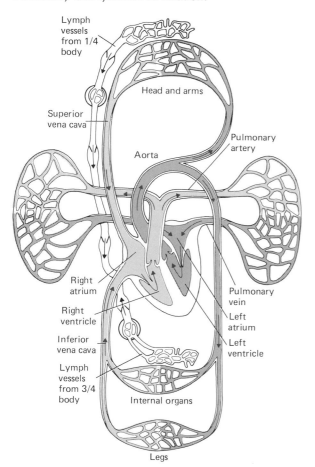

return the blood to the right atrium of the heart through the inferior and superior vena cava. This phase is called systemic circulation. The blood leaving the left ventricle goes through the aorta to the systems of the body. At the capillary level, fluids, nutrients, electrolytes, and minerals leave circulation and bathe all the cells of the body. The fluid is returned to the circulatory system by means of osmotic pressure within the blood and surrounding body tissues, and large vessels, known as veins, carry the blood back to the right side of the heart.

The contraction of the atrium and ventricles of the heart is termed *systole;* the resting phase is termed *diastole.* The heart of an average adult beats approximately 70–75 times per minute. The amount of blood squeezed out of the ventricle on each beat is called the stroke volume. Heart rate (beats per minute) multiplied by stroke volume (amount of blood per beat) equals cardiac output. The blood makes up about $\frac{1}{13}$ of the body weight, and at rest the heart pumps about the same quantity every minute. In an adult this is equivalent to between five and six liters of cardiac output.

Several concepts are important for understanding circulation. The heart is a double-pump organ functioning as one unit to send blood, in equal amounts, to the lungs and body system. The blood vessels transport blood to the tissues; allow for diffusion of fluids, nutrients, oxygen, and minerals out of circulation for the cells to use; and take in waste products of metabolism, including carbon dioxide. Blood flows from areas of higher pressure to areas of lower pressure. The heart can only pump out blood in proportion to the returning blood via venous return and lymphatic flow. Total blood is composed of about 40 to 45 percent red blood cells (erythrocytes), platelets, and white blood cells (leukocytes) and about 45 to 50 percent plasma, containing nutrients, minerals, electrolytes, and vitamins. Circulation is a major factor in respiration, because the blood carries oxygen to the cells and removes carbon dioxide. Blood volume is controlled by the intake and excretion of water. Finally, the blood is responsible for keeping most of the cells of the body supplied with oxygen and nutrients for maintenance and repair, as well as transporting waste products away from the cells and out of the body.

THE RESPIRATORY SYSTEM

Respiration is the process whereby oxygen is transported *to* the cells and carbon dioxide is transported *away* to be exhaled (see Fig. A.6). Oxygen and carbon dioxide are exchanged in two locations. Oxygen enters the blood through the pulmonary membrane of the lungs, and leaves the blood to enter the cells for metabolic use. Carbon dioxide takes the opposite path. It is produced by the cells, moves into the blood, and is transported to the lungs, where it passes through the pulmonary membrane to be exhaled.

External respiration (ventilation) is a simple mechanical process similar to a bellows in function. The ribs lift upward and outward and/or the diaphragm descends as it is contracted, creating a pressure that is negative relative to atmospheric pressure. Air rushes into the lungs. As the air comes in it is cleansed, moisturized, and warmed by the nasal and throat passages. In the lungs it is exposed to the most important part of the pulmonary tissue, the membrane, before diffusing into the capillaries of the pulmonary circulation.

As the ribs fall downward and inward, the diaphragm relaxes and rises. This creates pressure slightly greater than the atmospheric pressure, and air is exhaled. In the young adult this process is repeated about 12 to 20 times per minute at rest and amounts to approximately 6 to 10 liters of ventilation. During stren-

Figure A.6
The respiratory system.

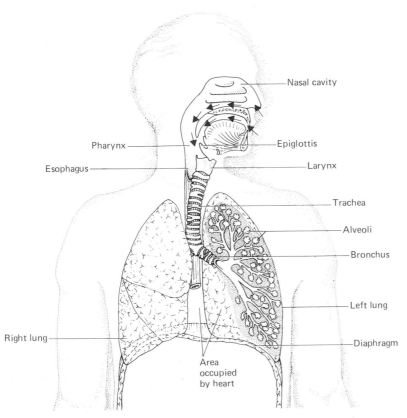

Nasal cavity

Pharynx

Esophagus

Epiglottis

Larynx

Trachea

Alveoli

Bronchus

Left lung

Right lung

Diaphragm

Area occupied by heart

uous activity, respiration may increase to about 50 breaths per minute and 150 liters of ventilation.

As oxygen diffuses through the pulmonary membrane, it is taken into the red blood cells and attached to molecules, called hemoglobin, which carry both oxygen and carbon dioxide. It remains attached until it reaches the metabolically active cells through the capillaries. At that point many of the molecules of oxygen will diffuse into the cells where they are used to produce energy units (ATP) from carbohydrates, fats, or proteins. One end product of this metabolic process is carbon dioxide, which then diffuses out of the cells into the blood, where it is transported back to the lungs to be exhaled. This process is termed *internal respiration*.

Respiration is automatically regulated, but it may be voluntarily modified for short periods of time. The control center of respiration is located in the medulla and lower pons of the brain. This center adjusts ventilation almost exactly to the demands of the body. Thus the relative pressure of oxygen and carbon dioxide remains fairly constant during rest and strenuous activity.

Factors affecting respiration include body metabolism, relative pressure of carbon dioxide, expansion of the lungs, collapse of the lungs, temperature, and the emotional state of the individual.

THE DIGESTIVE SYSTEM

The digestive system is a tubular structure beginning at the mouth and ending at the anus (see Fig. A.7). The alimentary canal permits simple passage of food; storage of food or waste material (feces); digestion of food (carbohydrates, fats, and proteins); and absorption of all the end products of digestion, including minerals, vitamins, and water.

Let's follow some food down the alimentary canal. First, the mouth and teeth grind food into smaller pieces, and then saliva softens and moisturizes it. Some other secretions help to initiate starch digestion, and mucus (a lubricant) is mixed with the food to facilitate its passage. Swallowing propels the food into the esophagus, which then moves the food through the system to the stomach.

The stomach has several functions. It acts as a temporary storage compartment, it further mixes the food until it becomes liquified, it continues the digestion of carbohydrates (starches), and it initiates the digestion of protein and fat by secreting protein-splitting and lipid-splitting enzymes. As the food gradually becomes liquified, it leaves the stomach and enters the small intestine (composed of the duodenum, jejunum, and ileum).

The food now is quite acidic, and almost immediately pancreatic secretions and bile (a fat emulsifier) from the gall bladder begin to enter the duodenum via the common bile duct to help neutralize the acid and to continue digestion of carbohydrates, protein, and fats.

The small intestine continues the movement of the liquified food with wavelike movements. As the food passes through this segment of the gastrointestinal tract, it is exposed to a folded, irregular surface and small hairlike projections of the interior wall of the gut, called villi. The irregular surface and the villi increase the surface area of the small intestine and allow for greater absorption of the minute particles of food. During this passage from the stomach to the large intestine, the small intestine secretes more digestive enzymes to assist in further neutralizing the acid. On its passage through the small intestine, much of the food is absorbed as carbohydrates, proteins, fats, water, vitamins, and minerals.

Upon entering the large intestine, the remaining substance is lubricated with mucus secretions and more water, and most is absorbed. The remaining 100 to 150 ml of substance (now called feces) is stored in the distal portion of the large intestine (colon) until it is eliminated by defecation.

In summary, the alimentary canal is responsible for selectively ingesting food, minerals, vitamins, and water, which are transported via the circulatory system to all cells of the body for immediate use or storage.

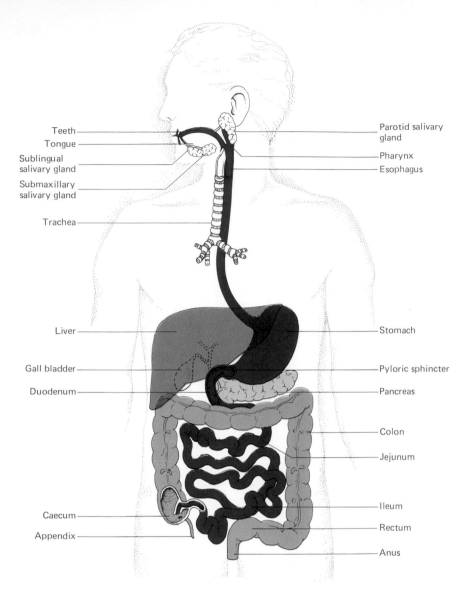

Teeth

Tongue

Sublingual
salivary gland

Submaxillary
salivary gland

Trachea

Liver

Gall bladder

Duodenum

Caecum

Appendix

Parotid salivary
gland

Pharynx

Esophagus

Stomach

Pyloric sphincter

Pancreas

Colon

Jejunum

Ileum

Rectum

Anus

Figure A.7
The digestive system.

THE ENDOCRINE SYSTEM

The endocrine, or hormonal, system is the chemical control mechanism for your bodily functions (see Fig. A.8). Hormones are chemical substances secreted into the body fluids (blood, lymph, or cerebrospinal fluid) that exert physiological effects on all cells of the body. The nervous system acts as the messenger in situations needing quick response, and it helps to regulate hormonal secretions for long-term bodily functions. The endocrine system helps to maintain optimal internal conditions for the body by bringing messages to the vital centers of action.

Specific cells or groups of cells located throughout the body secrete certain hormones. These include the pituitary, adrenal, thymus, thyroid, and parathyroid

530

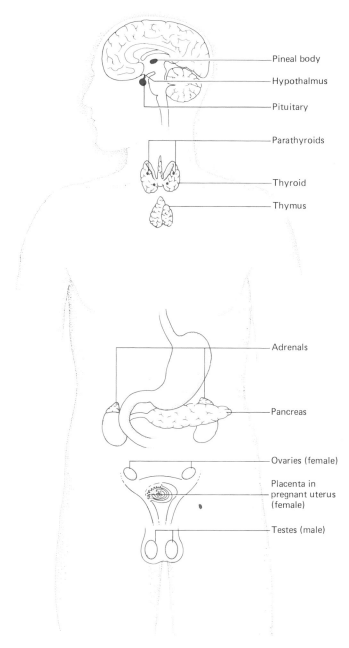

Figure A.8
The endocrine system.

glands, as well as the pancreas, ovaries, testes, kidneys, and pineal body. The hormones related to reproduction and sexual development are discussed in Chapter 12. Table A.1 on page 532 identifies the major hormones and their effects.

THE INTEGUMENTARY SYSTEM

The body covering, or integument, is composed of three layers of flattened cells (see Fig. A.9). The *epidermis* is the outside layer that people commonly think of as skin. Even though it continually sloughs off, it is tough, resistant to extreme temperature changes, and prevents excessive intake or loss of fluids.

The second layer, the *dermis,* supports and binds the epidermis to the underlying tissues. This layer is called the true skin; it contains blood vessels, nerve endings, oil and sweat glands, muscles, and hair follicles. The upper surface of the derma is rather irregularly shaped in conelike elevations called papillae. The *subcutaneous layer,* the deepest of the three layers of skin tissue, is supported by a thick layer of subcutaneous fatty tissue.

Because skin is living tissue, except for the epidermal layer, it must have a rich blood supply. Among its many functions, it serves as a heat-dissipating organ. This requires the service of many blood vessels, so that in times of excessive internal heat buildup the blood can act as a heat transport mechanism. As excessive heat is generated, either within the body as a result of exercise or outside of the body as a result of high temperature, the blood flow to the skin increases dramatically to help conduct more heat away from the body. Concurrently, the sweat glands begin to secrete fluid consisting of water, salts, and small quantities of urea (a waste product that is a component of urine). As the perspiration evaporates, more heat is dissipated. In this manner, increased blood flow, sweat secretion, and the evaporation of sweat help the body maintain a constant temperature. In extremely cold environments the fatty subcutaneous layer prevents excessive heat loss. To aid heat conservation, blood flow to the skin may

Table A.1
HORMONES AND THEIR EFFECTS

Hormone	Principal Effects	Secreted By
Adrenocorticotropic hormone (ACTH)	Stimulates the adrenal cortex	Pituitary
Thyrotropin (TSH)	Stimulates the thyroid gland	Pituitary
Follicle-stimulating hormone (FSH)	Stimulates production of egg cells by ovary and spermatozoa by testes	Pituitary
Luteinizing hormone (LH)	Helps maturation of egg-bearing follicles in ovary or stimulates production of testosterone (male hormone) in testes	Pituitary
Growth hormone	Governs normal growth and helps to regulate metabolism	Pituitary
Prolactin	Regulates breast development and milk production	Pituitary
Antidiuretichormone (ADH), or Vasopressin	Regulates absorption of water in the kidney	Neurohypophysis (part of the pituitary)
Oxytocin	Facilitates movement of sperm in Fallopian tube, stimulates uterine muscle in childbirth, stimulates secretion of milk by breasts	Neurohypophysis
Cortisol and similar hormones	Regulate metabolism of sugar, protein, fat, minerals, and water	Adrenal cortex (outer layer of adrenal gland)
Aldosterone and desoxycorticosterone	Regulate excretion and retention of minerals, particularly sodium and potassium, by kidneys	Adrenal cortex
Thyroid hormones	Regulate rate of body's metabolism	Thyroid
Estradiol 17-B ("Estrogen")	Regulates development of feminine characteristics and the menstrual-ovulatory cycle	Ovaries
Progesterone	Works with estrogen to regulate ovulation cycle and pregnancy. Estrogen-progesterone combinations, or similar agents, are the basis of birth-control pills	Ovaries
Testosterone	Regulates development of male characteristics and reproductive system	Testes
Insulin	Regulates utilization of sugar, proteins, and fats	Pancreas (Islets of Langerhans)
Glucagon	Helps to regulate utilization of sugar, antagonizes insulin	Pancreas (Islets of Langerhans)
Parathyroid hormone	Regulates calcium metabolism	Parathyroid glands
Thyrocalcitonin	Helps to regulate calcium metabolism	Thyroid
Adrenalin	Stimulates brain and heart rate, mobilizes sugar and fat	Adrenal medulla (inner layer of adrenal gland)
Noradrenalin	Increases force of heart contraction and constricts arterioles	Adrenal medulla
Releasing factors	Individual ones cause release of ACTH, TSH, LH, FSH, prolactin, and growth hormone by pituitary	Brain (hypothalamus)

Hormone	Principal Effects	Secreted By
Secretin	Stimulates pancreas to secrete chemicals needed for digestion of food	Lining of part of intestine
Cholecystokinin	Stimulates liver and pancreas to secrete chemicals for digestion of food	Lining of part of intestine
Gastrin	Stimulates stomach to secrete hydrochloric acid	Lining of part of stomach and intestine

From "Chemical Intervention" by Sherman M. Mellinkoff. Copyright © 1973 by Scientific American, Inc. All rights reserved.

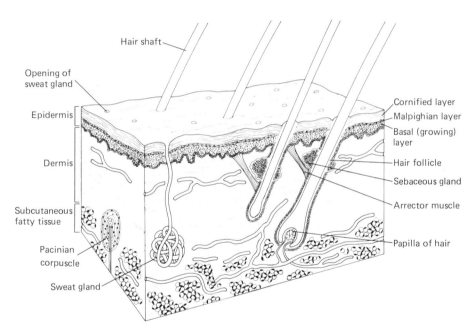

Figure A.9
The integumentary system.

be dramatically reduced so as not to lose body heat via the blood vessels.

Also located throughout the skin are receptors of touch, pain, heat, and cold.

The integumentary system is important in protecting the body from the invasion of many types of bacteria, an excessive increase or decrease in body temperature, and excessive absorption or loss of water. It also helps the kidneys control blood urea through excretion and keeps the organism informed of environmental changes, skin damage, and excessive pressure.

To summarize, the skin covers the other systems of the body, protects them, and may prevent serious injuries.

appendix B:
health emergencies,
accidents, and safety—
what you can do

In treating accident victims, every case is an emergency and requires action at or near the site of injury. The main concern is for the immediate care of the victim, and every adult should be capable of applying the principles of emergency first aid.

After approaching an accident victim, it is important to follow five steps:

1. *Establish an open airway.* Free respiration is essential to survival. Inhaled blood, mucus, or vomitus, or lower jaw injury permitting the tongue to drop back over the airway usually causes the blockage. If clearing the airway does not result in unaided breathing, artificial respiration must be administered.

2. *Control hemorrhage.* Severe bleeding must be controlled immediately.

3. *Prevent shock.* Rather than treating shock symptoms, steps should be taken to prevent shock from occurring.

4. *Splint fractures.* Any limb suspected of fracture should be splinted immediately, exactly where the victim is lying.

5. *Provide transportation of the injured.* Gentle, slow transportation should be provided.

The following pages will introduce some basic techniques that will enable you to administer help should the need arise.

RESCUE BREATHING

Heart attack, toxic gas poisoning, electric shock, drug overdose, brain concussion, fracture of the skull, certain neck fractures, drowning, and choking are among the injuries and ailments that may stop respiration. When breathing stops, seconds count, and lives can be saved providing that air enters the victim's lungs immediately. No more than 15 seconds should elapse in determining the need for artificial respiration and in preparing the victim. The majority of cases of cessation of breathing will not require external heart massage (CPR); however, when the heart has stopped completely, CPR is indicated. Performing CPR properly requires complete training. We do not recommend trying it unless you have taken a CPR course offered at your university or through the Red Cross or American Heart Association.

Artificial Respiration

Preparatory action for artificial respiration includes the following quick steps:

1. Clearing the victim's airway of foreign matter;
2. Choosing an individual to call a physician and rescue squad;
3. Extending the head fully to open air passages;

534

FOR ADULTS

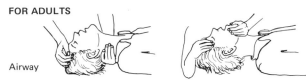

Airway

If you find a collapsed person, determine if victim is conscious by shaking the shoulder and shouting "Are you all right?" If no response, shout for help. Then open the airway. If victim is not lying flat on his back, roll victim over, moving the entire body at one time as a total unit.

To open the victim's airway, lift up the neck (or chin) gently with one hand while pushing down on the forehead with the other to tilt head back. Once the airway is open, place your ear close to the victim's mouth:

■ Look—at the chest and stomach for movement.
■ Listen—for sounds of breathing.
■ Feel—for breath on your cheek.

If none of these signs is present, victim is not breathing.
If opening the airway does not cause the victim to begin to breathe spontaneously, you must provide rescue breathing.

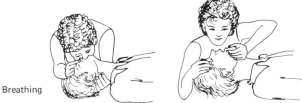

Breathing

The best way to provide rescue breathing is by using the mouth-to-mouth technique. Take your hand that is on the victim's forehead and turn it so that you can pinch the victim's nose shut while keeping the heel of the hand in place to maintain head tilt. Your other hand should remain under the victim's neck (or chin), lifting up.
Immediately give four quick, full breaths in rapid succession using the mouth-to-mouth method.

FOR INFANTS AND SMALL CHILDREN

Basic life support for infants and small children is similar to that for adults. A few important differences to remember are given below.

Airway

Be careful when handling an infant that you do not exaggerate the backward position of the head tilt. An infant's neck is so pliable that forceful backward tilting might block breathing passages instead of opening them.

Breathing

Don't try to pinch off the nose. Cover both the mouth and nose of an infant or small child who is not breathing. Use small breaths with less volume to inflate the lungs. Give one small breath every three seconds.

Figure B.1
Rescue breathing for adults, infants, and small children.

4. Loosening tight clothing and removing wet items as quickly as possible; and

5. Covering the victim with blankets, clothing, or newspapers to maintain body warmth.

Figure B.1 illustrates and describes the mouth-to-mouth method, which is the most effective and rapid method of restoring breathing.

A plastic breathing tube is available to provide more effective resuscitation. The mouthpiece used by the rescuer reduces the possibility of infection, and the breathing tube holes keep the victim's air passages open. It may be necessary to hold the tongue forward with the fingers while the tube is inserted. The long end of the tube is inserted into the mouth of adults, whereas the short end is designed for children over 3 years of age. The direct mouth-to-mouth-and-nose method must be used for children under the age of 3.

Hyperventilation

Under some circumstances an individual feels unable to get enough air to breathe. Chest pain or constriction may or may not accompany this feeling. The victim tries to compensate by overbreathing, which lowers carbon dioxide levels in the blood, leading to numbness and tingling in the hands and dizziness. This hyperventilation syndrome is most likely to occur when the individual is under stress or under the influence of alcohol. Symptoms are a direct result of the loss of additional carbon dioxide to the atmosphere from overbreathing. If the victim can remain calm enough and breathe into a paper bag for 5 to 15 minutes (bag over both nose and mouth), the symptoms will disappear as carbon dioxide levels are elevated. If in doubt, the victim should be transported to a physician's office.

CONTROL OF HEMORRHAGE

Bleeding is classified according to the three main sources from which it occurs—arteries, veins, and capillaries.

1. *Arterial bleeding.* Bright red blood may spurt from a wound; however, death is unlikely to occur unless a large artery is involved. Bleeding from the carotid (neck), axillary (armpit), brachial (inside of upper arm), or femoral (groin area) artery can produce death in three minutes or less. Arterial bleeding is extremely dangerous, because the force of blood flow through the arterial opening is so strong that the blood will not clot.

2. *Venous bleeding.* A steady flow of dark red blood, profuse at times, suggests that the source is a vein. Although it is easier to control venous bleeding than arterial bleeding, there is the danger of an air bubble or air embolism, particularly if a large vein is affected. Because the blood is being sucked toward the heart, air could enter the opening and interfere with the ability of the heart to pump blood.

3. *Capillary bleeding.* A general oozing of blood from tissue is not serious, and bleeding is easily controlled.

Controlling External Bleeding

When severe external bleeding occurs, the first step is to elevate the area of the body that is bleeding above the heart level. Once this is done, there are three basic methods of controlling hemorrhage: direct pressure, pressure points, and tourniquet, in that order. If bleeding is not controlled by direct pressure, pressure points are used. Only as a last resort and under certain unique circumstances is a tourniquet ever applied. Although direct pressure is a first step in most wounds, never apply direct pressure to a head injury because of the risk of pushing contaminates into the brain. Instead, apply a bandage and very light direct pressure, and utilize the pressure points.

1. *Direct pressure.* Place a heavy, sterile gauze over the wound, with the injured part flat against the floor or table. The edges of the wound should be placed tightly together (use adhesive or butterfly strips) before the compress is in place. Use the heel of the hand to apply just enough steady pressure to stop the bleeding. Too much pressure will obstruct the flow of blood to the rest of the limb, if an extremity is involved. If a pulse cannot be felt below the dressing, too much pressure is being exerted. If bleeding does not stop in several minutes, an artery may be involved and use of pressure points is indicated. Should bleeding increase, arterial bleeding is also suspected, because the venous return of blood back to the heart is being cut off and the arterial flow from the heart to the wound is not. Direct pressure is effective for most body parts, other than the head and neck, and should control most bleeding.

2. *Pressure points.* When a pressure dressing fails, bleeding can usually be controlled by strong finger pressure on the main artery of blood supply to the wounded part. Of the 22 pressure points (11 on each side), 6 are used to control external bleeding (see Fig. B.2). Pressure points represent the best method available to control bleeding body parts where a tourniquet would be dangerous or impossible to apply.

3. *Tourniquet.* Keep in mind that a tourniquet is a last resort and is rarely needed. Only in the case of a partially torn vessel would a tourniquet be indicated, and even then it would have to be applied immediately to prevent fatal bleeding. The use of a tourniquet is controversial; many physicians suggest that lay persons not be instructed in its use. It has been used too often with harmful effects, when firm, direct pressure or the pressure points could have controlled bleeding. For that reason, we will not describe it here, but recommend a first aid course for those who wish instruction.

Recognizing Internal Bleeding

Severe internal hemorrhage can result in death as rapidly as external bleeding. Common signs of internal bleeding are thirst, faintness, dizziness, cold and clammy skin, dilated pupils, irregular breathing, coughing up blood, and weak and irregular pulse—symptoms sim-

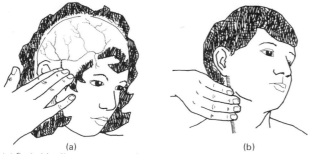

(a) Scalp bleeding: pressure on the temporal artery just in front of the ear.

(b) Head and neck bleeding: pressure on the common carotid artery through constriction against the vertebrae of the neck.

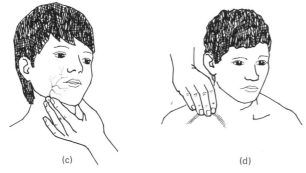

(c) Facial bleeding: pressure on the facial artery against the jawbone; may require pressure on both sides simultaneously.

(d) Armpit and chest wall bleeding: pressure on the subclavian artery as it passes behind the collarbone, downward with the thumb to press the artery against the first rib.

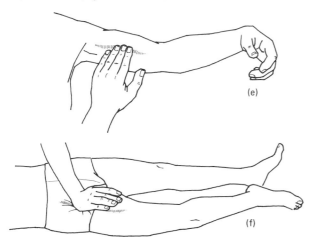

(e) Arm: pressure on the bracial artery against the bone midway between the shoulder and elbow.

(f) Leg: deep pressure on the femoral artery in the groin.

Figure B.2
Pressure points.

ilar to shock. Internal bleeding from an artery, vein, or capillary involves blood loss into the chest, abdominal, or pelvic cavities or into any organ contained therein. A tearing or bruising force, typical of automobile accidents or falls, often causes internal damage.

The color of the blood provides an indication of the injured site:

1. Lungs—Coughed-up blood is bright red and frothy.
2. Stomach—Vomited blood is bright red; if chronic over a longer period of time, blood may resemble coffee grounds.
3. Intestinal tract above the sigmoid colon—Stools are jet black.
4. Low in intestinal tract and recent—Blood in stools is bright red.
5. Bladder—Blood in the urine.

Intra-abdominal bleeding is characterized by vomiting, tenderness, and rigidity of the stomach muscles. Severe internal bleeding can be controlled only by surgery. Blood transfusions may be necessary at the hospital while surgery is arranged. Until medical assistance arrives, the victim must be kept still in a slightly reclined position or transported to a nearby hospital.

CHOKING

Many experts believe that the quickest and most effective method (some say the only method) of first aid for choking is the *Heimlich maneuver* (see Fig. B.3). The victim is grasped from behind in the "bear hug" position, with the fist of one hand placed just above the umbilicus and below the rib cage and covered by the other hand. A sharp, hard upward squeeze is given, forcing the diaphragm upward to compress the lungs. The air in the lungs will create an upward draft or pressure so great that the obstruction will often be spewed several feet. If the first attempt is unsuccessful, the squeeze is repeated until the obstruction is expelled. After the object is removed, mouth-to-mouth resuscitation is initiated if normal breathing does not occur.

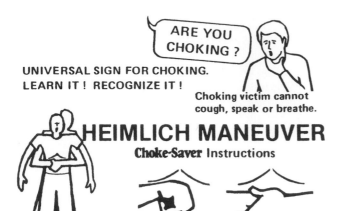

UNIVERSAL SIGN FOR CHOKING.
LEARN IT! RECOGNIZE IT!

**Choking victim cannot
cough, speak or breathe.**

HEIMLICH MANEUVER
Choke-Saver Instructions

- Have victim stand. Standing behind victim, rescuer places his arms around victim's waist.
- Make a fist. Place the thumb side against the victim's abdomen below the ribcage and just above the belly-button. (A)
- Cover your fist with your other hand and pull into the victim's abdomen with a **strong, quick upward thrust.** (B)
- Avoid squeezing victim's sides by keeping your elbows out.
- Object should pop out of victim's mouth.... if it doesn't **repeat maneuver immediately.**
- Victim should see a doctor as soon as possible.

If victim is sitting, have him stand immediately and apply maneuver as described above.

IF VICTIM COLLAPSES
or is too large for rescuer
to reach around...

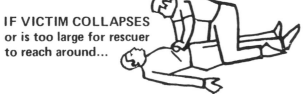

- Place the victim on the floor on his back, face up, head straight. Open mouth if victim is unconscious.
- Facing the victim, straddle victim's hips.
- Place the heel of one hand against the victim's abdomen below the ribcage and just above the belly-button.
- Place second hand directly on top of the other hand.
- Press into the victim's abdomen with a **strong, quick upward thrust.** Then check the mouth for expelled object and remove.
- Object should pop out of victim's mouth . . . if it doesn't **repeat maneuver immediately.**
- Victim should see a doctor as soon as possible.

Figure B.3
The Heimlich maneuver.
SOURCE: Blue Cross/Blue Shield of Massachusetts

SHOCK

Shock is one of the body's strongest natural reactions to disease and injury. It slows blood flow, acts as a natural tourniquet until the wound clots, and in a serious injury reduces pain and eases the body's agony when approaching death. The basic types of shock are *traumatic* (injury or loss of blood), *septic* (infection induced), and *cardiogenic* (from a heart attack). All three types can kill and repesent one of the greatest dangers for accident and heart attack victims; the severely burned; and those with broken or crushed bones, infection, and insect stings.

The body maintains a delicate balance between blood volume and the space the blood fills. When this balance is upset (as when an artery is severed, resulting in the loss of blood; or in the case of burns, where damaged tissue swells, space expands, and fluids are soaked up from the blood), shock may occur. When the heart or the circulatory system is affected, the shock mechanism may be triggered. The chain of events goes something like this: (1) injury causes a reaction in the adrenal glands, which inject epinephrine into the blood stream and the sympathetic nervous system; (2) blood vessels constrict, reducing the blood supply to body tissues through the capillaries; (3) breathing quickens and the heart rate increases in an attempt to pump more oxygen into the blood to the tissues; (4) inadequate oxygen is available to vital organs, such as the brain, liver, heart, lungs, and kidneys; and (5) tissue dies, the organ ceases functioning, and death occurs (see Fig. B.4).

Shock is much easier to prevent than to treat. Careful splinting of broken bones, careful handling, stopping a hemorrhage, and keeping the patient warm all go a long way toward prevention.

First Aid for Shock

Cold and clammy hands, weak and rapid pulse, low blood pressure, and shallow breathing are common signs of shock. Treatment for shock has changed in recent years. No longer is it recommended to lower the victim's head and elevate the feet. Until medical

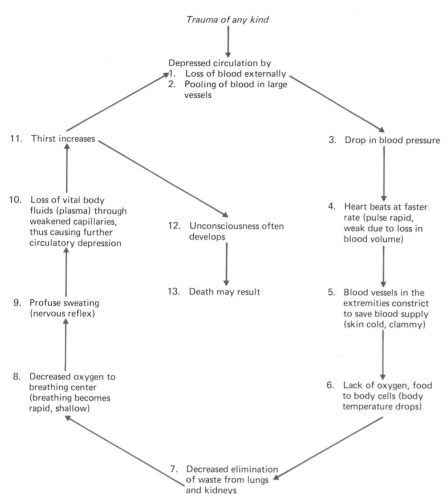

Trauma of any kind

Depressed circulation by
1. Loss of blood externally
2. Pooling of blood in large vessels

11. Thirst increases

3. Drop in blood pressure

10. Loss of vital body fluids (plasma) through weakened capillaries, thus causing further circulatory depression

12. Unconsciousness often develops

4. Heart beats at faster rate (pulse rapid, weak due to loss in blood volume)

13. Death may result

5. Blood vessels in the extremities constrict to save blood supply (skin cold, clammy)

9. Profuse sweating (nervous reflex)

8. Decreased oxygen to breathing center (breathing becomes rapid, shallow)

6. Lack of oxygen, food to body cells (body temperature drops)

7. Decreased elimination of waste from lungs and kidneys

Figure B.4
Continuous cycle of traumatic shock.

SOURCE: From Brennan, William T. and James W. Crowe, *Guide to Problems and Practices in First Aid and Emergency Care*, 4th, ed. © 1971, 1976, 1981 Wm. C. Brown Company Publishers, Dubuque, Iowa. Reprinted by permission.

help arrives, the recommended first aid treatment is to stop all bleeding, clear the mouth of vomit, keep the victim lying down, and cover the victim only enough to prevent loss of body heat.

FRACTURES

Splints can be applied by laying a board two feet longer than the leg along the side of the leg with its end butted against the groin. A bandage around the ankle and board completes a gentle traction, which will aid in preventing shock for a fractured thigh. Pillows and boards also make excellent splints for legs and knees. It is possible to bind the upper extremity to the body after using boards or magazines as splints for forearms or to bind the legs together for fractures of the thigh, if boards are available. Fig. B.5 demonstrates fixation splinting for the lower leg, lower arm, or wrist.

Great emphasis is placed on care of handling. If the victim is in no immediate danger, it is better to await medical personnel or others skilled in moving the injured. A patient should not be lifted by the knees

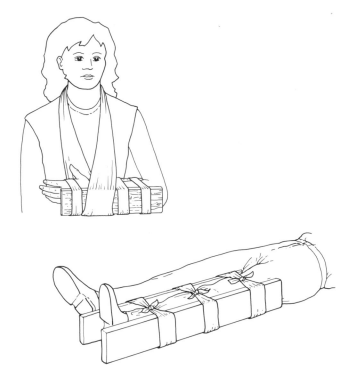

Figure B.5
Fixation splinting for the lower leg, lower arm, or wrist

and shoulders, allowing the spine to double. A blanket or five-person carry (four people lifting the patient by holding his or her clothes, while the fifth supports the head and neck) can be used to move the victim if absolutely necessary.

ORAL POISONING

Prevention and First Aid

If medications, insecticides, caustic cleaners, and organic solvents were stored out of the reach of young children, the majority of household poisonings would be prevented. The most common involve strong alkali solutions used in drain cleaners that are capable of destroying tissue on contact. Additional precautionary measures to consider are: (1) properly labeling all medical and chemical preparations, (2) avoiding the storage of chemicals in food containers, (3) avoiding taking medicine in the dark, (4) listing the purpose and dosage of medicines on the label, (5) washing the hands thoroughly after handling poisons, and (6) discarding prescription drugs after they have served their purpose.

Poisons enter the system by way of the mouth (most common), inhalation (for example, vapors or fumes from insecticides, leaky gas appliances, or exhaust systems on autos), injection (from insects), and absorption (directly through the skin). Poisons act in different ways once absorbed into the system: acids and alkalies burn and corrode tissue, sleeping pills and alcohol depress the central nervous system, insecticides produce extreme stimulation of the central nervous system, and cyanide and carbon monoxide prevent oxygen from being carried to tissues and cause an asphyxial death. Each type requires a different kind of emergency treatment. Table B.1 lists emergency procedures for various oral poisonings.

If you are confronted with a case of oral poisoning, do not panic. Quickly identify the ingested substance, then call the poison control center for advice. Do not start treatment before the substance is identified. If a hospital is nearby, you can bring the substance along to the emergency room. Two types of first aid are indicated: inducing vomiting and diluting or neutralizing the substance. It is essential to find out which treatment is appropriate for the particular kind of poison before proceeding. Vomiting can be induced by stimulating the back of the throat with a finger of using syrup of ipecac followed by water.

COMMON INJURIES AND THEIR TREATMENT

Many emergencies can be adequately and safely handled at home without the aid of a physician. Every adult should learn the proper treatment of minor ailments and injuries and be able to determine if and when a physician should be seen. Table B.2 provides guidelines for treating several common emergencies.

Table B.1
FIRST AID FOR ORAL POISONING

Emergency Situation: Known and Unknown Factors	Emergency First Aid
1. No knowledge of poison swallowed	Dilute with water or milk, search for original container, call poison control center to report symptoms and secure advice, transport to hospital or physician.
2. Aware that strong acid, alkali, or petroleum product was *not* swallowed; cannot locate container	Dilute with water or milk, induce vomiting (tickling back of throat with the index finger or administering syrup of ipecac or mustard and water), call poison control center, transport to medical help.
3. No knowledge of poison swallowed; presence of some of the following symptoms: burns around lips and mouth, breath odor (petroleum), unconsciousness, convulsions, exhaustion	Follow suggestions for (1), avoid administering anything orally to unconscious victim. Keep victim warm and seek medical help.
4. Strong acid (such as toilet bowl cleaner)	Dilute with water or milk; neutralize with milk of magnesia or weak alkali in water (1–2 glasses for children, 3–4 for adults); use milk, olive oil, or egg white as a demulcent without inducing vomiting.
5. Petroleum product (kerosene, gasoline, furniture polish, etc.)	Dilute with water or milk, do not use a neutralizing fluid or demulcent, call poison control center or physician for advice.
6. Alkali (drain cleaner)	Dilute with water or milk; neutralize with vinegar or lemon juice mixed in water; and use milk, olive oil, or egg white as a demulcent.
7. Inhaled poison gases (carbon monoxide)	Hold breath before entering closed garage or room, move victim to fresh air area, maintain an open airway, administer artificial respiration, call emergency rescue squad.
8. Unconscious victim	Keep airway open, administer artificial respiration, transport to medical help, deliver poison container.
9. Alcohol intoxication	Not needed if victim is breathing normally, has regular pulse. With signs of shock, irregular breathing, lack of response, maintain open airway, administer artificial respiration, keep warm, and transport.
10. Barbiturate (depressant) overdose—opium and morphine substances	Arouse with light slapping or cold compress; maintain open airway, administer artificial respiration if breathing ceases, keep warm, transport to hospital.
11. Hallucinogenic reaction (LSD, mescaline, psilocybin, morning glory seeds, and synthetic substances)	Protect from bodily harm; move to safe, quiet surroundings; transport to hospital.
12. Inhalant overdose (glue sniffing, paints and lacquers, gasoline, kerosene, nail polish, nail polish remover)	Administer artificial respiration if breathing stops, transport to hospital.
13. Stimulant overdose (Benzedrine, Dexedrine, Methedrine, ritalin)	Protect against injury, maintain open airway, administer artificial respiration if breathing stops, keep warm, transport to hospital.

Table B.2
COMMON INJURIES AND THEIR TREATMENT

Injury	Emergency Home Treatment	Need for a physician
Abrasion (with skin or layers scraped off)	Clean thoroughly with soap and warm water or hydrogen peroxide. Use bandage if wound oozes blood. Remove loose skin flaps with nail scissors if they are dirty; allow to remain if clean.	If all dirt and foreign matter cannot be removed If signs of infection occur
Animal bite	Catch the animal and arrange to have it observed for 15 days to be certain it does not develop rabies. Treat as a cut or puncture wound.	If a wild animal is involved If the animal's immunizations are not current If the observed animal develops rabies If the wound needs a physician's care
Ankle or knee sprain	Stop activity, apply ice pack immediately. Continue ice 3 times daily for 48 hours before switching to heat. Use crutches for 2 to 3 days if pain is severe when walking. Recovery should take this course: swelling and pain for 24–72 hours, decreasing symptoms for 6 to 10 days, full return to normal in 6 to 8 weeks.	If swelling and severe pain continue for more than 3 days If pain prevents any weight bearing If there is knee injury other than contusion If there is ligament or tendon damage
Broken bone	Look for evidence of a broken bone. Apply ice packs. Protect and rest the injured part for 72 hours. No additional damage is likely to occur if proper rest and protection are provided. Immobilize, call rescue squad, and transport to emergency room.	If the limb is cold, blue, or numb If the pelvis or thigh is involved If the limb is crooked, unusable If there is considerable bleeding and bruising If shock symptoms are present If pain lasts more than 72 hours
Burn	Diagnose the depth of the burn: first degree—superficial; second degree—deeper burns resulting in splitting of layers or blistering from scalding, sunburn, etc.; and third degree—destruction of all layers with damage to the deeper tissues. Apply cold compress for 5 to 10 minutes to reduce skin damage and pain; avoid rupturing blisters. Aspirin may be used for pain.	For all third-degree burns For second-degree burns involving an area greater than 25 to 35 sq in. If pain continues for more than 2 days
Dental injury	Chipped tooth—avoid hot and cold drinks; swelling of face due to abscessed tooth—apply ice pack; excessive bleeding of tooth socket after extraction—place gauze over socket and bite down, maintaining pressure; toothache—aspirin and ice packs may be used.	If victim has a chipped tooth, an abscessed tooth, excessive bleeding of socket, or a toothache
Fainting and dizziness	Lack of blood flow to the brain commonly occurs with increasing age and may result in a temporary loss of vision or lightheadedness. Avoid sudden changes in posture, reduce anxiety level.	If loss of consciousness occurs If room appears to be spinning If dizziness occurs frequently
Frostbite	Thaw rapidly in a warm water bath. Avoid rubbing frostbite with snow. Water should be comfortable to a normal, unfrozen hand (not over 104°F). When a flush reaches the fingers, remove the frostbitten part immediately. For an ear or nose, use cloths soaked in warm water.	Always see a doctor
Head injury	Apply ice bag to bruised area. Observe patient every 2 hours for the next 72 hours for alertness (unresponsiveness, deep sleep), unequal pupil size (one-fourth of population have unequal size all the time), and severe vomiting. Pressure inside skull may develop over a 72-hour period.	If there is bleeding from ears, eyes, or mouth If the victim has black eyes If there is unconsciousness, unequal pupil size, lethargy, or severe vomiting

Condition	Treatment	Call doctor
Infected wound (blood poisoning)	Bacterial infection in the blood stream, or septicemia. Keep area clean, changing the bandage twice daily. Soak and clean in warm water several times daily. Have patience—up to 10 to 12 days may be needed for normal healing.	If there is fever above 99.6°F. If there is thick pus, swelling since the second day
Insect bite/sting	Apply cold compress, use aspirin or other pain relievers. Identify the insect—black widow spiders have a glossy black body about one-half inch in diameter, red "hour glass" on abdomen. Bite produces sharp pain at the site; cramps appear within an hour and may involve the extremities and trunk. Breathing becomes difficult; nausea, vomiting, twitching, tingling sensations of the hand may occur.	If there is evidence of wheezing, difficulty in breathing, fainting, or hives or skin rash. For bite from a black widow spider. For severe local reaction
Minor cut	Clean the wound vigorously with soap and water or hydrogen peroxide, removing all dirt and foreign matter. Use a butterfly band-aid or steri-strip to bring the edges of the wound tightly together without trapping the fat or rolling the skin under. Avoid antiseptics; they may destroy tissue and retard healing and do not kill and wash away bacteria as effectively as soap and water.	For cuts on trunk or face, or deep cuts that may involve tendons, ligaments, blood vessels, or nerves. For blood pumping from a wound. For tingling or limb weakness. If signs of infection exist. For cuts that cannot be pulled together without trapping the fat
Nosebleed	Squeeze the nose between the thumb and forefinger just below the hard portion for 5 to 10 minutes while seated with the head back. Do not lie down. Apply cold compresses to the bridge of the nose and avoid blowing.	If it occurs frequently and is associated with a cold. If victim has a history of high blood pressure
Object in eye	Avoid rubbing—you could scratch the cornea. Close both eyes for several minutes to allow tears to wash out the foreign body. Grasp the lashes of the upper lid and draw out and down over the lower lid. If it feels like the foreign object is present but it is not, cornea scrape probably occurred and will heal in 24 to 48 hours. Using medicine dropper, flush eye with plain water. If speck is visible, touch lightly with moistened corner of handkerchief. If chemical was splashed in eye, dilute immediately by placing face under lukewarm shower with thick spray.	If the foreign object is on the eye itself. If it remains after washing. If the object could have penetrated the globe of the eye. If blood is visible in eye. If vision is impaired. If pain is present after 48 hours
Poison ivy and oak	After initial exposure, 12 to 48 hours may pass before a rash appears. If plant oil is removed from the skin with vigorous washing (2 to 3 times), a rash may be prevented. Apply cool compresses of Burrow's Solution. Cleanse the skin thoroughly. A hot bath will release histamine and cause intense itching; however, the cells of histamine will eventually be depleted and 6 to 8 hours of relief will follow.	If rash occurs without itching, redness, or exposure to oak or ivy. Contact may be from pets, clothing, or smoke from burning Rhus plants
Puncture wound	Let wound bleed as much as possible. Clean thoroughly with soap and water or hydrogen peroxide diluted to 3 percent. Soak the wound at least twice daily in warm water for 3 to 4 days to keep the skin puncture open and allow germs and foreign matter to drain.	If the wound is in the head, abdomen, or chest; danger of internal damage. If the object is still inside the wound. If the wound is deep, cannot be cleaned thoroughly, or a tetanus shot is needed
Sunburn	Apply cool compress using Aveeno or one-half cup baking soda in a tub of water. Avoid Vaseline and other lubricants the first day.	If there are abdominal cramps, dizziness, or second-degree burns

MEDIC ALERT

Approximately one in five persons has special medical conditions or is allergic to particular medications. If this individual is unable to speak, due to unconsciousness, shock, delirium, hysteria, or injury, rapid diagnosis and treatment, even by a physician, is not always possible. A diabetic could be diagnosed as intoxicated and go untreated, a shot of penicillin could kill an allergic victim, and those dependent upon life-saving medication could mistakenly be given improper doses or incorrect drugs. These and other individuals should wear a Medic Alert bracelet or necklace (see Fig. B.6). The Medic Alert symbol is recognized the world over. The bracelet or necklace contains the following vital information: the medical problem, file number, and telephone number of Medic Alert's central file. Information about a medical condition can be obtained in minutes via a collect telephone call 24 hours a day.

The 14 most common medical conditions that may require Medic Alert are asthma; diabetes; heart condition; taking anticoagulants; epilepsy; contact lenses; glaucoma; neck breather; implanted pacemaker; and allergy to penicillin, insect stings, sulfa, codeine, or tetanus antitoxin.

Medic Alert is a charitable, nonprofit organization. It was founded in 1956 by Marion C. Collins, M.D., and is currently endorsed by over 100 organizations, including the American Academy of Family Physicians, the International Associations of Fire Chiefs and Police Chiefs, the National Sheriffs' Association, and the National Association of Life Underwriters. The cost for a Medic Alert bracelet or necklace is as low as $10.00. For further information, write to Medic Alert Foundation International, Turlock, California 95380.

ACCIDENTS AND SAFETY

Although accident rates have declined slightly over the past 40 years, accidents remain a leading cause of death in the United States. In the general population accidents are the fourth leading cause of death, behind heart disease, cancer, and stroke. In the 1–24 age group accidents are the leading cause of death, and the accident rate for men is more than twice the rate for women.

Approximately one accidental death occurs every four minutes, with an accidental injury taking place every three or four seconds. As shown in Table B.3, motor vehicle accidents are the major cause of death at all age levels, followed by falls, drowning, fires and burns, ingestion of food and other small objects, poisoning, firearm accidents, and poisoning by gas. Each year approximately 50,000 deaths and millions of injuries are caused by motor vehicle accidents; about one person in two can be expected to be killed or injured in an auto accident during his or her lifetime. Home accidents cause the greatest number of injuries.

Factors Contributing to Accidents

Accidents are caused by the interaction of several factors and may not have a single cause. Although the layperson may view accidents as "acts of God," "fate," or simply "bad luck," only a small percentage of ac-

Figure B.6
Medic Alert symbol. The two sides of the Medic Alert bracelet (Medic Alert Foundation International).

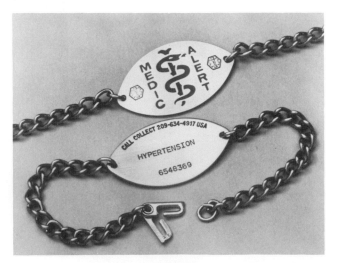

Table B.3
ACCIDENTAL DEATHS BY AGE, SEX, AND TYPE, 1978

Age and Sex	All Types	Motor Vehicle	Falls	Drown- ing	Fires, Burns	Ingest. of Food, Object	Fire- arms	Poison (Solid, Liquid)	Poison by Gas	% Male All Types
All Ages	105,561	52,411	13,690	7,026	6,163	3,063	1,806	3,035	1,737	70
Under 5	4,766	1,551	192	696	896	463	52	81	51	58
5 to 14	6,118	3,130	124	1,010	586	91	297	37	76	69
15 to 24	26,622	19,164	538	2,180	530	168	581	577	525	78
25 to 34	15,533	9,648	502	1,070	542	183	300	778	287	80
35 to 44	9,491	4,926	551	630	502	257	205	432	205	77
45 to 54	9,174	4,166	835	460	667	292	162	420	171	74
55 to 64	9,600	3,882	1,266	450	733	410	112	305	185	70
65 to 74	9,072	3,217	1,852	300	789	483	68	219	110	62
75 & over	15,185	2,727	7,830	230	918	716	29	186	127	47
Male	73,881	38,139	7,181	5,875	3,786	1,765	1,566	1,800	1,260	
Female	31,680	14,272	6,509	1,151	2,377	1,298	240	1,235	477	
Percent male	70	73	52	84	61	58	87	59	73	

SOURCE: National Safety Council, *Accident Facts*, 1981 Edition.

cidents can be attributed to the element of chance. Most often, accidents are caused by a combination of factors, such as individual neglect, attitude, psychological/emotional factors, personality, cultural factors, and environmental factors.

Changes in societal attitudes that eventually result in legislation to reduce speed limits; remove doors from discarded refrigerators; improve automobile design; or add fire alarms, fire escapes, and sprinkler systems to hotels and apartment buildings tend to occur only in the wake of highly publicized disasters or through the efforts of advocacy groups. When accidents are viewed as fate, prevention receives little attention or emphasis. The use of seat and shoulder belts by all occupants of motor vehicles all the time would probably save more than 10,000 lives each year. Yet only 25 percent of occupants use lap safety belts, and fewer than 3 percent use shoulder belts. The public's attitude about seat belts is relatively unchanged.

Various personality traits have been associated with high accident rates. Poor judgment, impulsiveness, overconfidence in one's ability, lack of patience, and an exaggerated opinion of one's importance may contribute to vehicle accidents, particularly in the 16–24 age group. Similar associations have been established for the accident-prone individual.

Cultural factors also contribute to accidents in the United States. As our society grows increasingly complex and competitive, the individual experiences more tension and strain. Divorce, inadequate parental guidance, widespread use of drugs and pills, and the worship of the automobile and of speed (auto races, boat races, airplane races, motorcycle races, bicycle races, etc.) all contribute to the accident rate in this country.

Physiological factors, such as poor coordination and motor skill, poor sight and hearing, or other physical handicaps, have little to do with the cause of accidents. Fatigue, however, does reduce reaction time, and thus contributes to accidents of all types. In addition, those who have certain diseases (epilepsy, heart disease, etc.) are somewhat more likely to be involved in an accident. Many over-the-counter and prescription drugs can cause drowsiness, and stimulants, depressants, and hallucinogens also drastically reduce performance, making the user more susceptible to all types of accidents. Even a low level of physical fitness is a contributing factor, particularly late in the day, when fatigue becomes evident. Perhaps the major drug contributing to accidents is alcohol, which is responsible for a large percentage of both automobile and occupational accidents. Among teenagers, use of alcohol and other drugs, such as quaaludes, frequently leads to automobile accidents.

Accident Prevention

Home and motor vehicle accidents don't always happen to other people. Unless you take some precautions, you too are likely to become involved before too long in a major accident of some type. The following suggestions may help avoid such an occurrence.

Preventing home accidents

- Fires

  1. Avoid smoking in bed or near flammable material.
  2. Avoid overloading electrical outlets.
  3. Check electrical equipment regularly, looking for frayed wires, unplugging appliances not in use, and making certain proper fuses are being used.
  4. Install a smoke alarm system in your home.
  5. Avoid keeping flammable liquids, such as paint and fuel, in your home.
  6. Wipe grease spills immediately and water down the area.
  7. Store matches, cigarette lighters, and heating and cooking appliances out of the reach of children.
  8. Inspect attics, garages, and cellars carefully for potential firetraps.
  9. Develop and rehearse a plan of action in case of a fire that requires leaving the home through an exit other than the doors; go through the procedure with the entire family.
  10. Keep emergency fire numbers and a fire extinguisher accessible.

- Poisoning (see p. 540)

- Falls

  1. Keep a close watch on infants at all times.
  2. Keep floors uncluttered and well lit. Check handrails near stairs for sturdiness.
  3. Check ladders carefully before each use; place them carefully and avoid climbing beyond the third rung from the top under any conditions.
  4. Clean ice and snow from porches and steps.
  5. Consider use of rubber matting to avoid slipping in hallways, on porches, and in bathtubs.

- Suffocation

  1. Do not allow infants to sleep on pillows.
  2. Discard plastic bags (such as those accompanying clothes from the cleaners) immediately.
  3. Remove doors and lids from all discarded large objects (refrigerators, coolers, trunks).
  4. Inspect toys carefully and throw away items with loose objects or stuffing that could result in choking if swallowed.
  5. Practice the proper first aid procedure (Heimlich maneuver) for choking with the entire family (see p. 538).

- Drowning

  1. Learn to swim in one of the many programs available to the public (YMCA and YWCA clubs, American Red Cross, youth centers, etc.).
  2. Learn proper boat safety and exercise caution at all times. If your boat capsizes, cling to it rather than trying to swim to shore.
  3. Don't swim alone in unattended areas and don't swim at night. Don't leave a child alone in a children's pool, no matter how shallow.
  4. Swim near the shore.
  5. Be certain the water is deep enough before diving.
  6. Before entering the water to rescue a victim in difficulty, throw out a life preserver or rope.

Gun accidents

1. Avoid storing loaded weapons in the house; keep under lock and key and hidden from children.

2. Unload your weapon while cleaning; avoid showing off with guns.

3. If you must have a gun in your home, learn how to use it properly. Practice in a safe area until you feel comfortable with the weapon.

4. Never point a gun at another person.

Preventing Motor Vehicle Accidents

● Automobiles, trucks, and buses

1. The automobile is slowly becoming a more safe vehicle, although it remains a deadly weapon at high speeds. Several changes in safety standards and design either have already taken place or will eventually occur to improve the safety of the automobile: elimination of sharp parts on the dashboard and other interior parts, seat and shoulder belts, strategic location of rupture-resistant gas tanks, energy-absorbing bumpers, collapsible steering columns, padded interiors, air bags, outside rearview mirrors, larger and sturdier tires, door safety catches, removal of protruding hub-cap ornaments, emergency brake systems, energy-absorbing frames, engines that deflect downward rather than into the driver in a head-on collision, and roll bars to prevent the roof from collapsing during a roll-over. Additional changes are needed.

2. Don't drive while under the influence of alcohol or any other drug.

3. Have your car inspected periodically; check brakes, lights, and engine between inspection dates.

4. Buckle up, even if you are only going "up the street." Insist that all passengers in your car use seat and shoulder belts.

5. Obey speed limits; avoid driving too fast or too slow.

6. Keep a safe distance from the car ahead of you (one car length for every 10 mph of speed).

7. Leave for your destination in plenty of time to avoid rushing and tension.

8. Use the proper lane before turning; signal your intentions.

9. Yield to other drivers.

10. Stay in the right lane except to pass.

11. Don't drive when emotionally upset.

12. Learn and follow good seeing habits: Aim high in steering by looking far ahead of the path your car will follow; keep your eyes moving; get the big picture by scanning in front, to the sides, and behind you; make sure others see you by communicating with your brake lights, headlights, horn, car position, and turn signals; and always leave yourself an out or escape path.

● Motorcycles

1. Follow the suggestions listed under automobiles, trucks, and buses.

2. Use an approved helmet and eye protection device, and insist on all passengers wearing the same.

3. Inspect your motorcycle regularly and keep the rearview mirror clean and properly positioned.

4. Practice riding your motorcycle in a field or desolate area before entering a highway.

5. Don't borrow a motorcycle you are not used to; habits are difficult to break, and mechanical handling varies from one motorcycle to another.

6. Wear long pants and a leather jacket to reduce injury in case of a fall.

7. Keep headlights on at all times to aid other motorists in seeing you.

8. Use a proper muffler to keep the noise level low and unalarming to other motorists.

9. Avoid changing lanes unless absolutely necessary; remember, you are difficult for the motorist to see.

10. Avoid riding in a driver's blind spot (at the right or left rear of the car).

11. Avoid riding between the lines of moving cars.

12. Ride in the left car-wheel track of a lane.

appendix C: a guide to nutritive value*

This guide was designed to relate the nutritive value of food to individual nutritional needs and to compare the nutritive value of commonly eaten foods. The standard used for these comparisons is the U.S. Recommended Daily Allowance (U.S. RDA).

UNDERSTANDING THE U.S. RECOMMENDED DAILY ALLOWANCE (U.S. RDA)

The U.S. RDA is the standard used in nutrition labeling. It is based on the Recommended Dietary Allowances (RDAs) set by the National Research Council. The RDAs are judged by the Council to be adequate for nearly all healthy persons and generous for most.

U.S. RDA
Protein	65 grams[1]
Vitamin A	5000 International Units
Vitamin C	60 milligrams

*SOURCE: Adapted from "A Guide to Nutritive Value," An Extension Publication of the Division of Nutritional Sciences, New York State College of Human Ecology, Cornell University, Ithaca, New York. Reprinted with permission.

[1]65 grams is the U.S. RDA for a mixed diet of animal and plant proteins; 45 grams is the U.S. RDA for a diet of mainly animal-proteins: meat, fish, poultry, eggs, and milk.

Thiamin	1.5 milligrams
Riboflavin	1.7 milligrams
Calcium	1 gram
Iron	18 milligrams

The U.S. RDA for these nutrients is the *highest* RDA for all sex–age categories. For many individuals, the U.S. RDAs are higher than recommended by the National Research Council for their sex and age:

- Table C.2 adjusts the U.S. RDA to fit individual nutrient needs. To illustrate: a five-year-old needs only 50 percent of the U.S. RDA for protein. Thus two cups of milk furnishing 40 percent of the U.S. RDA almost meet the child's protein needs.

- Table C.3 lists recommended calorie allowances. Calorie needs depend on age, sex, size, and activity. Body weight is the best measure of adequacy; weight gains indicate excess calories.

OTHER NUTRIENTS IN FOODS

Many nutrients other than those listed in this chart are important. No single food, not even one that is highly enriched, provides all the nutrients needed for optimum health. Thus, eating a variety of foods is wise.

Table C.1
PERCENTAGE U.S. RDA OF SOME COMMON FOODS[1] (BOLDFACE INDICATES SIGNIFICANT SOURCES OF NUTRIENTS)

Food	Amount or Description	Metric weight (grams)	Calories	Protein	Vitamin A	Vitamin C	Thiamin	Riboflavin	Calcium	Iron
Milk and milk products										
Milk, whole; yogurt	1 cup	(240)	160	**20**	6	2	6	25	30	—
Skim, unfortified; buttermilk	1 cup	(240)	90	**20**	—	2	6	25	30	—
Modified skim (99% fat free), fortified	1 cup	(240)	120	**25**	10	2	6	25	30	—
Evaporated, undiluted	½ cup	(120)	160	**20**	8	2	4	25	30	—
Nonfat dry solids, fortified	3 tbsp; 1 cup reconstituted	(23; 240)	90	**20**	10	2	6	25	30	—
Milkshake, chocolate	10 ounces (1 cup whole milk)	(345)	400	**25**	15	2	6	**35**	**40**	4
Cheeses: cheddar; American; Swiss; processed	1 ounce (1¼" cube)	(30)	115	**15**	6	—	2	8	**20**	—
Cheese, cottage creamed	½ cup	(115)	120	**30**	4	—	2	**15**	10	—
Ice cream (10% fat)	½ cup	(115)	130	6	6	—	2	8	10	—
Milk pudding, vanilla	½ cup	(130)	140	10	4	—	2	**12**	**15**	—
Cream, half-half	¼ cup	(60)	80	4	6	—	—	6	6	—
Vegetables										
Important Sources of Vitamins A and/or C[2]										
Broccoli	½ cup cooked	(75)	20	4	**40**	**120**	6	**10**	**8**	4
Brussels sprouts; green pepper	½ cup cooked; 1 medium pepper	(75; 90)	25	4	10	**110**	4	4	2	6
Cabbage; cauliflower	½ cup raw; ½ cup cooked	(90)	15	2	2	**50**	2	2	4	2
Carrots	½ cup cooked or raw	(80)	30	2	**150**	10	4	2	2	2
Greens: beet; chard; collards; kale; mustard; spinach; turnip	½ cup cooked	(100)	20	2	**100**	**50**	6	**10**	**10[3]**	**8**
Plantain, green or ripe	½ cup cooked	(100)	140	2	**25**	10	4	2	—	2

1. References: *Composition of Foods,* Agriculture Handbook No. 8, USDA, 1963; *Nutritive Value of American Foods in Common Units,* Agriculture Handbook No. 456, USDA, 1975; *Food Values of Portions Commonly Used,* Bowes and Church, Lippincott, 1970; *Tabla de Composición de alimentos de use corrente en Puerto Rico,* Reguero and Santiago, University of Puerto Rico, 1974; California Prune Advisory Board, 1973.

2. Highest vitamin A content is found in darker yellow-orange and green vegetables and fruits.

3. Some calcium in spinach, swiss chard, or beet greens may combine with a plant acid and may not be absorbed.

Table C.1 *(continued)*

Food	Amount or Description	Metric weight (grams)	Calories	Protein	Vitamin A	Vitamin C	Thiamin	Riboflavin	Calcium	Iron
Squash, winter; pumpkin; calabaza	½ cup cooked	(100)	60	2	**90**	**20**	4	6	2	4
Sweet potato; yam, yellow	½ cup cooked	(100)	120	2	**120**	**20**	4	4	2	4
Tomatoes, raw; canned; juice	1 small; ½ cup	(100)	20	2	**15**	**35**	4	2	—	4
Other Vegetables										
Asparagus	½ cup cut pieces	(80)	15	2	**15**	**30**	8	8	2	4
Beans, lima	½ cup cooked	(80)	95	**10**	4	**20**	**10**	4	4	**10**
Beans, snap	½ cup cooked	(60)	15	2	8	**15**	4	4	4	4
Beets; onions	½ cup cooked	(80)	30	2	—	8	2	2	—	2
Celery; cucumber; radishes	½ cup sliced	(50)	10	—	—	8	—	—	—	—
Corn	½ cup cooked; 1 5-inch ear	(80; 140)	85	4	6	8	2	4	—	4
Lettuce, crisp head; loose leaf	1 cup shredded	(55)	8	—	8	8	2	4	—	4
Peas, green	½ cup cooked	(80)	65	8	**10**	**25**	**15**	6	2	8
Turnips; rutabaga	½ cup cooked	(80)	20	2	6	**25**	2	2	2	2
Mushrooms	½ cup cooked	(120)	20	4	—	2	—	**15**	—	2
Potatoes, white	One: 4 per lb	(100)	85	2	—	**25**	6	2	—	4
Potatoes, white, mashed	½ cup, milk and butter added	(100)	90	4	—	**20**	6	4	2	2
Squash, summer; zucchini; crookneck	½ cup cooked	(100)	15	2	8	**15**	4	4	2	2
Viandas[4]	½ cup cooked	(100)	90–130	2	4	4	4	2	—	4
Important sources of vitamins A and/or C[3]										
Apricots, canned in syrup	½ cup	(130)	110	—	**35**	6	—	2	—	2
Cantaloupe	¼ (5 inch diameter)	(230)	40	—	**90**	**70**	2	2	—	2
Grapefruit, white (edible portion); juice	½ (4 inch diameter); ½ cup	(120)	50	—	—	**70**	4	2	2	2
Mangos, raw	½ cup sliced	(80)	55	—	**80**	**45**	2	2	—	2
Orange (edible portion); juice	1 (2½ inch diameter); ½ cup	(120)	65	—	4	**100**	6	2	4	2
Peaches, raw	One: 4 per lb	(100)	40	—	**25**	**15**	2	4	—	2
Strawberries, raw; frozen, sweetened	1 cup	(150; 250)	60; 250	—	2	**150**	2	6	4	8
Watermelon	1 cup diced	(160)	40	2	**20**	**20**	4	2	2	4
Other Fruits										
Apples; applesauce, sweetened	One: 3 per lb; 1 cup	(150; 240)	85; 200	—	2	**10**	2	2	—	4

Food	Amount	Weight (g)	Calories	Protein	Vit. A	Vit. C	Thiamin	Riboflavin	Niacin	Calcium	Iron
Bananas	1 medium; 1 cup sliced	(175)	100	2	4	20	2	4	4	—	4
Blueberries; raspberries	½ cup unsweetened	(65)	40	—	—	25	—	—	—	—	2
Canned fruit in syrup: cocktail; pears	½ cup	(120)	80	—	2	6	2	2	2	—	2
Grapes	½ cup	(75)	60	—	—	6	2	2	2	—	2
Pears	One: 2½ per lb	(180)	100	—	—	10	2	2	4	—	2
Pineapple, raw	½ cup diced	(75)	40	—	4	20	4	4	—	—	2
Prunes, dried; juice	5 medium; ½ cup	(30; 120)	80; 120	—	10	2	—	2	2	2	10
Raisins, seedless	⅓ cup; 1½ oz package	(45)	120	—	—	—	—	2	2	2	8

Meat, fish, poultry, eggs, legumes

Food	Amount	Weight (g)	Calories	Protein	Vit. A	Vit. C	Thiamin	Riboflavin	Niacin	Calcium	Iron
Beef; veal; lamb	3 ounces cooked, lean only	(90)	180–225	**50**	—	—	4	4	20	—	15
Chicken, fried	1 drumstick and thigh	(125)	250	**50**	—	—	4	10	25	—	8
Chicken; turkey	3 ounces, no skin	(90)	180	**50**	—	—	4	10	20	—	8
Fish: clams; shrimp	3 ounces meat, no fat/breading	(90)	100	**50**	—	—	4	6	10	2	**15**[5]
haddock; perch; cod	3 ounces, no fat added	(90)	100	**50**	—	—	4	6	10	—	6
tuna, canned	3 ounces, in water; in oil	(90)	110; 170	**50**	10	—	4	6	10	—	6
Hamburg	3 ounces, cooked	(90)	250	**45**	—	—	4	10	20	—	15
Hot dogs; bologna; cold cuts	1 hot dog; 2 ounces	(60)	160	15	—	—	6	6	6	—	6
Liver	2 ounces, no fat added	(60)	135	35	**500**	30	15	**120**	45	—	25
Pork; ham	3 ounces cooked, lean only	(90)	300	**45**	—	—	**40**	10	25	—	15
Pork sausage, cooked	1 link: 16 per lb	(20)	95	6	—	—	4	2	4	—	2
Eggs	1 large	(50)	80	15	**10**	—	4	**8**	—	2	6
Legumes: dried beans; peas	1 ounce dried; ½ cup cooked	(30; 90)	125	15	—	—	10	4	4	4	15
Peanut butter; nuts	2 tbsp peanut butter; ¼ cup	(30)	190	15	—	—	4	4	15	4	4

Cereal products, whole grain/enriched[6]

Food	Amount	Weight (g)	Calories	Protein	Vit. A	Vit. C	Thiamin	Riboflavin	Niacin	Calcium	Iron
Bread; toast; bagel	1 slice; ½ bagel	(25)	70	4	—	—	6	4	6	4	8
Cereals: oatmeal; wheat	1 cup cooked	(240)	110	4	—	—	10	4	10	4	6
ready-to-eat	1 ounce	(30)	100			refer to label on package					
Corn grits; corn meal	1 cup cooked	(240)	125	4	2	—	8	4	4	—	6
Hamburg roll	1 medium	(40)	120	6	—	—	10	6	10	6	10
Spaghetti; macaroni; noodles; rice	1 cup cooked	(150–200)	200	8	—	—	15	6	8	2	8

4. Yautia (white tanier), name (white yam), malanga (taro, dasheen), yuca (cassava). Yuca has somewhat more vitamin C than listed.

5. Clams provide 30 percent iron.

6. Values for thiamin, riboflavin, and iron are based on enrichment levels specified by FDA, October 1973.

Note: Some figures represent judgments made to help the user identify the most dependable sources of individual nutrients.

Table C.2
PERCENT OF U.S. RDA FOR YOU (BY AGE)

	Children			Women				Men
	4–6	7–10	11–18	19–50	51+	Preg-nant	Nurs-ing	19+
Protein	50	55	85	75	75	+50[1]	+35[1]	90
Vitamin A	50	70	100	80	80	100	120	100
Vitamin C	70	70	75	75	75	100	135	75
Thiamin	60	80	100	75	70	+20[1]	+20[1]	100
Riboflavin	65	75	110	85	65	+20[1]	+30[1]	110
Calcium	80	80	120	80	80	120	120	80
Iron	60	60	100	100	60	100	100	60

[1]To be added to the percentage for females of appropriate age.

Table C.3
RECOMMENDED CALORIE ALLOWANCES

	Ages	Calorie Allowance
Children	4–6	1800
	7–10	2400
Women[1]	11–14	2400
	15–22	2100
	23–50	2000
	51+	1800
Men	11–14	2800
	15–22	3000
	23–50	2700
	51+	2400

[1]Add 300 calories for pregnancy, 500 for lactation.

Note: Tables 1 and 2 are adapted from *Nutrition Labeling; Tools for Its Use,* USDA, Agriculture Information Bulletin No. 382, 1975.

USING THE GUIDE

Percentages of the U.S. RDA are shown for seven major nutrients: protein, vitamin A, vitamin C, thiamin, riboflavin, calcium, and iron. Food energy is expressed as calories.

Percentages are given to the nearest 2 percent up to 10 percent; to the nearest 5 percent up to 50 percent; and to the nearest 10 percent above 50 percent. A dash indicates only a trace or none of the nutrient.

Numbers given are averages compiled from tables of food composition. When several foods are listed on the same line, the figures may not fit equally well all the foods included. Important differences are explained in footnotes.

Highly significant sources of a nutrient are indicated by boldface type. In general this designation is merited if a serving of food contains 10 percent or more of the U.S. RDA. Less than 10 percent is considered significant when more than one serving daily is common (for example, vitamin A in milk). Obviously, if the amount eaten is large enough, foods may be significant for some nutrients even though not differentiated here.

No differentiation is used in the iron column because judging which foods are especially significant is more complex for iron than for other nutrients. The amount of iron absorbed from foods varies with the types of food eaten and the individual's needs for iron. The U.S. RDA assumes an average availability of 10 percent of food iron. Present knowledge indicates that iron in meat, fish, poultry, and soybeans is *more* than 10 percent available; iron in eggs, whole grains, nuts, and dried beans is *less.*

The percentage of protein contributed by foods depends on whether the food comes from plants or

Table C.4
CALORIE VALUES

Description	Amount	Calories	Description	Amount	Calories
Bacon, crisp	2 slices	100	Donuts, Danish	1 medium	150–175
Beverages			Gelatin dessert	½ cup	80
Beer	12 oz	150	Gravy	2 tablespoons	80
Carbonated, sweetened	12 oz	130–150	Jam, jelly, syrup, molasses,	1 tablespoon	50–60
Liquor 70–100 proof	1½ oz	100–120	honey	1 tablespoon	50–60
Dry wine	3 oz	75	Oils	1 tablespoon	125
Sweet wine: sherry, port	3 oz	120	Pie	⅙ of 9-in. pie	350–400
Butter, margarine	1 tablespoon	100	Popcorn with oil	1 cup	40
Cake, angel	2 × 3 × 1½ in.	120	Potato chips	10 2-in. chips	110
Cake, shortened, frosted.	3 × 3 × 2 in.	400	Potatoes, French fried	10 fries	140
Candy bar, milk chocolate	1 oz	145	Pretzels	10 3-in. sticks	25
Cookies, chocolate chip	2	100	Salad dressings		
Crackers, saltine	1	15–20	French	1 tablespoon	70
Cream			Mayonnaise	1 tablespoon	100
Heavy	1 tablespoon	55	Salad dressing	1 tablespoon	65
Sour	1 tablespoon	25	Sherbet	½ cup	130
Cream cheese	1 in. cube	60	Sugar	1 teaspoon	15

animals. Animal protein is more efficiently used than plant protein. Thus 45 grams is the U.S. RDA basis for estimating the percent of protein in meat, fish, poultry, milk, and eggs. Sixty-five grams is the basis for cereals, legumes, and other vegetables.

Calorie values of several foods not included in the chart are listed in Table C.4. In general these foods have relatively few nutrients in relation to calories. For food mixtures the exact calorie value depends on ingredients used, especially amounts of fat or sugar.

health improvement contract

Throughout this text we've presented you with a good deal of information and asked you to complete activities aimed at helping you learn how to make informed health-related decisions. At this point it seems appropriate to ask you, what have you learned and how will you use that knowledge to become healthier? To answer, consult the questionnaire you completed at the beginning of this book. Now that you have expanded your knowledge about health and about yourself, which of your health behaviors do you wish to change? Which are you willing to work at changing?

The purpose of the contract below is to help you commit yourself to behavioral change related to your health. If you are willing to make this change, complete the contract and consult it periodically to renew your commitment to healthier behavior.

I _____ am concerned about my health. Consequently, I have analyzed my behavior and have concluded that some of the ways I behave need changing. I have decided to commit myself to the following behavioral changes:

1. _____
2. _____
3. _____
4. _____
5. _____

If in two months I have broken this contract, I will deprive myself of the following two privileges:

1. _____
2. _____

_____   _____
Signature   Date

glossary

abortion Termination of a pregnancy before the fetus or embryo is able to exist on its own.

abscess A collection of pus.

accommodation The automatic adjustment of the shape of the lens of the eye for seeing at different distances.

acetone A chemical frequently found in the urine of diabetics.

acne A skin disorder characterized by eruptions appearing on the face, neck, chest, and back usually associated with adolescence but also occurring in adulthood.

actual user effectiveness How effective a method of contraception is when used in real life (non-laboratory) situations.

acuity The ability to discriminate fine details of an object.

acupuncture A pain-relieving method using needles inserted at special points in the body.

acute The sudden onset of pain or disease, continuing for a short time.

additives Substances added to foods to improve the taste or alter or preserve the foods.

adipose tissue Body fat.

adrenal glands Two glands located at the upper part of the kidneys which secrete hormones that affect body functions such as heart rate, respiratory rate, and blood pressure.

adrenocorticotropic hormone A hormone secreted by the pituitary gland which activates the adrenal glands.

aerobic Activity rated by the amount of oxygen necessary to perform an exercise bout through the intake of atmospheric oxygen for fuel.

affective disorders A category of mental disorders in which people act inappropriately joyful, sad, or both.

alcoholic One who uses alcohol compulsively. The body craves the alcohol, and withdrawal symptoms will manifest themselves should alcohol not be available.

Alcoholics Anonymous An organization comprised of recovered alcoholics devoted to helping other alcoholics stop drinking alcoholic beverages.

alienation A feeling of being separated from the society in which one lives. Not being able to relate to others, control one's destiny, or accept societal norms.

all-or-none law The law that a muscle fiber will contract completely or not at all.

allergic hypersensitivity reactions Harmful allergic reactions.

allergy A hypersensitivity of the body to a specific substance such as a food, pollen, or dust. The body may react to this substance by sneezing, coughing, developing a rash, or in other ways.

alveoli Small air sacs at the end of each bronchiole in the lungs where the exchange of oxygen and carbon dioxide takes place.

ambisexual A sexual orientation in which a person is attracted to people of both sexes.

amino acid A protein building block needed for the body to function well.

amniocentesis Extraction and analysis of amniotic fluid from a pregnant woman's uterus.

amniotic fluid The fluid surrounding the fetus in the uterus.

amphetamines Drugs that increase metabolic rate and decrease appetite. Sometimes termed "uppers."

ampulla Part of the vas deferens where sperm meets seminal vesicle fluids.

anaerobics Exercise of short, intense duration such as a 100-meter dash that is performed in the absence of oxygen.

androgyny The blending of masculine and feminine characteristics in one person.

anemia A condition marked by reduced or deficient red corpuscles of the blood causing paleness of the skin and shortness of breath.

angina pectoris Insufficient blood supply and oxygen to a portion of the heart muscle resulting in chest pain and tissue damage.

angiogram X-ray viewing of a blood vessel following injection of a dye.

antabuse A drug used to treat alcoholics which causes nausea if the user ingests alcohol.

antacids An over-the-counter drug designed to eliminate indigestion.

antagonistic drugs Drugs that have opposite effects on the body. When one drug increases heartbeat and another one decreases heartbeat, the drugs are said to be antagonistic.

antibody A protein substance produced in the body that will neutralize an antigen.

antibiotic A synthetic compound used to control bacterial diseases.

antigens Invading foreign molecules that cause the body to produce antibodies.

antihistamine A chemical substance that retards the production of histamines released by the body in allergic reactions.

antiperspirant A drug used to help control body odor by reduced sweating.

antisocial personality A mental disturbance characterized by a history of chronic antisocial behavior and a lack of long-range purpose, a moral sense, and feelings of anxiety and guilt.

anxiety A psychological state of extreme worry or fear.

anxiety disorders Mental disturbance in which high levels of anxiety are experienced.

aorta The largest artery in the body that receives oxygen-rich blood from the left ventricle and distributes it to the entire body through a system of arteries.

apathy A state of mind characterized by not caring.

aphasia Speech and language difficulties caused by left brain injury.

appetite A psychological urge to eat.

arteriosclerosis A condition in which the arteries have hardened, become thick, and lost elasticity.

artery A blood vessel that carries blood away from the heart.

artificial insemination Sperm introduced into a woman's vagina from a syringe to help her become pregnant. Used when a couple is experiencing difficulty in conceiving a child.

aspirin A drug commonly used to relieve cold symptoms of headache, body ache, pain, inflammation, or fever.

assertiveness Expressing yourself and satisfying your own needs. Feeling good about this and not hurting others in the process.

asymptomatic Absence of any evidence of the disease.

atherosclerosis Condition in which arterial walls contain deposits of either soft, spongy, or hard calcified substances to produce narrowing or blocking.

atopy Reaginic antibody dependent reaction, the most common form of allergy.

atrophy The withering away of normal body tissue.

attitude A predisposition or tendency to behave in a particular way.

authoritarianism Rigid adherence to conventional middle class values, unquestioning attitude toward authorities, and stereotypical thinking.

autogenic training A means of learning general body relaxation through the use of imagery and the feeling of heaviness and warmth in the body's limbs.

autohypnotic Bringing about a highly relaxed state of mind and body by oneself.

autonomic nervous system (ANS) The involuntary portion of the nervous system.

autonomy Independence. Doing and being on one's own. Not governed by others.

barbiturates Drugs that slow down body functioning. Sometimes termed "downers."

basal metabolism The amount of calories expended daily while in a resting (not sleeping) state.

basic food groups Four major categories: milk, meat, vegetables and fruits, and bread and cereals.

behaviorism A psychological theory concerned with how one behaves rather than the underlying causes of behavior.

behavior therapist Psychological counselors who focus upon changing the client's behavior, without seeking underlying causes.

benign tumors Harmless, irregular growth of cells generally not dangerous to life or health.

bereavement Honoring the death of a loved one.

Better Business Bureau Supplies information on businesses, investigates advertising misinformation, and mediates disputes between consumers and businesses.

biodegradable Material that disintegrates over time when discarded and attacked by invading bacteria.

biofeedback A method to provide information about the functioning of the autonomic nervous system—muscular contractions, brain-wave patterns, blood pressure, body part temperature, heart rate, etc.

biopsy Examination of surgically removed tissue.

birth control pill An oral form of contraception that prevents ovulation.

blackout The inability to remember significant periods of time when under the influence of alcohol. Analogous to the amnesia reaction, only brought about by alcohol. Considered one of the signs of alcoholism.

blood alcohol level (BAL) The amount of alcohol in the blood, expressed in percentage of total blood.

blood pressure The amount of force exerted by the blood against the walls of the arteries when the heart is contracting (systolic) or resting (diastolic).

body language What the position of the body can indicate to others. Various body positions reflect feeling and thought that are not expressed verbally.

bonding The closeness and psychological attachment that occurs between parents and their newborn children.

brachial Refers to the arm above the elbow.

brain death A determination of death by the cessation of brain activity.

brand name The name of a drug given by the manufacturer of the drug. Not the drug's pharmacological name.

breech birth A birth in which the fetus is positioned buttocks first rather than head first.

bulbocavernosa muscle A muscle in the penis that contracts during ejaculation.

caesarean section The removal of a newborn from the mother through an incision in the mother's abdomen.

caffeine A stimulant drug present in coffee, tea, cola drinks, and some other sodas.

calcium A mineral that is the main component of the bones and teeth.

calculus Hardened plaque on the teeth.

caloric balance A condition achieved when the calories taken in from food exactly equal caloric expenditure (calories of basal metabolism, calories of work metabolism, and calories lost in excreta).

calorie A unit used to measure the amount of heat released from food; one calorie supplies the quantity of heat required to raise the temperature of one kilogram of water one degree centigrade.

cancer A group of diseases characterized by wildly, rapidly, and abnormally growing cells which may eventually damage organs.

capillaries The smallest blood vessels in the body that link the arterial and venous blood systems and provide oxygen and nutriments to body tissues.

carbohydrates Organic compounds composed of carbon, hydrogen, and oxygen, including starches, sugars, and cellulose.

carbon dioxide Gaseous waste material eliminated by the body during exhalation.

carbon monoxide A colorless, odorless yet poisonous gas.

carcinogens Substances that have been shown to produce cancerous cells.

carcinomas Cancer involving the lungs, digestive organs, reproductive organs, and tissue lining body cavities.

cardiac output The amount of blood ejected into the circulatory system minute by minute (a function of heart rate and stroke volume).

cardiovascular Referring to the functioning of the heart and circulatory system.

carotid pulse The pulse taken in the neck as the blood pressure through the carotid artery.

carrier An individual who harbors a pathogenic organism within his or her body and is capable of passing it on to others.

cartilage Fibrous connective tissue between the surfaces of movable and immovable joints.

cellulite A label given to lumpy deposits of fat that commonly appear on the back and front of the legs and on the buttocks in overweight individuals; it is actually just fat.

central nervous system The brain and the spinal cord.

cerebral palsy A disease affecting the motor area of the brain, resulting in loss of control of the voluntary muscles.

cerebrovascular accident (CVA) A stroke. See stroke.

cervical cap A contraceptive device covering the cervix to prevent sperm from entering the uterus during coitus.

cervix The mouth of the uterus. The cervix is adjacent to the vagina.

Chamber of Commerce Liaison between the business community and consumers.

chemotherapy Treatment involving the administration of chemicals that act unfavorably on the causative organism.

chiropractic Adjustment of the vertebrae to treat disease.

chlamydia trachomatis A bacterium which causes non-gon-ococcal urethritis.

chloasma Patchy, irregular darkening of the skin. This can be a result of using birth control pills. Also called the "mask of pregnancy."

cholesterol A chemical substance found in animal fats that is believed to play a part in clogging the arteries.

chorionic gonadotropic hormone A hormone produced by the placenta once a zygote is implanted in it. The detection of this hormone in a woman's urine is used to determine pregnancy.

chronic The slow onset of disease that persists for a long period of time.

chronic bronchitis Inflammation of the bronchial tubes often resulting from smoking cigarettes and characterized by constant coughing and expectorating mucus.

circadian rhythm A natural biological cycle of various bodily functions. For example, see the menstrual cycle.

claudication Leg pain during exercise occurring from atherosclerosis that partially blocks the arteries to the leg.

client-centered therapy Counseling designed to help the client understand and deal with problems; uses such methods as unconditional positive regard.

climacteric Menopause.

climax Orgasm. The height of sexual tension resulting in muscular contractions.

clitoris An external structure of the female reproductive system which is homologous (similar) to the male penis. The most sensitive structure in the female body due to its large number of nerve endings.

co-alcoholic The family of the alcoholic.

cocaine A stimulant drug made from coca leaves.

codeine A pain-killing drug used for relief from coughs and pain.

coitus Sexual intercourse.

coitus interruptus A method of contraception involving the withdrawal of the penis from the vagina just prior to ejaculation.

collateral blood vessels Blood vessels developing around a blocked artery that compensate in part for the loss of blood supply to the heart.

colon The large intestine.

colostrum A thin liquid secreted by the mammary glands for three or four days following birth.

condom A contraceptive device placed over the penis to prevent sperm from entering the vagina.

confirmation A response showing acceptance by the person you are communicating with.

congenital Existing at birth.

congenital heart disease Inborn heart defects.

congestive heart failure Fluid buildup in the tissues of the legs and lungs in individuals with reduced heart function.

conjugal love A kind of domestic, calm, solid comforting love relationship.

conjunctivitis (pink eye) Inflammation of the eye characterized by burning, itching, and a discharge.

Consumer Product Safety Commission The federal agency responsible to protect the public from unsafe products.

contraception Preventing the sperm from fertilizing the ovum, or from successfully implanting on and being nourished by the endometrial lining of the uterus.

conversion disorders A category of mental disturbance where individuals experience physical symptoms without any known organic causes.

coping Responding and dealing with situations which require a reaction.

coronary arteries The blood vessels that supply the heart muscle with blood.

coronary collaterilization Newly developed branches of the coronary arteries that may provide an alternative means of supplying sections of the heart with blood when a coronary artery blockage occurs.

coronary thrombosis Blockage of a coronary blood vessel due to a clot.

corpora spongiosa Part of the penis.

corpora cavernosa The part of the penis (in men) or clitoris (in women) that becomes engorged with blood during sexual stimulation, causing erection.

corpus luteum The yellow body of cells formed from the Graafian follicle in the ovary following release of an ovum.

corticotropin-releasing factor (CRF) A hormone released by the hypothalamus in response to a stressor. This hormone activates the pituitary gland.

cortisol A hormone secreted from the cortex of the adrenal gland which increases blood fats, glucose, and body-core temperature, while reducing white-blood-cell count and protein stores.

cough suppressants Medications that inhibit coughing.

Cowper's gland A gland that lubricates the male urethra.

critical threshold of training A heart rate during exercise approximately 60 percent of the distance between the resting and maximum rates.

cunnilingus Oral stimulation of the female genitalia.

cystic fibrosis A hereditary disease of children characterized by either absence or malformation of the excretory duct of the exocrine glands; affected organs may be the liver, pancreas, sweat glands, testicles, lungs, and throat.

dandruff The normal loss of epidermal cells in the form of dry, white scales.

decongestants Medication to shrink swollen membranes which result from the common cold.

defense mechanisms Unconscious attempts at dealing with anxiety-provoking stimuli; may take a variety of forms.

dehydration The excessive loss of water from body tissues.

deodorant A cosmetic product used to mask body odor by providing a stronger, pleasant smell.

depressants Drugs which depress the central nervous system.

dextromethorphan A drug contained in cough medicine.

diabetes An illness caused by the insufficient production of the hormone insulin.

diabetic coma Insufficient insulin in the blood causing fainting and vomiting.

diaphragm A contraceptive device consisting of a shallow cap covering the cervix so as to prevent sperm from entering the uterus during coitus.

diastolic blood pressure The pressure of the blood against the walls of the arteries. This pressure is considered high when it exceeds 90 mm. Hg.

diethylstilbestrol (DES) A chemical which is included in the ''morning-after'' contraceptive pill. Prior to the discovery that it is related to the development of vaginal cancer, DES was given to women to prevent miscarriages.

dilation Enlargement or expansion of an organ.

dilation and curettage (d and c) The widening and opening of the cervix and the insertion of an instrument to scrape the lining of the uterus.

disability insurance Private health insurance designed to provide income during periods of sickness or injury.

disease A disability that is caused by incorrect functioning of a body part or system.

disorganized schizophrenia A form of mental disturbance characterized by hallucination, delusion, strange thought and behavior patterns, and occasional violent activity and gestures.

distress That stress which is harmful; for example, stress resulting from fear of heights.

diuretic A chemical substance that increases the secretion and discharge of urine and body fluids.

diverticulosis Outward ballooning of the intestinal wall in the descending colon.

divorce The legal declaration of the termination of a marriage.

dominant inheritance Harmful gene is dominant and can be transmitted by only one parent.

dosage The amount of a drug taken.

douching A method of contraception in which a solution is injected into the vagina to flush out semen.

Down's syndrome A genetic disorder caused by the presence of an extra chromosome and causing mental retardation.

drug abuse The use of chemical substances in such a way as to cause extensive physiological or psychological harm to the user.

drug misuse Using medically prescribed drugs improperly; for example, taking too large a dosage or mixing drugs that don't work well together.

dysfunctional Anything that prevents something or someone from behaving effectively.

dyspareunia Painful intercourse.

early pregnancy test (EPT) A do-it-yourself pregnancy test that indicates the presence or absence of human chorionic gonadotropin hormone in the urine.

ectoderm The outer cell layer of the embryo, from which the skin, sense organs, and nervous system are formed.

edentulism Loss of teeth.

ego A term used in psychoanalysis referring to that part of the psyche that controls the pleasure seeking of the id.

ejaculation The act of male orgasm resulting in expulsion of semen.

Electra complex Described by Freud as a girl's love of her father. This begins at age three.

electrocardiogram (ECG or EKG) Graphic record of the electrical currents emitted from heart contractions.

electrolysis A method of permanently removing unwanted body hair by injecting an electric needle into the root of the hair follicle and turning on low current.

electrolytes Compounds in solution in the human body capable of producing electric current.

embalming Treating the body of a dead person by replacing the blood with various chemicals to make the body appear more presentable.

embolus A clot that breaks free from a vessel wall and travels in the bloodstream until it reaches an area it is unable to pass.

embryo The fertilized ovum from the point of fertilization until the third month of pregnancy.

emollient cream A common ingredient of most skin creams.

emotional health The ability to control one's feelings so that they are used to enhance living and human relationships.

emotional lability Loss of emotional control.

emotions Feelings. Sometimes referred to as affect. Examples of emotions are love, hate, fear, and anger.

emphysema Swelling and inflammation of tissue resulting in tearing of the alveoli and decreased lung efficiency.

encephalitis Inflammation of the brain.

endemic A disease that is somewhat restricted to an area or community.

endocardium The inner layer of tissue separating the heart muscle from the blood.

endocrine Glands or organs that secrete substances into the blood and lymph.

endoderm The inner cell layer of the embryo, from which the digestive and glandular systems and the lungs are formed.

endometriosis The presence of endometrial tissue in places where it is not normally found. Sometimes a cause of infertility.

endometrium Innermost layer of the uterus. Has an abundance of blood vessels and is partly discharged during menstruation.

epidemic An infectious disease spreading to large numbers of people in the same geographical area.

epidemiology The study of the causes and means of controlling disease.

epididymus A duct at the top of the testis where sperm are stored and nourished.

epiglottis Skin attached to the entrance of the windpipe that covers the windpipe to prevent food or liquid from entering during swallowing.

epilepsy A neurological condition resulting in seizures.

epinephrine Also termed adrenalin, this hormone is secreted by the medulla (inner section) of the adrenal gland. It increases heart rate, respiratory rate, blood pressure, and perspiration.

episiotomy An incision in the vaginal opening made by a physician during the birth of a baby. The purpose of this incision is to prevent tearing of the vaginal tissue during the birth process.

erythrocyte A red blood corpuscle that carries hemoglobin and oxygen.

estrogen A hormone produced by the ovaries that affects the development of secondary sex characteristics (breast, body hair, etc.) and the menstrual cycle.

estrogen replacement therapy The administration of synthetic estrogen to replace the decrease of estrogen production in women after menopause.

ethics Standards of conduct and moral judgment.

etiology The course of the development of an illness or disease.

eustress Stress that is helpful and positive, for example, the stress caused by news of a promotion.

evacuation and curettage A method of abortion where the products of conception are scraped prior to vacuuming them out.

excitement phase The first phase in the human sexual response, marked by stimulation and arousal.

existential therapy A form of therapy which involves helping a patient choose behaviors consistent with the patient's values.

expectorants Medications which liquify and loosen secretions so they may be coughed up.

extended family A group of people considering themselves a family encompassing more than just parents and their children. Relatives and friends may be a part of an extended family.

external locus of control A belief that, regardless of what one might do, one's fate will be determined by other people or other events.

Fallopian tubes Ducts that connect the uterus to the ovaries in the female reproductive system.

familial hypercholesterolemia (FH) A dominant genetic disease resulting in cholesterol levels 5–12 times the normal level and the inability of the body to regulate cholesterol at normal levels.

family therapy A form of therapy in which a therapist works with the client and the client's family to change the family dynamics.

fats Food components that store energy and vitamins in the body.

fat-soluble vitamins Vitamins not easily eliminated from the body but rather stored in the fatty tissues.

Federal Trade Commission The federal agency responsible for approving the manufacture and sale of drugs.

fellatio Oral stimulation of the male genitals.

fertility control Either preventing pregnancy from occurring (as by contraception) or aiding in the fertilization and successful uterine implantation of the zygote.

fertilization When the ovum is impregnated by a sperm.

fetal alcohol syndrome A set of physical and mental defects found in babies born to women who are heavy users of alcohol.

fetishism A compulsion in which sexual arousal is brought about by a specific object.

fetus The unborn in the womb from the third month of pregnancy until birth.

fiber A nonnutritive substance in food which combines with water to form stools and aid in digestion.

fibrin A sticky substance that combines with blood cells to form a blood clot in the healing of a cut.

fimbria Fingerlike projections at the end of the Fallopian tubes in the female reproductive system.

flashbacks Hallucinations caused by drugs used in the past.

fluorides Mineral salts added to drinking water for the prevention of tooth decay.

follicle-stimulating hormone (FSH) A sex hormone produced by the pituitary gland.

Food and Drug Administration (FDA) The nation's food taster and enforcer of the Federal Food, Drug, and Cosmetic Act designed to protect consumers, manufacturers, and dealers.

foreplay Sexual and affectionate behavior occurring just prior to sexual intercourse.

frustration An unpleasant emotional feeling that results from the inability to satisfy one's desires, impulses, etc.

functional heart murmur A soft murmur heard in a normal heart due to the rapid circulation of blood across normal heart valves.

fundus The part of the uterus closest to the Fallopian tubes.

general adaptation syndrome (GAS) The name given by Hans Selye to the complex of bodily reactions in response to a stressor. This syndrome consists of three stages: alarm reaction, resistance, and exhaustion.

generic drug One not registered or protected by a trademark.

generic name Refers to the chemical ingredient of a drug, not the brand name.

genetic counseling Professional advice regarding the probability of inherited conditions being present in one's offspring.

genetics The study of hereditary factors and their transmission during the life of an individual.

gerontology The study of aging.

gestation The period of time from conception to birth.

gingivitis Gum inflammation resulting in bleeding gums, pain, and foul odor.

glaucoma A disease characterized by the pressure within the eye being higher than normal and potentially damaging to the retina or cornea.

glucose Sugar which can be used by the body for energy.

glycogen The form in which excessive sugar is stored in the body.

gonadotropins Sex hormones.

gonococcus The bacterium which causes gonorrhea.

gonorrhea A sexually transmitted disease which is caused by a bacterium and produces a pus-like discharge from the penis in men. The symptoms in women may go unnoticed.

Graafian follicle The follicle in the ovary that releases a mature egg and secretes estrogen.

grief A strong feeling of loss accompanying the death of a loved one.

group therapy A form of therapy in which a group of people with somewhat similar problems all meet together with a therapist.

habituation Becoming used to a stimulus after experiencing it a lot.

hair follicle A small cavity in the skin where hair develops.

halitosis Chronic unpleasant breath odor.

hallucinogen A drug capable of causing the user to see, hear, or smell something that is not actually present.

hay fever An allergic reaction to house dust, pollen, or mold spores.

hazard The potential of a chemical to produce injury under conditions of use.

health education A process which may consist of formal instruction, mass communication, or informal learning concerned with health content. Health education is designed to help the person being educated to make effective and appropriate health-related decisions.

health maintenance organization (HMO) A comprehensive medical insurance plan that covers both treatment and prevention for a fixed pre-paid monthly fee.

heart attack Death of heart muscle due to an occlusion or insufficient blood supply that fails to meet the oxygen needs of the heart muscle.

heart murmur Vibration within the heart that can be heard through a stethoscope that is generally a result of the rushing of blood across an abnormal heart valve.

heat exhaustion Collapse due to water loss and electrolyte imbalance.

heat stroke Failure of the body to regulate heat after exposure to high temperatures.

hematoma An effusion of blood under the skin caused by rupture of tissue from trauma.

hemoglobin Pigment of the red blood cells that transport oxygen.

hemorrhage Excessive bleeding from a blood vessel.

hemostasis Stoppage of blood to a body part.

hemiplagia Paralysis on one side of the body.

hepatitis A viral inflammation of the liver.

hernia Protrusion of a part of an organ through an abnormal opening.

heroin A narcotic drug derived from morphine.

herpes simplex A viral skin disease similar in appearance to a blister. Occurs in two forms: herpes, type 1, and herpes, type 2. Herpes type 2 is a sexually transmitted disease.

Hodgkin's disease Cancer of the lymph glands.

holistic health Viewing a person as one entity and responding to his or her health in this way. Thus the family of a person with hypertension might be counseled on environmental and nutritional factors, a social worker might help find ways to subsidize the medical bills, etc.

homeostasis A state of bodily equilibrium. The body is functioning as it was designed to function.

homosexual A person who has a sexual preference for those of the same sex.

hormone A chemical substance secreted from a body gland and carried to an organ or tissue where it has a specific effect.

hospice A facility designed to care for the dying patient in a homelike setting.

host The organism upon or within which a parasite lives.

hot flashes Sudden sensations of heat often associated with menopause.

human chorionic gonadotropin A hormone whose presence in a woman indicates she is pregnant.

hunger A physiological need of the body for food.

hymen A thin tissue separating the vestibule from the vagina.

hyperglycemia High blood glucose levels.

hyperlipidemia A high level of lipoproteins in the blood.

hyperplasia New fat cell formation.

hypersomnia The inability to sleep.

hypertension Often termed high blood pressure, hypertension exists when the systolic blood pressure exceeds 140 mm Hg and/or the diastolic blood pressure exceeds 90 mm Hg.

hypertrophy Unusual enlargement of a tissue or organ.

hyperventilation Excessive or accelerated breathing causing a reduction in blood carbon dioxide levels.

hypnotherapy Using hypnosis in a therapeutic setting.

hyposensitization See immunotherapy.

hypothalamus The part of the brain that activates the pituitary gland. Responsible for the homeostasis of body.

hysterotomy A method of abortion involving an abdominal incision and removal of the products of conception through this incision.

id A term used in psychoanalysis referring to that part of the psyche that is the source of all instinctive energy. The id is always seeking pleasure.

identity A sense of oneself. Knowing who and what one is. Understanding one's assets and liabilities.

identity diffusion An unclear view of one's values, beliefs, and other aspects of uniqueness.

immunity Resistance of the body to a particular disease or infection.

immunotherapy The stimulation of the body's own defense system to attack cancer cells.

impotence The inability of the male to maintain an erection long enough to have sexual intercourse.

incest Sexual intercourse with a member of one's immediate family.

incubation period The time between the initial infection and the appearance of its first symptoms.

induced abortion The purposeful termination of a pregnancy.

induced labor A method of abortion where an injection of saline solution induces premature labor and the expulsion of the products of conception.

infarct Tissue death to a body part due to lack of oxygen.

infectious hepatitis (Type A) A viral inflammation of the liver caused by fecal contamination of food or the environment.

infectious mononucleosis A viral infection with long-lasting symptoms of fever, sore throat, headache, and fatigue.

infertility An inability to conceive a child after trying for a year's time.

influenza (flu) Viral infection of the respiratory tract resulting in chills, fever, sore throat, and weakness.

insomnia Difficulty in sleeping.

insulin Manufactured in the pancreas, this substance helps the body metabolize sugar for use in the body. Diabetes occurs when there is not enough insulin to handle the sugar in the body.

insulin shock The condition that results when there is too much insulin in the blood.

interferon A cell protein active against many viruses, some bacteria, rickettsia, and chlamydiaceae.

internal locus of control A belief that one can determine for oneself one's own fate. Belief that what one does will directly affect one's life.

interstitial-cell-stimulating hormone (ICSH) A sex hormone that stimulates the testes to manufacture testosterone.

intervertebral disk A cushionlike pad separating each two vertebral bodies in the spinal column.

intoxication A condition characterized by poor judgment, slurred speech, poor balance, and a general lack of control resulting from alcohol's depressant effect on the brain.

intrauterine device (IUD) A contraceptive device placed within the uterus.

in vitro fertilization Fertilization of the ovum outside of the woman's body.

iron One of the body's essential minerals.

ischemia Inadequate blood supply (oxygen) to a body part.

isotonic training Muscle contraction with the muscle actually shortening against resistance to produce visible work (moving an object through a range of motion).

ketosis A condition brought about by restricted carbohydrate intake resulting in excessive acetones or other ketones being secreted by the liver—stored fat becomes more available for energy aiding in the loss of body fat.

kilocalorie A unit representing 1,000 calories.

labia majora Two large outer folds surrounding the external structure of the female reproductive system.

labia minora Two thin folds of tissue inside the labia majora.

labor The birth process.

lactic acid The waste product produced from anaerobic metabolism or use or glucose or glycogen.

laetrile A derivative of apricot pits used in the treatment of cancer. There is no evidence of its effectiveness.

Lamaze method Natural childbirth. Childbirth without medication to decrease the mother's pain.

laparoscopy A female sterilization procedure in which the Fallopian tubes are cut and tied through two small incisions in the abdomen.

lead poisoning (plumbism) Accumulation of lead in the human body that can lead to brain damage, mental retardation, miscarriage, and death.

lesbian A female homosexual.

leukemia Malignant overgrowth of blood-forming organisms characterized by the overproduction of white corpuscles.

lifestyle The manner in which people live. Their eating habits, sexual behavior, use of drugs, things they spend money on, etc.

ligaments A band of tissue connecting bones or supporting viscera.

lipid Refers to all fats and fatty substances.

lipoproteins Circulating proteins that become attached to blood lipids.

living will Written instructions that when death is near no artificial means should be employed to save the signer's life.

locus of control One's perceptions of whether or not one controls events or is controlled by them.

lumbar The lower back area.

luteinizing hormone (LH) A sex hormone produced in the pituitary gland.

lymphatic system Channels and other structures for the circulation of "lymph" (yellow fluid) throughout the body.

lymphocyte A type of white blood cell formed in the lymph glands that makes up about one-fourth to one-half of the white cells in the blood. This substance fends off harmful bacteria.

lyse To decompose or break down.

lysergic acid diethylamide (LSD) A hallucinogenic drug.

macrominerals Minerals that the body needs in large amounts.

macrophage A type of cell that assists in ingesting and destroying foreign substances that are capable of harming the body.

major medical insurance Insurance paying for nearly all of the major medical expenses not covered by hospitalization or surgery insurance plans.

major tranquilizers Tranquilizers used to manage certain forms of mental illness.

malignant Life-threatening irregular growth of cells.

manic-depressive disorder A mental disturbance characterized by sharp mood swings between severe depression and suicidal feelings and inappropriate elation.

marijuana A psychoactive drug made from the crushed leaves and flowers of the cannabis sativa plant.

masturbation Self-stimulation of the genitals usually resulting in orgasm.

maximum oxygen uptake (MO₂) The amount of oxygen one is capable of utilizing at the tissue level during vigorous exercise.

Medicaid Federal-state health program providing free medical treatment to the needy of all ages.

medic alert symbol A bracelet or neck chain that calls attention to a specific medical problem.

Medicare A federally administered public health insurance program, financed mainly through Social Security, providing partial payment for hospitalization and medical costs for individuals over 65 years of age.

meditation A relaxation technique which either uses focused attention upon something repetitive or something unchanging.

megavitamins Vitamins taken in extremely large doses.

melanin A brown-black pigment occurring naturally in the skin.

menarche When a female first starts to menstruate. Usually anywhere between 9 and 14 years of age.

menopause Cessation of menstruation and ovulation. Usually occurs between 45 and 55 years of age.

menses The menstrual period.

menstruation The cyclical discharge of the endometrium and unfertilized ovum through the vagina.

mental health A state in which one is able to meet life with sufficient mental and emotional skill to exist satisfactorily. This concept is related to the specific society in which it is being studied. What is considered mental health in one society may be considered mental illness in another.

mercury A metal contaminant found in the environment that is related to cancer and other illnesses.

mesoderm The middle cell layer of the embryo, from which the muscular, circulatory, and excretory systems are formed.

metabolic rate The number of calories burned while the body is at rest but not sleeping.

metabolism The chemical transformations of the body; conversion of food into body tissue, muscle contraction, and maintenance of chemical machinery.

metastasis The spread of cancer cells from their initial site to other parts of the body.

methadone A synthetic drug used to withdraw addicts from heroin or to maintain them on methadone rather than heroin.

microorganism One-celled organisms that cause disease.

minerals Components of various hormones, enzymes, and other substances that help regulate chemical reactions in cells.

Minimata disease A neurological disease caused by mercury poisoning.

minor tranquilizers Tranquilizers used to treat anxiety and muscle tension.

monoclonal antibodies Synthetic antibodies made to seek out malignant cells.

monounsaturated fats Oils such as peanut and olive oil which are chemically between saturated and polyunsaturated fats.

morbidity The number of people who become ill from a disease.

mortality The number of people who die from a disease.

motility Ability of the sperm to swim.

multiple sclerosis (MS) A chronic degenerative disease of the central nervous system generally affecting individuals 20–40 years of age, characterized by weakness, loss of coordination, and loss of speech and vision and other autonomous functions.

mumps A viral infection resulting in swelling of the parotid glands.

muscular dystrophy Progressive weakness and withering away of the muscles.

mutant A genotype containing a mutation.

myometrium The middle layer of the uterine wall. Has contractile qualities.

myotonia Muscle tension.

narcolepsy A condition of the nervous system that produces sleep many times daily without warning.

narcotic A drug derived from opium that depresses the central nervous system.

natural family planning A method of birth control involving the identification of ovulation by interpreting the woman's cervical mucus pattern and then abstaining from coitus during her fertile period.

necrosis Death of body tissue.

nicotine An oily acrid poison found in tobacco leaves.

nongonococcal urethritis (NGU) An infection of the urinary tract not caused by the gonococcus.

normlessness A factor of alienation that pertains to a lack of rules, regulations, and standards to which one ascribes and by which one is willing to live.

nuclear family A family comprised of parents and their children. Sometimes termed the conjugal family.

obesity A higher than normal proportion of body fat.

obsessive-compulsive disorders A form of mental disturbance involving constant repetition of particular acts in anxiety-provoking situations.

Oedipus complex Described by Freud as a boy's sexual attraction to his mother and jealousy of his father.

open marriage A form of marriage in which both partners are permitted to participate in sexual liaisons with other people.

opiates Drugs synthesized from opium that have a narcotic effect.

oral-genital sex Contact between the mouth of one sexual partner and the genitalia of the other sexual partner.

organic foods Foods grown without the use of insecticides or synthetic fertilizers.

orgasm The height of sexual tension resulting in muscular contractions and, in the male, ejaculation. Associated with intense sexual pleasure.

orgasmic dysfunction The inability of a woman to experience orgasm.

orgasmic phase The third phase in the human sexual response, marked by involuntary muscular contraction in both partners and ejaculation in the male.

over-the-counter medicine Medicine that can be purchased without a physician's prescription.

ovulation The period of time during the menstrual cycle when the ovary releases an ovum.

ovulation method A natural means of contraception whereby the time of ovulation is determined from the woman's cervical mucus pattern.

ovum An egg deposited from an ovary.

oxygen debt The difference between the amount of oxygen needed to perform an exercise task and the actual amount of oxygen taken in.

oxygen uptake The process of inhaling atmospheric oxygen, diffusing it into the blood, and utilizing it at the tissue level.

pandemic Worldwide epidemic of a disease.

Pap smear Diagnostic examination of secretions from the uterus or lungs to detect abnormal cells.

paranoid personality A mental disturbance characterized by a pervasive and unwarranted suspiciousness and mistrust of people.

paranoid schizophrenia A mental disturbance characterized by general suspiciousness and mistrust of people, hallucinations, inappropriate affect, and occasional hostility and violence.

parotid glands Large serous salivary glands located below and in front of each ear.

pathogen A disease-producing agent.

patient's bill of rights Standards that member hospitals follow in offering patients responsible and ethical care and treatment.

pedophilia Sexual relations between an adult and a child.

peer group One's friends and associates. Peer groups have been found to have a profound influence on health-related behavior.

penis The external organ in the male reproductive system through which sperm are ejaculated.

pepsin Digestive enzyme in gastric juice responsible for the breaking down of protein.

perimetrium Outermost layer of the uterine wall. Has elastic qualities.

periodontal diseases Diseases of the gums, spreading to the sockets containing teeth.

peristalsis Rhythmical muscular movements of the digestive tract aiding transport of food from the mouth to the stomach.

petting Sexually stimulating another without actual sexual intercourse.

pH Refers to the degree of acidity or alkalinity in a solution (pH of 7 is neutral, values from 0–7 indicate acidity, 7–14 indicate alkalinity).

phagocyte A special kind of white blood cell that engulfs and digests bacteria.

phencyclidine (PCP) A depressant that acts as a psychedelic in large doses.

phenobarbital A drug used to control epilepsy in some patients.

phobic disorders Abnormal fear of a particular situation or object. A form of mental disturbance.

physical dependence Sometimes termed an addiction. Refers to the body needing a drug to feel right.

physiological Referring to the functioning of the body.

pink eye Conjunctivitis in the eye.

pituitary gland An endocrine gland located at the base of the brain which secretes hormones which control body growth, metabolism, and other body functions.

placenta A membrane which filters the blood of the pregnant woman to the fetus or embryo.

plaque Strands of fibrous tissue that attach to the inside of arteries to form soft and mushy (if mostly fat particles) or hard (if scar tissue) atheromatous buildup. Also refers to bacteria that form on the teeth.

plateau phase The second phase in the human sexual response, marked by intensified sexual arousal.

platelet Small cell-like structures in the blood involved in blood coagulation and the formation of blood clots.

polygamy A system permitting a person to have more than one husband or wife at once.

polygenic (multifactorial) inheritance The interaction of several genes causing a genetic disease.

polyunsaturated fats Derived from vegetables, lean poultry, fish, and cereal.

potency How powerful a drug's effects are. The more potent, the less the dose needed to obtain the effect.

potentiation When the effect of two or more drugs taken together is greater than the sum of the two drugs taken separately.

powerlessness The feeling of not being in control of one's own destiny.

precancerous An abnormal state of a tissue that tends to become malignant.

pre-ejaculatory fluid Fluid from the penis prior to ejaculation occurring. This fluid contains some sperm and, if allowed to enter the vagina, is capable of resulting in pregnancy.

premature ejaculation The inability of the male to prevent ejaculation long enough, when inserted in the female's vagina, to satisfy her sexually.

prenatal Existing or occurring before birth.

prescription medicine Any drug that cannot be purchased without a doctor's authorization.

primary care physician The family physician who treats common illnesses and injuries and makes referrals to specialists whenever necessary.

primary prevention That part of health education concerned with preventing illness and/or disease before it begins.

progesterone A hormone produced by the ovaries which affects the menstrual cycle and stimulates the mammary glands during pregnancy.

progressive relaxation A means of learning general body relaxation by first contracting, then relaxing, various muscles in the body.

prolactin A pituitary hormone that activates the mammary glands to produce milk.

prostate A gland surrounding the male urethra.

protein A basic food component critical to all living things.

psyche The mind.

psychedelics A category of psychoactive drugs.

psychodrama Therapy which requires the patient to act out events and feelings which are believed to be related to the patient's problems.

psychogenic Originating in the mind.

psychological Referring to the functioning of the psyche or mind.

psychological dependence Sometimes termed a habit. Refers to needing a drug to function although no known physiological basis for this need can be determined.

psychosocial Concerned with psychological and sociological factors.

psychosomatic illness A physical ailment aided in development by the state of the mind. The mind changes the body chemistry so that the illness can better develop.

psychotherapy Treatment for psychological disorders based on Freudian theory.

pyloric valve The valve separating the stomach from the duodenum (the first part of the small intestine).

quacks People who misrepresent their products or services.

quickening Fetal movements which can be felt by the pregnant woman. Usually occurs during the second trimester in first pregnancies.

radial pulse The pulse taken at the wrist.

radioactive isotopes Chemicals ingested orally that are designed to seek out and destroy malignant tissue.

rape Sexual penetration of an individual against her or his will.

rational emotive therapy A counseling method to help patients give up their self-defeating thoughts.

recessive inheritance Inheritance pattern in which a harmful gene is recessive and two genes, one from each parent, are necessary to transmit the gene.

reflective listening Paraphrasing what a person just said so as to let him or her know that you listened and understood the communication. Sometimes termed active listening.

relabeling Changing the description or value ascribed to something—for example, from good to bad. Used to manage anxiety.

remission Disappearance of the signs and symptoms of a disease.

resolution phase The fourth stage in the human sexual response, marked by dissipation of sexual tension.

reverse tolerance A condition where less of a drug is needed to get high.

Reyes syndrome An acute upper respiratory illness in children associated in some cases with the child's reaction to aspirin.

rheumatic heart disease Disease of one or more heart valves from scarring that occurs from acute rheumatic fever.

rheumatoid arthritis Chronic inflammation of the joints.

rhythm method A contraceptive method which includes abstinence for the period of time during the menstrual cycle when fertilization might occur.

role ambiguity An occupational stressor involving the job expectations being unclear or ill-defined.

role conflict An occupational stressor involving two supervisors having different and conflicting expectations of a worker.

role expectation What one expects from someone who has a certain job, title, or other form of classification.

role insufficiency An occupational stressor occurring when a worker's background is not adequate to do the job.

role overload An occupational stressor involving too much work in too short a period of time.

romantic love A total absorption of intimate partners with each other; often develops into conjugal love.

rooming-in Having the baby living in the mother's hospital room rather than spending most of the time in a hospital nursery.

rubella German measles.

sarcoma Cancer involving bones, muscles, ligaments, and other connective tissue.

saturated fats Chemically an alcohol with enough similarities to be a fat: found in animal products and strongly linked to plaque buildup in the arteries.

sciatica Pain in the buttocks, hip, thigh, leg, or foot at the site of the great sciatic nerve.

scrotum Baglike structure in the male reproductive system containing the testes.

sebaceous gland A sweat gland.

secondary prevention That part of health education concerned with early detection of illness and/or disease and return to optimal health.

self-actualization Realizing one's full potential. Being all that one is capable of being. Cited by Abraham Maslow as the highest of all needs.

self disclosure Revealing personal information about oneself.

self-esteem The extent to which a person believes himself or herself to be valuable and of worth.

self-talk Method of managing anxiety wherein one dialogues with oneself regarding a realistic view of the anxiety provoking stimulus.

semen The male ejaculate, which contains fluids from the seminal vesicles, prostate gland, and Cowper's gland, as well as sperm.

seminal vesicles Glands that secrete a substance that nourishes sperm.

seminiferous tubules Small tubes in the testes that produce sperm.

serum hepatitis (Type B) A viral inflammation of the liver transmitted by unclean needles or bodily secretions.

sex flush A darkening of the skin resulting from sexual tension. A direct result of a lot of blood accumulating in an area.

sex hormones Those hormonal secretions that affect the development of secondary sex characteristics, gender, or sexual functioning.

sex-linked inheritance Traits carried by genes on the X chromosome that lack corresponding genes on the Y chromosome.

sex roles Behaviors and tasks society expects of men and women respectively.

sex role stereotyping Assigning behaviors, characteristics, personality types, and chores based upon sex.

sexual anesthesia The inability to experience erotic pleasure from sexual contact. Previously called frigidity.

sexual deviations Sexual behavior directed at objects rather than people or coitus performed under bizarre circumstances.

sexual harassment Sexual advances made by someone of power or authority who threatens sanctions unless sex is agreed to.

sexual response The physiological cycle that occurs during sexual arousal.

sexually transmitted diseases (STDs) Diseases contracted through sexual contact.

shyness Being afraid of people; especially people who are emotionally threatening, strangers about whom one is uncertain or wants to impress, or people who wield power.

sickle cell anemia A type of anemia characterized by sickle-shaped red blood corpuscles.

situational adaptability Being flexible in one's communications from one situation to another.

skinfold measures A procedure to estimate total body fat by measuring the thickness of two layers of skin and the fatty tissue attached.

smooth muscle Involuntary muscle or nonstriated spindle-shaped fibers such as that of the intestines and blood vessels.

social isolation A factor of alienation that pertains to the lack of important people in one's life with whom one can discuss concerns and problems.

sperm Cells produced in the seminiferous tubules of the male reproductive system and ejaculated through the penis.

spermicidal suppositories A spermicidal chemical inserted in the vagina which dissolves into a thick sperm-killing barrier.

spermicides Chemical substances that kill sperm. Spermicides are used with diaphragms, condoms, intrauterine devices, and alone to prevent fertilization of the ovum.

sphygmomanometer An instrument used to measure blood pressure.

spirochete The bacterium which causes syphilis.

spontaneous abortion Termination of a pregnancy from internal causes rather than by outside intervention.

squeeze technique A method developed by William Masters and Virginia Johnson to prevent premature ejaculation.

staphylococci A type of bacteria responsible for staph infections.

starch A complex carbohydrate.

statutory rape Unlawful sexual intercourse with a female minor.

sterilization A procedure that makes one incapable of contributing to conception. In males vasectomy is the usual form; in females tubal ligation.

sternum The breast bone in the center of the chest.

stethoscope An instrument which magnifies sound and is used to hear the heart beat and the blood flow through blood vessels.

stimulants Drugs that result in body functions being increased. Sometimes termed "uppers" or "pep pills," these drugs stimulate the central nervous system.

strength The amount of force you can apply to a particular muscle group.

streptococcus A type of bacteria capable of causing acute forms of disease.

stress The nonspecific reaction of the body to any demand made upon it.

striated muscle Skeletal muscle.

stroke A lack of blood to the brain resulting from the blockage or the rupture of a blood vessel.

stroke volume The amount of blood ejected by the heart per beat.

subcutaneous Beneath the skin, such as the location of body fat.

suction curettage A method of abortion where the products of conception are vacuumed out.

sunscreen A lotion designed to keep out some of the sun's ultraviolet rays.

superego A term used in psychoanalysis to represent that part of the psyche that is the conscience. The superego helps the ego to control the pleasure seeking of the id.

susceptible hosts The segment of a population that contracts a disease endemic to the area.

synergism The more potent action which occurs when two drugs are taken together. The effect is greater than the sum of the effects of the two drugs ingested on separate occasions.

syphilis A sexually transmitted disease which occurs in four progressive stages. If untreated causes organ damage and even death.

systematic desensitization A technique to treat anxiety which involves becoming less anxious with small components of the anxiety-provoking stimulus until one can manage the anxiety altogether.

systolic blood pressure The pressure of the blood as it is forced out of the heart. This pressure is considered high when it exceeds 140 mm Hg.

tachycardia Rapid heart rate.

target heart rate The exercise heart rate needed to produce an increase in aerobic conditioning.

tars Thick dark-colored substances consisting of a mixture of hydrocarbons and their derivatives.

Tay-Sachs disease A hereditary disease caused by the absence of an enzyme needed to break down fats.

tendon A fibrous cord by which a muscle is attached to a bone or other structure.

tertiary prevention That part of health education concerned with preventing further illness and/or disease in people who are well along in an ill or diseased state.

testes The two organs in the male scrotum that produce sperm and testosterone.

testosterone A male sex hormone.

Tetrahydrocannabinol (THC) The psychoactive ingredient in marijuana. THC can now be synthesized (developed in the laboratory).

theoretical effectiveness How effective a method of contraception is when used under controlled laboratory conditions.

tolerance The body getting used to a drug so that more and more is needed to obtain the desired reaction.

toxemia Pregnancy-induced hypertension. May include other symptoms such as swelling.

toxicity The potential capacity of a chemical to harm living organisms.

toxic shock syndrome (TSS) A serious disease characterized by flu-like symptoms in the early stages and more serious symptoms later. Thought to be related to use of tampons.

toxin A poisonous substance formed during the growth of pathogenic bacteria.

trace minerals Minerals the body needs in very small amounts.

trade name A name given to a drug by the manufacturer.

transaction management The ability of two individuals to control their communication rather than be controlled by it.

transactional analysis A system of analyzing people's interactions.

transcendental meditation A means of relaxation in which a Sanskrit word (mantra) is focused upon resulting in general body relaxation.

transitory ischemic attack (TIA) A mild stroke that occurs when the brain is deprived of adequate blood supply for a short period of time.

trauma A wound or injury causing an alteration in tissue.

triglycerides Fatty chemicals of glycerol and fatty acids linked to atherosclerosis.

trimester A three-month period during the term of pregnancy.

tubal ligation Sterilizing the female by cutting and tying the Fallopian tubes.

Type A behavior pattern A complex of personality traits which has been related to the development of coronary heart disease. These traits are aggressiveness, competitiveness, impatience, a harrying sense of time urgency, and free-floating hostility.

Type B behavior pattern A complex of personality traits believed to be possessed by those not likely to develop coronary heart disease. These personality traits are the opposite of those possessed by Type A behavior pattern people.

umbilical cord The cord connecting the fetus or embryo to the placenta.

urea A constituent of urine and blood.

urethra The canal through which urine, and semen in the male, is discharged.

uterus The female reproductive organ in which a fertilized egg is implanted and grows into a fetus.

vaccine A solution of dead bacteria that is introduced into the body to stimulate the production of antibodies.

vagina The passage in the female genitalia leading from the external orifice to the uterus.

vaginismus An involuntary tightening of the muscles in the vagina so that the penis may not enter or, if it does, only with a good deal of pain.

value Something about which one feels very strongly. Something held in high esteem. Different from a belief, opinion, or attitude in its degree of worth.

varicose veins Veins stretched, elongated, and folded due to nonfunction of vein valves.

vas deferens The duct that carries the sperm from the epididymus to the ejaculatory duct.

vasa efferentia The duct through which the sperm pass from the testes to the epididymus.

vasectomy A male sterilization procedure in which the vas deferens is cut and tied.

vasocongestion Increased blood flow to a particular area of the body.

vector The entity transmitting the disease.

vein Blood vessels that transport blood toward the heart.

vertebra One of the 33 spinal-column bones.

vestibule The part of the female genitalia containing the vaginal and urethral openings.

virus The smallest known parasitic organism that enters a living cell.

warm-down Slow, easy exercise for 5-10 minutes immediately following a vigorous exercise effort to allow the body to slowly return to its normal state.

water-soluble vitamins Vitamins which combine with water and which are easily eliminated from the body.

withdrawal syndrome A constellation of bodily conditions associated with the elimination of a drug. These conditions may include a great deal of perspiration, loss of appetite, pain, anxiety, tremors, convulsions, etc.

work hypertrophy A conditioning process whereby one's conditioning level temporarily declines after exercise, but during recovery tissue rebuilds beyond the original level of conditioning.

World Health Organization (WHO) International health agency of the United Nations formed to improve world health and control of communicable diseases.

photo credits

Page	Source
235	Culver Pictures, Inc.
242	Movie Star News
253	Carol Palmer
254	Grant Heilman Photography
258	American Lung Association
270	The Museum of Modern Art/Film Stills Archive
277	Bruce Kliewe/Jeroboam
279	Joel Gordon
282	United Press International Photo
284	Ellis Herwig/Stock, Boston
286	The Washington Post
290	The Museum of Modern Art/Film Stills Archive
292	Christopher Brown/Stock, Boston
300	Jeff Albertson/Stock, Boston
302	Mitchell Payne/Jeroboam
303	Robert Levin/Black Star
307	Stephen J. Sherman
308	Bettye Lane
316	The Museum of Modern Art/Film Stills Archive
318	Creative Media Group, Inc., Charlottesville, Va.
324	Jean Boughton
331	Patricia Hollander Gross/Stock, Boston
334	Florence Sharp
337	Abigail Heyman/Archive
339	Florence Sharp
344	Movie Star News
347	Boston Globe Photo
350	Richard Feldman
352	Mimi Forsyth/Monkmeyer Press
354	Michael Malyszko/Stock, Boston
357	Jim Ritscher/Stock, Boston
364	Richard Feldman
372	The Bettmann Archive
379	Ken Heyman
382	Jon Rawle/Stock, Boston
384	American Heart Association
386	Boston Globe Photo
389	Wide World Photos
396	The Museum of Modern Art/Film Stills Archive
400	Grant Heilman Photography
401	Burk Uzzle/Magnum Photos
409	Ira Wyman
412	United Press International Photo
415	Peck-Sun Lin, Tufts Univ.
416	President's Committee on Mental Retardation
418 (a)	J. Heslop-Harrison, Univ. College of Wales
(b)	F. Dan Hess, Purdue
424	Museum of Modern Art/Film Stills Archive
426	Lee D. Simon
429 (a)	James G. Hirsch, Rockefeller Univ.
(b)	Peck-Sun Lin, Tufts Univ.
432	World Health Organization
435	World Health Organization
439	N.Y.S. Health Department, Public Health Education Unit
442	Center for Disease Control
452	The Bettmann Archive
459	Richard Feldman
465	The Bettmann Archive
467	The Bettmann Archive
470	Richard Feldman
476	Movie Star News
479	Richard Feldman
481	Bohdan Hrynewych/Stock, Boston
486	Virginia Commonwealth University
488	Ken Heyman
492	Richard Feldman
500	The Bettmann Archive
503	Ellis Herwig/Stock, Boston
509	Grant Heilman Photograph
511	Stephen J. Sherman
514	Wide World
516	Boston Globe Photo

index